Clinical Handbook of Interstitial Lung Disease

Clinical Handbook of Interstitial Lung Disease

Edited by

Muhunthan Thillai
Cambridge Interstitial Lung Disease Unit
Royal Papworth Hospital, Cambridge, United Kingdom

David R Moller
Department of Medicine, Division of Pulmonary and
Critical Care Medicine, Johns Hopkins University School
of Medicine, Baltimore, Maryland, USA

Keith C Meyer
Department of Medicine, Division of Allergy, Pulmonary,
Critical Care and Sleep Medicine, University of Wisconsin School
of Medicine and Public Health, Madison, Wisconsin, USA

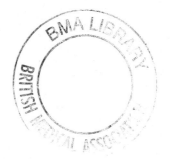

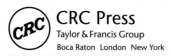

CRC Press
Taylor & Francis Group
Boca Raton London New York

CRC Press is an imprint of the
Taylor & Francis Group, an **informa** business

CRC Press
Taylor & Francis Group
6000 Broken Sound Parkway NW, Suite 300
Boca Raton, FL 33487-2742

© 2018 by Taylor & Francis Group, LLC
CRC Press is an imprint of Taylor & Francis Group, an Informa business

No claim to original U.S. Government works

Printed on acid-free paper by Ashford Colour Press Ltd.

International Standard Book Number-13: 978-1-4987-6825-2 (Paperback)
978-1-138-29670-1 (Hardback)

Visit the Taylor & Francis Web site at
http://www.taylorandfrancis.com

and the CRC Press Web site at
http://www.crcpress.com

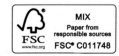

We dedicate this book to our patients and research volunteers for their courage and support, to our families and to our mentors.

Muhunthan Thillai dedicates this book to his mentor Donald Mitchell, to his wife Abi and to his family Raj, Anushya, Kiruthikah, Krishnan and Ambika.

David Moller dedicates this book with love, to his wife Teresa and our family Stephanie, Christopher, Ryan, Kristen and Avery.

Keith Meyer especially dedicates this book to all the patients who have trusted his guidance and given him important lessons about coping with interstitial lung disease and to his wife, Emily Auerbach, and his children and grandchildren.

Contents

Foreword

The *Clinical Handbook of Interstitial Lung Disease*, edited by Drs. Thillai, Moller, and Meyer, provides a comprehensive, thoughtful, and in depth review of the complexity of interstitial lung disease (ILD), with a broad perspective provided by 60 authors with expertise in ILD. The book is extensively referenced, and provides insights suited not only for trainees but for clinicians and academicians at all levels with an interest in ILD.

More than 200 ILDs have been identified, and a logical approach requires the analysis of clinical, radiographic, and histological patterns that may establish a precise and definitive diagnosis. The first few chapters provide an overview of the evolving classification schema of ILD, the disparate histological patterns of ILD, the use of thoracic imaging [particularly high-resolution thin-section computed tomographic scanning (HRCT)] to diagnose and follow ILDs, and clinical evaluation of patients with suspected ILD. These initial chapters, as well as those that follow, are replete with superb color photomicrographs and HRCT scans to illustrate the salient findings of these various ILDs. The major patterns (both radiographic and histologic) are discussed, including: acute and chronic lung injury; airway-centered (bronchiolocentric); alveolar filling (e.g., alveolar hemorrhage, pulmonary alveolar proteinosis, organising pneumonia); nodular patterns (e.g., sarcoidosis, granulomatosis with polyangiitis, silicosis, Langerhans cell histiocytosis (LCH), infections, malignancy); cystic patterns [(e.g., lymphangioleiomyomatosis (LAM), LCH, lymphocytic interstitial pneumonia (LIP)]; and mixed patterns. Further, the salient features of the idiopathic interstitial pneumonias (IIPs) are illustrated and discussed, with in-depth discussion of usual interstitial pneumonia (UIP) and nonspecific interstitial pneumonia (NSIP)

patterns. Throughout the book, the pathogenetic mechanisms are discussed in detail, including genetic associations and polymorphisms and external factors (inhaled irritants or allergens, smoking, environmental factors) that may influence clinical expression and course of ILD. Over the past 30 years, several genetic mutations have been implicated in familial and sporadic ILDs. Initial epidemiological studies identified mutations in surfactant C and A proteins, and subsequent studies identified a variety of genetic abnormalities (e.g., telomerase mutations, polymorphisms of MUC5B premeter gene, etc.). Differences in the function of specific genetic loci affecting host defense, cell adhesion, and DNA may be central to the pathogenesis and clinical expression of idiopathic pulmonary fibrosis (IPF) and other ILDs. Investigations using peripheral blood mononuclear cell (PBMC) or alveolar epithelial cells in IPF and other ILDs suggest that specific genetic profiles may be critical to the evolution of the disease process, resulting in a rapid or slow disease progression, with associated differences in survival. A better understanding of genetic risk factors for IPF and other ILDs may lead to improved phenotyping of disease and more targeted therapies.

Clinical approach to ILD includes careful occupational history, exposures (drugs, inhaled antigens), demographics (age, gender), in addition to physical exam and radiographic tests. Blood tests may be critical to identify specific causes of ILD such as connective tissue disease (CTD) or hypersensitivity pneumonia (HP). The role of invasive techniques including bronchoscopy with bronchoalveolar lavage (BAL), endobronchial ultrasound-guided biopsies (EBUS), and surgical lung biopsy are discussed. Several authors emphasize the limitations, as well as risks, associated with these biopsy procedures, and present specific approaches and recommendations. The diagnosis of ILD is not always straightforward, and collaboration among disciplines (e.g., clinicians, radiologists, pathologists) may be critical to narrow and establish the diagnosis. Three chapters (chapters 8–10) provide in-depth discussion of IPF, the most common of the ILDs, including epidemiology, clinical features, diagnostic approach, and management of this disorder. In the chapters that follow, the major types of ILD are discussed. Separate chapters review specific entities including: hypersensitivity pneumonitis; IIPs other than IPF; eosinophilic interstitial lung disorders; ILD associated with CTD; sarcoidosis (both pulmonary and extrapulmonary); smoking-related ILD; drug-induced and iatrogenic ILD; occupational ILD; pulmonary vasculitis and alveolar hemorrhage syndromes; cystic lung diseases; pulmonary alveolar proteinosis; childhood ILD, and other rare ILDs. Within each chapter, sections on pathogenesis, epidemiology, clinical, radiographic, and pathological features, and management are discussed in depth. Specific aspects of ILD are addressed in separate chapters regarding: comorbidities; diagnosis and management of critical illness in patients with ILD; and role of lung transplantation for ILD.

This book provides an outstanding perspective of the evolving field of ILD, and heightens the imagination for future strategies to develop more targeted therapies. One of the strengths of this book is the plethora of images (histological and radiographic) and comprehensive figures and tables throughout. The references cited in this book are extensive, and allow the reader to easily retrieve the key sentinel articles in the field. This book is an outstanding review not only for Fellows and trainees, but for clinicians and academicians with an interest in ILD.

Joseph P. Lynch, III, M.D., FCCP, FERS
Holt and Jo Hickman Endowed Chair of Advanced Lung Disease and Lung Transplantation
Professor of Clinical Medicine, Step IX
Division of Pulmonary, Critical Care Medicine Allergy, and Clinical Immunology
The David Geffen School of Medicine at UCLA
Los Angeles, CA

Contributors

Traci Adams, MD
Department of Medicine
University of Texas Southwestern
Dallas, Texas

Adam L Anderson, MD
Division of Pulmonary and Critical Care Medicine
Washington University School of Medicine
St. Louis, Missouri

Deborah Assayag, MD, MAS, FRCPC
Department of Medicine
McGill University
Montreal, Canada

Kaïssa de Boer, BSc, MD, FRCPC
Department of Medicine
Division of Respirology
The Ottawa Hospital
University of Ottawa
Ottawa, Canada

Philippe Bonniaud
CHU Dijon Bourgogne
Hôpital François Mitterrand
Dijon, France

Kevin K Brown, MD
Department of Medicine
Autoimmune Lung Center
National Jewish Health
Denver, Colorado

Damian AD Bruce-Hickman
Department of Advanced Internal Medicine
National University Hospital Singapore
Singapore
and
Department of Neuroscience
University College London Medical School
London, United Kingdom

Andrew Bush, MBBS (HONS), MA, MD, FRCP, FRCPCH, FERS
Imperial College London
and
National Heart and Lung Institute
and
Royal Brompton Harefield
NHS Foundation Trust
London, United Kingdom

Philippe Camus
Hôpital Le Bocage
Dijon, France

William YC Chang, BA, BMBCh, MA, PhD, MRCP
Respiratory Medicine Department
Nottingham University Hospitals
NHS Trust
Nottingham, United Kingdom

Bridget F Collins, BA, MD
Department of Medicine
Center for Intestinal Lung Diseases
University of Washington Medical Center
Seattle, Washington

Vincent Cottin, MD, PhD
Hospices Civils de Lyon
Hôpital Louis Pradel
Centre de Référence National des Maladies Pulmonaires Rares
Service de Pneumologie
and
Claude Bernard University Lyon 1
Lyon, France

J Scott Ferguson, MD, FACP, FCCP
Department of Medicine
Division of Allergy, Pulmonary, Critical Care and Sleep Medicine
University of Wisconsin School of Medicine and Public Health
Madison, Wisconsin

Christine Fiddler, BSc, MBCHB, PhD, MRCP
Cambridge ILD Service
Royal Papworth and Addenbrooke's Hospital
Cambridge, United Kingdom

Aryeh Fischer, MD
Department of Medicine
Division of Rheumatology
Autoimmune and Interstitial Lung Disease Program
University of Colorado School of Medicine
Aurora, Colorado

Stephen K Frankel, MD, FCCM, FCCP
Department of Medicine
National Jewish Health
Denver, Colorado

Junya Fukuoka, MD, PhD
Department of Pathology
Graduate School of Biomedical Sciences
Nagasaki University Faculty of Medicine
Nagasaki, Japan

Helen Garthwaite
University College
London Hospitals
NHS Trust
London, United Kingdom

Craig Glazer, MD, MSPH
Department of Medicine
University of Texas Southwestern
Dallas, Texas

Amanda T Goodwin
Division of Respiratory Medicine
Nottingham University Hospitals NHS Trust
University of Nottingham
Nottingham, United Kingdom

Bibek Gooptu, BSc, MBBChir, PhD, AFHEA, MRCP
Leicester ILD Service and NIHR
Leicester Biomedical Research
Centre – Respiratory
Institute for Lung Health
Glenfield Hospital
and
Leicester Institute of Structural and Chemical
Biology
and
Divisions of Infection
Immunity and Inflammation and Molecular and
Cell Biology
University of Leicester
Leicester, United Kingdom

Melissa Heightman
University College London Hospitals
NHS Trust
London, United Kingdom

Richard J Hewitt, MBBS, BSc, MRCP
NIHR Academic Clinical Fellow in
Respiratory Medicine
Imperial College Healthcare NHS Trust
London, United Kingdom

Ling-Pei Ho, MD, PhD, FRCP
Oxford Interstitial Lung
Disease Service
Oxford Center for Respiratory Medicine
University of Oxford
Oxford, United Kingdom

Florence Jeny
University Paris
Assistance Publique Hôpitaux de Paris
Hôpital Avicenne
Bobigny, France

Marc A Judson
Department of Medicine
Division of Pulmonary and Critical
Care Medicine
Albany Medical College
Albany, New York

Jeffrey P Kanne, MD
Department of Radiology
Thoracic Imaging
University of Wisconsin School of Medicine
and Public Health
Madison, Wisconsin

Rebecca C Keith, BA, MD
Pulmonary Critical Care Medicine
Department of Medicine
National Jewish Health
Denver, Colorado
and
University of Colorado School of
Medicine
Aurora, Colorado

Joyce S Lee, MD, MAS
Department of Medicine
Division of Pulmonary Sciences and Critical
Care Medicine
University of Colorado Denver
Aurora, Colorado

Kevin O Leslie, MD
Department of Pathology
Mayo Clinic
Arizona, Minnesota

and

Mayo Clinic College of Medicine
Rochester, Minnesota

Toby M Maher, MB, MSc, PhD, FRCP
NIHR Respiratory Biomedical Research Unit
Royal Brompton Hospital
and
Fibrosis Research Group
National Heart and Lung Institute
Imperial College
London, United Kingdom

Matthieu Mahévas
University Paris Est Créteil
Centre de Référence des Cytopénies Autoimmunes
de l'adulte and Assistance Publique
Hôpitaux de Paris
Hôpital Henri Mondor
Créteil, France

Lisa A Maier, MD, MSPH
Division of Environmental and Occupational
Sciences
National Jewish Health
Denver, Colorado

and

Colorado School of Medicine and Public Health
Aurora, Colorado

Maria Daniela Martin, MD
Department of Radiology
Thoracic Imaging
University of Wisconsin School of Medicine and
Public Health
Madison, Wisconsin

Susan K Mathai, MD
Department of Medicine
Division of Pulmonary Sciences and Critical Care
Medicine
University of Colorado School of Medicine
Aurora, Colorado

Annyce S Mayer, MD, MSPH
National Jewish Health
Denver, Colorado

and

Colorado School of Public Health
Aurora, Colorado

Keith C Meyer, MD, MS
Department of Medicine
Division of Allergy, Pulmonary, Critical Care
and Sleep Medicine
University of Wisconsin School of Medicine
and Public Health
Madison, Wisconsin

David R Moller, MD
Department of Medicine
Division of Pulmonary and Critical Care
Medicine
Johns Hopkins University School of Medicine
Baltimore, Maryland

Cliff Morgan, BM, FRCA, FFICM
Royal Brompton and Harefield NHS Foundation
Trust
Royal Brompton Hospital
London, United Kingdom

Teng Moua, MD
Division of Pulmonary and Critical
Care Medicine
Mayo Clinic
Rochester, Minnesota

Steven D Nathan, MD, FCCP
Advanced Lung Disease and Lung Transplant
Program
Department of Medicine
INOVA Fairfax Hospital
Falls Church, Virginia

Hilario Nunes
University Paris
Assistance Publique Hôpitaux de Paris
Hôpital Avicenne
Bobigny, France

Amy L Olson, MD, MSPH
Department of Medicine
Interstitial Lung Disease Program and
Autoimmune Lung Center
National Jewish Health
Denver, Colorado

Helen Parfrey, BA, MA, BM, BCh, PhD, FRCP
Cambridge ILD Service
Royal Papworth and Addenbrooke's Hospitals
Cambridge, United Kingdom

Jasvir S Parmar, BM, PhD, FRCP, FFICM
Royal Papworth Hospital NHS Foundation Trust
University of Cambridge
Cambridge, United Kingdom

Ganesh Raghu, MD, FACP, FCCP
Department of Medicine
Center for Intestinal Lung Diseases
University of Washington Medical Center
Seattle, Washington

Tonya Russell, BS, MD
Division of Pulmonary and Critical Care
Medicine
Washington University School of Medicine
St. Louis, Missouri

Jay H Ryu, MD
Division of Pulmonary and Critical Care
Medicine
Mayo Clinic College of Medicine and Science
Rochester, Minnesota

David A Schwartz, MD
Department of Medicine
Division of Pulmonary Sciences and Critical Care
Medicine
University of Colorado School of Medicine
Aurora, Colorado

Adrian Shifren, MD
Division of Pulmonary and Critical Care Medicine
Washington University School of Medicine
St. Louis, Missouri

Joshua J Solomon, MD, FCCP
Department of Medicine
Autoimmune Lung Center
National Jewish Health
Denver, Colorado

Jeffrey J Swigris, MS, DO
Department of Medicine
Interstitial Lung Disease Program and
Autoimmune Lung Center
National Jewish Health
Denver, Colorado

Angela M Takano, MD
Department of Pathology
Singapore General Hospital (SGH)
and
Duke-NUS Medical School
National University of Singapore
Singapore

Muhunthan Thillai, MBBS, MRCP, PhD
Cambridge Interstitial Lung Disease Unit
Royal Papworth Hospital
Cambridge, United Kingdom

Claudia Valenzuela, MD
Hospital Universitario de la Princesa
Madrid, Spain

Dominique Valeyre, MD
University of Paris
Assistance Publique Hôpitaux de Paris
Hôpital Avicenne
Bobigny, France

Athol Wells, MBChB, FRACP, MD, FRCP, FRCR
Interstitial Lung Disease Unit
Royal Brompton Hospital
London, United Kingdom

Melissa Wickremasinghe, BSc, PhD, FRCP
Imperial College London
Imperial College Healthcare NHS Trust
London, United Kingdom

Henry Yung, MB, BChir, MRCP
Royal Papworth Hospital
Papworth Everard, United Kingdom

Zulma Yunt, MD
Department of Medicine
Interstitial Lung Disease Program and
Autoimmune Lung Center
National Jewish Health
Denver, Colorado

Introduction

The intention of writing this book is to provide readers a comprehensive overview of the lung disease entities that we recognize as the differing forms of interstitial lung disease (ILD). Our understanding and characterization of these disorders and recognition of the features which differentiate the specific forms of ILD has evolved rapidly over the past few decades. Whilst these advances have necessitated changes in classification schemes and terminology, new knowledge of the genetics and histopathologic manifestations of specific forms of ILD have improved our ability to provide prognoses to patients, develop therapies that specifically target individual forms of ILD (such as idiopathic pulmonary fibrosis – IPF) and provide personalized medicine to our patients. Providing the best care to patients with ILD depends on the recognition of clues from their clinical presentation combined with a careful physical examination, the use of state-of-the-art thoracic imaging, and the use of tissue sampling, when needed, to identify diagnostic histopathologic patterns and optimize the likelihood of making an accurate and confident diagnosis.

In the ideal setting, clinicians, thoracic radiologists, and lung pathologists should review all clinical, radiological, and histopathologic data together for any patient with a complex presentation of ILD to reach a consensus diagnosis and provide the best practice for their patients. In the near future, specific biomarkers will become validated that may be useful both in diagnosis and therapeutic management of ILD. Additionally, our evolving understanding of the genetic underpinnings and the role of epigenetic factors in disease risk and disease behaviour will undoubtedly improve our ability to provide better and safer therapies for specific forms of ILD. Our evolving knowledge of ILDs can also be used to construct better placebo-controlled, randomized clinical trials to identify effective therapies for specific forms of ILD, as has been recently accomplished with novel anti-fibrotic therapies for IPF.

It is our hope that this book will enhance our readers' knowledge of the various aspects of the disorders we recognize as specific forms of ILD, and inspire them to engage in meaningful clinical and translational research. Those who provide care to patients with ILD will find this book useful in both their ability to diagnose ILD in the clinic and the provision of appropriate therapies to their patients. We are greatly indebted to our authors who were gracious enough to contribute their chapters, and we believe that this compendium of knowledge and clinical wisdom will provide a firm foundation for all clinicians who diagnose and manage patients with ILD.

Muhunthan Thillai
David R Moller
Keith C Meyer
December 2017

An overview of the classification and diagnosis of interstitial lung disease

KEITH C MEYER

HISTORICAL BACKGROUND AND EVOLUTION OF TERMINOLOGY

Recognition of the existence of interstitial lung disease (ILD) dates back more than 100 years when Sir William Osler described 'cirrhosis of the lungs' and recognized the diversity of its forms and the difficulty of classifying these disorders (1). Various terminologies were coined over the span of the twentieth century as various leaders in the field described patients whose lungs displayed changes of interstitial inflammation and fibrosis. Hamman and Rich (1944) described four cases of rapidly progressive, diffuse alveolar wall thickening without identifiable cause, which led to use of the term, 'Hamman–Rich syndrome' for either acute-onset or chronic fibrotic ILD. Subsequently, diffuse pulmonary fibrosis was linked to forms of connective tissue disease (CTD) and other causes, such as exposure to organic or inorganic dusts and pneumotoxic drug reactions, but many forms remained unexplained by any associations. Terms such as 'chronic idiopathic interstitial fibrosis', 'diffuse

fibrosing alveolitis' or 'idiopathic pulmonary fibrosis' were used to designate fibrotic ILD of unknown aetiology, and these disorders were thought to occur as a consequence of alveolar wall inflammation ('alveolitis'). The term 'diffuse fibrosing alveolitis' was coined by Scadding (2) to describe widespread fibrotic change beyond the level of the terminal bronchioles, and Scadding subdivided entities according to known or unknown associations and patterns of fibrosis (Figure 1.1). Liebow and Carrington (3,4) published a classification system for chronic idiopathic interstitial pneumonias that was based on histopathologic changes; one of the five subgroups that they described was termed 'usual' interstitial pneumonia (UIP), and the Hamman–Rich syndrome was felt to be an acute form of UIP (Figure 1.1).

The classification systems proposed by Scadding or Liebow and Carrington were quite similar, but clinicians tended to overlook histopathologic variations and termed 'chronic idiopathic fibrosing ILD' as 'cryptogenic fibrosing alveolitis' (Europeans) or 'idiopathic pulmonary fibrosis' (United States). Katzenstein and Myers (5) re-examined Liebow's

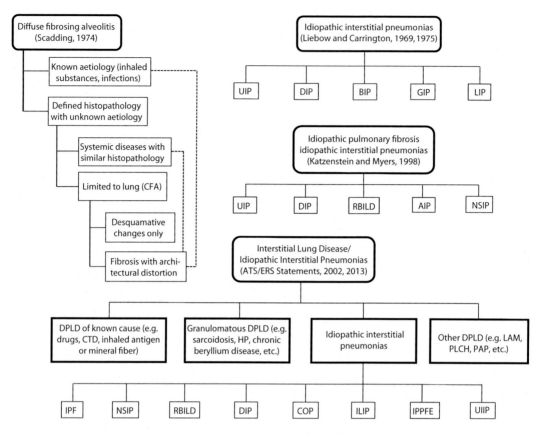

Figure 1.1 Evolution of classification systems for interstitial lung disease and forms of idiopathic interstitial pneumonia. (Abbreviations: AIP = acute interstitial pneumonia; BIP = bronchiolitis interstitial pneumonia; CFA = cryptogenic fibrosing alveolitis; COP = cryptogenic organizing pneumonia; CTD = connective tissue disease; DIP = desquamative interstitial pneumonia; DPLD = diffuse parenchymal lung disease; GIP = giant cell interstitial pneumonia; HP = hypersensitivity pneumonia; ILIP = idiopathic lymphoid interstitial pneumonia; IPF = idiopathic pulmonary fibrosis; IPPFE = idiopathic pleuropulmonary fibrosis; LAM = lymphangioleiomyomatosis; NSIP = non-specific interstitial pneumonia; PLCH = pulmonary Langerhans cell histiocytosis; RBILD = respiratory bronchiolitis interstitial lung disease; UIIP = undifferentiated interstitial pneumonia; UIP = usual interstitial pneumonia.)

classification system and refined the histopathology-based system by adding two new categories (non-specific interstitial pneumonia [NSIP] and respiratory-bronchiolitis-associated ILD [RBILD]) while revising/retaining some of Liebow's categories (UIP and desquamative interstitial pneumonia [DIP]): acute interstitial pneumonia (AIP) was coined as a term for the Hamman–Rich syndrome (Figure 1.1). Their scheme recognized giant cell interstitial pneumonia (GIP) as caused by hard-metal exposure and considered lymphoid interstitial pneumonia (LIP) as a lymphoproliferative disorder, while bronchiolitis interstitial pneumonia (BIP) was recognized as an intraluminal (rather than interstitial) process that could take the

form of organizing pneumonia (aka bronchiolitis obliterans organizing pneumonia [BOOP]) or diffuse alveolar damage (DAD). They also correlated their histopathologic pattern-based classification system with clinical features and natural history.

With the evolution of ongoing clinical and pathologic investigations of ILD from the late twentieth century to the present era combined with the advent of thoracic high-resolution computed tomography (HRCT) imaging, schemes for the classification of ILD that melded clinical syndromes, histopathologic changes and HRCT imaging together to define specific diagnostic entities were formulated (6–10). However, it also became apparent that histopathologic patterns could have overlap among clinical entities (e.g. a UIP pattern can be idiopathic and consistent with a diagnosis of idiopathic pulmonary fibrosis [IPF], or a UIP pattern can be associated with CTD accompanied by lung involvement). Finally, classification schemes will undoubtedly change as we identify causative genomic and epigenetic determinants that appear to be operant in risk and causation of the myriad forms of ILD (11–15), and understanding the genomics of ILD will likely lead to improved, personalized therapies.

CURRENT CLASSIFICATION SYSTEMS FOR ILD

The pantheon of more than 200 forms of ILD can be classified in a variety of ways. An updated consensus classification system (Figure 1.1) forged by expert opinion (while using a multidisciplinary approach that combined clinical characteristics with histopathologic and HRCT patterns) segregated the various forms of ILD into four major categories while focusing on the category of IIPs was published in 2002 (6) and updated in 2013 (7). Alternative approaches that also focus on the combination of etiologies, clinical presentation and findings, radiologic imaging patterns and histopathologic characteristics can also be used to represent a clinically useful classification system (Tables 1.1 and 1.2). Forms of ILD can be differentiated by acute (e.g. acute interstitial pneumonia [AIP]) versus chronic onset (e.g. UIP), disorders that tend to be more responsive to anti-inflammatory/immunosuppressive therapies (e.g. sarcoidosis, hypersensitivity pneumonitis [HP], CTD-associated ILD, interstitial pneumonia with autoimmune features [IPAF], cryptogenic organizing pneumonia [COP]) versus those unlikely to respond to such therapy (e.g. UIP, pneumoconioses), disorders that may remit with appropriate therapy but have a propensity to relapse (e.g. COP), disorders linked to exposures (e.g. pneumoconioses, HP), lung-limited disorders (e.g. IIPs) versus those linked to extrapulmonary disease processes (e.g. sarcoidosis, CTD-associated ILD), those caused by therapeutic interventions for pulmonary or non-pulmonary disorders (e.g. iatrogenic ILD due to drug reactions or radiation therapy) and those that are caused by inherited gene variants (e.g. Hermansky–Pudlak syndrome).

Regardless of the classification system utilized to characterize and define the various forms of ILD,

Table 1.1 Classification of interstitial lung disease (diffuse parenchymal lung disease)

1. Idiopathic interstitial pneumonia
   - Idiopathic pulmonary fibrosis (i.e. idiopathic usual interstitial pneumonia)
   - Non-specific interstitial pneumonia (NSIP)
   - Desquamative interstitial pneumonia (DIP)
   - Respiratory bronchiolitis-associated interstitial lung disease (RBILD)
   - Acute interstitial pneumonia (AIP)
   - Cryptogenic organizing pneumonia (COP)
   - Lymphocytic interstitial pneumonia (idiopathic)
   - Pleuro-parenchymal fibroelastosis (idiopathic)
   - Non-classifiable interstitial pneumonia (NCIP)
2. Connective tissue disease associated
   - Rheumatoid arthritis
   - Systemic sclerosis (scleroderma)
   - Anti-synthetase syndromes
   - Sjögren syndrome
   - Systemic lupus erythematosus
   - Ankylosing spondylitis
3. Primary disease related
   - Sarcoidosis
   - Pulmonary Langerhans cell histiocytosis (PLCH)
   - Lymphangioleiomyomatosis (LAM)
   - Eosinophilic lung disease related (e.g. eosinophilic pneumonia)
   - Chronic aspiration
   - Pulmonary alveolar proteinosis (PAP)
   - Amyloidosis
   - Inflammatory bowel disease associated
   - Hepatic disease associated (e.g. primary biliary cirrhosis, viral hepatitis)
   - Mimics of ILD (infection or malignancy associated)
4. Iatrogenic
   - Drug induced
   - Radiation pneumonitis/fibrosis
5. Inhalational exposure related (occupational or environmental)
   - Hypersensitivity pneumonitis (organic antigen inhalation)
     - Acute/subacute
     - Chronic fibrosing

(Continued)

Table 1.1 (*Continued*) Classification of interstitial lung disease (diffuse parenchymal lung disease)

- • Inorganic dust/fibre/fume related
  - • Pneumoconiosis (e.g. asbestosis, silicosis, hard metal lung disease)
  - • Other (e.g. berylliosis, chronic beryllium disease, gaseous phase agents)
6. Inherited lung disease
   - • Familial interstitial pneumonia (FIP)
   - • Hermansky–Pudlak syndrome (HPS)
   - • Other (e.g. metabolic storage diseases)
7. Miscellaneous disorders
   - • Interstitial pneumonia with autoimmune features (IPAF)
   - • Diffuse alveolar haemorrhage (e.g. Goodpasture syndrome)
   - • Idiopathic diffuse alveolar haemorrhage
   - • Acute fibrinous and organizing pneumonia (AFOP)
   - • Bronchiolocentric pattern of interstitial pneumonia

considerable overlap will continue to exist among various observations used to differentiate many of these disorders from one another. Despite such overlap, however, findings such as Velcro-like crackles on chest auscultation, which are usually detected in patients with IPF but may be present with other ILD with advanced fibrosis, can narrow the differential diagnosis. Other examples include finding a UIP radiologic and/or histopathologic pattern, which can be seen not only in IPF but also other ILD such as CTD-associated ILD, chronic HP, asbestosis or drug reactions, or by detecting a significant lymphocytosis in bronchoalveolar lavage fluid (BALF), which essentially rules out IPF but implicates other entities such as sarcoidosis, acute HP or cellular NSIP, and can considerably narrow a differential diagnosis and help attain an ultimate, confident diagnosis. One must put all the data together to navigate through various levels of potential overlap among characteristics of specific entities to arrive at a consensus clinical–radiologic–pathologic diagnosis that is consistent with the specific disease at hand.

IDIOPATHIC INTERSTITIAL PNEUMONIAS

The usage and definition of the term 'idiopathic pulmonary fibrosis' have changed considerably since it was initially used by clinicians to signify cases of pulmonary fibrosis of unknown cause (16). In the decades leading up to statements and clinical practice guidelines published over the past two decades, cases with overlapping clinical features and imaging characteristics (e.g. non-IPF forms of IIP, chronic HP, CTD-associated ILD, IPAF) were typically lumped together and assigned a diagnosis of IPF (or cryptogenic fibrosing alveolitis [CFA]) by clinicians despite the heterogeneity of histopathologic findings and clinical features. As the most common form of IIP encountered in the clinic, the term 'IPF' has been retained but is now specifically defined according to the key features of a consistent clinical presentation, the presence of a confident UIP pattern on HRCT imaging, exclusion of other potential diagnoses, and, if needed, a UIP pattern on lung biopsy specimens if the HRCT does not adequately identify a typical UIP pattern (17). However, a definitive diagnosis may not be forthcoming despite obtaining HRCT imaging and an adequately sampled lung biopsy specimen, and a multidisciplinary discussion may be required to facilitate interobserver agreement and reach a consensus diagnosis (18–21). A search for evidence of CTD is also essential, as UIP, NSIP, AIP or DIP patterns can be seen when patients have CTD-associated ILD (22) or an interstitial pneumonia with autoimmune features (IPAF) for which criteria for a specific CTD diagnosis are not met (23). Making an accurate diagnosis of a specific form of IIP can be even more challenging when clinical and laboratory data are present that suggest a diagnosis of CTD but criteria for a specific CTD are not met. Patients with this situation can be classified as having IPAF, but if the only finding is a positive anti-nuclear antibody or rheumatoid factor without any other criteria for a diagnosis of CTD or IPAF, a diagnosis of an idiopathic IIP (e.g. IPF) can still be assigned and maintained (although some patients may develop criteria for a diagnosis of CTD as their disease evolves over time).

The updated statement on multidisciplinary classification of the IIPs (7) recognizes that some cases that appear to be consistent with an IIP diagnosis may not satisfy criteria that allow diagnosis as a specific form of IIP. Circumstances in which a final diagnosis may not be reached include a lack of adequate clinical, radiologic or pathologic data to allow a specific diagnosis to be rendered or major discordance among clinical, radiologic and pathologic findings that preclude reaching a specific

Table 1.2 Classification according to disease characteristics

Characteristic	ILD diagnosis or complication
Associated with smoking	RBILD, DIP, PLCH, IPF, CPFE, NSIP
Associated with occupational, environmental, medication or radiation exposures	Inorganic dust pneumoconiosis, HP (e.g. bird protein, grain dust, humidifiers, hot tubs), drug-induced pneumonitis (e.g. amiodarone, methotrexate, nitrofurantoin), radiation pneumonitis, infection
Frequent pleural involvement	CTD-ILD (RA, SLE), PPFE
Rapid onset and/or worsening	AIP, drug-induced pneumonitis, acute HP, acute EP, COP, DAD, DAH, acute lupus pneumonitis, AFOP, AEIPF
Associated with GERD, dysphagia	CTD-ILD (especially scleroderma), IPF, aspiration pneumonitis/fibrosis
Predisposition to relapse	COP
Responsive to anti-inflammatory or immunosuppressive therapy	Acute HP, COP, sarcoidosis, cellular NSIP, CTD-associated ILD
Poor response to anti-inflammatory or immunosuppressive therapy	IPF, fibrotic NSIP, AEIPF, AIP
Lung-limited disorders	IIP (e.g. IPF, idiopathic NSIP, RBILD, DIP, AIP, COP, idiopathic PPFE, idiopathic LIP), familial interstitial pneumonia/fibrosis, inhalation-related ILD, PAP, PLCH, EP, drug/radiation-induced ILD
Disorders frequently associated with extrapulmonary organ system involvement	Sarcoidosis, CTD-ILD, Hermansky–Pudlak syndrome, LAM, malignancy
Associated with advanced age	IPF, RA-associated ILD

Abbreviations: AEIPF = acute exacerbation of idiopathic pulmonary fibrosis; AFOP = acute fibrinous and organizing pneumonia; AIP = acute interstitial pneumonia; COP = cryptogenic organizing pneumonia; CPFE = combined pulmonary fibrosis and emphysema; CTD-ILD = connective tissue disease-associated interstitial lung disease; DAD = diffuse alveolar damage; DAH = diffuse alveolar haemorrhage; DIP = desquamative interstitial pneumonia; EP = eosinophilic pneumonia; GERD = gastro-oesophageal reflux disease; HP = hypersensitivity pneumonitis; IIP = idiopathic interstitial pneumonia; IPF = idiopathic pulmonary fibrosis; LAM = lymphangioleiomyomatosis; LIP = lymphoid interstitial pneumonia; NSIP = non-specific interstitial pneumonia; PAP = pulmonary alveolar proteinosis; PLCH = pulmonary Langerhans cell histiocytosis; PPFE = pleuro-parenchymal fibroelastosis; RA = rheumatoid arthritis; RBILD = respiratory bronchiolitis interstitial lung disease; SLE = systemic lupus erythematosus.

diagnosis. One example of when this situation may exist is when previous therapies (e.g. corticosteroids) may have altered subsequent radiologic imaging characteristics or histologic findings obtained at the time a patient undergoes a diagnostic evaluation for suspected IIP.

GENETICS OF ILD: POTENTIAL IMPACT ON CLASSIFICATION AND TERMINOLOGY

Many forms of ILD/pulmonary fibrosis have recently been linked to specific inherited gene mutations and polymorphisms (Table 1.3), and an evolving understanding of genomics has also identified numerous epigenetic mechanisms that are associated with the pathogenesis of many forms of ILD (11–15). Telomere dysfunction, polymorphisms for the *MUC5B* gene, and a variety of single-nucleotide polymorphisms for genes such as *TOLLIP* or *TLR3* have been associated with both disease risk and behaviour for patients with IPF. Ongoing studies are likely to discover many other genetic factors that are associated with various ILD diagnoses and identify specific genotype–phenotype relationships that modulate the natural history of disease and/or interact

Table 1.3 Fibrotic disorders linked to gene mutations or polymorphisms

Clinical disorder	Abnormal gene(s) and expression patterns	Proposed mechanisms of pathogenesis
Familial or sporadic PF	MUC5B, TOLLIP, TLR3, ATP11A, DSP, DPP9, SPPL2C	Host defense impairment
Familial or sporadic PF	TERC (AD), TERT (AD), RTEL1, PARN, OBRFC1	Telomere shortening/dysfunction DNA repair
Familial PF	SFTPA1 (AD), SFTPA2 (AD), SFTPC (AD), SFTPB (AD), NKX2-1 (AD), ABCA3 (AD)	Surfactant dysfunction
Familial or sporadic PF	ELMOD2	Disruption of signalling pathways
Hermansky–Pudlak syndrome (subtypes HPS1, HPS2 and HPS4)	HPS1 (AR), HPS4 (AR), AP3B1	Intracellular protein trafficking Cytoplasmic organelle dysfunction Surfactant dysfunction
Dyskeratosis congenita	DKC1 (XLR), TERC (AD), TERT (AD), TINF2 (AD)	Telomere shortening/dysfunction

Abbreviations: AD = autosomal dominant inheritance pattern; AR = autosomal recessive inheritance pattern; PF = pulmonary fibrosis; XLR = X-linked recessive inheritance pattern.

with environmental risk factors to increase risk of developing a specific ILD entity. As useful bio-markers of disease and genomics of ILD progress, classification systems are likely to change in accordance with new discoveries in the field.

CURRENT APPROACH TO MAKING A CONFIDENT ILD DIAGNOSIS

A systematic approach (24) is required to accurately diagnose specific forms of ILD (Figure 1.2). Most patients present with new onset of symptoms such as dyspnoea on exertion, cough and/or fatigue, but asymptomatic or relatively asymptomatic patients with earlier stages of disease may be identified when interstitial abnormalities are an incidental finding on thoracic imaging obtained for other indications. A careful and comprehensive interview that includes whether there is a history of medication/drug exposures (e.g. amiodarone, nitrofurantoin, methotrexate), occupational or environmental exposures or a history of CTD should be obtained and can provide important clues to an ultimate diagnosis. Physical examination may reveal basilar 'Velcro-like' crackles on lung auscultation, the presence of digital clubbing, or other findings that are suggestive of specific forms of ILD such as IPF. Laboratory testing (pulmonary function testing,

CTD serologies, other testing as appropriate) combined with the history, physical examination and routine chest radiographic imaging (postero-anterior and lateral view x-rays) may be adequate to establish a reasonably confident ILD diagnosis.

If additional diagnostic testing is needed, a non-contrast, HRCT that is performed at full inspiration with both supine and prone positioning and expiratory views can provide essential diagnostic information. If HRCT scan results show a definite radiologic pattern of UIP (subpleural and basilar predominant changes, reticular pattern, honeycomb change with or without traction bronchiectasis and absence of features that are inconsistent with a UIP pattern), a confident diagnosis of IPF can be made if clinical features do not suggest the presence of a non-IPF ILD diagnosis such as ILD associated with CTD-ILD.

If a confident ILD diagnosis cannot be made via findings from the clinical presentation and evaluation combined with HRCT imaging results, invasive testing must be considered to secure a diagnosis. Bronchoscopy is relatively safe, and bronchoalveolar lavage (BAL) and/or endoscopic lung biopsies may provide very useful information that can be diagnostic, especially when combined with other clinical data and HRCT imaging. However, bronchoscopy may be perceived as unlikely to secure a diagnosis, especially if a form of IIP is suspected to be present.

Progression to a more invasive type of lung biopsy without performing bronchoscopy may be

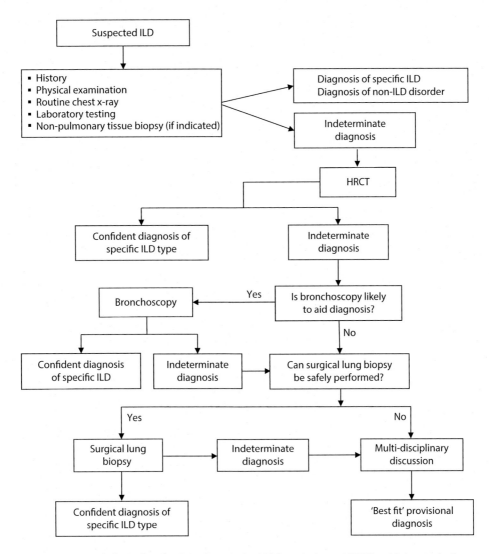

Figure 1.2 A suggested algorithm for ILD diagnosis. (Abbreviations: HRCT = high-resolution computed tomography of the thorax; ILD = interstitial lung disease.)

reasonable, and such may be required if bronchoscopy is performed but does not provide diagnostic findings. Obtaining a surgical lung biopsy (SLB), which is usually performed via a video-assisted thorascopic surgery (VATS) approach, remains the procedure of choice at most centres if other diagnostic testing cannot allow a confident diagnosis to be made. However, patients at high risk for serious complications if a SLB is performed may not be good candidates to undergo the procedure, and patients should thoroughly understand the potential risks and benefits of SLB. Ideally, multidisciplinary discussions among clinicians, radiologists, and pathologists (if tissue biopsies are obtained)

should be held to attain an ultimate, 'best fit' diagnosis. Bronchoscopic lung cryobiopsy (BLC), which can retrieve much larger tissue specimens than endoscopic transbronchial biopsies, may become an alternative to SLB, but the utility of BLC remains to be determined (25).

SUMMARY

Classification schemes that encompass and distinguish among the various forms of ILD have evolved tremendously over recent decades and will continue to change as our knowledge of these disorders, especially their genetic and genomic underpinnings and causative/modulatory epigenetic factors, evolves. Nonetheless, such classification schemes continue to have some degree of redundancy and overlap. When clinicians encounter a patient with signs and symptoms of ILD, a systematic approach that evaluates the combination of clinical features, potential risk factors and exposures, appropriate laboratory testing, measurements of lung function, thoracic imaging characteristics and, if needed, histopathologic patterns in adequately sampled lung biopsy specimens is likely to lead to a confident diagnosis of a specific form of ILD. The currently used ILD classification systems will continue to evolve and change as useful biomarkers and genetic factors that are indicative of specific disorders are discovered and incorporated into diagnostic algorithms and classification schemes that point to causation as well as potential responses to specific therapies.

REFERENCES

1. Osler W. *The Principles and Practice of Medicine.* New York, NY: Appleton; 1892.
2. Scadding JG. Diffuse pulmonary alveolar fibrosis. *Thorax.* 1974;29:271–81.
3. Liebow AA, Carrington DB. The interstitial pneumonias. In: Simon M, Potchen EJ, LeMay M, eds. *Frontiers of Pulmonary Radiology.* New York, NY: Grune & Stratton; 1969:102–41.
4. Liebow AA. Definition and classification of interstitial pneumonias in human pathology. *Prog Respir Res.* 1975;8:1–33.
5. Katzenstein ALA, Myers JL. *Am J Respir Crit Care Med.* 1998;157:1301–15.
6. American Thoracic Society/European Respiratory Society International Multidisciplinary Consensus Classification of the Idiopathic Interstitial Pneumonias. *Am J Respir Crit Care Med.* 2002;165:277–304.
7. Travis WD, Costabel U, Hansell DM et al. An official American Thoracic Society/ European Respiratory Society statement: Update of the international multidisciplinary classification of the idiopathic interstitial pneumonias. *Am J Respir Crit Care Med.* 2013;188(6):733–48.
8. Collard HR, King TE Jr. Diffuse lung disease: Classification and evaluation. In: Baughman RP, du Bois RM, eds. *Diffuse Lung Disease: A Practical Approach.* 2nd ed. New York, NY: Springer; 2012:85–100.
9. Gomez AD, King TE Jr. Classification of diffuse parenchymal lung disease. In: Costabel U, du Bois RM, Egan JJ, eds. *Diffuse Parenchymal Lung Disease, Progress in Respiratory Research.* Basel: Karger; 2007;36:2–10.
10. Leslie KO. My approach to interstitial lung disease using clinical, radiological and histopathological patterns. *J Clin Pathol.* 2009;62:387–401.
11. Devine MS, Garcia CK. *Clin Chest Med.* 2012;33:95–110.
12. Mathai SK, Schwartz DA, Warg LA. Genetic susceptibility and pulmonary fibrosis. *Curr Opin Pulm Med.* 2014;20:429–35.
13. Chu SG, El-Chemaly S, Rosas IO. Genetics and idiopathic interstitial pneumonias. *Semin Respir Crit Care Med.* 2016;37:321–30.
14. Mathai SK, Yang IV, Schwarz MI, Schwartz DA. Incorporating genetics into the identification and treatment of idiopathic pulmonary fibrosis. *BMC Med.* 2015;13:191.
15. Yang IV, Schwartz DA. Epigenetics of idiopathic pulmonary fibrosis. *Transl Res.* 2015;165:48–60.
16. Meyer KC. Idiopathic pulmonary fibrosis: A historical perspective. In: Meyer KC, Nathan SD, eds. *Idiopathic Pulmonary Fibrosis: A Comprehensive Clinical Guide.* New York, NY: Humana Press, Springer; 2014:1–8.
17. Raghu G, Collard HR, Egan JJ et al. An official ATS/ERS/JRS/ALAT statement: Idiopathic pulmonary fibrosis: Evidence-based guidelines for diagnosis and management. *Am J Respir Crit Care Med.* 2011;183:788–824.
18. Flaherty KR, King TE Jr, Raghu G et al. Idiopathic interstitial pneumonia: What is the effect of a multidisciplinary approach to diagnosis? *Am J Respir Crit Care Med.* 2004;170:904–10.
19. Walsh SL, Wells AU, Desai SR et al. Multicentre evaluation of multidisciplinary team meeting agreement on diagnosis

in diffuse parenchymal lung disease: A case-cohort study. *Lancet Respir Med.* 2016;4:557–65.

20. Meyer, KC. Multidisciplinary discussions and interstitial lung disease diagnosis: How useful is a meeting of the minds? *Lancet Respir Med.* 2016;4:529–31.

21. Jo HE, Glaspole IN, Levin KC et al. Clinical impact of the interstitial lung disease multidisciplinary service. *Respirology.* 2016;21(8):1438–44.

22. Swigris JJ, Brown KK, Flaherty KR. The idiopathic interstitial pneumonias and connective tissue disease-associated interstitial lung disease. *Curr Rheumatol Rev.* 2010;6:91–98.

23. Fischer A, Antoniou KM, Brown KK et al. An official European Respiratory Society/ American Thoracic Society research statement: Interstitial pneumonia with autoimmune features. *Eur Respir J.* 2015;46:976–87.

24. Meyer KC. Diagnosis and management of interstitial lung disease. *Translat Respir Med.* 2014;2:4. doi: 10.1186/2213-0802-2-4. eCollection 2014.

25. Patel NM, Borczuk AC, Lederer DJ. Cryobiopsy in the diagnosis of interstitial lung disease. A step forward or back? *Am J Respir Crit Care Med.* 2016;193:707–9.

2

Histopathology of interstitial lung disease: A pattern-based approach

ANGELA M TAKANO, JUNYA FUKUOKA AND KEVIN O LESLIE

INTRODUCTION

Interstitial lung diseases encompass a diverse group of more than 200 separate entities affecting the lung parenchyma. Because these conditions are multilobar and frequently bilateral in distribution on imaging, the term 'diffuse parenchymal lung disease' (DPLD) has been suggested as both more appropriate and less restrictive at the microscopic pathology level. Today the diagnosis of DPLD requires correlation of clinical, radiologic and histopathologic features for clinical relevance.

The hurdles facing the general surgical pathologist confronted with DPLD are many. Most importantly, the rarity of the individual diseases combined with the infrequency of surgical lung biopsy make the appropriate management of them nearly impossible in general pathology practice. Also notable is the complex terminology applied over the years, nomenclature that has been optimized in recent years by the efforts of the American Thoracic Society and European Respiratory Society (ATS/ERS) (1). Finally, the fact that many of these diseases have multiple causes, ranging from drug exposure to autoimmune disease, adds a layer of nuance to the interpretation that lies beyond the comfort zone of most general pathologists. Histopathologically, these diverse diseases are most often characterized by varying degrees of inflammation, repair and fibrosis; the exact histological picture presented in a lung biopsy specimen depends on the timing of the biopsy in relationship to the onset of the disease as well as the possibility that multiple injuries have accumulated over time or are occurring simultaneously (2). The final histopathologic features resulting from such complex interactions are generally difficult to decode without a proper pattern approach, which must be applied together with adequate clinical information and a basic understanding of the radiologic findings.

In this chapter we discuss the six histopathologic patterns of interstitial lung disease (ILD) and their correlation with ILD diagnoses as well as with thoracic high-resolution computed tomography (HRCT) imaging.

PATTERN I: ACUTE LUNG INJURY

This is the first histopathologic pattern to be considered because these instances are most often associated with an acute clinical presentation. Such conditions need immediate intervention (such as the case of diffuse alveolar haemorrhage with capillaritis) and can portend a high mortality rate (such as diffuse alveolar damage in cases of acute respiratory distress syndrome), or both (3). The pattern of acute lung injury is characterized by the presence of one or more of the following elements: *interstitial oedema, intra-alveolar fibrinous exudates, reactive type 2 pneumocytes, hyaline membranes, tissue necrosis, intra-alveolar blood, haemosiderin-laden macrophages and intra-alveolar eosinophils.*

The duration of symptoms is generally hours to days, and sometimes up to a few weeks before the time of biopsy. Clinically, the patients present with breathlessness, fever, chills and night sweats, the intensity and combination of which depend on the type and intensity of injury.

Radiologically, they present with bilateral infiltrates with different degrees of compromise of the lung parenchyma, which varies from patchy opacities to so-called lung 'white-out', where there is complete opacification of both lung fields (Figure 2.1).

Several specific histopathologic entities fall under this umbrella of 'acute lung injury' and correspond to clinical–radiological presentations. These are presented below.

DIFFUSE ALVEOLAR DAMAGE

The main histopathologic feature is the presence of intra-alveolar hyaline membranes with a spectrum of changes depending on the phase of the injury. Diffuse alveolar damage (DAD) is the histopathologic manifestation of many types of acute alveolar injury caused by diverse agents and mechanisms (Table 2.1). In some instances, however, the cause of the injury remains unknown. The idiopathic type of DAD corresponds to the clinical presentation of acute interstitial pneumonia (AIP) (4). Because infections figure prominently in the list of causes, special stains for organisms, including immunohistochemical stains for viruses, if available, must be performed as part of the standard workup of the biopsy. The clinical presentation of this type of injury is typically the acute respiratory distress syndrome (ARDS). Patients with ARDS present with an abrupt onset of refractory respiratory failure with typical bilateral ground glass opacities

(a)

(b)

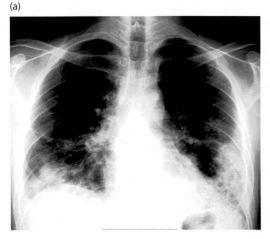
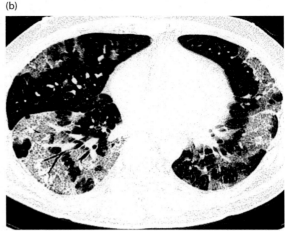

Figure 2.1 (a) Antero-posterior chest x-ray of acute lung injury showing bilateral, predominantly peripheral, somewhat asymmetrical consolidation with air bronchograms. (b) HRCT image of the same case shows bilateral ground glass opacification and consolidation with irregular dilatation of bronchi and bronchioles.

Table 2.1 Causes of DAD

1. Pulmonary infections (viral, bacterial, mycobacterial and fungal pneumonia)
2. Sepsis
3. Post-transplantation
4. Connective tissue diseases manifesting in the lung (myositis related, systemic lupus erythematosus)
5. Acute exacerbation of chronic interstitial pneumonias
6. Drug toxicity
7. Toxic inhalants
8. Radiation pneumonitis
9. Traumatic injury
10. Acute interstitial pneumonia
11. Idiopathic

producing a 'white-out' radiological pattern with air bronchograms (5). The histologic changes of DAD can be further divided into three phases: (1) exudative, (2) proliferative and (3) repair.

Exudative phase

This phase lasts for approximately 1 week from the initial injury (point zero, in experimental models). The process begins with congestion of the alveolar capillaries, exudation, interstitial oedema, and collapse of the involved alveoli ('congestive atelectasis') (6). This is followed by formation of

'hyaline membranes' composed of fibrin mixed with sloughed-off epithelial cells and secretory proteins. Variable degrees of alveolar haemorrhage, interstitial lymphoid infiltrates and early proliferation of type II alveolar pneumocytes can be seen (7) (Figure 2.2).

Proliferative phase

This phase begins in the second week following a single injury and lasts for 1 or 2 weeks. It consists of marked type II pneumocyte proliferation beneath the hyaline membranes, and differentiation toward type I pneumocytes in order to cover up the denudation that the alveolar surfaces suffered during the exudative phase, while 'pushing-off' some hyaline membranes into the alveolar lumen. In some instances, however, the epithelium incorporates the hyaline membranes into the interstitium, where they can participate in a fibrotic process (6). Type II pneumocyte hyperplasia can also be accompanied by marked squamous metaplasia, so extreme as to simulate a malignancy (Figure 2.3).

Repair phase

This phase is characterized by proliferation of connective tissue cells such as fibroblasts and myofibroblasts, with deposition of collagen with the purpose to regenerate damaged basement membranes. Extension of the fibrosis into the alveolar

(a)

(b)

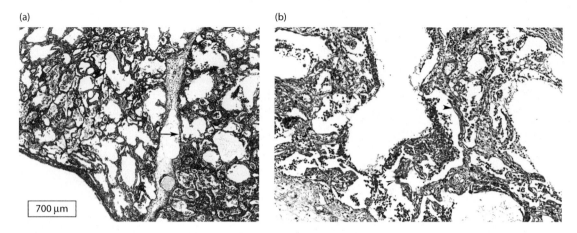

700 µm

Figure 2.2 Diffuse alveolar damage, exudative phase. **(a)** Diffuse abnormality showing widening of alveolar ducts, which causes simplification of the lung structure (*asterisks*) and dilatations of inter-lobular septa (*arrow*), key findings of this phase. **(b)** Higher magnification highlights the presence of hyaline membrane (*arrowheads*) along with interstitial oedema and mild interstitial cellular infiltration. Surrounding alveolar sacs were collapsed and form 'thick septa' (*asterisk*).

ducts gives rise to 'rings' of fibrosis (8). In some cases, there can be marked intra-alveolar plugs of fibroblasts, in a similar manner to that seen in organizing pneumonia. This pattern has been described in cases of bleomycin-induced acute lung injury, with complete recovery of lung function (Figure 2.4).

It is important to point out that in spite of the diffuse nature of this pathologic process, histo-pathologic findings in biopsy material may not be completely uniform and may be quite variable from field to field. Immunocompromised patients who present with an acute interstitial lung disease,

frequently show DAD in their lung biopsies. In this instance, infectious causes and drugs are the most common culprits. In patients with end-stage idiopathic pulmonary fibrosis (IPF), DAD can be superimposed, a manifestation that is known as acute exacerbation of IPF (9) (Figure 2.5). A variant of acute injury recently described is 'acute fibrin-ous and organizing pneumonia' (AFOP). This vari-ant was described in patients with acute respiratory failure. The biopsy material in these cases shows intra-alveolar 'ball-like' collections of fibrin with-out eosinophils, formation of hyaline membranes, and little organization. Minimal intra-alveolar and

(a)

(b)

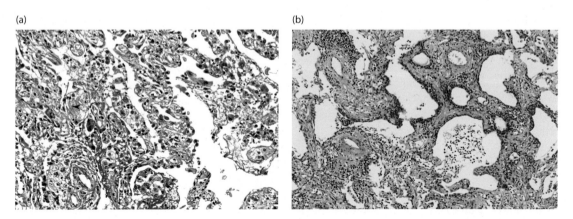

Figure 2.3 Proliferative phase of DAD. **(a)** Residual hyaline membranes become faint and incorpo-rated to alveolar septa (*arrowhead*). Type 2 cell proliferation is a characteristic finding of this phase. **(b)** Squamous metaplasia is a frequent event of DAD and starts to appear in the proliferative phase, which may last for a long period.

(a) (b)

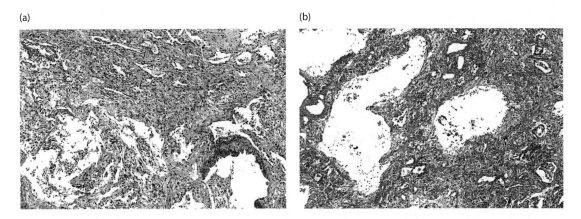

Figure 2.4 Repair phase of DAD. **(a)** Proliferation of myofibroblasts as seen in organizing pneumonia appears in a diffuse manner. It affects both airspace and alveolar septa, often with architectural destruction. **(b)** Young fibrosis developing to replace hyaline membranes, which may produce 'rings' of fibrosis around the dilated alveolar ducts.

(a) (b)

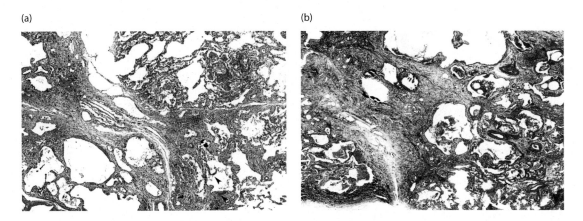

Figure 2.5 Acute exacerbation of IPF. **(a)** Coexistence of chronic dense fibrosis and any phase of DAD is the typical presentation. In these images, the left side shows dense fibrosis while the right side shows the exudative phase of DAD. Note the presence of hyaline membranes (*arrowheads*). **(b)** The presence of chronic dense fibrosis can be highlighted by azan trichrome staining.

interstitial inflammatory infiltrates are present. When patients with AFOP required mechanical ventilation, the mortality rate was similar to that seen in patients with DAD (10).

ACUTE INJURY WITH NECROSIS

If the lung biopsy material of a patient with acute respiratory distress shows manifestations of acute lung injury accompanied by necrosis, infectious causes have to be considered first in the differential diagnosis, regardless of the results of special stains. Other possible differential diagnoses include granulomatosis with polyangiitis (GPA), necrotizing sarcoidosis, infarction, malignant tumour and Churg–Strauss syndrome (Figure 2.6).

ACUTE EOSINOPHILIC PNEUMONIA

This presentation of acute respiratory failure is characterized by the presence of increased numbers of interstitial and intra-alveolar eosinophils with features of exudative and proliferative DAD (11) (Figure 2.7). This finding is extremely important because this serious condition responds well to corticosteroids. A complicating factor for

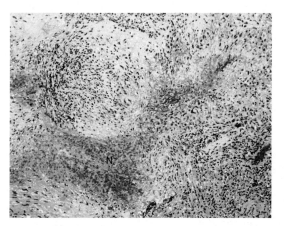

Figure 2.6 Churg–Strauss: Eosinophilic microabscess. Geographic necrosis (N) with an eosinophilic appearance centrally, is characteristic but not required for the diagnosis. Palisaded histiocytes are present, reminiscent of granulomatosis with polyangiitis (Wegener granulomatosis).

diagnosis occurs when even a single dose of corticosteroid is given prior to biopsy, as this can virtually eliminate eosinophils from the tissue. There are many conditions associated with Acute eosinophilic pneumonia (AEP) (Table 2.2).

DIFFUSE ALVEOLAR HAEMORRHAGE

Diffuse alveolar haemorrhage (DAH) consists of extensive extravasation of blood and fibrin into the alveolar spaces, and DAH is a common manifestation of pulmonary vasculitis/capillaritis. The

Table 2.2 Causes of AEP

1. Cigarette smoking (recent onset)
2. Inhaled drugs (heroin, cannabis)
3. Toxic inhalants (Scotchguard)
4. Heavy dust exposure (World Trade Center)
5. Drugs (antibiotics, antimalarials, antidepressants)
6. Parasites (*Toxocara*, *Strongyloides*)

clinical presentation varies from asymptomatic with incidental radiological findings to severe respiratory failure. Histologically, the presence of intra-alveolar red blood cells together with fibrin, organization and siderophages is good evidence of haemorrhage, as opposed to presence of blood alone due to procedural trauma, which is frequent in transbronchial biopsies. Also, not all alveolar haemorrhage or haemoptysis is immune mediated (e.g. lobar haemorrhage with bronchiectasis), but when haemorrhage is present bilaterally on imaging, the probability of an immune origin increases. It is important to note the presence of neutrophilic margination in small capillaries, because it often is a hallmark of biopsy-related injury. This finding should be differentiated from capillaritis, since the latter is an important diagnostic histopathologic feature in the majority of instances of DAH, corresponding to immune-mediated alveolar haemorrhage syndromes. The use of Prussian blue stain for iron highlights the presence of haemosiderin in macrophages; however, the typical appearance of the haemosiderin granules should be thick, golden brown and refractile, in contrast to the dusty type

(a)

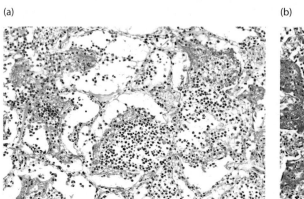

(b)

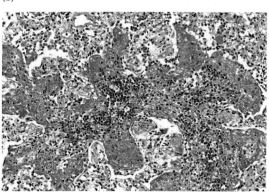

Figure 2.7 Acute eosinophilic pneumonia. **(a, b)** Various levels of airspace fibrin and/or hyaline membrane present with eosinophilic abscess. Basic pulmonary architecture is often preserved. Pink alveolar macrophages, which are often seen in chronic eosinophilic pneumonia, are faint or absent.

Table 2.3 Possible causes of diffuse alveolar haemorrhage (DAH)

1. Airway injury (bronchitis, bronchiolitis)
2. ANCA-associated vasculitis (GPA, EGPA, MPA)
3. Connective tissue disease related (SLE, RA, MCTD, myositis related, Behçet)
4. Idiopathic pulmonary haemosiderosis
5. Goodpasture syndrome
6. Pauci-immune idiopathic glomerulonephritis
7. Coagulation disorders
8. Drug toxicity/inhalations
9. Acute lung transplant rejection
10. Cardiac disease related (mitral stenosis, endocarditis, heart failure)
11. Radiation pneumonitis
12. Diffuse alveolar damage

DAH may occasionally present with one or more episodes of haemoptysis, which helps to substantiate the evidence of true alveolar haemorrhage; however, up to one third of patients with DAH do not show this symptom (12). Once it has been decided that the intra-alveolar red blood cells constitute an immune-mediated process, it is important to suggest all the possible causes and mechanisms involved to develop a differential diagnosis and narrow down possible causes, mainly with serologic studies (13) (Table 2.3). These vasculitides associated with immune alveolar haemorrhage are generally systemic, injuring organs like the kidneys, in the form of glomerulonephritis (Table 2.4). Such diseases can also affect the lung in a limited manner, for example isolated pulmonary capillaritis and a limited form of GPA. The histopathologic manifestations in these cases are alveolar haemorrhage, infiltration of alveolar walls with neutrophils corresponding to capillaritis, and in some instances, there may be marked overlap with the histopathology of DAD (Figure 2.8).

The presence of capillaritis portends a risk of massive haemoptysis and constitutes a medical emergency. The pathologist should communicate this finding immediately to the treating clinician.

of pigment seen in smokers' lungs (which can also contain some iron). Alveolar haemorrhage shows variable (and sometimes dramatic) airspace organization, and this element helps verify the clinical significance of the haemorrhagic process. Patients with

Table 2.4 Systemic vasculitides that can affect the lung

1. Large vessel vasculitis (LVV)
   a. Takayasu arteritis (TA)
   b. Giant cell arteritis (GCC)
   c. Medium vessel vasculitis (MVV)
   d. Polyarteritis nodosa (PAN)
   e. Kawasaki disease (KD)
2. Small vessel vasculitis (SVV)
   a. ANCA-associated vasculitis (AAV)
      i. Microscopic polyangiitis (MPA)
      ii. Granulomatosis with polyangiitis (GPA; known before as Wegener granulomatosis)
      iii. Eosinophilic granulomatosis with polyangiitis (EGPA; Churg–Strauss syndrome)
   b. *Immune complex SVV*
      i. Anti-glomerular basement membrane disease (anti-GBM, Goodpasture syndrome)
      ii. Cryoglobulinemic vasculitis (CV)
      iii. IgA vasculitis (Henoch–Schönlein purpura)
      iv. Hypocomplementemic urticarial vasculitis (HUV, anti-C1q vasculitis)
3. Variable vessel vasculitis (VVV)
   a. Behçet's disease
   b. Cogan syndrome
4. Vasculitis associated with systemic disease or probable aetiology
   a. *Systemic diseases*: rheumatoid arthritis (RA), systemic lupus erythematosus (SLE), etc.
   b. *Probable aetiology*: hepatitis C virus-associated cryoglobulinemic vasculitis, hepatitis B virus–associated vasculitis, drug-induced vasculitis, etc.

(a)

(b)

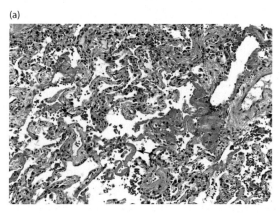
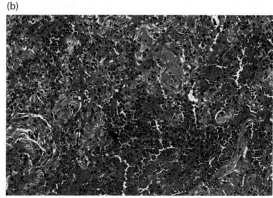

Figure 2.8 Alveolar haemorrhage showing areas of diffuse alveolar damage (DAD). **(a)** Alveolar haemorrhage can be overshadowed by DAD. Presence of hyaline membrane (arrows) without conspicuous haemorrhagic change or capillaritis may lead to a wrong diagnosis. **(b)** Note the presence of severe alveolar haemorrhage and capillaritis (*arrowhead*) in the same case.

Chronic and recurrent presentations of DAH are associated with airspace organization (organizing pneumonia) and interstitial fibrosis. In the histologic context of alveolar haemorrhage, clinical correlation is paramount to support the diagnosis of a true alveolar haemorrhage syndrome with presence, for example, of anaemia, haemoptysis, rashes, renal involvement, eye, ear, nose, sinus and neurologic symptoms. The status of serologic markers associated with different pulmonary vasculitic syndromes such as anti-neutrophil cytoplasmic antibodies (ANCA) in its two forms: cytoplasmic subtype or c-ANCA (PR3-ANCA specificity) and perinuclear or p-ANCA (MPO-ANCA specificity), anti-glomerular basement membrane antibody (anti-GBM), anti-nuclear antibodies (ANA), rheumatoid factor (RF), anti-phospholipid antibodies, creatine kinase (CK), urinalysis and urinary sediment cytology, among others. If these tests have not been performed, it is recommendable to suggest ordering these studies for completion of clinical evaluation in a case of DAH. Immunofluorescence studies on lung tissue are no longer a standard of practice for diagnosis in the patient with suspected DAH.

PATTERN II: FIBROSIS

This histopathologic pattern is subordinate to acute injury, because, although interstitial fibrosis is a hallmark of irreversible damage and may portend a serious prognosis, it is rarely a medical emergency. Suffice it to say that collagen deposition with structural remodelling is always first attended by some level of prior acute injury, and for this reason when both acute injury and fibrosis are present in the same biopsy, attention should first be focused on the acute disease. Regarding the approach to therapy for pulmonary fibrosis, the horizon looks promising, but much work is still required given limited therapies, none of which can reverse fibrosis at this juncture (14). This pattern is characterized by the presence of collagen deposition in the parenchyma with variable architectural distortion and alveolar loss. The fibrotic process has different secondary features depending on the particular histopathological entity involved. These include the 'temporal heterogeneity' of usual interstitial pneumonia (non-uniform fibrosis with presence of normal lung, ongoing fibrosis in areas, intercalated with areas of established collagen fibrosis), the uniform alveolar fibrosis of non-specific interstitial pneumonia, the airway-centred scarring of chronic hypersensitivity pneumonitis, the isolated stellate scars of Langerhans cell histiocytosis, and various non-specific patterns of fibrosis, including those biopsies with only advanced remodelling and scar (microscopic honeycombing only).

FIBROSIS WITH TEMPORAL HETEROGENEITY: USUAL INTERSTITIAL PNEUMONIA

Usual interstitial pneumonia (UIP) is the prototype of chronic interstitial pneumonia with a

(a)

(b)

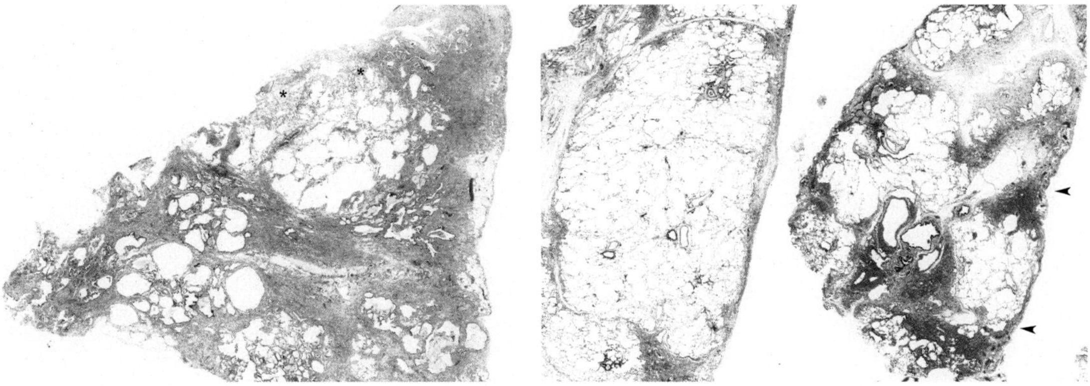

Figure 2.9 Classical usual interstitial pneumonia (UIP). **(a)** Presence of pinkish dense fibrosis that completely destroys the basic lung architecture is seen directly in subpleural areas and areas around interlobular septa. Uninvolved normal lung parenchyma is seen in the central parts of the lobules (*asterisks*). **(b)** Peripheral accentuation of the disease is easier to recognize in the early lesions of UIP (*arrowheads*).

non-uniform pattern of fibrosis. The main histopathologic feature of UIP is the presence of intercalated areas of architecturally altered lung with dense scarring alternating with areas of normal lung parenchyma creating a 'heterogeneous patchwork pattern' at low magnification (15). This fibrotic process shows a peripheral acinar pattern that translates as a subpleural and paraseptal predominant location, better appreciated on low-power magnification (Figure 2.9). Another defining feature of UIP is the presence of honeycomb cysts that represent marked remodelling of the acinus, with complete replacement of the parenchyma by dilated mucin-filled spaces of different sizes and shapes lined by respiratory epithelium and a fibrotic wall that surrounds the spaces. The mucin-filled cysts are associated with variable inflammation and occasionally, multinucleated giant cells. Finally, the last feature required for a definitive diagnosis of UIP pattern, is the presence of fibroblastic foci (FF) (16). These are discrete convex or partially concave areas of active fibroplasia that are located at the interface between the fibrotic and the normal lung and represent an 'advancing front' in this fibrosing process. The FF are composed of fibroblasts and myofibroblasts in a myxoid stroma rich in proteoglycans highlighted by connective tissue stains such as the Movat's pentachrome stain (17). FF are frequently covered by a layer of reactive type II epithelial cells. In the current model of IPF pathogenesis, type I alveolar pneumocytes appear to be the initial target of injury, followed by

proliferation of type II pneumocytes with secretion of cytokines and growth factors that promote myofibroblastic activation and proliferation as well as synthesis of collagen leading to pulmonary fibrosis (18) (Figure 2.10). UIP is the histopathologic pattern associated with idiopathic pulmonary fibrosis (IPF). HRCT studies typically show peripheral bibasilar reticulation with honeycombing (Figure 2.11). Additionally, UIP can show minimal lymphoplasmacytic infiltrates that should not form large lymphoid aggregates (or follicles) or demonstrate extensive pleuritis, since these features would point to collagen vascular disease associated interstitial lung disease, which can mimic a UIP-like histomorphology. Another pertinent feature arguing against UIP is the presence of poorly formed granulomas, since this finding together with some degree of bronchiolocentricity would point to the possibility of chronic hypersensitivity pneumonitis producing a UIP-like pattern of fibrosis (Table 2.5). The 'patchwork' of fibrosis in UIP can be simulated by airway-centred fibrosis (such as chronic hypersensitivity pneumonitis), so recognizing the anatomic distribution of disease is essential to making an accurate diagnosis in this setting.

UNIFORM ALVEOLAR WALL FIBROSIS: NON-SPECIFIC INTERSTITIAL PNEUMONIA

This is a homogeneous pattern of interstitial fibrosis with or without chronic inflammation in

(a)   (b)

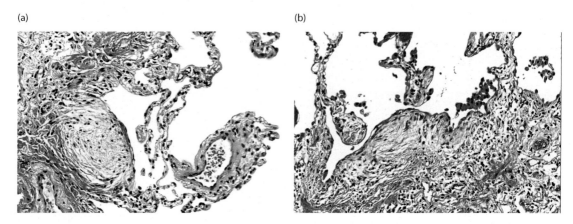

Figure 2.10 Fibroblastic focus. **(a, b)** Presence of a dome-shaped proliferation of myofibroblasts covered by enlarged pneumocytes in the continuous zone between dense fibrosis and normal lung.

(a)   (b)

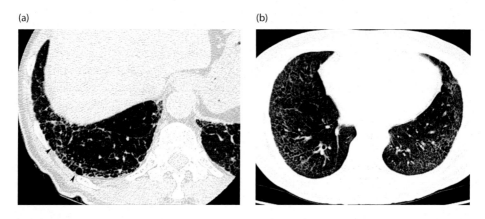

Figure 2.11 **(a, b)** HRCT images of IPF. Both images show bibasilar reticular shadows (*arrows*) with cystic changes called 'honeycomb cysts' (*arrowheads*).

Table 2.5 Pertinent histological features arguing against usual interstitial pneumonia (UIP)

1. Severe lymphoplasmacytic infiltration away from honeycombing
2. Marked lymphoid follicles with germinal centres
3. Scattered foci of granuloma
4. Predominant airway-centred distribution
5. Features of acute lung injury (airspace fibrin, hyaline membrane, clear organizing pneumonia)
6. Marked pleuritis
7. Presence of asbestos bodies
8. Extensive fibroelastosis
9. Extensive and atypical epithelia suggestive of carcinoma

which there is a tendency to preserve the original alveolar architecture instead of forming confluent scars. The parenchymal alterations can be subtle, as to be hardly detectable on low-power magnification (Figure 2.12). NSIP is a common manifestation of the systemic collagen vascular diseases, chronic drug reactions and some cases of hypersensitivity pneumonitis. HRCT findings consist of ground glass opacities and reticulations, and honeycombing is typically absent at initial presentation (Figure 2.13). In 1994, Katzenstein and Fiorelli reported NSIP as an idiopathic form of fibrotic and inflammatory interstitial pneumonia that did not fulfill the existing criteria for other interstitial lung diseases such as AIP, UIP, desquamative interstitial pneumonia (DIP) and respiratory bronchiolitis interstitial lung disease (RBILD), as originally described by Leibow in his classification of

(a)

(b)

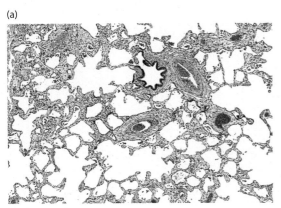
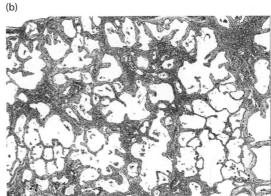

Figure 2.12 Non-specific interstitial pneumonia (NSIP). **(a)** Mild cellular and fibrotic changes are seen diffusely in the alveolar septa. Basic architecture is well preserved. **(b)** A case of fibrotic NSIP. Diffuse fibrosis showing pinkish thickening of alveolar septa is seen without breakdown of lung architecture. Areas of completely normal lung are not identified.

the idiopathic interstitial pneumonias (IIPs) (19). NSIP was defined as a temporally uniform process, meaning that the pathologic changes seemed to be of uniform 'age' throughout the lung parenchyma without a spectrum of changes from normal to markedly fibrotic, or from old injury to new, as is the case in UIP. The original description of this disease considered three subgroups: groups I, II and III, encompassing cellular, cellular and fibrotic and predominantly fibrotic subtypes, respectively.

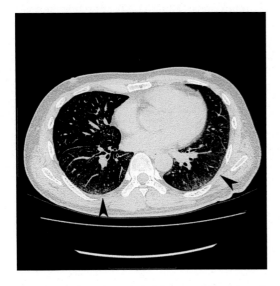

Figure 2.13 HRCT image of NSIP. Wide areas of ground glass change with reticulation are seen in both lungs. No definite honeycomb cysts are identified. Subpleural sparing is a frequent finding (*arrowheads*).

We discuss the cellular variant of NSIP together with histopathologic pattern III. The main feature of the fibrotic variant is collagen deposition in the interstitium with preservation of the overall architecture, presence of a few fibroblast foci, and absent or minimal honeycomb change. In a follow-up study of NSIP, it was shown that patients with cellular variants of NSIP had better 5- and 10-year survival than those with fibrotic variants. In this same study, patients with UIP had a worse 5-year survival than patients with fibrotic NSIP (20).

AIRWAY-CENTRED FIBROSIS

This pattern of scarring is best appreciated at low magnification. It consists of nodular and linear branching areas of fibrosis around bronchioles. In some advanced cases, the fibrotic process can extend beyond the centrilobular areas and be tethered to subpleural/paraseptal areas, making it occasionally difficult to distinguish from the fibrosis of UIP (Figure 2.14). Peribronchiolar metaplasia (PBM) frequently accompanies airway-centred fibrosis (ACF). We discuss PBM further in pattern VI. The differential diagnosis of this pattern of fibrosis includes inhalational injury for example by cigarette smoke, inhaled dusts, aspiration injury in gastroesophageal reflux, chronic hypersensitivity pneumonitis (CHP), and rarely, collagen-vascular diseases such as rheumatoid arthritis (21) (Table 2.6). An idiopathic form of bronchiolocentric inflammation and fibrosis has been described (22). HRCT findings include

(a)

(b)

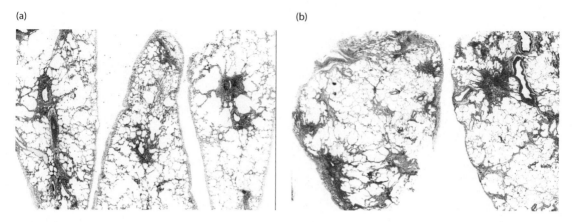

Figure 2.14 Airway-centred interstitial fibrosis simulating UIP. **(a)** Patchy fibrosis around bronchovascular bundles is obvious in the earlier phase. **(b)** Airway-centred fibrosis progresses, involving peripheral zones of pulmonary lobules, which simulate patchy fibrosis of UIP.

Table 2.6 Differential diagnosis of airway-centred fibrosis

1. Hypersensitivity pneumonitis (HP)
2. Gastroesophageal reflux disease (GERD)
3. Cigarette smoking
4. Collagen-vascular disease
5. Inhalation of toxic fumes (e.g. chemicals used for cleaning)
6. Idiopathic

reticular infiltrates, ground glass opacities, peribronchovascular opacities, centrilobular nodules and mosaic attenuation due to air trapping. The distribution of HRCT findings can help point to the possible aetiology involved. For example, inhalational diseases tend to involve mid and upper zones, while autoimmune disorders tend to involve the lower lobes and the lung periphery.

ISOLATED STELLATE SCARS

Healed lesions of Langerhans cell histiocytosis (LCH) can appear as acellular parenchymal fibrous scars with a stellate architecture. These lesions may coexist with active LCH, or be incidental findings in a biopsy or resection taken for another disease, such as lung carcinoma. When stellate fibrotic foci are numerous, one should consider smoking-related interstitial lung disease (SRILD) (Figure 2.15). HRCT findings in such cases would include reticulation and emphysema (in contrast to the HRCT of LCH in the subacute stage where cysts and nodules dominate).

NON-SPECIFIC PATTERNS OF FIBROSIS INCLUDING 'MICROSCOPIC HONEYCOMBING ONLY': HONEYCOMB LUNG

A wide variety of chronic lung diseases may result in complete destruction of the pulmonary lobular architecture with fibrosis and formation of microscopic honeycombing. Some patterns of fibrosis are completely non-specific and consist only of scars, most often secondary to intrapulmonary abscesses and infarctions. 'Honeycomb lung' does not correspond to a specific disease, but to a morphologic appearance of the lung parenchyma affected by this process. A biopsy showing only honeycomb changes and no preserved parenchyma can only be diagnosed as 'lung with advanced microscopic honeycomb remodeling' (Figure 2.16). The history and location of the honeycomb cysts may be helpful in the differential diagnosis. If the patient is above 60 years of age and the HRCT shows basal and bilateral subpleural reticulations, the most likely diagnosis would be UIP/IPF.

PATTERN III: CELLULAR INFILTRATES

This pattern is characterized by diffuse presence of chronic inflammatory cells (lymphocytes and plasma cells) within alveolar walls, and it is a very common feature among all DPLD. Other possible accompanying features are well or poorly formed

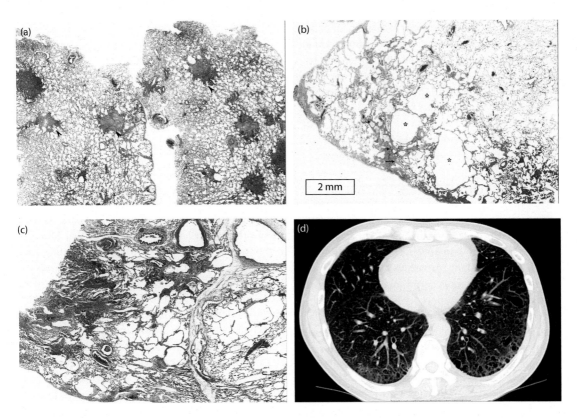

Figure 2.15 Airway-centred interstitial fibrosis (ACIF). **(a)** ACIF that is strongly suggestive of scarred Langerhans cell histiocytosis (LCH) (arrowheads). In some cases, a diagnosis of LCH can be given based on the architecture of ACIF alone, without immunohistochemical proof of Langerhans cells. **(b, c)** ACIF can also be seen in smoking-related ILD. Most cases are associated with periacinar emphysema (asterisks) (fibrosis with arrows). Some cystic spaces may be called 'airspace enlargement with fibrosis (AEF)'. **(d)** HRCT image of the same case. The combination of reticular fibrosis and emphysema is a characteristic change.

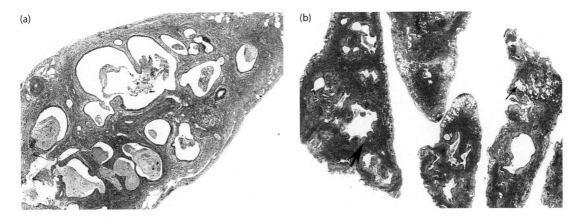

Figure 2.16 Fibrotic lung disease with honeycomb change. **(a)** Advanced microscopic honeycombing in a case of UIP. Microscopic honeycomb cysts are dilated airspaces filled with mucus and inflammatory cells and lined by columnar ciliated epithelium. **(b)** A case with less advanced honeycomb change (*thick arrow*) to differentiate it from dilated bronchioles (*thin arrow*) in UIP.

granulomas, as well as different degrees of fibrosis. These patterns seldom occur in a pure manner. For example cellular infiltrates of NSIP occur frequently in association with some degree of interstitial fibrosis. The cellular infiltrates pattern can be further subdivided into secondary patterns as follows: *pure cellular interstitial pneumonia, cellular infiltrates with poorly formed granulomas and cellular infiltrates with well-formed granulomas.*

PURE CELLULAR INTERSTITIAL PNEUMONIA: CELLULAR NSIP

This pattern of DPLD is aptly named because the process is indeed non-specific. Many pathologic processes in the lung can show cellular interstitial infiltrates. The most common are healing viral pneumonias, drug reactions, collagen vascular disease related, hypersensitivity pneumonitis, the late phase of diffuse alveolar damage and even low-grade lymphoproliferative diseases such as marginal zone extranodal B-cell lymphoma (Figure 2.17) (23). NSIP was described by Katzenstein and Fiorelli in 1994 in 64 patients (19). The authors described three variants of the disease (types I–III). Type I or cellular NSIP demonstrated temporally uniform interstitial lymphocytic and plasma cell infiltrates that were generally more marked than the degree of accompanying fibrosis (Figure 2.18). A degree of alveolar pneumocyte hyperplasia was present in these cases, as well as some foci of OP. In their series, some cases were 'idiopathic', while others had a previous diagnosis of connective tissue disease or hypersensitivity pneumonitis. In some, autoimmune disease developed after the diagnosis

of interstitial pneumonia (19). The entity of idiopathic NSIP was granted a provisional status in the 2002 International Multidisciplinary Consensus Committee Report, but was finally accepted as a defined idiopathic clinicopathologic chronic interstitial pneumonia in the 2013 update of this document (23).

CELLULAR INFILTRATES WITH POORLY FORMED GRANULOMAS: HYPERSENSITIVITY PNEUMONITIS

The prototype of this category is hypersensitivity pneumonitis (HP), known also as extrinsic allergic alveolitis. HP is a hypersensitivity reaction limited to the lung, resulting from inhalational exposure to aerosolized organic antigen. The clinical presentation of HP is dominated by subacute and chronic manifestations, each with different histopathology and HRCT findings. The acute form exists and occurs after exposure to large quantities of the inhaled antigen and may present with features of acute lung injury with DAD pattern (rarely subjected to biopsy). The subacute form is the most commonly recognized in biopsy material and consists of mild lympho-plasmacytic interstitial inflammatory infiltrates with centrilobular and peribronchovascular accentuation, together with non-necrotizing poorly formed granulomas or small aggregates of multinucleated interstitial giant cells (Figure 2.19). In some cases, the granulomas can be sparse or replaced by Schaumann bodies or concentric calcifications. Other less common granulomatous interstitial pneumonias are also considerations such as granulomatous and

(a)

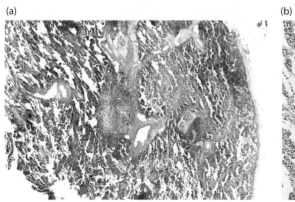

(b)

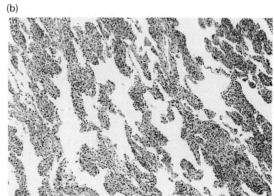

Figure 2.17 Cellular interstitial infiltrates. **(a, b)** Interstitial lymphoplasmacytic infiltrates in a case of marginal zone extranodal B cell lymphoma result in widening of the interstitium without fibrosis.

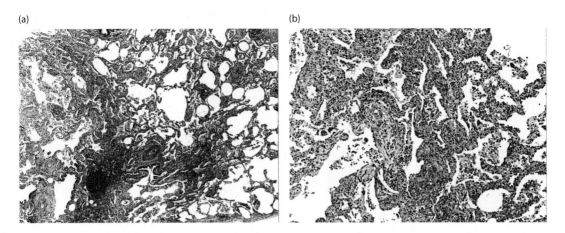

Figure 2.18 Non-specific interstitial pneumonia, cellular variant. **(a)** Scanning magnification demonstrates spatial and temporal homogeneous involvement by interstitial lymphoid infiltrates and occasional lymphoid aggregates. **(b)** Interstitial widening by a cellular lymphoid infiltrate with no significant fibrosis.

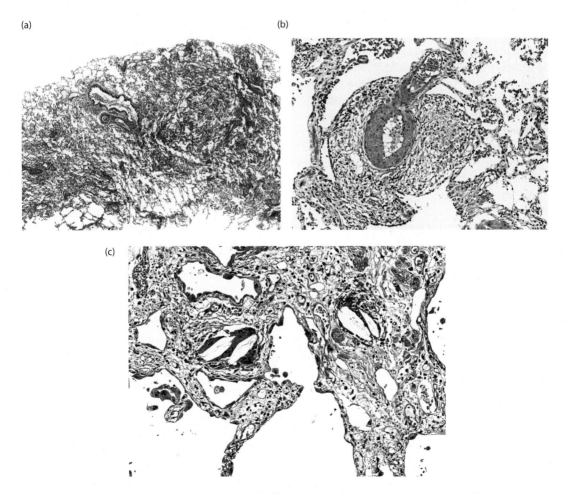

Figure 2.19 Hypersensitivity pneumonitis. **(a)** Diffuse interstitial lymphoplasmacytic infiltrates with peribronchovascular accentuation. **(b)** Loose collections of histiocytes in the interstitium (poorly formed granulomata). **(c)** Cholesterol cleft granulomata.

(a)

(b)

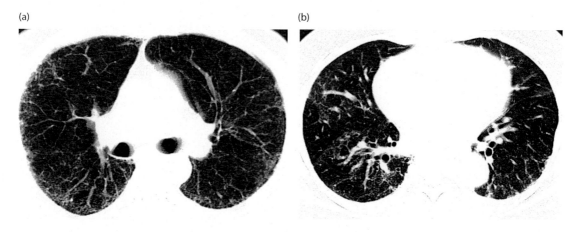

Figure 2.20 Hypersensitivity pneumonitis. **(a, b)** HRCT scan shows mosaic attenuation, a typical manifestation of air trapping.

lymphoid interstitial pneumonia (GLIP) in common variable immunodeficiency (24). HRCT findings can help in the diagnosis of subacute HP by pointing to a predominant upper and mid-upper lobe location of ground glass opacities as poorly defined centrilobular nodules and mosaic attenuation/air trapping (25) (Figure 2.20). Sarcoidosis is always considered in the differential diagnosis of pneumonitis with granulomas; however, the granulomas of sarcoidosis are well formed and generally surrounded by a fibrous cuff, and they tend to form coalescent nodules. Sarcoidosis is discussed within Pattern V: Nodules.

CELLULAR INFILTRATES WITH WELL-FORMED GRANULOMAS: HOT TUB LUNG

This pattern is typically seen in exposure to *Mycobacterium avium* complex (MAC), which contaminates the water in hot water soaking tubs (hot tubs). The bioaerosol exposure produces a form of hypersensitivity pneumonitis, rather than a true infection by mycobacteria (26). The disease has been hence named 'hot tub lung'. The histologic features are presence of non-necrotizing well-formed granulomas in peribronchiolar areas as well as within air spaces: alveolar ducts and alveoli. Rarely, the granulomas of hot tub lung can show some degree of necrosis, especially when other species of atypical mycobacteria are at play (Figure 2.21). HRCT findings in these patients are centrilobular bilateral nodular opacities with upper lobe predominance and extensive compromise of

the parenchyma, in many cases indistinguishable from the findings in extrinsic allergic alveolitis in subacute phase (Figure 2.22). Another entity showing this histopathologic pattern is subacute/chronic aspiration pneumonia. In aspiration pneumonia there are foreign-body multinucleated giant cells, mostly within the bronchioles and airways, surrounding foreign-body material (27).

PATTERN IV: ALVEOLAR FILLING

The main feature of this pattern is filling of alveolar spaces by cellular or non-cellular material. Alveolar filling can be a component of many interstitial lung diseases, so to qualify as the 'dominant' pattern, acute injury (pattern I) and fibrosis (pattern II) should not be present.

The cellular material may consist of immature fibroblasts, macrophages, neutrophils, erythrocytes, siderophages, amorphous proteinaceous material and even bone. Many DPLD cause alveolar filling, manifested radiologically and macroscopically as diffuse or patchy parenchymal consolidation.

Typical examples of these consolidative processes are organizing infections, pulmonary haemorrhage, desquamative interstitial pneumonia (DIP), pulmonary alveolar proteinosis (PAP) and chronic eosinophilic pneumonia (CEP), among others. Only few are histologically characteristic, such as PAP, in which there is intra-alveolar accumulation of amorphous granular material

(a)

(b)

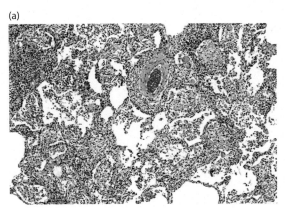

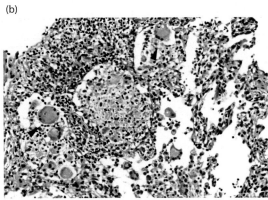

Figure 2.21 Hot tub lung. **(a)** Interstitial lymphocytic infiltrates with interstitial and intra-alveolar non-necrotizing granulomas. **(b)** Loose granulomas (arrowheads) composed of multinucleated giant cells and epithelioid histiocytes.

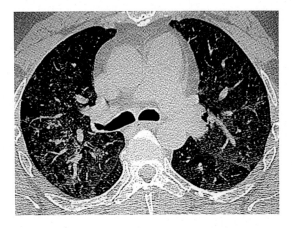

Figure 2.22 Hot tub lung HRCT scan shows patchy area of ground glass attenuation with air trapping.

corresponding to lipoproteins, due to a dysfunction in the metabolism of surfactant by the alveolar macrophages. Another entity that is histologically typical is CEP due to the conspicuous presence of eosinophils, which are not dominant in other lesions.

IMMATURE FIBROBLASTS: ORGANIZING PNEUMONIA

This histopathological pattern consists of plugs of immature (tissue culture-like) fibroblasts within alveolar ducts and respiratory bronchioles. These 'Masson bodies' appear typically pale pink to grayish on haematoxylin and eosin (H&E) stains due to their myxoid matrix rich in acid

mucopolysaccharides. The plugs contain a variable amount of inflammatory cells within and in the surrounding interstitium. The Masson bodies extend from alveolus to alveolus and often involve respiratory bronchioles, forming an interconnected and branching pattern of buds, and thus, were historically described as 'bourgeons conjunctifs' (Figure 2.23). In addition, there may be hyperplastic type 2 alveolar pneumocytes as well as variable intra-alveolar collections of foamy macrophages representing a form of obstructive pneumonia (28). This process was reported as bronchiolitis obliterans organizing pneumonia (BOOP) by Epler et al. (29); however, the ATS/ERS Consensus Classification suggested the use of organizing pneumonia alone, to avoid confusion with the term 'obliterative' or 'constrictive' bronchiolitis, which corresponds to a completely different entity (30). The OP pattern is used by pathologists today in a more generic descriptive way, because it can be seen associated to many entities; for example, it is frequently seen at the edges of tumours, in organizing infections, in chronic infections, in drug reactions, etc. (Table 2.7). An OP pattern is seen commonly in organizing acute lung injury of any aetiology and can cause some indecision as to whether it represents a pattern I of acute lung injury, or a pattern IV of intra-alveolar filling. The clinical presentation is very important to decide which one is the predominant process. For example, an acutely ill patient will point to a pattern I together with additional histological findings such as fibrinous exudates and hyaline membranes. A pure OP histological pattern with a subacute presentation will be more in

(a)

(b)

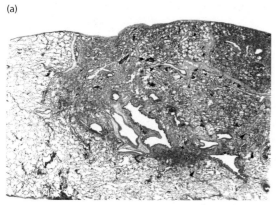
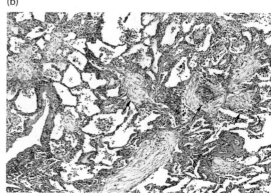

Figure 2.23 Organizing pneumonia. **(a)** Alveolar filling pattern with Masson bodies (*arrowheads*). **(b)** Masson bodies composed of loose collections of fibroblasts, some containing inflammatory cells within (*arrows*).

Table 2.7 Conditions associated with an OP pattern

1. Cryptogenic organizing pneumonia (COP)
2. Organizing infections
3. Organizing diffuse alveolar damage
4. Eosinophilic pneumonia (EP)
5. Hypersensitivity pneumonitis (HP)
6. Aspiration pneumonia
7. Collagen vascular diseases (CVDs)
8. Peripheral reaction to lesions such as tumours, infarcts, infections

Table 2.8 Conditions associated with a DIP pattern

1. Idiopathic desquamative interstitial pneumonia (DIP)
2. Respiratory bronchiolitis interstitial lung disease (RB-ILD)
3. Langerhans cell histiocytosis (LCH)
4. Eosinophilic pneumonia (EP)
5. Drug reactions (Amiodarone)
6. Pneumoconioses (hard metal disease, asbestosis, talcosis)
7. Lipidoses (Gaucher disease, Niemann–Pick)
8. Obstructive pneumonia (intra-alveolar foamy macrophages)
9. Chronic alveolar haemorrhage
10. Infections (intra-alveolar collections of histiocytes)

keeping with a pattern IV. The initial descriptions of idiopathic BOOP typically showed a subacute clinical presentation. The idiopathic type of OP is known clinically as cryptogenic organizing pneumonia (COP). HRCT findings are bilateral peribronchial and subpleural areas of consolidation.

MACROPHAGES: DESQUAMATIVE INTERSTITIAL PNEUMONIA

The pattern consists of numerous intraalveolar macrophages with mild inflammatory interstitial infiltrates. Desquamative interstitial pneumonia (DIP), is in fact, a misnomer, since there are no cells 'desquamated' into the lumens, and it originated from the original description by Liebow, who interpreted the intralumenal cells as desquamated type II pneumocytes. Eventually, ultrastructural analysis demonstrated the true identity of these cells (31). There are many conditions associated

with a DIP pattern (Table 2.8). The specific features of the macrophages in these different conditions can help to indicate the possible diagnosis. For example, foamy macrophages are seen in amiodarone toxicity, storage diseases, obstructive and lipoid pneumonias; smoker's macrophages with dusty and delicate light-brown pigment are seen in RBILD; and multinucleated histiocytes are seen in hard metal pneumoconiosis, described by Leibow as giant cell interstitial pneumonia (GIP). RBILD, DIP and LCH are diseases that occur exclusively in smokers, and hence, can show overlapping features. DIP and RBILD have been recently reclassified by the ERS/ATS as smoking-related interstitial lung diseases within the larger category of major idiopathic interstitial pneumonia (23).

ALVEOLAR FILLING WITH EOSINOPHILIC MATERIAL: PULMONARY ALVEOLAR PROTEINOSIS

Pulmonary alveolar proteinosis (PAP) is the prototype of this histopathologic pattern. It consists of filling of amorphous granular eosinophilic material within alveolar spaces with occasional larger anucleate ovoid eosinophilic structures, probably representing dead macrophages (Figure 2.24a). Some macrophages and cholesterol clefts can sometimes be seen within the material. PAP is strongly periodic acid Schiff (PAS)-positive after digestion with diastase, and this finding is useful to differentiate it from pulmonary oedema. Compromise of the alveoli is generally diffuse in the biopsy material; however, it can also be patchy. Generally, there is only mild fibrosis with minimal inflammatory infiltrates. The eosinophilic material consists of accumulated lipoproteins due to defective clearance by the alveolar macrophages that require granulocyte–macrophage colony-stimulating factor (GM-CSF) to metabolize surfactant. In the primary types of PAP, 'autoimmune PAP', there is production of anti-GM-CSF antibodies that cause the dysfunction of the macrophages. There are many causes of PAP: primary, hereditary and secondary (Table 2.9). HRCT shows a rather typical pattern known as 'crazy-paving' in some cases (Figure 2.24b).

RED BLOOD CELLS AND HAEMOSIDERIN-LADEN MACROPHAGES: ALVEOLAR HAEMORRHAGE

This is a typical example of an entity that shares two patterns. We classified DAH under pattern I because it conveys a real sense of urgency that must be adopted in such cases. DAH is a medical emergency that needs to be treated immediately. But also consider that the presence of intra-alveolar red blood cells could be secondary to a tumour, infection, bronchiectasis or vascular anomaly, and haemorrhage may be localized rather than diffuse.

ALVEOLAR FILLING WITH NEUTROPHILS

A typical example of this pattern, is, in fact, acute infectious bronchopneumonia, characterized by alveolar filling with neutrophils.

ALVEOLAR FILLING WITH MICROLITHS: PULMONARY ALVEOLAR MICROLITHIASIS

Pulmonary alveolar microlithiasis (PAM) is a rare disease with a typical intra-alveolar accumulation of calcified bodies with concentric laminations and radial striations.

The disease has been known since the early 1900s (32), and an extensive description of it appeared in the Italian medical literature later (33). PAM is

(a)

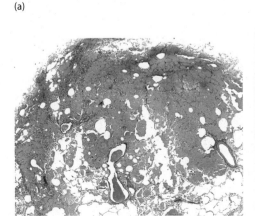

(b)

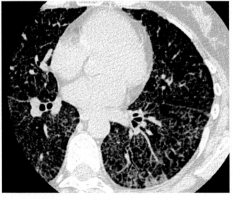

Figure 2.24 Pulmonary alveolar proteinosis. **(a)** Extensive eosinophilic intra-alveolar exudates. **(b)** HRCT image showing a crazy-paving pattern.

Table 2.9 Causes of PAP

1. Auto-immune (presence of anti-GM-CSF antibodies, >90% of cases)
2. Secondary
    a. Myeloproliferative disorders
    b. Myelodysplastic disorders
    c. Haematolymphoid neoplasias
    d. Haematologic conditions such as aplastic anaemia, Fanconi's anaemia, congenital dyserythropoietic anaemia, post stem cell and bone marrow transplantation
    e. Non-haematologic malignancies such as lung cancer, thymoma, melanoma, mesothelioma, glioblastoma
    f. Dusts and fume inhalation such as silica, titanium, aluminium, indium, cotton/linen, wood, flour, chlorine gas, gasoline, plastics, NO_2
    g. Drugs such as sirolimus, imatinib mesylate, mycophenolate mofetil, cyclosporine, busulphan, dasatinib
    h. Autoimmune disorders such as Hermansky–Pudlak syndrome, Sjogren syndrome, ANCA-related vasculitis, granulomatosis and polyangiitis (GPA), juvenile dermatomyositis
    i. Immunodeficiencies such as IgA deficiency, HIV infection, hypogammaglobulinemia, agammaglobulinemia, HIV infection, GATA-2 deficiency, dendritic cell monocyte B and NK lymphoid (DCML) syndrome
3. Genetic
    a. Mutations involving production of surfactant such as surfactant protein B (SFTPB), surfactant protein C(SFTPC), ATP binding cassette 3(ABCA3), NK2 homeobox1(NKX2-1)
    b. Mutations involving the GM-CSF receptor such as CSF2RA and CSF2RB
    c. Mutation involving soluble carrier family 7 member 7 (SLC7A7) causing lysinuric protein intolerance

considered to be an autosomal recessive disease. A responsible gene mutation has been discovered in the *SLC34A2* gene, which encodes a sodium-phosphate co-transporter in patients with PAM (34).

Histologically, the airspaces are filled by numerous concentrically laminated bodies with radial striations composed of calcium and phosphorus, as well as minor amounts of magnesium and iron. The microliths are generally uniform in size, varying from 250 μm to 1 mm in diameter. Occasionally they compromise the alveolar walls with some degree of interstitial fibrosis and inflammation (35) (Figure 2.25).

PATTERN V: NODULES

Non-neoplastic nodules may form in the lung parenchyma by either cellular (inflammatory) or stromal proliferations with collagen deposition, or combinations of both, and such nodules have a tendency to delineate rather discrete areas, as opposed to parenchymal consolidations that involve large irregular, less defined areas. These nodules can be small or large, well formed or poorly formed, single or multiple, separate or confluent. The cellular proliferations may be of diverse type, such as lymphoid, epithelial, histiocytic, benign or malignant. The stromal proliferations with collagen deposition, on the other hand, can appear stellate, round or of indistinct shape. The majority of nodules in the lungs, especially single nodules, actually represent neoplasms, mostly malignant, but it is not the purpose of this chapter to discuss neoplastic diseases (Table 2.10).

Table 2.10 Causes of nodular lesions in the lung

1. Sarcoidosis
2. Langerhans cell histiocytosis (LCH)
3. Granulomatosis and polyangiitis (GPA)
4. Silicosis
5. Tumours
    a. Carcinoma
    b. Sarcoma
    c. Lymphoma
    d. Others such as melanoma
6. Infections

(a)
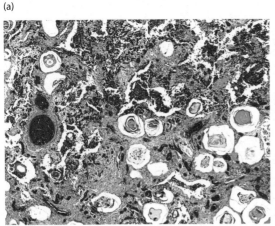

(b)
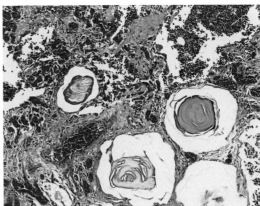

Figure 2.25 Pulmonary alveolar microlithiasis (PAM). **(a)** Low magnification shows the interstitial fibrosis that is common in PAM as well as the microcalcifications. **(b)** Close-up image of the calcifications with concentric laminations.

The main types of nodules that we encounter in the differential diagnosis of interstitial lung diseases are nodules with granulomatous inflammation, nodules with mineral dusts and macrophages, granulomatosis with polyangiitis (GPA), nodules with stellate scars and Langerhans cells. It is important to examine the slides at low power magnification, as in all ILDs, to determine the predominant anatomic compartment location of these nodules, since this finding will help to narrow the differential diagnosis. The use of special stains is important to uncover causative organisms, such as mycobacteria and fungi, as well as cultures of fresh tissue, and occasionally, polymerase chain reaction (PCR) in formalin-fixed paraffin-embedded (FFPE) tissue for identification of mycobacteria (36).

Table 2.11 Nodular lesions with granulomatous inflammation

1. Infections
   a. *Mycobacterium tuberculosis*
   b. Non-tuberculous mycobacteria (NTM)
   c. Fungal infections
2. Non-infectious
   a. Sarcoidosis
3. Pneumoconioses
   a. Talcosis
   b. Berylliosis
4. Foreign-body aspiration
   a. Food particles
   b. Pills

NODULES WITH GRANULOMATOUS INFLAMMATION: SARCOIDOSIS

Diverse interstitial lung diseases present with non-necrotizing or necrotizing granulomas as histopathologic manifestations (Table 2.11).

The most important features to be determined at the beginning of the histologic analysis of nodules of granulomatous inflammation are the anatomic location and the type of granulomas. For example, in sarcoidosis and berylliosis, the granulomas are present within lymphatic routes and tend to be well formed, which means tight aggregates of epithelioid histiocytes, multinucleated giant cells and few lymphoid cells (37). Frequently, these granulomas are surrounded by concentric lamellar eosinophilic collagen, which may completely replace the granulomas (38). Sarcoid-type granulomas are by definition non-necrotizing and show more of a hyaline or sometimes fibrinoid appearance, which probably represents a degenerative change (Figure 2.26). Schaumann bodies are haematoxyphilic inclusions in the cytoplasm of multinucleated giant cells, also called conchoidal bodies, due to their shell-like undulated edge. These inclusions have been described in sarcoidosis, but in fact, are present in many different diseases. The same is true for asteroid bodies, which are star-shaped eosinophilic inclusions in the multinucleated giant cells. Randomly located multiple tiny nodules, especially if necrotizing, are associated with infectious

(a)
(b)

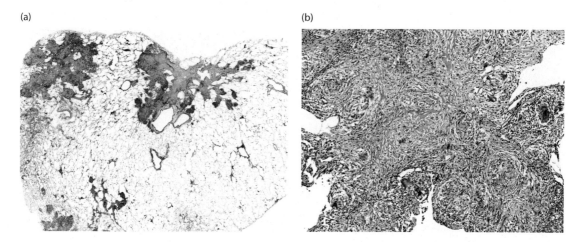

Figure 2.26 Sarcoidosis. **(a)** Confluent interstitial peribronchovascular granulomas. **(b)** Higher magnification of non-necrotizing interstitial granulomas surrounded by hyaline fibrosis.

granulomas, such as *Mycobacterium tuberculosis*, in some regions of the world, while non-tuberculous mycobacteria (NTM) infection is more common in the United States. Miliary-type granulomas with necrosis in immunocompetent hosts should raise the question of exposure to MAC that contaminates the water in hot water soaking tubs and produces a subtype of HP due to inhalation of this bioaerosol containing *Mycobacterium avium-intracellulare* (MAI), as discussed earlier in the pattern of cellular infiltrates section. Granulomatous inflammation of perivascular location containing polarizable foreign bodies consistent with talc or other foreign material is typical of use of an intravenous drug that has been adulterated with contaminants such as talc, or the intravenous injection of solubilized crushed tablet medication containing substances such as microcrystalline cellulose and crospovidone. Some inclusions such as oxalate crystals seen in multinucleated giant cells must not be confused with foreign bodies, seen for example, in cases of aspiration, as we discussed previously in the section Pattern III.

NODULES WITH MINERAL DUSTS AND MACROPHAGES: SILICOSIS

Variably fibrotic nodules of pneumoconioses such as silicosis and silicatosis are rarely seen in lung biopsy material examined by the pathologist. These nodules have a whorled collagenous appearance, and contain polarizable silicates, which are aluminium and magnesium salts of silica.

Nodules due to remote exposure tend to be completely devoid of peripheral histiocytic infiltration, while more recent exposures are associated with nodules having a slightly stellate appearance at the periphery due to lymphohistiocytic infiltrates (Figure 2.27).

The presence of polarizable foreign material in the lung is not by itself, sufficient for a diagnosis of pneumoconiosis, since all urban dwellers have small amounts of silica, silicates and carbon pigment just from environmental exposure. The radiologic examination is a key component in the diagnosis of pneumoconiosis together with a history of exposure to the offending agent (39).

NODULE AND STELLATE SCARS WITH LANGERHANS CELLS: LANGERHANS CELL HISTIOCYTOSIS

The early phase of Langerhans cell histiocytosis (LCH) is characterized by round or stellate airway centred nodules containing a mixture of Langerhans cells, eosinophils, lymphoplasmacytic cells and pigmented alveolar macrophages. The Langerhans cells are ovoid with a grooved nucleus and stain typically for S-100, CD1a and langerin (40). Eosinophils are variable and may be hard to find. The early lesions can become cystic and rupture in the pleura, causing a pneumothorax (Figure 2.28). Late lesions become hypocellular resulting in stellate scars with little or no residual LCs.

(a) (b)

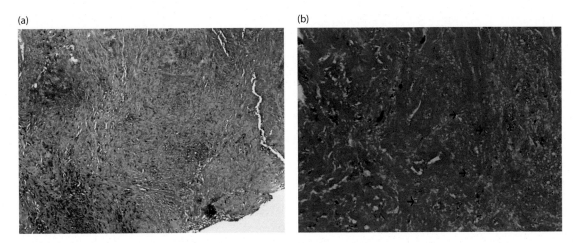

Figure 2.27 Silicotic nodule **(a)** composed of whorled collagen fibres and lymphohistiocytic infiltrates at the periphery. **(b)** Higher magnification shows refractile crystals (*arrows*).

(a) (b)

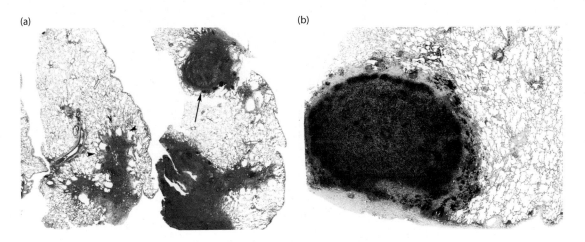

Figure 2.28 Langerhans cell histiocytosis. **(a)** Large confluent solid areas (*arrow*) and nodules with 'stellate' edges (*arrowhead*). **(b)** Higher-power view of a single nodule.

PATTERN VI: MINIMAL CHANGES

Minimal changes refer to some surgical biopsy cases of clinically manifested DPLD that may appear 'normal' at low power magnification, however clinical–radiologic correlation and the use of special stains such as van Gieson's stain to highlight elastic layers of damaged airways and subtle vascular changes, should uncover the particular lesions (Table 2.12).

Within this pattern we consider small airways disease, vascular or lymphatic pathology and cysts.

Table 2.12 Lesions that appear as minimal changes

1. Pulmonary oedema
2. Pulmonary emboli
3. Airway disease (mainly bronchiolar)
4. Pulmonary vascular disease such as plexiform arteriopathy of pulmonary hypertension
5. Lymphatic disease such as lymphangiomatosis
6. Langerhans cell histiocytosis (LCH)
7. Lymphangioleiomyomatosis (LAM)
8. Subtle interstitial infiltrate
9. Early diffuse alveolar damage (DAD)

MINIMAL CHANGES WITH SMALL AIRWAY DISEASE: CONSTRICTIVE BRONCHIOLITIS

The aetiologies of small airway disease are rather varied in nature (Table 2.13) and may be difficult to detect microscopically. Histologic features include lymphoplasmacytic infiltrates in the bronchiolar wall, muscular hypertrophy and collagen deposition along with changes in the lumen that range from minimal peribronchiolar nodular scarring to complete obliteration of the bronchiolar lumen and replacement of the bronchiole by a scar surrounded by smooth muscle, as evidenced by elastic stains (Figure 2.29). Another disease process that may appear as a 'minimal change' is peribronchiolar scarring with metaplastic bronchiolar epithelium extending into the adjacent alveoli, called peribronchiolar metaplasia or lambertosis (Figure 2.30). The majority of these entities present radiologically with characteristics of obstruction to airflow, as evidenced by the HRCT pattern of mosaic attenuation and air-trapping (41). Peribronchiolar metaplasia, on the other hand, can present

Table 2.13 Aetiology of small airways disease

1. Primary bronchiolitis
   a. Acute bronchiolitis
      i. Infections such as viruses, mycoplasma
      ii. Asthma
      iii. Inflammatory bowel disease
      iv. Collagen vascular disease
      v. Aspiration
   b. Constrictive bronchiolitis
      i. Post-infectious
      ii. Chronic lung allograft rejection
      iii. Graft-versus-host disease (GVHD)
      iv. Drugs such as penicillamine, CCNU
      v. Inhaled/ingested toxins
      vi. Neuroendocrine cell hyperplasia
      vii. Idiopathic
      viii. Diffuse panbronchiolitis
2. Secondary bronchiolitis
   a. Respiratory bronchiolitis interstitial lung disease (RB-ILD)
   b. Airway-centred interstitial fibrosis; peribronchiolar metaplasia
   c. Hypersensitivity pneumonitis (HP)
   d. Cryptogenic organizing pneumonia (COP)

(a)

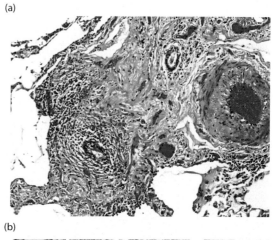

(b)

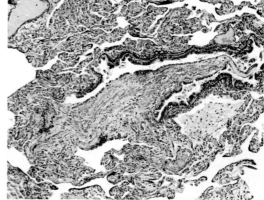

Figure 2.29 Constrictive bronchiolitis. **(a)** High-power image shows a pulmonary arteriole with an adjacent collagenous scar and residual lumen of the paired bronchiole. **(b)** Elastic stain of a similar case shows partial replacement of the bronchiolar wall by fibrous tissue.

clinically and radiologically as a typical ILD and has been recently described as a rare histologic pattern of idiopathic interstitial pneumonia by the 2013 ATS/ERS classification of IIPs (23,42).

MINIMAL CHANGES WITH VASCULAR OR LYMPHATIC PATHOLOGY: PLEXIFORM ARTERIOPATHY OF PULMONARY HYPERTENSION

Chronic fibrosing lung disease is generally associated with changes in the architecture of the vasculature and airways, and these changes should be differentiated from prototypical alterations of

(a)

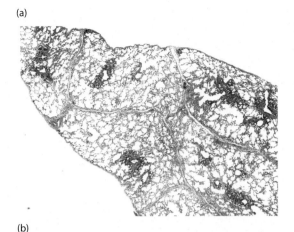

(b)

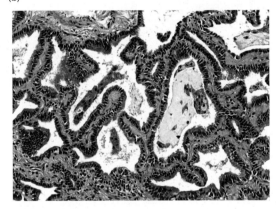

Figure 2.30 Peribronchiolar lung scarring. **(a)** Low-power image shows peribronchiolar fibrosis. **(b)** High-power magnification highlights foci of lambertosis or peribronchiolar metaplasia that imitates a neoplastic proliferation.

specific diseases, such as pulmonary hypertension with its characteristic plexiform arteriopathy.

MINIMAL CHANGES WITH CYSTS: LYMPHANGIOLEIOMYOMATOSIS

The cysts of lymphangioleiomyomatosis (LAM) are very delicate, and the specimens have to be handled correctly to be able to show these abnormalities. It is recommended to remove the staples and shake the wedges before fixation to allow distension of the alveolar spaces for adequate recognition of the lesions. The use of immunohistochemistry (IHC), such as staining for HMB45, Melan-A, oestrogen and progesterone, is helpful in highlighting the fascicles of delicate elongated cells diagnostic of LAM.

TRANSBRONCHIAL BIOPSY MATERIAL

The pattern approach can also be used in transbronchial biopsy with a concentrated examination of specific features (Table 2.14).

Table 2.14 Features to focus on while examining transbronchial lung biopsy specimens for diffuse parenchymal lung diseases (DPLD) and their possible causes

1. Evidence of diffuse alveolar damage (DAD)
   a. Idiopathic (acute interstitial pneumonia)
   b. Alveolar haemorrhage syndrome
   c. Infections
   d. Drug reactions
   e. Acute radiation reaction
   f. Acute allergic reaction (hypersensitivity pneumonitis)
   g. Toxic inhalants
   h. Shock
2. Features of organizing pneumonia pattern (OP)
   a. Cryptogenic organizing pneumonia (COP)
   b. Organizing infections
   c. Organizing diffuse alveolar damage
   d. Eosinophilic pneumonia (EP)
   e. Hypersensitivity pneumonitis (HP)
   f. Aspiration pneumonia
   g. Collagen vascular diseases (CVD)
   h. Peripheral reaction to lesions such as tumours, infarcts, infections
3. Presence of tissue eosinophilia
   a. Acute eosinophilic pneumonia (AEP)
   b. Hypereosinophilic syndrome
   c. Churg–Strauss syndrome
   d. Asthma
   e. Parasitic and fungal infections
   f. Cigarette smoking
   g. Drug reaction
4. Presence of diffuse alveolar haemorrhage (DAH)
   a. Idiopathic pulmonary haemosiderosis
   b. Goodpasture syndrome (anti-glomerular basement membrane [GBM] antibody syndrome)
   c. Vasculitides (e.g. granulomatosis with polyangiitis [GPA])
   d. Isolated capillaritis

(Continued)

Table 2.14 (*Continued*) Features to focus on while examining transbronchial lung biopsy specimens for diffuse parenchymal lung diseases (DPLD) and their possible causes

    e. Collagen vascular diseases (e.g. systemic lupus erythematosus [SLE])
    f. Antiphospholipid syndrome
    g. Pulmonary veno-occlusive disease
    h. Behçet syndrome
    i. Immunoglobulin A nephropathy
    j. Bronchiectasis
    k. Mitral stenosis
    l. Acute lung allograft rejection
5. Presence of chronic interstitial inflammatory infiltrates
    a. Non-specific interstitial pneumonia (NSIP)
    b. Hypersensitivity pneumonitis (HP)
    c. Lymphoid interstitial pneumonia (LIP)
    d. Lymphoid interstitial pneumonia in human immunodeficiency virus (HIV) infection
    e. Low-grade lymphoproliferative diseases
    f. Hypersensitivity to drugs
    g. Resolving infection
6. Presence of granulomatous inflammation
    a. Granulomatous infection
    b. Sarcoidosis
    c. Pneumoconiosis
    d. Excipient lung disease
    e. Aspiration pneumonia
    f. Granulomatosis and polyangiitis (GPA)

CONCLUSION

The algorithmic approach to the histopathologic diagnosis of ILD, using six main patterns of disease at very low magnification, is an extremely useful and practical approach to the diagnosis of these diverse diseases encountered by pathologists. This protocol, followed by clinical–radiologic correlation will result in the most accurate interpretation of histologic findings. It is expected that the patterns will overlap in many instances. However, identification of the predominant pattern based on clinical importance is paramount.

REFERENCES

1. Nicholson, AG. Classification of idiopathic interstitial pneumonias: Making sense of the alphabet soup. *Histopathology*. 2002;41(5):381–91.
2. Leslie K, Colby T, Lynch D. Anatomic distribution and histopathologic patterns of interstitial lung disease. In: Schwarz MI, King TE, eds. *Interstitial Lung Disease*. 5th ed. Shelton, CT: People's Medical Publishing; 2011:35–60.
3. Cardinal-Fernandez P, Bajwa EK, Dominguez-Calvo A, Menéndez JM, Papazian L, Thompson BT. The presence of diffuse alveolar damage on open lung biopsy is associated with mortality in patients with acute respiratory distress syndrome: A systematic review and meta-analysis. *Chest*. 2016:149(5):1155–64.
4. Olsen J, Colby T, Elliot C. Hamman-Rich syndrome revisited. *Mayo Clin Proc*. 1990;65(12):1538–48.
5. Zompatori M, Ciccarese F, Fasano L. Overview of current lung imaging in acute respiratory distress syndrome. *Eur Respir Rev*. 2014;23(134):519–30.
6. Corrin B, Nicholson AG. Acute alveolar injury and repair. In: Corrin B, Nicholson AG, eds. *Pathology of the Lungs*. 3rd ed. London, UK: Churchill Livingston; 2011:135–53.
7. Nicholson, AG, Rice, AJ. Interstitial lung diseases. In: Hasleton P, Flieder DB, eds. *Spencer's Pathology of the Lung*. 6th ed. Cambridge, UK: Cambridge University Press; 2013:366–408.
8. Fukuda Y, Ishizaki M, Masuda Y, Kimura G, Kawanami O, Masugi Y. The role of intraalveolar fibrosis in the process of pulmonary structural remodeling in patients with diffuse alveolar damage. *Am J Pathol*. 1987;126(1):171–82.
9. Hyzy R, Huang S, Myers J, Flaherty K, Martinez F. Acute exacerbation of idiopathic pulmonary fibrosis. *Chest*. 2007 November 1;132(5):1652–58.
10. Beasley MB, Franks TJ, Galvin JR, Gochuico B, Travis WD. Acute fibrinous and organizing pneumonia: A histological pattern of lung injury and possible variant of diffuse alveolar damage. *Arch Pathol Lab Med*. 2002;126(9):1064.
11. Tazelaar HD, Linz LJ, Colby TV, Myers JL, Limper AH. Acute eosinophilic pneumonia:

Histopathologic findings in nine patients. *Am J Respir Crit Care Med.* 1997;155(1):296.

12. de Prost N, Parrot A, Picard C, Ancel PY, Mayaud C, Fartoukh M, Cadranel J. Diffuse alveolar haemorrhage: Factors associated with in-hospital and long-term mortality. *Eur Respir J.* 2010;35(6):1303–11.

13. Colby TV, Fukuoka J, Ewaskow SP, Helmers R, Leslie KO. Pathologic approach to pulmonary haemorrhage. *Ann Diagn Pathol.* 2001;5(5):309–19.

14. Kottmann RM, Hogan CM, Phipps RP, Sime PJ. Determinants of initiation and progression of idiopathic pulmonary fibrosis. *Respirology.* 2009;14(7):917–33.

15. Katzenstein AL. Idiopathic interstitial pneumonia. In: Katzenstein AL, eds. *Katzenstein and Askin's Surgical Pathology of Non-Neoplastic Lung Disease.* 4th ed. New York, NY: Elsevier Health Sciences; 2006:51–61.

16. Raghu G, Collard HR, Egan JJ, Martinez FJ, Behr J, Brown KK et al. An official ATS/ERS/JRS/ALAT statement: Idiopathic pulmonary fibrosis: Evidence-based guidelines for diagnosis and management. *Am J Respir Crit Care Med.* 2011;183(6):788–824.

17. Corrin B, Nicholson AG. Diffuse parenchymal disease of the lung. In: Corrin B, Nicholson AG, eds. *Pathology of the Lungs.* 3rd ed. London, UK: Churchill Livingstone; 2011:263–326.

18. Nho RS. Current concept for the pathogenesis of idiopathic pulmonary fibrosis (IPF). *Clin Res Pulmonol.* 2013;1:1008.

19. Katzenstein AL, Fiorelli RF. Nonspecific interstitial pneumonia/fibrosis. Histologic features and clinical significance. *Am J Surg Pathol.* 1994;18(2):136–47.

20. Travis WD, Matsui K, Moss J, Ferrans VJ. Idiopathic nonspecific interstitial pneumonia: Prognostic significance of cellular and fibrosing patterns: Survival comparison with usual interstitial pneumonia and desquamative interstitial pneumonia. *Am J Surg Pathol.* 2000;24(1):19–33.

21. Kuranishi LT, Leslie KO, Ferreira RG, Coletta EAN, Storrer KM, Soares MR, de Castro Pereira CA, Airway-centered interstitial fibrosis: Etiology, clinical findings and prognosis. *Respir Res.* 2015;16:55.

22. Yousem SA, Dacic S. Idiopathic bronchiolocentric interstitial pneumonia. *Modern Pathol.* 2002;15(11):1148–53.

23. Travis WD, Costabel U, Hansell DM, King J, Talmadge E, Lynch DA et al. An official American Thoracic Society/European Respiratory Society statement: Update of the international multidisciplinary classification of the idiopathic interstitial pneumonias. *Am J Respir Crit Care Med.* 2013;188(6):733–48.

24. Rao N, Mackinnon A, Routes JM. Granulomatous and lymphocytic interstitial lung disease: A spectrum of pulmonary histopathologic lesions in common variable immunodeficiency-histologic and immunohistochemical analyses of 16 cases. *Human Pathol.* 2015;46(9):1306–14.

25. Selman M, Pardo A, King J, Talmadge E. Hypersensitivity pneumonitis: Insights in diagnosis and pathobiology. *Am J Respir Crit Care Med.* 2012;186(4):314.

26. Hanak V, Golbin JM, Ryu JH. Causes and presenting features in 85 consecutive patients with hypersensitivity pneumonitis. *Mayo Clinic Proc.* 2007;82(7):812–16.

27. Mukhopadhyay S, Katzenstein AA. Pulmonary disease due to aspiration of food and other particulate matter: A clinicopathologic study of 59 cases diagnosed on biopsy or resection specimens. *Am J Surg Pathol.* 2007;31(5):752–59.

28. Katzenstein AL. Acute lung injury patterns: Diffuse alveolar damage and bronchiolitis obliterans-organizing pneumonia. In: Katzenstein AL, ed. *Katzenstein and Askin's Surgical Pathology of Non-Neoplastic Lung Disease.* 4th ed. New York, NY: Elsevier Health Sciences; 2006:36–39.

29. Epler GR, Colby TV, McLoud TC, Carrington CB, Gaensler EA. Bronchiolitis obliterans organizing pneumonia. *N Engl J Med.* 1985;312(3):152–58.

30. American Thoracic Society, European Respiratory Society. American Thoracic Society/European Respiratory Society International Multidisciplinary Consensus Classification of the Idiopathic Interstitial Pneumonias. *Am J Respir Crit Care Med.* 2002;165(2):277–304.

31. Katzenstein AL. Idiopathic interstitial pneumonia: Classification and diagnosis. In: Churg A, Katzenstein AL, eds. *Lung: Current Concepts (Monographs in Pathology)*. Philadelphia, PA: Lippincott Williams & Wilkins; 1993:1–31.

32. Harbitz F. Extensive calcification of the lungs as a distinct disease. *Arch Internal Med.* 1918;XXI(1):139–46.

33. Mariani B, Montanini N, Torelli G. Microlitiasipolmonareendoalveolarediffusa. *Annalidell'Istituto Carlo Forlanini.* 1947;10(2):179–99.

34. Huqun, Izumi S, Miyazawa H, Ishii K, Uchiyama B, Ishida T et al. Mutations in the SLC34A2 gene are associated with pulmonary alveolar microlithiasis. *Am J Respir Crit Care Med.* 2007;175(3):263–68.

35. Fukuoka J, Leslie KO. Chronic diffuse lung diseases. In: Leslie KO, Wick MR, eds. *Practical Pulmonary Pathology: A Diagnostic Approach.* 2nd ed. Philadelphia, PA: Elsevier Saunders; 2011:213–76.

36. Mukhopadhyay S, Gal AA. Granulomatous lung disease: An approach to the differential diagnosis. *Arch Pathol Lab Med.* 2010;134(5):667–90.

37. Mukhopadhyay S, Aubry M. Pulmonary granulomas: Differential diagnosis, histologic features and algorithmic approach. *Diagn Histopathol.* 2013;19(8):288–97.

38. Cheung OY, Muhm JR, Helmers RA, Aubry M, Tazelaar HD, Khoor A, Leslie KO, Colby TV. Surgical pathology of granulomatous interstitial pneumonia. *Ann Diagn Pathol.* 2003;7(2):127–38.

39. Wright JL, Churg A. Diseases caused by metals and related compounds, fumes and gases. In: Churg A, Francis HY, eds. *Pathology of Occupational Disease.* New York, NY: IGAKU-SHOIN Medical; 1988:56–61.

40. Suri HS, Yi ES, Nowakowski GS, Vassallo R. Pulmonary Langerhans cell histiocytosis. *Orphanet J Rare Dis.* 2012;7:16.

41. Ryu J. Classification and approach to bronchiolar diseases. *Curr Opin Pulm Med.* 2006;12(2):145–51.

42. Fukuoka J, Franks TJ, Colby TV, Flaherty KR, Galvin JR, Hayden D, Gochuico BR, Kazerooni EA, Martinez F, Travis WD. Peribronchiolar metaplasia: A common histologic lesion in diffuse lung disease and a rare cause of interstitial lung disease: Clinicopathologic features of 15 cases. *Am J Surg Pathol.* 2005;29(7):948–54.

3

Using thoracic imaging to diagnose ILD

MARIA DANIELA MARTIN AND JEFFREY P KANNE

Imaging plays a central role in the diagnosis and management of diffuse lung diseases (DLDs), both for establishing a diagnosis and for determining causes of worsening signs or symptoms. In some instances, imaging may be sufficient to establish a definitive diagnosis without biopsy or further clinical workup.

RADIOGRAPHY

Chest radiography (CXR) is usually the initial imaging test performed when a patient is suspected of having DLD. Radiography is relatively inexpensive, easy to obtain and perform, and employs relatively low levels of ionizing radiation (typical effective dose for postero-anterior [PA] and lateral radiographs is 0.1 mSv). Radiography provides information on lung volumes and can often indicate the presence, extent and nature of DLD. However, with rare exception, radiography is insufficient to establish a definitive radiologic diagnosis.

COMPUTED TOMOGRAPHY

Computed tomography (CT) is the preferred imaging examination for patients with known or suspected DLD. The high spatial resolution of CT, the inherent contrast between air and soft tissue, and the ability to obtain volumetric imaging data make CT ideal for imaging the lungs. High-resolution CT (HRCT) of the chest is a technique that uses thin (<1.5 mm) slice thickness and a high-spatial frequency reconstruction kernel to optimize spatial resolution for lung imaging. However, with modern CT technology, the distinction between standard CT and HRCT has all but disappeared. The vast majority of CT scanners in use today can perform volumetric CT scans of the chest during a single breath hold typically shorter than 8 seconds and construct contiguous thin-section, high-resolution images in multiple planes. Expiratory and prone images can be obtained as needed (1). A variety of radiation dose reduction techniques allow for minimized patient radiation exposure while optimizing imaging quality. High-quality volumetric, thin-section CT scans of the chest can be performed with effective doses between 2 and 5 mSv, far lower than the standard-resolution chest CT that has been replaced by HRCT imaging.

PATTERN APPROACH TO CT OF DIFFUSE LUNG DISEASE

The diagnosis of DLD on chest CT usually hinges on the pattern and distribution of abnormalities. Distribution not only applies to the transaxial dimension but also the craniocaudad dimension.

Predominant patterns of DLD on CT are as follows:

- Linear
- Nodular
- Increased attenuation
- Decreased attenuation
- Cystic

LINEAR PATTERN

A linear pattern can be subcategorized into septal and reticular patterns. A septal pattern (Figure 3.1) is characterized by thickening, and thus visibility, of the interlobular septa. Lung oedema is the most common cause of a septal pattern and usually results in symmetric, basal and posterior predominance of smooth septal thickening. Pleural effusions often accompany a septal pattern in the setting of lung oedema. Lymphangitic carcinomatosis can also result in a septal pattern

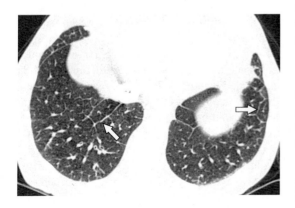

Figure 3.1 Lung oedema. HRCT image shows smooth septal thickening (*arrows*) in both lung bases.

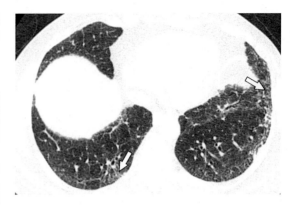

Figure 3.2 Usual interstitial pneumonia. HRCT image shows subpleural reticulation (*arrows*) in both lung bases.

on CT. Unlike oedema, septal thickening in lymphangitic carcinomatosis is more likely to be randomly distributed and have a more nodular or beaded appearance.

Common causes of a septal pattern include

- Lung oedema
- Lymphangitic carcinomatosis

Uncommon causes of a septal pattern include

- Pulmonary veno-occlusive disease
- Storage diseases such as Niemann–Pick disease
- Lymphangiectasia

A reticular pattern usually is the result of interstitial fibrosis, most commonly the usual interstitial pneumonia (UIP) (Figure 3.2).

Common causes of a reticular pattern include

- Usual interstitial pneumonia
- Nonspecific interstitial pneumonia
- Fibrotic hypersensitivity pneumonitis

Uncommon causes of a reticular pattern include

- Sarcoidosis
- Hard metal pneumoconiosis
- Asbestosis
- Familial interstitial pneumonia

NODULAR PATTERN

A nodular pattern can be subcategorized into centrilobular, perilymphatic and random distributions. Centrilobular nodules are fairly evenly

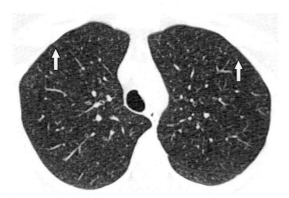
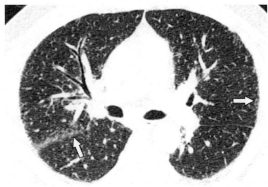

Figure 3.3 Hypersensitivity pneumonitis. HRCT image shows diffuse, poorly defined centrilobular nodules (*arrows*).

Figure 3.4 Sarcoidosis. HRCT image shows a perilymphatic pattern of diffuse nodules with nodules clustering along the pleural surfaces (*arrows*).

spaced, do not abut pleural surfaces and do not contact large vessels and airways (Figure 3.3). A pattern of well-defined centrilobular nodules with or without branching centrilobular opacities (tree-in-bud) is most often the result of cellular bronchiolitis, usually due to infection or aspiration. When centrilobular nodules are poorly defined or ground-glass attenuation, respiratory bronchiolitis and hypersensitivity pneumonitis are common. Because the lobular pulmonary artery is located adjacent to the terminal bronchiole, pulmonary arteriolar disease, albeit rarely, can also manifest as a centrilobular pattern.

Common causes of a centrilobular pattern are

- Well defined (with or without tree-in-bud opacities)
  - Infectious bronchiolitis
  - Aspiration
- Ground-glass attenuation
  - Hypersensitivity pneumonitis
  - Respiratory bronchiolitis

Uncommon causes of a centrilobular pattern are

- Well defined
  - Follicular bronchiolitis
  - IV drug use (excipient lung disease)
  - Endovascular metastases
- Ground-glass attenuation
  - Pulmonary capillary haemangiomatosis
  - Severe pulmonary hypertension

A perilymphatic pattern is characterized by nodules located primarily along the pulmonary lymphatics, particularly along the pleural surfaces, interlobular septa, centrilobular core and large bronchovascular structures. Sarcoidosis is the most common cause of a perilymphatic pattern (Figure 3.4). The micronodules of silicosis and coal worker's pneumoconiosis also have a perilymphatic distribution, but they tend to be rounder and smoother in contrast to the irregular shapes encountered with sarcoidosis.

Common causes of a perilymphatic pattern include

- Sarcoidosis
- Lymphangitic carcinomatosis

Uncommon causes of a perilymphatic pattern include

- Silicosis
- Coal worker's pneumoconiosis
- Berylliosis

A random pattern of diffuse lung nodules reflects haematogenous spread of infection or tumour (Figure 3.5). Miliary pattern is a term used to describe diffuse, randomly distributed tiny (<4 mm) nodules. Mycobacteria and endemic fungi are the most common causes of miliary infection, and patients are often immunocompromised. The nodules with miliary metastases tend to be more heterogeneous than the nodules of miliary infection. Diffuse idiopathic pulmonary neuroendocrine cell hyperplasia (DIPNECH) is characterized by patchy air trapping and scattered randomly distributed nodules.

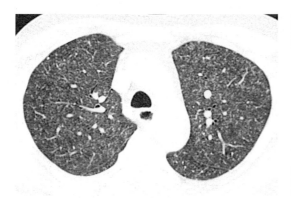

Figure 3.5 Disseminated tuberculosis in kidney transplant recipient. HRCT image shows diffuse, randomly distributed tiny (miliary) nodules.

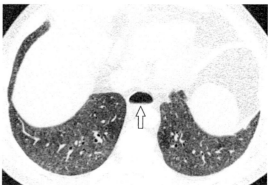

Figure 3.6 Non-specific interstitial pneumonia in a patient with systemic sclerosis. HRCT image shows diffuse ground-glass opacity in the lower lobes. Note the fluid level in the lower oesophagus (*arrow*).

Common causes of a random pattern include

- Disseminated infection
  - Tuberculosis
  - Endemic fungus
    - Histoplasmosis
    - Coccidioidomycosis
    - Blastomycosis
  - Varicella-zoster virus
- Metastases

A rare cause of a random pattern is

- Diffuse idiopathic pulmonary neuroendocrine cell hyperplasia (DIPNECH)

INCREASED ATTENUATION

Increased attenuation of the lung parenchyma can be divided into ground-glass opacity (GGO) and consolidation. It is not uncommon for GGO and consolidation to coexist, as they represent a continuum of altered lung attenuation.

Ground-glass opacity

GGO describes a subtle or hazy increase in lung attenuation with preservation of the underlying structures including vessels, airways and interlobular septa.

GGO is the result of volume averaging of a process below the spatial resolution of CT, whether it be primarily affecting the airspaces or the pulmonary interstitium. Any process that fills the alveoli with fluid or cells in its early stage can result in GGO. Similarly, infiltration of the interstitium, such as with an inflammatory or fibrotic process, can also cause GGO. Increased capillary blood volume can also lead to increased attenuation of the lung, which is referred to as mosaic perfusion.

GGO can be the manifestation of acute or chronic processes and may be subtle or occult on CXR, which is why HRCT plays a pivotal role in diagnosis of DLD (Figure 3.6). A detailed clinical history including the duration of symptoms is imperative for making an accurate diagnosis or narrowing the differential diagnosis. The distribution of GGO is also important for narrowing the differential diagnosis.

Common causes of GGO include

- Acute
  - Oedema
  - Aspiration
  - Infection (especially *Pneumocystis*, viral, *Mycoplasma*)
  - Haemorrhage
- Subacute or chronic
  - Organizing pneumonia (related to infection, drug toxicity, etc.)

Uncommon causes of GGO include

- Acute
  - Diffuse alveolar damage
  - Acute exacerbation of DLD
  - Acute eosinophilic pneumonia
  - Hypersensitivity pneumonitis
  - Radiation pneumonitis
- Subacute or chronic
  - Nonspecific interstitial pneumonia
  - Hypersensitivity pneumonitis

- Lymphoid interstitial pneumonia
- Smoking-related diffuse lung disease
- Chronic eosinophilic pneumonia
- Sarcoidosis
- Pulmonary alveolar proteinosis
- Vasculitis
- Lung adenocarcinoma

Common pitfalls in the diagnosis of GGO and information that can help are as follows:

- The attenuation value of air is 1000 Hounsfield units (HU). Normal lung parenchyma attenuation in full inspiration ranges from 700–900 HU and decreases approximately 100–300 HU in expiration. Familiarity with these values can help identify artifacts and normal physiologic variation of lung attenuation (2).
- Falsely increased attenuation of the lung on contrast-enhanced CTs → Evaluation for DLD should not use intravenous contrast; compare lung to tracheal air column. The attenuation of air in the trachea and the lung parenchyma will both show an artefactual increase in the presence of IV contrast.
- Expiration: Normal lungs are usually high attenuation in the expiratory phase → Evaluate the posterior tracheal wall for flattening or anterior bowing, which is seen in expiration.
- Dependent atelectasis → An AP gradient is nearly always seen, and the sagittal reformations often show the gradient well (a flat dependent line is often seen). If in doubt, prone images can be obtained, and the GGO will disappear if it is caused by atelectasis.
- Thicker slices → It is difficult to detect GGO when thicker slices (>1.5 mm) are used. Also, clusters of tiny nodules, as sometimes encountered with sarcoidosis, can mimic ground-glass opacity when thicker slices are used.
- GGO involves the entire lung → Compare lung parenchyma density to the tracheal air column (measurement of attenuation should not include vessels). If lung attenuation is increased compared to the trachea, it is likely abnormal. Routine use of the same window and level settings can also help the reader recognize abnormal lung attenuation.
- Body habitus or technique can result in artefactual GGO → Compare the attenuation of the tracheal air column to that of lung

parenchyma; if the tracheal air column appears 'gray' rather than black, the GGO is likely artefactual. The attenuation of tracheal air and the lung parenchyma will both show an artefactual increase in density, similar to the administration of IV contrast.

Crazy-Paving

Crazy-paving describes an area of GGO with superimposed septal lines. This pattern was described originally in cases of pulmonary alveolar proteinosis (PAP). However, many other diseases can cause a crazy-paving pattern (3). Crazy-paving can be the only finding (typical of PAP) or more commonly coexists with ground-glass opacity, consolidation, or both. The differential diagnosis for crazy-paving is similar to that of GGO.

Causes of crazy-paving include

- Infection (*Pneumocystis*, viral, *Mycoplasma*, and bacterial)
- Oedema
- Haemorrhage
- Diffuse alveolar damage
- Organizing pneumonia
- Lipoid pneumonia
- Sarcoidosis
- Pulmonary alveolar proteinosis (primary or secondary)
- Neoplasm (adenocarcinoma or lymphoma)
- Radiation-induced injury

Ancillary CT findings, a good clinical history (e.g. chronicity of the symptoms) and physical examination aid in narrowing the differential diagnosis.

Consolidation

Consolidation represents an area of homogeneous increased lung attenuation that obscures the underlying structures, with the possible exception of airways (air bronchograms).

Similar to GGO, consolidation can be caused by processes that primarily affect the airspaces, the interstitium or both, although alveolar processes, such as those caused by infection and aspiration, are by far more common (Figure 3.7). Any condition that replaces the alveolar air with fluid, cells, tissue or external substances can result in

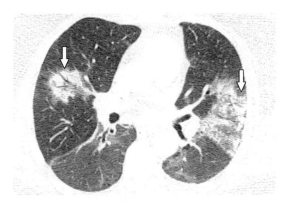

Figure 3.7 Cryptogenic organizing pneumonia. HRCT image shows bilateral discrete foci of lung consolidation (*arrows*), which contain air bronchograms. A peripheral or peribronchial distribution of discrete lung consolidation is commonly the result of organizing pneumonia.

consolidation. Similarly, an advanced interstitial process leading to fibrosis can cause consolidation. In those cases, there are usually other findings on HRCT that should be taken into consideration when evaluating an area of consolidation, since it is usually caused by confluent disease. Exceptions can occur, such as a superimposed acute process or malignancy on a background of DLD.

The clinical presentation and anatomic distribution of consolidation help narrow the differential diagnosis.

Common causes of consolidation include

- Acute
  - Common
    - Infection
    - Aspiration
    - Oedema
  - Uncommon
    - Diffuse alveolar damage
    - Haemorrhage
    - Acute eosinophilic pneumonia
- Chronic
  - Common
    - Organizing pneumonia
    - Cancer (especially invasive mucinous adenocarcinoma)
  - Uncommon
    - Sarcoidosis
    - Lipoid pneumonia
    - Lymphoma and other lymphoproliferative diseases

- Chronic eosinophilic pneumonia
- Hypersensitivity pneumonitis
- Radiation-induced injury
- Vasculitis

Rare causes of processes in the lung with higher attenuation opacities and calcifications include amiodarone toxicity, hard metal pneumoconiosis, alveolar microlithiasis, dendriform pulmonary ossification, talcosis and pulmonary metastatic calcification.

DECREASED ATTENUATION

Decreased attenuation occurs when the lung parenchyma is darker or more lucent than normal, usually from reduced perfusion or gas trapping. Comparing it to the trachea, the lung should always have higher attenuation. Diseases that cause low attenuation include those that destroy the lung parenchyma such as emphysema, those causing mosaic perfusion including chronic pulmonary embolism, and cystic lung disease, the latter of which is discussed separately.

Destruction of the lung parenchyma

Common:

- Smoking-related emphysema (centrilobular, paraseptal)
- Emphysema related to α-1-antitripsin deficiency (panlobular)

Uncommon:

- Pulmonary laceration
- Inflammatory pneumatoceles

If advanced, distinguishing emphysema from lung cysts can be challenging. Helpful clues to distinguish between the two are given in Table 3.1.

Mosaic perfusion (mosaic oligemia)

To understand this term, one needs to understand that the attenuation of the lung parenchyma is partially related to the circulating blood in the pulmonary vessels. Mosaic perfusion refers to the heterogeneous appearance of the lung with alternating areas of different attenuation caused by a shift in lung perfusion by a disease. Both airway

Table 3.1 Helpful clues to distinguish emphysema from lung cysts

Emphysema	Cysts
No clear walls	Well-defined walls that are usually thin
Destroys pulmonary architecture	Displaces adjacent structures (vessels and airways) without destroying them
Often has a central dot, which represents the remaining lobular pulmonary artery	No central structures

and vascular diseases can cause mosaic perfusion, although airway causes are by far more common. The areas of different attenuation can be lobular, segmental or larger.

When encountering heterogeneous lung attenuation, the first distinction that should be made is what area of the lung is abnormal. In mosaic perfusion, the dark lung is abnormal and underperfused. Careful review starts with evaluation of the size of the pulmonary arteries in the areas of decreased attenuation. If mosaic perfusion is present, the pulmonary arteries are usually smaller in the lucent areas. In case of a vascular process, the arteries may be stenosed or occluded. With airway diseases, decreased ventilation to a focal area of the lung causes hypoxia-induced reflex vasoconstriction and subsequently decreased lung

perfusion. Identifying smaller vessels in the lucent lung is not always straightforward. A blinded study reported that a small vessel was identified in the lucent lung only in 68% of cases of vascular or airways diseases (4). Sometimes there are other clues that suggest the underlying diagnosis such as thickened or dilated airways in the lucent lung in cases of airways disease or secondary signs of pulmonary hypertension in vascular causes. Also, lobular areas of lucent lung are more commonly seen with airways disease, whereas vascular aetiologies tend to cause larger areas of decreased perfusion (e.g. segmental, lobar or larger) (Figures 3.8 and 3.9).

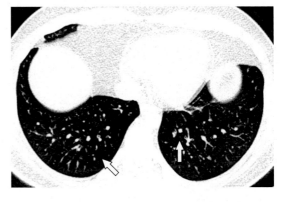

Figure 3.8 Long-standing asthma. HRCT image shows mosaic perfusion in the lower lobes with areas of decreased attenuation (*arrows*). Mild bronchial wall thickening suggest airways disease as the underlying aetiology.

(a) (b)

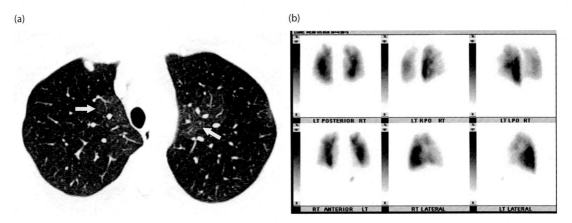

Figure 3.9 Chronic thromboembolic pulmonary hypertension. **(a)** HRCT image shows mosaic perfusion in the upper lobes with areas of increased attenuation (*arrows*) containing larger pulmonary vessels. **(b)** Nuclear medicine perfusion scan shows multiple wedge-shaped perfusion defects in the lung periphery. Ventilation scan (not shown) was normal.

Expiratory images are extremely useful in distinguishing airways from vascular disease. Small airways disease will show air trapping on expiratory images, which means that the lucent areas will stay lucent on expiratory images and the remaining lung will become denser. If all of the lung parenchyma (including the lucent areas) increase in attenuation and decrease in volume on expiratory images, then the aetiology is vascular.

Common airways causes of mosaic perfusion include

- Asthma
- Bronchiectasis
- Constrictive bronchiolitis

Uncommon airways causes of mosaic perfusion include

- Cystic fibrosis
- Hypersensitivity pneumonitis
- DIPNECH

Common vascular causes of mosaic perfusion include

- Acute or chronic pulmonary thromboembolism

Uncommon vascular causes of mosaic perfusion include

- Pulmonary hypertension (especially chronic thromboembolic pulmonary hypertension)
- Large vessel vasculitis

If the pulmonary artery size is normal in the areas of decreased lung attenuation, and there are no other signs indicative of an airway or vascular process, the true abnormality is likely in the areas of increased attenuation (GGO), with relatively lucent areas representing normal lung. This will lead towards the differential diagnosis of ground-glass opacities. Ancillary findings encountered with GGO include reticulation, nodules or consolidation. GGO can be stable, resolve or change over time. Heterogeneous lung parenchyma that remains stable over multiple exams is probably true mosaic perfusion. It is worth mentioning that some authors use the term 'mosaic attenuation pattern' when referring to a heterogeneous appearing lung parenchyma of unknown cause.

CYSTIC PATTERN

A lung cyst is defined as any round circumscribed space that is surrounded by an epithelial or fibrous wall of variable thickness, usually <2 mm. Cysts usually contain air but can be filled with liquid or solid material (5). Diseases mimicking lung cysts include emphysema and cystic bronchiectasis, as discussed in the previous section. For bronchiectasis, volumetric HRCT or multiplanar images can help in connecting the dilated cystic spaces to the airways, as well as showing other areas of bronchiectasis and thickened airways.

Lung cysts are a known incidental finding in elderly individuals. Their incidence increases with age and lower body mass index. Incidence of lung cysts varies, but several older population studies have shown incidences ranging up to 25% (6). They are uncommon in younger people and typically should not be seen in individuals younger than 50 years (7). This is helpful since many cystic lung diseases are seen in younger people.

Cystic lung disease is usually radiographically occult unless advanced, in which case lung volumes can be large with fine reticular opacities, which reflect overlapping cyst walls. Advanced cystic disease can be confused with emphysema on CXR and HRCT.

HRCT is the study of choice for the evaluation of suspected or known cystic lung disease (Figure 3.10). Clinical information is very valuable and aids in arriving to an accurate diagnosis.

Common causes of cystic lung disease are

- Incidental (usually elderly patients; usually not a negligible finding if patient is <50 years old)

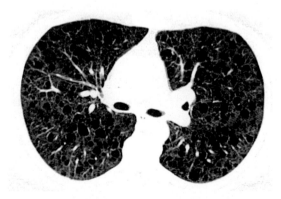

Figure 3.10 Lymphangioleiomyomatosis. HRCT image shows diffuse, fairly uniform thin-walled cysts.

- Pulmonary Langerhans cell histiocytosis (PLCH)
- Bullae

Uncommon causes of cystic lung disease are

- Lymphangioleiomyomatosis (LAM)
- Tuberous sclerosis complex (TSC)
- Birt–Hogg–Dubé syndrome (BHD)
- Lymphoid interstitial pneumonia (LIP)
- Amyloidosis and light-chain deposition disease (LCDD)
- Pneumatoceles (such as in *Pneumocystis* infection)
- Barotrauma
- Cystic metastasis
- Tracheobronchial papillomatosis
- Neurofibromatosis
- Proteus syndrome
- Honeycombing (UIP)

As with any lung disease, distribution is important. Lower lobe predominant cysts are more common in LIP, whereas upper lobe distribution and sparing of the costophrenic sulci and anterior tips of the lungs favour PLCH. Diffuse distribution favours LAM. The shapes of the cysts can slightly vary. For instance, cysts in LAM tend to be round, thin walled and homogeneous as opposed to PLCH, in which cysts tend to be irregular, varying in shape and wall thickness. LIP, amyloid and LCDD have identical appearances, likely reflecting the underlying commonality of lymphoproliferation and abnormal protein deposition. These diseases usually present with fewer cysts than LAM and PLCH, and the cysts tend to be perivascular, with often a dot associated to their walls representing an adjacent vessel. BHD cysts are usually basal predominant, larger, of different shapes and associated with pleural surfaces and interlobular septa.

Another common and confusing finding in cystic lung disease is the presence of lung nodules. For instance, PLCH can present with upper lobe predominant nodules, some of which may have subtle central lucency. LAM can be associated with small benign nodules in approximately 10% of cases, a condition known as multifocal micronodular pneumocyte hyperplasia (MMPH). LIP can also present with nodules, both solid and ground glass, and these may be the precursor lesions of the cysts or reflect amyloid deposition. It is worth noticing that if a solid nodule enlarges in a patient with LIP,

lymphoma should be considered. Patients with LIP can also have interlobular septal thickening and GGO. In HIV patients with GGO and a few lung cysts, both LIP and *Pneumocystis* pneumonia should be considered, although the clinical presentations usually are different.

Other clinical features that can affect the differential diagnosis of cystic lung disease include

- Non-smokers → PLCH almost always excluded
- LAM → Almost exclusively in women. Can be associated with angiomyolipomas
- Tuberous sclerosis complex → Can be associated with subependymal giant cell tumours and angiomyolipomas
- Associated with renal tumours → TSC and BHD
- Skin lesions → BHD
- Lymphoma → can be associated with LIP
- Multiple myeloma → can be associated with amyloidosis and LCDD
- Autoimmune disease or HIV → LIP
- Family history of lung cysts or recurrent pneumothorax → LAM, BHD
- Subpleural distribution → Exclude honeycombing (fibrosis) versus paraseptal emphysema

CONCLUSION

HRCT is pivotal in the evaluation of patients with known or suspected DLD. Although CT manifestations of some DLDs are protean and overlap, others are quite specific. Interpretation of HRCT of the chest requires that several conditions must be met in order to arrive at an accurate diagnosis. First, in order to avoid diagnostic errors, familiarity with the normal structures and their subtle variations related to physiology is needed. Second, one needs an organized approach to the interpretation of HRCT that includes the recognition of true pathology, its distribution and change over time. Third, a detailed clinical history including the chronology of the patient's symptoms and note of any exposures or underlying systemic illness should be provided. Last, it is important to remember that a multidisciplinary approach is usually needed in order to reach an accurate diagnosis, including close collaboration between pulmonologists, radiologists and pathologists familiar with these uncommon and complex diseases.

REFERENCES

1. Brett ME, Richard WR. *Fundamentals of High-Resolution Lung CT: Common Findings, Common Patterns, Common Diseases, and Differential Diagnosis.* Philadelphia, PA: Wolters Kluwer Lippincott Williams & Wilkins; 2013.
2. Müller NL, Silva CIS. Imaging of the Chest. New York, NY: Saunders; 2008.
3. Rossi S, Erasmus J, Volpacchio M, Franquet T, Castiglioni T, McAdams HP. Crazy-paving pattern at thin-section CT of the lungs: Radiologic-pathologic overview. *RadioGraphics.* 2003;23(6):1509–19.
4. Arakawa H, Webb WR, McCowin M, Katsou G, Lee KN, Seitz RF. Inhomogeneous lung attenuation at thin-section CT: Diagnostic value of expiratory scans. *Radiology.* 1998;206(1):89–94.
5. Hansell DM, Bankier AA, MacMahon H, McLoud TC, Muller NL, Remy J. Fleischner society: Glossary of terms for thoracic imaging. *Radiology.* 2008;246:697–722.
6. Copley SJ. Morphology of the aging lung on computed tomography. *J Thorac Imaging.* 2016;31(3):140–50.
7. Trotman-Dickenson B. Cystic lung disease: Achieving a radiologic diagnosis. *Eur J Radiol.* 2014;83:39–46.

4

Genetics and genomics of idiopathic pulmonary fibrosis

SUSAN K MATHAI AND DAVID A SCHWARTZ

INTRODUCTION

Interstitial lung diseases (ILDs), also known as diffuse parenchymal lung diseases, refer to a diverse set of pathologies affecting the tissue and space around the alveoli. Idiopathic pulmonary fibrosis (IPF), the most common form of the idiopathic interstitial pneumonias (IIPs), is characterized by relentless scarring of the lung parenchyma and by a poor prognosis. Median survival from the time of diagnosis is 3 years (1,2), and there are few available treatments and no known cure (3–6). Despite decades of research, the aetiology of IPF remains a topic of controversy with many hypotheses focusing on aberrant behaviour of injured alveolar epithelial cells (7). However, more recent investigations have identified numerous rare variants (8–10), common genetic variants (11–13), transcriptional changes (14–17) and epigenetic changes (18) associated with IPF, leading to new hypotheses regarding disease pathogenesis. This chapter focuses on our current understanding of the genetics and genomics of IPF, how these discoveries have changed our understanding of the disease, how genetics and genomics might influence patient management and how they could influence future studies in the field.

USING CLUES FROM FAMILIAL DISEASE TO UNDERSTAND IPF

Early studies investigating potential genetic influences in the development of IPF utilized subjects with familial pulmonary fibrosis (or, familial interstitial pneumonia, FIP), defined as pulmonary fibrosis in individuals with two or more relatives also affected by an IIP. Early studies utilized twins and family aggregation of cases (19) because investigators had observed that a family history of pulmonary fibrosis was a risk factor for an IPF diagnosis (20–22). These early observational studies suggested that there was a familial risk for the disease, and the first disease-associated gene variants were identified in surfactant protein genes among FIP patients (23–27). Specifically, studies of families with pulmonary fibrosis identified a heterozygous coding mutation in surfactant protein C (SFTPC) (23), numerous coding and noncoding variants in SFPTC (24) and two rare coding mutations in surfactant protein A that segregated with disease and that were not found in controls (26,27).

Investigators also focused on rare familial syndromes associated with pulmonary fibrosis, such as Hermansky–Pudlak syndrome, a genetically heterogeneous autosomal recessive disorder (28) characterized by pigmentation defects, leucocyte dysfunction and pulmonary fibrosis caused by defects in numerous intracellular protein trafficking genes such as AP3B1 (29). Similarly, pulmonary fibrosis is part of the phenotype of dyskeratosis congenital (DC), a syndrome characterized by aplastic anaemia, myelodysplastic syndrome, skin hyperpigmentation, nail dystrophy and fibrosis of the lung and liver (30,31). Numerous genetic mutations are thought to be causal for this disorder, including mutations in telomere-related genes, such as DKC1, a gene involved in the stabilization of telomeres (8,30,31). Based on the numerous telomere-related mutations associated with DC, telomeropathy was (and continues to be) investigated as a potential driving mechanism for fibrosis. Studies of FIP cases and their kindred identified germline mutations in the telomerase

genes, telomerase reverse transcriptase (TERT) and telomerase RNA component (TERC), in up to one-sixth of pulmonary fibrosis families (8,32). Intriguingly TERT and TERC mutations were present in cases of both familial and sporadic IPF and were associated with shorter leucocyte telomeres compared to age-matched family members without the same mutations (32).

These studies linking specific mutations to measurable differences in telomere phenotype (i.e. telomere length) suggested that these mutations are altering gene function, strengthening the causal connection between genotype and phenotype. More recent studies utilizing exome sequencing of FIP subjects by Cogan and colleagues have described rare variants in genes encoding telomere elongation helicase 1 (RTEL1) polyadenylation-specific ribonuclease deadenylation nuclease (PARN) associated with FIP (9,10). Subjects with genetic variants in these genes had shortened telomeres in their peripheral blood mononuclear cells (PBMCs), though the specific mechanism through which PARN mutations affect telomere length remains to be described (9,10). In addition, telomere length has been associated with survival in IPF (33). The consistent findings of telomere-related mutations associated with pulmonary fibrosis (both disease status and severity) argue that telomere pathways are important in the pathogenesis of IPF. Indeed, mouse models for loss of function of telomere-related genes suggest that impaired telomerase function impairs the injury response in the lung (34). Further mechanistic studies will be needed in order to understand the means by which telomere shortening leads to pulmonary fibrosis and to identify potential therapeutic targets in this pathway.

MUC5B IN IPF

Though FIP studies built support for the hypothesis that pulmonary fibrosis and IPF were diseases in which genetic factors play a significant role, more recent studies have identified numerous common genetic variants (defined as a minor allele frequency [MAF] >0.05) associated with IPF. In 2011, Seibold and colleagues used genome-wide linkage analysis followed by sequencing to conclude that a single-nucleotide polymorphism (SNP) rs35705950 on the p-terminus of chromosome 11 within the promoter region of the MUC5B gene is strongly associated with both FIP and sporadic IPF (defined as IPF cases with no known family history of the disease) (11).

MUC5B encodes mucin 5B, a glycosylated macromolecular component of mucus secretions. *MUC5B* is the major gel-forming mucin in mucus and a major contributor to lubricating saliva, normal lung mucus, cervical mucus and innate immune function (35). rs35705950 is located in a highly conserved region of the gene, and Seibold and colleagues found that heterozygous (GT) and homozygous (TT) subjects had increased odds ratios (OR) for developing disease—6.8 (95% confidence interval [CI], 3.9–12) and 20.8 (95% CI, 3.8–113.7) for FIP and 9 (95% CI, 6.2–13.1) and 21.8 (95% CI, 5.1–93.5) for IPF, respectively, indicating the strength of this individual SNP's influence on disease risk (11). This initial study showed that the MAF was 0.338 in FIP subjects and 0.375 in IPF subjects, while the MAF was 0.091 in the control subjects genotyped—the risk allele had similar frequency in FIP and sporadic IPF, illustrating that rs35705950's influence on risk of disease is similar for IPF and FIP (11).

Additionally, an IPF diagnosis was associated with a greater than 14-fold increase in *MUC5B* gene expression in lung tissue regardless of genotype, but the presence of the minor allele (T) was associated with a 37.4-fold increase in gene expression even in unaffected (control) individuals (11). *MUC5B* has also been found in honeycomb cysts, one of the characteristic pathologic findings of IPF (36).

This association between the minor allele at rs35705950 and IPF has been validated in seven independent non-Hispanic white (NHW) cohorts (12,13,37–41), and this variant remains the strongest and most replicated single genetic risk factor for IPF. However, as the MAF in control subjects from the Seibold report in 2011 and follow-up cohort studies illustrate, the *MUC5B* promoter variant is relatively common in the general NHW population, found in 19% of those without any evidence of disease (42). Since IPF is observed in a small percentage of the NHW population, the *MUC5B* promoter variant alone is insufficient to cause disease. There may be interplay between rs35705950 and other genetic or environmental factors contributing to the development of disease; these gene-by-gene and gene-by-environment relationships are an active area of research (43).

Adding to its strength as a genetic risk factor for IPF, the *MUC5B* promoter polymorphism appears

to be specific to risk of IPF and fibrotic IIPs. Studies examining cohorts with ILD secondary to systemic sclerosis (38,39), asbestosis, sarcoidosis (38), acute lung injury or acute respiratory distress syndrome (ARDS), chronic obstructive pulmonary disease (COPD) and asthma have failed to show association between disease and rs35705950 genotype (44). Furthermore, rs35705950 may be significant in populations outside of NHWs—the *MUC5B* promoter polymorphism is a strong genetic risk factor for IPF in the Mexican population (OR = 7.36, $P = 0.0001$), yet is rare in a Korean cohort (45). Among Asians, the minor allele frequency for the *MUC5B* promoter variant rs35705950 is low; however, the rs35705950 variant had a significantly higher prevalence in IPF cases compared to healthy controls in both Japanese and Chinese populations (41,46). The prevalence of the rs35705950 variant across difference ethnic groups may reflect disease prevalence in these groups—it has been observed that NHWs appear to be at higher risk of developing IPF than Hispanics and Asians, and the disease is thought to be rare in African populations (47). Correspondingly, the *MUC5B* promoter polymorphism is not present when measured in Sub-Saharan African populations (http://www.ncbi.nlm.nih.gov/SNP/snp_ref. cgi?rs=35705950). Therefore, though its relationship to IPF was first described in studies of NHWs, the rs35705950 may be important in the development of pulmonary fibrosis in other ethnic groups, as well; the examination of IPF-associated genetic variants in a wider array of racial and ethnic groups will be critical to the understanding of how genetic variants confer risk of disease across racial and ethnic backgrounds.

BEYOND IPF: RS35705950 AND INTERSTITIAL LUNG ABNORMALITIES

A study examining the Framingham Heart Study cohort found that the MAF for rs35705950 variant in the NHW population was 10.5%, and so correspondingly 19% of the population had one or more copies of the risk variant (42). The odds of interstitial lung abnormalities (ILAs), defined as nondependent changes affecting more than 5% of any lung zone (including ground-glass or reticular abnormalities, diffuse centrilobular nodularity, nonemphysematous cysts, honeycombing or traction bronchiectasis) were 2.8 times greater for each copy of the rs35705950 variant (42), suggesting that the variant may have a relationship to pre-clinical forms of pulmonary fibrosis. Though it is not clear that ILAs are always precursor lesions for pulmonary fibrosis, other studies of this and similar cohorts suggest that ILAs are associated with increased all-cause mortality and with mortality specifically due to respiratory diseases such as pulmonary fibrosis (48). Moreover, the Framingham Heart Study observations showed that the rates of definite radiographic evidence of pulmonary fibrosis in individuals over 50 years of age may be 2%, higher than had been previously reported in the literature (42,49). The associations between the rs35705950 variant and FIP, IPF, as well as 'pre-fibrotic' ILA lesions are intriguing because they suggest that genetic markers may guide interventions for the earlier detection of fibrosis in asymptomatic subjects, opening the door to the possibility of preventative IPF care (42,50).

OTHER COMMON GENETIC VARIANTS AND IPF

Though rs35705950 is the most well-studied common genetic variant associated with IPF, other disease-associated common variants have recently been discovered (Table 4.1). The development of cost-effective high-throughput variant screening mechanisms allowed genome-wide association studies (GWASs) to be performed on subjects with IPF and other IIPs. In 2013, Fingerlin and colleagues published a case–control GWAS in 1,616 fibrotic IIP and 4,683 control subjects, followed by a replication study of 876 cases and 1,890 controls (12). This large genome-wide study confirmed disease associations with *TERT* (chromosome 5p15), *MUC5B* (11p15) and the 3q26 region near *TERC*; however, it also identified seven new loci associated with fibrotic IIP, including *FAM13A* (4q22), *DSP* (6p24), *OBFC1* (10q24), *ATP11A* (13q4), *DPP9* (19p13) and regions on chromosomes 7q22 and 15q14-15 (12). Examining the reported biological function of the genes in the disease-associated loci suggests that host defense (*MUC5B* and *ATP11A*), cell-cell adhesion (*DSP* and *DPP9*) and DNA repair (*TERT*, *TERC* and *OBFC1*) could be pathways critical to disease pathogenesis (12,43,50,51). These genetic loci, excluding the *MUC5B* variant, account for

approximately one-third of disease risk, emphasizing the importance that genetic predisposition is playing in this disease (12,17,50). Once again, as was observed with the *MUC5B* promoter polymorphism, the ORs for the loci identified in this study did not differ in *post hoc* analyses comparing FIP and sporadic IPF cohorts (12,43). Furthermore, the same was true when comparing non-IPF fibrotic IIPs to the cases of IPF, illustrating that genetic risk factors for all fibrotic IIPs may be similar and adding to the growing evidence that FIP and IPF are genetically similar conditions.

An additional GWAS performed in subjects with IPF compared to non-diseased controls confirmed the association of the *MUC5B* promoter variant with IPF, but also identified further risk alleles, including one in Toll-interacting protein (*TOLLIP*) and signal peptidase-like 2C (*SPPL2C*) as risk loci (13). Importantly, this study not only identified risk variants, but also drew connections between specific variants (rs5743890) in *TOLLIP* and differential mortality from disease (13,52).

RARE VARIANTS AND COMMON VARIANTS

Despite individual studies describing associations between rare and common variants and IPF, future studies focused on the genetics of ILD need to address the potential interactions between variants in disease pathogenesis and risk. Individual rare variants that have been described, particularly telomerase mutations, are frequently associated with dramatic phenotypes (53); indeed, telomerase mutations often lead to multiple clinically significant organ abnormalities (e.g. cirrhosis, bone marrow dysfunction, premature greying, in addition to pulmonary fibrosis) (8,53). Yet, though the common variants in *MUC5B* and the other loci are strongly associated with disease, they appear to have smaller effect sizes (43,50). Due to the varying methodologies utilized to discover the association of rare versus common variants and disease (Table 4.1), careful study of the interaction between rare and common variants in determining an individual's risk of disease has yet to be performed. Future studies will be important in parsing the relative contributions of genetic variants and will be critical in the rational integration of genetic information into clinical care of ILDs.

Table 4.1 Genes and variants associated with idiopathic pulmonary fibrosis

Genes	Gene product functions	Mutation(s)/variant(s)	Type of study	Type of variant	References
SFTPC	Lung surfactant	1. IVS4 + 1,G > A 2. Leu188Gly 3. 10 sequence variants 4. Met71Val, Ile73Thr, IVS4 + 2, T > C 5. Gly100Ser	Targeted sequencing	Rare variants	1. Nogee et al. (2001) 2. Thomas et al. (2002) 3. Lawson et al. (2004) 4. Van Moorsel et al. (2010) 5. Ono et al. (2011)
SFTPA	Lung surfactant	G231 V, F198S	Linkage analysis, targeted sequencing	Rare variants	Wang et al. (2009)
TERT	DNA repair	1. Numerous coding variants 2. K902N 3. Leu55Gln, IVS1 + 1G > A, codon 112 del C, IVS9-2 A > C, Thr1110Met 4. R865C, V144M, P33S, R486C, V747fsX766, R865H 5. rs2736100, rs2853676	1–4. Targeted sequencing 5. GWAS	1. Rare variants 2. Rare variant 3. Rare variants 4. Rare variants 5. Common variants	1. de Leon et al. (2010) 2. Armanios et al. (2005) 3. Armanios et al. (2007) 4. Tsakiri et al. (2007) 5. Fingerlin et al. (2013); Wei et al. (2014)
TERC	DNA repair	1. 98 G > A 2. r.37 A > G 3. rs1881984	1–2. Targeted sequencing 3. GWAS	1–2. Rare variants 3. Common variant	1–2. Armanios et al. (2007) 3. Fingerlin et al. (2013)
PARN	DNA repair	Numerous (splicing and coding)	Exome sequencing	Rare variant	Stuart et al. (2014)
RTEL1	DNA repair	Numerous coding	Exome sequencing	Rare variant	Stuart et al. (2014); Cogan et al. (2015)
DKC1	DNA repair	1Thr405Ala mutation	Targeted sequencing	Rare variant	Kropski et al. (2014)

(Continued)

Table 4.1 (Continued) Genes and variants associated with idiopathic pulmonary fibrosis

Genes	Gene product functions	Mutation(s)/variant(s)	Type of study	Type of variant	References
MUC5B	Host defense	rs35705950	Linkage study; GWAS	Common variant	Seibold et al. (2011); Zhang et al. (2011); Stock et al. (2013); Borie et al. (2013); Noth et al. (2013); Fingerlin et al. (2013); Wei et al. (2014); Horimasu et al. (2015)
TOLLIP	Host defense	rs111521887, rs5743894, rs5743890	GWAS	Common variant	Noth et al. (2013)
SPPL2C	Protease	rs17690703	GWAS	Common variant	Noth et al. (2013)
DSP	Cell–cell adhesion	rs2076295	GWAS	Common variant	Fingerlin et al. (2013)
FAM13A	Unknown	rs2609255	GWAS	Common variant	Fingerlin et al. (2013)
OBFC1	DNA repair	rs11191865	GWAS	Common variant	Fingerlin et al. (2013)
ATP11A	Host defense	rs1278769	GWAS	Common variant	Fingerlin et al. (2013)
Chromosomal region 7q22	Unknown	rs4727443	GWAS	Common variant	Fingerlin et al. (2013)
Chromosomal region 15q14-15	Unknown	rs2034650	GWAS	Common variant	Fingerlin et al. (2013)
DPP9	Cell–cell adhesion	rs12610495	GWAS	Common variant	Fingerlin et al. (2013)

Abbreviation: GWAS = genome-wide association study.

Note: Common variant defined as those with minor allele frequency (MAF) >0.05.

CURRENT KNOWLEDGE OF GENE EXPRESSION DIFFERENCES IN IPF

GENE EXPRESSION PROFILING: LUNG TISSUE

Numerous gene expression studies have been done utilizing lung tissue of subjects with IPF to attempt to understand the processes that could be driving disordered repair and fibroproliferation. An early study utilizing microarrays to perform gene expression analyses on lung tissue examined lungs with the usual interstitial pneumonia (UIP) pattern (histopathology characteristic of, but not exclusive to, IPF) compared to non-diseased control lung tissue and found clear distinction between gene expression patterns in UIP versus control lungs (54). This study was limited in terms of application to IPF, since two of the five UIP lung tissue samples came from individuals with diagnosed autoimmune diseases, in which UIP is considered secondary to their systemic disease and therefore is not diagnostic of IPF (54). Genes related to smooth muscle proteins, complement, chemokines (such as numerous matrix metalloproteases, specifically matrix metalloprotease 7 [MMP7]) were upregulated in fibrotic lung, although inflammatory genes were not differentially expressed (54).

The diagnosis of IPF versus other forms of IIP holds prognostic and therapeutic implications, and other gene expression studies focused on employing genomic methods to distinguish between different IIPs in order to tease apart biological mechanisms specific to IPF. A 2005 study compared lung tissue microarray data from 15 IPF subjects, 12 with hypersensitivity pneumonitis (HP), and 8 with nonspecific interstitial pneumonia (NSIP)-like patterns (14). Gene expression patterns distinguished IPF from HP, with IPF lung strongly expressing genes related to extracellular matrix (e.g. collagens), muscle-specific genes, cell motility, and contraction, consistent with the active tissue remodelling and reorganization thought to be prominent in fibrotic lungs (14). Other epithelial cell-related genes (keratins, mucins) were also noted among differentially expressed genes in IPF, and similar to the earlier study, 'typical' inflammatory genes were notably absent in IPF compared to HP (14).

A larger study of lung tissue from 26 subjects with various IIPs and 9 control subjects utilized microarrays to discover 558 differentially expressed transcripts in the diseased lungs (15). The genes identified included a number that are involved in extracellular matrix (ECM) turnover, ECM structure, ECM degradation, and cell adhesion (15). This study also compared different forms of IIP, finding that FIP cases clustered together in terms of gene expression patterns and generally had more extreme expression differences when compared to controls than did other IIPs (15). Transcriptionally, non-specific interstitial pneumonia (NSIP) cases and IPF, though clinically quite distinct, did not differ dramatically.

Other studies of gene expression profiles in lung tissue have also attempted to use genome-scale gene expression data to identify genes and pathways active during 'acute exacerbations' of IPF (IPF-AE), periods of accelerated decline in respiratory function that occur in patients with stable or less rapidly progressive disease (47,55). Globally, the gene expression profile of lung tissue from IPF-AE subjects is nearly identical to that of stable IPF when both were compared to control samples, but when compared directly, 579 genes, many related to stress responses, were significantly differentially expressed (55). Even in the direct comparison of IPF-AE to stable IPF, inflammatory genes were not differentially expressed, arguing against a direct role for inflammation or acute viral infection in IPF-AE pathogenesis. Alpha-defensin gene expression and plasma alpha-defensin levels were elevated in IPF-AE, suggesting that these could be potential biomarkers in this disease and that epithelial cells are important in IPF-AE processes (55).

In a larger study of lung tissue, different IPF disease phenotypes were associated with specific gene expression signatures. Yang and colleagues utilized microarray analysis of lung tissue from 50 control subjects and 119 IPF subjects to discover that the expression of cilium genes identified two unique clinical phenotypes of IPF; the findings were then validated in an independent group of IPF lung tissue samples ($n = 111$) (16). Those with high cilium gene expression levels showed more microscopic honeycombing on pathology and had elevated tissue expression of *MUC5B* and *MMP7* (16). These results suggest that IPF is a heterogeneous disease consisting of at least two phenotypes differentiated by their expression of cilium genes in the lung, implicating cilia in disease pathogenesis and also implicating the airway epithelia in fibrogenesis within at least one sub-phenotype of this disease (16). The clinical ramifications of these sub-phenotypes remain to be examined in prospective studies.

GENE EXPRESSION PROFILING: PERIPHERAL BLOOD

Though the use of lung tissue to characterize gene expression profiles in IPF is logical given that the disease primarily affects this organ, there is significant interest in utilizing the peripheral blood to diagnose or prognosticate disease, since peripheral blood is readily available with routine phlebotomy (an outpatient procedure), while obtaining lung tissue requires an invasive procedure (either bronchoscopy or surgical lung biopsy).

A study utilizing the microarray-derived peripheral blood mononuclear cell (PBMC) gene expression profiles from IPF subjects (discovery $n = 45$, replication $n = 75$) allowed investigators to develop a model to predict poor clinical outcomes, defined as death or lung transplantation (56). A signature of 52 genes was associated with shorter transplant-free survival (TFS) in their cohorts, many of which were involved in T-cell signalling (56). In addition, utilizing CD28, ICOS, LCK and ITK gene expression quantifications in addition to age, sex and percent predicted forced vital capacity (a measure of lung function), a proportional hazards model was able to predict TFS—indeed, the gene expression factors improved the model's prediction capabilities when compared to the clinical parameters alone (56).

A follow-up study performed by the same investigatory team utilized their previously described PBMC microarray dataset (56) to identify potential prognostic predictor genes and then utilized an unbiased analytic technique 'Weighted Gene Co-expression Network Analysis' (WGCNA) to find groups of genes whose expression patterns suggested co-regulation (57). These gene modules were then associated with pulmonary function and clinical outcome (57). The resulting functional genomic model illustrated diagnostic (IPF versus control) and prognostic utility. It also suggested down-regulation of immune system pathways were predictive of poor prognosis (57). This is consistent with the finding that immunosuppressive therapy (e.g. prednisone, azathioprine) can worsen the clinical course for IPF patients (5).

Another study by Meltzer and colleagues examined microarray data utilizing RNA from peripheral whole blood to derive a 108-gene signature to distinguish IPF from normal controls (17) that had a sensitivity of 70% and specificity of 100% (accuracy 77%), though was not useful in predicting disease severity. Notable genes highlighted in this analysis included granulin (GRN) and matrix metalloprotease 9 (MMP9), a gene whose protein product has been implicated in prior studies of IPF (17,58).

Though these predictive models derived from gene expression data are not routinely used in clinical care, their reported prognostic power suggests that they could be useful not only at the laboratory bench or to generate hypotheses, but in the clinic to aid in directing therapy for and in diagnosing individual patients.

CURRENT KNOWLEDGE OF EPIGENETIC FACTORS IN ILD PATHOGENESIS

Epigenetics refers to characteristics and changes to the genome that affect gene function without changes in nucleotide sequence, such as DNA methylation, histone acetylation and micro-RNAs (miRNAs). Epigenetics are influenced by both the environment/exposures (59,60) and by genetics (61,62). Therefore, they are of particular interest in diseases such as pulmonary fibrosis and ILD because environmental exposures, such as cigarette smoking (59,63,64), in addition to sex and age, which are known to cause alterations in the epigenome, are risk factors for disease (65–70). IPF is a disease in which genetic and environmental factors are paramount – therefore, epigenetic modifications are a mechanism through which genetic (71) and environmental factors can be mediated (65).

EPIGENETIC MECHANISMS STUDIED IN IPF

Methylation of cytosine residues in CpG dinucleotides is thought to be the simplest form of epigenetic regulation (65). DNA methyltransferases are the enzymes responsible for adding methyl groups to these dinucleotides, while other enzymes actively demethylate DNA. Traditionally, it is thought that DNA methylation of 'CpG islands' in promoter regions of genes leads to 'silencing', or decreased transcription, of the gene. Methylation also occurs within genes and can be important in regulating transcription as well as splicing (61,65). Acetylation of histone tails regulates gene expression by altering DNA accessibility to RNA polymerase and transcription factors (65).

EPIGENETIC STUDIES IN IPF

IPF is a disease influenced by genetics (11,12,43), demographic risk factors such as age and sex (2,47), and environmental factors such as smoking and other inhaled exposures (47,71)—all factors that are known to modulate the epigenome (59,63,64). It is therefore unsurprising that epigenetic marks have been associated with IPF.

Studies targeting DNA methylation and histone modification have been shown to regulate genes and miRNAs that have been implicated in pathogenesis of IPF (65,70,72–74). These genes and miRNAs include cyclooxygenase-2 (72,73), chemokine IFN-gamma-inducible protein 10 (IP-10) (75), Thy-1 (CD90) (76,77), p14 alternative reading frame (ARF) (78), alpha-smooth muscle actin (79,80) and miR-19~92 cluster (81). Other molecular processes thought to be important in IPF pathogenesis, such as fibroblast apoptosis (82), cell senescence (83) and innate immunity (84), also show evidence of epigenetic regulation (65).

On a genome-wide level, DNA methylation studies illustrate that IPF lung tissues may have characteristic methylation profiles. Early studies utilizing methylation arrays with probes targeting CpG islands and promoters revealed differential methylation patterns in IPF lung tissue compared with non-diseased lung tissue (85,86). A similar genome-wide study of IPF fibroblasts, a potential effector cell for disease, showed significant global methylation differences (87).

A more comprehensive study of IPF lung tissue performed by Yang and colleagues examined 4.6 million CpG sites across the genome in 94 subjects with disease and 67 controls and identified 2,130 significantly differentially methylated regions (DMRs). Sixty percent of these DMRs are located in CpG island shores, comparable to other studies in cancers (18,65,88). In addition, 738 of the DMRs were associated with significant gene expression changes, enriched for the traditional inverse relationship between expression and methylation (18). Intersection of the set of 2,130 DMRs with the genetic loci identified by the two GWAS in IPF (12,13) also revealed significant methylation changes within five of these loci, including *TOLLIP* and *DSP* (18). These findings illustrate a global alteration in the methylation profile of the IPF lung tissue, links between gene expression and differential methylation, as well as links between disease-associated genetic loci and DMRs. The majority of the findings in this study utilized whole lung tissue, but specific analysis of the *CASZ1* transcription factor found that the gene was hypermethylated and had reduced gene expression in lung tissue as well as in type II alveolar epithelial cells from IPF subjects (18).

FUTURE DIRECTIONS IN IPF EPIGENETICS

Future analysis could include cell-specific examination of DNA methylation and gene expression in order to make more mechanistic inferences about DMRs and disease pathogenesis and would allow examination of histone modifications to add dimension to understanding of epigenetics and lung disease (65). Also, as more specific disease-associated genetic loci are identified, studies will be able to target these regions for epigenetic study to understand the relationship between sequence variation, epigenetic marks and disease.

In terms of therapeutic implications of epigenetic findings in IPF, examples from oncology suggest that the epigenome could be a target for intervention. DNA methyltransferases have been approved for haematologic abnormalities such as myelodysplastic syndrome (89) and have been investigated as therapeutic options for solid malignancies (90). Generally, DNA methyltransferases lack genome location specificity, but locus-specific genome editing technologies are an active area of research (65,91,92), suggesting that epigenome editing could be a future therapeutic avenue in IPF.

HOW GENOMIC INVESTIGATIONS PLAY A KEY ROLE IN OUR CLINICAL UNDERSTANDING OF AND ABILITY TO TREAT ILD

PHENOTYPE AND GENETIC VARIANTS

Not only have specific genetic variants been linked to disease risk, but they have now been linked to distinct disease phenotypes.

Retrospective analysis of survival after lung transplantation suggests that the carriers of telomerase mutations have greater incidence of post-transplant complications than do historical controls, with the difference driven by haematological complications signalling the systemic nature of their telomere-related abnormalities (93). Current practice does not include telomerase sequencing as part of an individual's consideration for lung transplantation, but these preliminary findings suggest need for further study.

In terms of the common *MUC5B* promoter polymorphism, retrospective analysis of large clinical trials data has illustrated that IPF subjects with the risk variant (T allele) had improved survival when compared to wild-type subjects (GG genotype) in the same cohorts, independent of age, sex, lung function and treatment status (45). Including the rs35705950 genotype in modelling outcomes improved predictive accuracy of the model (45). Similarly, the disease-associated *TOLLIP* variant described by Noth and colleagues was also found to be associated with differential survival; however, in the case of rs5743890, although the minor allele (G) was associated with decreased disease severity within diseased subjects, minor-allele carriers with disease had increased mortality risk (13).

Interestingly, a retrospective analysis of the PANTHER-IPF clinical trial data showed that when *TOLLIP* (rs5743890/rs5743894/rs5743854/rs3750920) and *MUC5B* (rs35705950) variants were examined, of those who received N-acetylcysteine (NAC), individuals with TT genotype for rs3750920 (*TOLLIP*) had decreased risk of the trial's composite endpoint (death, transplantation, hospitalization or greater than 10% decrease in FVC) (52), while the CC genotype at rs3750920 was associated

with an increased risk of the composite endpoint. These findings suggest that though NAC has not been shown to be efficacious in treating IPF in general (94), it is possible that a subset of patients defined by their rs3750920 (*TOLLIP*) genotype could benefit from the drug (52).

Though these initial retrospective studies suggest strongly that genetic variants could be useful in prognosticating for patients, the relationships between genotypes and survival are likely to be complex and need to be validated in rigorous prospective trials. Such future studies will be necessary to understand the extent of potential phenotypic differences between IPF patients who have different disease-associated genetic variants. At this time, though the studies described point to genotype–phenotype relationships, the appropriate clinical use of these results remains unknown, and the cumulative effects of specific variants are also yet to be understood fully.

BENCH TO BEDSIDE: GENOTYPING IN THE CLINIC?

Though we have presented examples of associations between genotype and disease prognosis, genotyping of individuals with IPF is not part of routine clinical care at this time. For one, prospective studies in this area are lacking. Furthermore, no definitive evidence exists to date to suggest that genotype should be used to determine selection of approved IPF therapies (pirfenidone [3], nintedanib [4] or lung transplantation [95]) for an individual patient. Currently, therapeutic decision making should be based on published, well-described risks and benefits, all of which have been studied independently of genotype (3,4).

However, future clinical studies will need to take into account phenotypic variation between specific genotypes, since they appear to affect primary outcomes (such as mortality and response to treatment) frequently utilized in clinical trials (52,96). Failure to control for genotype (e.g. *MUC5B* promoter polymorphism) would be similar to failing to control for other factors such as age, sex and baseline lung function, all of which are known to influence clinical outcomes (50). In addition, further understanding of genotype–phenotype relationships and gene–gene interactions are likely to shape how knowledge of genetic variants is to be used in the clinical practice of treating and counselling patients with ILD.

HOW SCREENING FOR INHERITED ILD WILL LIKELY EVOLVE AND BE INCORPORATED INTO CLINICAL PRACTICE

IPF has a poor prognosis and unpredictable clinical course, and there are no approved medications for the disease that are proven to alter mortality – but existing treatments slow disease progression (3,4). Therefore, earlier diagnosis of the disease is critical – yet given the relatively low prevalence of IPF, it is not a disease for which clinicians routinely screen their patients. The growing evidence for genomic methods of assessing disease risk may prompt the pulmonary community to consider targeted mechanisms for high-yield screening.

As was the case in the early studies regarding genetic risk and IPF, our initial insights on this come from the world of FIP. It is well known that first-degree relatives of patients with pulmonary fibrosis are at elevated risk of developing lung abnormalities, but the clinical significance of these radiographic and pathologic abnormalities was unclear (21). In the 1980s, studying relatives of autosomal dominant FIP led to the discovery that those without clinically apparent disease had bronchoalveolar lavage (BAL) fluid with excess inflammatory cells. Twenty-seven years later, repeat evaluation of these study subjects revealed interim development of radiographic evidence of ILD, as well as measurable pulmonary function impairment (97). This initial study was small in sample size but illustrated that subtle pulmonary abnormalities and alveolar inflammation in FIP relatives could progress to overt pulmonary fibrosis – and, importantly, that this disease may have an extended lead-time, during which individuals could be screened and diagnosed prior to loss of significant functional lung parenchyma (21,97).

More recent extensive phenotyping of FIP relatives has revealed evidence of dysfunction in numerous pathways associated with pulmonary fibrosis, such as reduced telomere length, endoplasmic reticulum stress and elevated MUC5B levels in the BAL (98). These findings were observed in relatives with and without pathologic evidence of pulmonary fibrosis, suggesting again that molecular signatures can help identify those at risk for progression to clinically evident disease. A third of these FIP relatives, an 'at-risk' cohort, had pathologic evidence of histologically abnormal lung tissue, and 14.7% had radiographic evidence of early interstitial lung disease (98). Additional studies will be required to determine the clinical significance of these findings in FIP relatives and of the asymptomatic interstitial lung abnormalities noted in the Framingham Heart Study, described above (42).

Developing a means of targeted screening for at-risk individuals incorporating genomic discoveries and testing its efficacy in preventing IPF morbidity and mortality will be a focus of future research; however, given the elevated risk of IPF in FIP family members, avoidance of disease-associated exposures (such as tobacco smoke) and vigilance for the development of respiratory symptoms are warranted (50).

CONCLUSIONS

Genetic and genomic discoveries in the field of IPF have led investigators to new hypotheses regarding disease pathogenesis and potential therapeutic targets; however, numerous questions persist. The mechanisms through which gene expression changes, epigenetic marks and genetic variants interact in the pathogenesis of fibrosing ILD remain poorly understood. The consideration of genetic risk factors for IPF will undoubtedly lead to improved disease phenotyping and more targeted clinical care. Most importantly, such knowledge could facilitate a shift from a palliative to a preventative focus in the clinical care of patients with this progressive and incurable disease.

REFERENCES

1. Raghu G, Collard HR, Egan JJ, Martinez FJ, Behr J, Brown KK et al. An Official ATS/ERS/JRS/ALAT Statement: Idiopathic pulmonary fibrosis: Evidence-based guidelines for diagnosis and management. *Am J Respir Crit Care Med.* 2011;183(6):788–824.

2. Olson AL, Swigris JJ, Lezotte DC, Norris JM, Wilson CG, Brown KK. Mortality from pulmonary fibrosis increased in the United States from 1992 to 2003. *Am J Respir Crit Care Med.* 2007;176(3):277–84.

3. King TE, Bradford WZ, Castro-Bernardini S, Fagan EA, Glaspole I, Glassberg MK et al. A phase 3 trial of pirfenidone in patients with idiopathic pulmonary fibrosis. *N Engl J Med.* 2014;370(22):2083–92.

4. Richeldi L, du Bois RM, Raghu G, Azuma A, Brown KK, Costabel U et al. Efficacy and safety of nintedanib in idiopathic pulmonary fibrosis. *N Engl J Med.* 2014;370(22):2071–82.

5. Raghu G, Anstrom KJ, King TE, Lasky JA, Martinez FJ. Prednisone, azathioprine, and N-acetylcysteine for pulmonary fibrosis. *N Engl J Med.* 2012;366(21):1968–77.

6. The Idiopathic Pulmonary Fibrosis Network. Randomized trial of acetylcysteine in idiopathic pulmonary fibrosis. *N Engl J Med.* 2014;370(22):2093–2101.

7. King TE, Pardo A, Selman M. Idiopathic pulmonary fibrosis. *Lancet.* 2011;378(9807):1949–61.

8. Armanios MY, Chen JJ-L, Cogan JD, Alder JK, Ingersoll RG, Markin C et al. Telomerase mutations in families with idiopathic pulmonary fibrosis. *N Engl J Med.* 2007;356(13):1317–26.

9. Stuart BD, Choi J, Zaidi S, Xing C, Holohan B, Chen R et al. Exome sequencing links mutations in PARN and RTEL1 with familial pulmonary fibrosis and telomere shortening. *Nat Genet.* 2015;47(5):512–17.

10. Cogan JD, Kropski JA, Zhao M, Mitchell DB, Rives L, Markin C et al. Rare variants in RTEL1 are associated with familial interstitial pneumonia. *Am J Respir Crit Care Med.* 2015;191(6):646–55.

11. Seibold MA, Wise A, Speer M, Steele M, Brown K, Lloyd JE et al. A common MUC5B promoter polymorphism and pulmonary fibrosis. *N Engl J Med.* 2011;364(16):1503–12.

12. Fingerlin TE, Murphy E, Zhang W, Peljto AL, Brown KK, Steele MP et al. Genome-wide association study identifies multiple susceptibility loci for pulmonary fibrosis. *Nat* ⁿt. 2013;45(6):613–20.

13. Noth I, Zhang Y, Ma S-F, Flores C, Barber M, Huang Y et al. Genetic variants associated with idiopathic pulmonary fibrosis susceptibility and mortality: A genome-wide association study. *Lancet Respir Med.* 2013;1(4):309–17.

14. Selman M, Pardo A, Barrera L, Estrada A, Watson SR, Wilson K et al. Gene expression profiles distinguish idiopathic pulmonary fibrosis from hypersensitivity pneumonitis. *Am J Respir Crit Care Med.* 2006;173(2):188–98.

15. Yang IV, Burch LH, Steele MP, Savov JD, Hollingsworth JW, McElvania-Tekippe E et al. Gene expression profiling of familial and sporadic interstitial pneumonia. *Am J Respir Crit Care Med.* 2007;175(1):45–54.

16. Yang IV, Coldren CD, Leach SM, Seibold Ma, Murphy E, Lin J et al. Expression of cilium-associated genes defines novel molecular subtypes of idiopathic pulmonary fibrosis. *Thorax.* 2013;68(12):1114–21.

17. Meltzer EB, Barry WT, Yang IV, Brown KK, Schwarz MI, Patel H et al. Familial and sporadic idiopathic pulmonary fibrosis: Making the diagnosis from peripheral blood. *BMC Genomics.* 2014;15(1):902.

18. Yang IV, Pedersen BS, Rabinovich E, Hennessy CE, Davidson EJ, Murphy E et al. Relationship of DNA methylation and gene expression in idiopathic pulmonary fibrosis. *Am J Respir Crit Care Med.* 2014;190:1263–72.

19. Javaheri S, Lederer DH, Pella JA, Mark GJ, Levine BW. Idiopathic pulmonary fibrosis in monozygotic twins: The importance of genetic predisposition. *Chest.* 1980;78(4):591–4.

20. Solliday N, Williams J, Gaensler E, Coutu R, Carringon C. Familial chronic interstitial pneumonia. *Am Rev Respir Dis.* 1973;108(2):193–204.

21. Bitterman PB, Rennard SI, Keogh BA, Wewers MD, Adelberg S, Crystal RG. Familial idiopathic pulmonary fibrosis. Evidence of lung inflammation in unaffected family members. *N Engl J Med.* 1986;314(21):1343–7.

22. García-Sancho C, Buendía-Roldán I, Fernández-Plata MR, Navarro C, Pérez-Padilla R, Vargas MH et al. Familial

pulmonary fibrosis is the strongest risk factor for idiopathic pulmonary fibrosis. *Respir Med.* 2011;105(12):1902–7.

23. Nogee LM, Dunbar AE, Wert SE, Askin F, Hamvas A, Whitsett JA. A mutation in the surfactant protein C gene associated with familial interstitial lung disease. *N Engl J Med.* 2001;344(8):573–9.

24. Lawson WE, Grant SW, Ambrosini V, Womble KE, Dawson EP, Lane KB et al. Genetic mutations in surfactant protein C are a rare cause of sporadic cases of IPF. *Thorax.* 2004;59(11):977–80.

25. Fernandez BA, Fox G, Bhatia R, Sala E, Noble B, Denic N et al. A Newfoundland cohort of familial and sporadic idiopathic pulmonary fibrosis patients: Clinical and genetic features. *Respir Res.* 2012;13(1):64.

26. Maitra M, Wang Y, Gerard RD, Mendelson CR, Garcia CK. Surfactant protein A2 mutations associated with pulmonary fibrosis lead to protein instability and endoplasmic reticulum stress. *J Biol Chem.* 2010;285(29):22103–13.

27. Wang Y, Kuan PJ, Xing C, Cronkhite JT, Torres F, Rosenblatt RL et al. Genetic defects in surfactant protein A2 are associated with pulmonary fibrosis and lung cancer. *Am J Hum Genet.* 2009;84(1):52–9.

28. Wei ML. Hermansky-Pudlak syndrome: A disease of protein trafficking and organelle function. *Pigment Cell Res.* 2006;19(1):19–42.

29. Gochuico BR, Huizing M, Golas Ga, Scher CD, Tsokos M, Denver SD et al. Interstitial lung disease and pulmonary fibrosis in Hermansky-Pudlak syndrome type 2, an adaptor protein-3 complex disease. *Mol Med.* 2012;18:56–64.

30. Vulliamy TJ, Marrone A, Knight SW, Walne A, Mason PJ, Dokal I. Mutations in dyskeratosis congenita: Their impact on telomere length and the diversity of clinical presentation. *Blood.* 2006;107(7):2680–5.

31. Armanios M, Chen J-L, Chang Y-PC, Brodsky Ra, Hawkins A, Griffin Ca et al. Haploinsufficiency of telomerase reverse transcriptase leads to anticipation in autosomal dominant dyskeratosis congenita. *Proc Natl Acad Sci U S A.* 2005;102(44):15960–4.

32. Tsakiri KD, Cronkhite JT, Kuan PJ, Xing C, Raghu G, Weissler JC et al. Adult-onset pulmonary fibrosis caused by mutations in telomerase. *Proc Natl Acad Sci U S A.* 2007;104(18):7552–7.

33. Stuart BD, Lee JS, Kozlitina J, Noth I, Devine MS, Glazer CS et al. Effect of telomere length on survival in patients with idiopathic pulmonary fibrosis: An observational cohort study with independent validation. *Lancet Respir Med.* 2014;2(7):557–65.

34. Alder JK, Barkauskas CE, Limjunyawong N, Stanley SE, Kembou F, Tuder RM et al. Telomere dysfunction causes alveolar stem cell failure. *Proc Natl Acad Sci.* 2015;112(16):5099–5104.

35. Roy MG, Livraghi-Butrico A, Fletcher AA, McElwee MM, Evans SE, Boerner RM et al. Muc5b is required for airway defence. *Nature.* 2014;505(7483):412–6.

36. Seibold MA, Smith RW, Urbanek C, Groshong SD, Cosgrove GP, Brown KK et al. The idiopathic pulmonary fibrosis honeycomb cyst contains a mucocilary pseudostratified epithelium. *PLoS One.* 2013;8(3):e58658.

37. Zhang Y, Noth I, Garcia JGN, Kaminski N. A variant in the promoter of MUC5B and idiopathic pulmonary fibrosis NT5E mutations and arterial calcifications. *N Engl J Med.* 2011;364(16):1576–7.

38. Stock CJ, Sato H, Fonseca C, Banya WaS, Molyneaux PL, Adamali H et al. Mucin 5B promoter polymorphism is associated with idiopathic pulmonary fibrosis but not with development of lung fibrosis in systemic sclerosis or sarcoidosis. *Thorax.* 2013;68(5):436–41.

39. Borie R, Crestani B, Dieude P, Nunes H, Allanore Y, Kannengiesser C et al. The MUC5B variant is associated with idiopathic pulmonary fibrosis but not with systemic sclerosis interstitial lung disease in the European Caucasian population. *PLoS One.* 2013;8(8):e70621.

40. Wei R, Li C, Zhang M, Jones-Hall YL, Myers JL, Noth I et al. Association between MUC5B and TERT polymorphisms and different interstitial lung disease phenotypes. *Transl Res.* 2014;163(5):494–502.

41. Horimasu Y, Ohshimo S, Bonella F, Tanaka S, Ishikawa N, Hattori N et al. MUC5B promoter polymorphism in Japanese patients with idiopathic pulmonary fibrosis. *Respirology*. 2015;20(3):439–44.

42. Hunninghake GM, Hatabu H, Okajima Y, Gao W, Dupuis J, Latourelle JC et al. MUC5B promoter polymorphism and interstitial lung abnormalities. *N Engl J Med*. 2013;368(23):2192–2200.

43. Mathai SK, Schwartz DA, Warg LA. Genetic susceptibility and pulmonary fibrosis. *Curr Opin Pulm Med*. 2014;20(5):429–35.

44. Yang IV, Schwartz DA. Epigenetics of idiopathic pulmonary fibrosis. *Transl Res*. 2015;165(1):48–60.

45. Peljto AL, Selman M, Kim DS, Murphy E, Tucker L, Pardo A et al. The MUC5B promoter polymorphism is associated with idiopathic pulmonary fibrosis in a Mexican cohort but is rare among Asian ancestries. *Chest*. 2015;147(2):460–4.

46. Wang C, Zhuang Y, Guo W, Cao L, Zhang H, Xu L et al. Mucin 5B promoter polymorphism is associated with susceptibility to interstitial lung diseases in Chinese males. *PLoS One*. 2014;9(8):e104919.

47. Ley B, Collard HR. Epidemiology of idiopathic pulmonary fibrosis. *Clin Epidemiol*. 2013;5:483–92.

48. Putman RK, Hatabu H, Araki T, Gudmundsson G, Gao W, Nishino M et al. Association between interstitial lung abnormalities and all-cause mortality. *JAMA*. 2016;315(7):672.

49. Raghu G, Weycker D, Edelsberg J, Bradford WZ, Oster G. Incidence and prevalence of idiopathic pulmonary fibrosis. *Am J Respir Crit Care Med*. 2006;174(7):810–6.

50. Mathai SK, Yang IV, Schwarz MI, Schwartz DA. Incorporating genetics into the identification and treatment of idiopathic pulmonary fibrosis. *BMC Med*. 2015;13(1):191.

51. Yang IV, Fingerlin TE, Evans CM, Schwarz MI, Schwartz DA. MUC5B and idiopathic pulmonary fibrosis. *Ann Am Thorac Soc*. 2015;12 (Suppl 2):S193–9.

52. Oldham JM, Ma SF, Martinez FJ, Anstrom KJ, Raghu G, Schwartz DA et al. ͡P MUC5B, and the response to

53. Armanios M, Blackburn EH. The telomere syndromes. *Nat Rev Genet*. 2012;13(10):693–704.

54. Zuo F, Kaminski N, Eugui E, Allard J, Yakhini Z, Ben-Dor A et al. Gene expression analysis reveals matrilysin as a key regulator of pulmonary fibrosis in mice and humans. *Proc Natl Acad Sci U S A*. 2002;99(9):6292–7.

55. Konishi K, Gibson KF, Lindell KO, Richards TJ, Zhang Y, Dhir R et al. Gene expression profiles of acute exacerbations of idiopathic pulmonary fibrosis. *Am J Respir Crit Care Med*. 2009;180(2):167–75.

56. Herazo-Maya JD, Noth I, Duncan SR, Kim S, Ma S-F, Tseng GC et al. Peripheral blood mononuclear cell gene expression profiles predict poor outcome in idiopathic pulmonary fibrosis. *Sci Transl Med*. 2013;5(205):205ra136.

57. Huang Y, Ma S-F, Vij R, Oldham JM, Herazo-Maya J, Broderick SM et al. A functional genomic model for predicting prognosis in idiopathic pulmonary fibrosis. *BMC Pulm Med*. 2015;15(1):147.

58. Cabrera S, Gaxiola M, Arreola JL, Ramírez R, Jara P, D'Armiento J et al. Overexpression of MMP9 in macrophages attenuates pulmonary fibrosis induced by bleomycin. *Int J Biochem Cell Biol*. 2007;39(12):2324–38.

59. Jirtle RL, Skinner MK. Environmental epigenomics and disease susceptibility. *Nat Rev Genet*. 2007;8(April):253–62.

60. Wan ES, Qiu W, Baccarelli A, Carey VJ, Bacherman H, Rennard SI et al. Cigarette smoking behaviors and time since quitting are associated with differential DNA methylation across the human genome. *Hum Mol Genet*. 2012;21(13):3073–82.

61. Bell JT, Pai AA, Pickrell JK, Gaffney DJ, Pique-Regi R, Degner JF et al. DNA methylation patterns associate with genetic and gene expression variation in HapMap cell lines. *Genome Biol*. 2011;12(1):R10.

62. Zhang D, Cheng L, Badner JA, Chen C, Chen Q, Luo W et al. Genetic control of individual differences in gene-specific methylation in human brain. *Am J Hum Genet*. 2010;86(3):411–9.

63. Buro-Auriemma LJ, Salit J, Hackett NR, Walters MS, Strulovici-Barel Y, Staudt MR et al. Cigarette smoking induces small airway epithelial epigenetic changes with corresponding modulation of gene expression. *Hum Mol Genet.* 2013;22(23):4726–38.

64. Liu F, Killian JK, Yang M, Walker RL, Hong Ja, Zhang M et al. Epigenomic alterations and gene expression profiles in respiratory epithelia exposed to cigarette smoke condensate. *Oncogene.* 2010;29(25):3650–64.

65. Helling BA, Yang IV. Epigenetics in lung fibrosis. *Curr Opin Pulm Med.* 2015;21(5):454–62.

66. Fraga MF, Ballestar E, Paz MF, Ropero S, Setien F, Ballestar ML et al. Epigenetic differences arise during the lifetime of monozygotic twins. *Proc Natl Acad Sci U S A.* 2005;102(30):10604–9.

67. Heyn H, Li N, Ferreira HHJ, Moran S, Pisano DG, Gomez A et al. Distinct DNA methylomes of newborns and centenarians. *Proc Natl Acad Sci U S A.* 2012;109(26):10522–7.

68. Ong ML, Holbrook JD. Novel region discovery method for Infinium 450 K DNA methylation data reveals changes associated with aging in muscle and neuronal pathways. *Aging Cell.* 2014;13(1):142–155.

69. Issa J. Aging and epigeneric drift: A vicious cycle. *J Clin Invest.* 2014;124(1):24–9.

70. Selman M, Pardo A. Stochastic age-related epigenetic drift in the pathogenesis of idiopathic pulmonary fibrosis. *Am J Respir Crit Care Med.* 2014;190(12):1328–30.

71. Taskar VS, Coultas DB. Is idiopathic pulmonary fibrosis an environmental disease? *Proc Am Thorac Soc.* 2006;3(4):293–8.

72. Coward WR, Watts K, Feghali-Bostwick Ca, Knox A, Pang L. Defective histone acetylation is responsible for the diminished expression of cyclooxygenase 2 in idiopathic pulmonary fibrosis. *Mol Cell Biol.* 2009;29(15):4325–39.

73. Coward WR, Feghali-Bostwick CA, Jenkins G, Knox AJ, Pang L. A central role for G9a and EZH2 in the epigenetic silencing of cyclooxygenase-2 in idiopathic pulmonary fibrosis. *FASEB J.* 2014;28(7):3183–96.

74. Sanders YY, Hagood JS, Liu H, Zhang W, Ambalavanan N, Thannickal VJ. Histone deacetylase inhibition promotes fibroblast apoptosis and ameliorates pulmonary fibrosis in mice. *Eur Respir J.* 2014;43(5):1448–58.

75. Coward WR, Watts K, Feghali-bostwick CA, Jenkins G, Pang L. Repression of IP-10 by interactions between histone deacetylation and hypermethylation in idiopathic pulmonary fibrosis. *Mol Cell Biol.* 2010;30(12):2874–86.

76. Sanders YY, Pardo A, Selman M, Nuovo GJ, Tollefsbol TO, Siegal GP et al. Thy-1 promoter hypermethylation: A novel epigenetic pathogenic mechanism in pulmonary fibrosis. *Am J Respir Cell Mol Biol.* 2008;39(5):610–8.

77. Sanders YY, Tollefsbol TO, Varisco BM, Hagood JS. Epigenetic regulation of Thy-1 by histone deacetylase inhibitor in rat lung fibroblasts. *Am J Respir Cell Mol Biol.* 2011;45(1):16–23.

78. Cisneros J, Hagood J, Checa M, Ortiz-Quintero B, Negreros M, Herrera I et al. Hypermethylation-mediated silencing of p14ARF in fibroblasts from idiopathic pulmonary fibrosis. *AJP Lung Cell Mol Physiol.* 2012;303(4):L295–303.

79. Hu B, Gharaee-kermani M. Epigenetic regulation of myofibroblast differentiation by DNA methylation. *Am J Pathol.* 2010;177(1):21–8.

80. Hu B, Gharaee-Kermani M, Wu Z. Essential role of MeCP2 in the regulation of myofibroblast differentiation during pulmonary fibrosis. *Am J Pathol.* 2011;178(4):1500–8.

81. Dakhlallah D, Batte K, Wang Y, Cantemir-Stone CZ, Yan P, Nuovo G et al. Epigenetic regulation of mir-17~92 contributes to the pathogenesis of pulmonary fibrosis. *Am J Respir Crit Care Med.* 2013;187(4):397–405.

82. Huang SK, Scruggs AM, Donaghy J, Horowitz JC, Zaslona Z, Przybranowski S et al. Histone modifications are responsible for decreased Fas expression and apoptosis resistance in fibrotic lung fibroblasts. *Cell Death Dis.* 2013;2(4):e621–8.

83. Sanders YY, Liu H, Liu G, Thannickal VJ. Free radical biology and medicine epigenetic mechanisms regulate NADPH oxidase-4 expression in cellular senescence. *Free Radic Biol Med.* 2015;79:197–205.

84. Hogaboam CM, Murray L, Martinez FJ. Epigenetic mechanisms through which toll-like receptor – 9 drives idiopathic pulmonary fibrosis progression. *Proc Am Thorac Soc.* 2012;9(3):172–6.

85. Sanders YY, Ambalavanan N, Halloran B, Zhang X, Liu H. Altered DNA methylation profile in idiopathic pulmonary fibrosis. *Am J Respir Crit Care Med.* 2012;186(6):525–35.

86. Rabinovich EI, Kapetanaki MG, Steinfeld I, Gibson KF, Pandit KV, Yu G et al. Global methylation patterns in idiopathic pulmonary fibrosis. *PLoS One.* 2012;7(4):e33770.

87. Huang SK, Scruggs AM, Mceachin RC, White ES, Peters-golden M. Lung fibroblasts from patients with idiopathic pulmonary fibrosis exhibit genome-wide differences in DNA methylation compared to fibroblasts from nonfibrotic lung. *PLoS One.* 2014;9(9):e107055.

88. Irizarry RA, Ladd-acosta C, Wen B, Wu Z, Montano C, Onyango P et al. The human colon cancer methylome shows similar hypo- and hypermethylation at conserved tissue-specific CpG island shores. *Nat Genet.* 2009;41(2):178–86.

89. Kaminskas E, Farrell A, Abraham S, Baird A, Hsieh L, Lee S et al. Report from the FDA approval summary: Azacitidine for treatment of myelodysplastic syndrome subtypes. *Clin Cancer Res.* 2005;11(8):3604–9.

90. Juergens RA, Wrangle J, Vendetti FP, Murphy SC, Zhao M, Coleman B et al. Combination epigenetic therapy has efficacy in patients with refractory advanced non–small cell lung cancer. *Cancer Discov.* 2011;1(7):598–607.

91. Di Ruscio A, Embralidze A, Benoukraf T, Amabile G, Goff L, Terragni J et al. DNMT1-interacting RNAs block gene-specific DNA methylation. *Nature.* 2013;503(7476):371–6.

92. Heller EA, Cates HM, Peña CJ, Herman JP, Walsh JJ. Locus-specific epigenetic remodeling controls addiction- and depression-related behaviors. *Nat Neurosci.* 2014;17(12):1720–7.

93. Silhan LL, Shah PD, Chambers DC, Snyder LD, Riise GC, Wagner CL et al. Lung transplantation in telomerase mutation carriers with pulmonary fibrosis. *Eur Respir J.* 2014;44(1):178–87.

94. The Idiopathic Pulmonary Fibrosis Network. Randomized trial of acetylcysteine in idiopathic pulmonary fibrosis. *N Engl J Med.* 2014;370:2093–2101.

    ⁻haffer JM, Singh SK, Reitz Ba, Zamanian
    ʰdi HR. Single- vs double-lung

    transplantation in patients with chronic obstructive pulmonary disease and idiopathic pulmonary fibrosis since the implementation of lung allocation based on medical need. *JAMA.* 2015;313(9):936.

96. Peljto AL, Zhang Y, Fingerlin TE, Ma S-F, Garcia JGN, Richards TJ et al. Association between the MUC5B promoter polymorphism and survival in patients with idiopathic pulmonary fibrosis. *JAMA.* 2013;309(21):2232–9.

97. El-Chemaly S, Ziegler SG, Calado RT, Wilson Ka, Wu HP, Haughey M et al. Natural history of pulmonary fibrosis in two subjects with the same telomerase mutation. *Chest.* 2011;139(5):1203–9.

98. Kropski JA, Pritchett JM, Zoz DF, Crossno PF, Markin C, Garnett ET et al. Extensive phenotyping of individuals at risk for familial interstitial pneumonia reveals clues to the pathogenesis of interstitial lung disease. *Am J Respir Crit Care Med.* 2015;191(4):417–26.

99. Thomas AQ, Lane K, Phillips J, Prince M, Markin C, Speer M et al. Heterozygosity for a surfactant protein C gene mutation associated with usual interstitial pneumonitis and cellular nonspecific interstitial pneumonitis in one kindred. *Am J Respir Crit Care Med.* 2002;165:1322–1328.

100. Van Moorsel CHM, Van Oosterhout MFM, Barlo NP, De Jong P a., Van Der Vis JJ, Ruven HJT, Van Es HW, Van Den Bosch JMM, Grutters JC. Surfactant protein C mutations are the basis of a significant portion of adult familial pulmonary fibrosis in a dutch cohort. *Am J Respir Crit Care Med.* 2010;182:1419–1425.

101. Ono S, Tanaka T, Ishida M, Kinoshita a, Fukuoka J, Takaki M et al. Surfactant protein C G100S mutation causes familial pulmonary fibrosis in Japanese kindred. *Eur Respir J* 2011;38:861–869.

102. de Leon AD, Cronkhite JT, Katzenstein AL a, Godwin JD, Raghu G, Glazer CS et al. Telomere lengths, pulmonary fibrosis and telomerase (TERT) Mutations. *PLoS One* 2010;5:e10680.

103. Kropski JA, Mitchell DB, Markin C, Polosukhin VV, Choi L, Johnson JE et al. A novel dyskerin (DKC1) mutation is associated with familial interstitial pneumonia. *Chest* 2014;146:e1–7.

5

Clinical evaluation of the patient with suspected ILD

KAÏSSA DE BOER AND JOYCE S LEE

INTRODUCTION

Interstitial lung disease (ILD) comprises a heterogeneous group of lung diseases of over 150 aetiologies. Challenges in generating a diagnosis arise due to the overlapping clinical, radiological and pathological features, which many forms of ILD share. Thus, the clinical history, including drug history, organic and inorganic substance exposure history and other potential disease manifestations, is vital to attaining a diagnosis and requires careful data gathering to delineate the underlying aetiology.

While certain subtypes of ILD, such as lymphoid interstitial pneumonia, are considered to be rare, the question of whether a patient may have an ILD is not an infrequently encountered scenario in clinical practice. Based on Danish national registry data from 1995 to 2005, using

International Classification of Diseases, Tenth Revision (ICD-10) codes to identify a new diagnosis of ILD, the incidence rate for ILD was 32.57 per 100,000 person-years (95% CI, 31.94–32.30) (1). Further, the incidence of ILDs seems to be increasing over time (1–3).

Regarding idiopathic pulmonary fibrosis (IPF), one of the more common forms of ILD, a recent study using an Italian healthcare database from 2005 to 2010 reported the prevalence of IPF to be 12.6–35.5 adjusted per 100,000 person-years, depending on the case definition used (4). In the United States, recent Medicare data on patients with IPF estimated the annual incidence of IPF to be 93.7 cases per 100,000 person-years (95% CI 91.9–95.4) between 2001 and 2011, with an annual cumulative prevalence that increased over that time period to 494.5 cases per 100,000 people in 2011 (3). These epidemiologic trends may, in part, be a reflection of increased awareness of ILD in the setting of newly available novel anti-fibrotic therapies (5–7) or increased detection through the use of low-dose computed tomography scanning for lung cancer screening (8,9). However, these registry data studies do support the fact that ILD is not uncommonly encountered in clinical practice and remains an important consideration when evaluating a patient with chronic cough or progressive dyspnoea.

Further, failure to consider a diagnosis of ILD may result in delays in diagnosis, treatment and/or access to novel therapies as part of clinical research trials. In a patient questionnaire designed to better understand patient experiences relating to diagnosis and management, 54.6% reported a minimum of a 1-year delay in diagnosis, with more than a third of patients seeing three or more physicians before a diagnosis was established (10). As the landscape for treatment options for ILDs expands, and with improved outcomes in lung transplantation (11,12), it behooves the practicing clinician to consider ILD in the differential diagnosis, striving for earlier diagnosis in these patients. Finally, the diagnosis of ILD is not made in isolation, but rather through consensus after multidisciplinary discussion (MDD) with clinicians, radiologists and pathologists who have expertise in the field of ILD (13–15).

COMPREHENSIVE BASELINE ASSESSMENT FOR INITIAL EVALUATION OF PATIENTS WITH SUSPECTED ILD

The initial assessment of a patient with suspected ILD aims to address several key issues:

1. Confirm the presence of ILD and the specific type of ILD.
2. Determine the disease severity and the tempo of disease progression.
3. Assess the patient's quality of life and baseline functioning.
4. Provide patient education on their underlying disease.
5. Determine if pharmacologic treatment should be initiated.

6. Consider lung transplant referral and/or clinical trial enrollment where appropriate.
7. Assess for the presence of associated comorbidities and consider treatment.
8. Review the non-pharmacologic management of ILD for all patients, including the need for long-term oxygen, vaccinations, weight management, regular exercise, and enrollment in a formal pulmonary rehabilitation programme.

The initial evaluation of a patient with suspected ILD requires an integrated approach. The first clinic visit necessitates a thorough history and physical examination, not only to discern the underlying aetiology of their disease, but also to address many of the issues listed above. Figure 5.1 provides a template for approaching the undifferentiated patient with suspected ILD. While this list is difficult to complete in a single appointment, it stresses the need for these patients to have close serial longitudinal follow-up with their pulmonologist and ILD care team to provide ongoing, comprehensive care.

HISTORY

The history portion of the initial evaluation of a patient with suspected ILD aims to determine the aetiology of the ILD or, in cases where no clear aetiology is established, exclude any potential alternative aetiologies prior to confirming a diagnosis of an idiopathic interstitial pneumonia (IIP).

ILD-SPECIFIC SYMPTOMS

Patients with ILD often experience progressive breathlessness and a chronic non-productive cough. Limitation in exercise tolerance or when travelling to altitude may provide earlier clues of an underlying ILD. Quantifying the level of dyspnoea using tools such as the medical council dyspnoea scale (MRC) can assist clinicians in following a patient's disease progression over time, approximates disease severity (16) and conveys insight on prognosis (17). Further, in patients with IPF, the level of dyspnoea has been independently associated with a greater number of comorbidities, including depression (18).

Wheeze is an uncommon clinical manifestation in ILD, suggesting small airways involvement, as

Demographics

Age at diagnosis:

Sex: M | F   Ethnicity:

Social History

Smoker: Current | Former | Never   Pack years:

Occupation:

Clinical History

Clinical presentation:

Quantify degree of impairment:

Symptoms of connective tissue disease†: Y | N   Comments

Past Medical History

List relevant:

Exposures*

Asbestos: Y | N Comment:
HP exposure: Y | N Comment:
Occupation: Y | N Comment:
Hobbies: Y | N Comment:
Other:

Family History

ILD: Y | N Comment:
CTD: Y | N Comment:

Medications‡

Amiodarone: Y | N Comment:
Nitrofurantoin: Y | N Comment:
Chemotherapy: Y | N Comment:
Radiation: Y | N Comment:
Other:

Physical Exam

Resting Oxygen saturation:
Crackles: Y | N
Clubbing: Y | N
Signs of pulmonary hypertension: Y | N
Signs of connective tissue disease: Y | N Comment:

Pulmonary Function Testing:

Date	FVC L (% predicted)	FEV_1 L (% predicted)	FEV_1/FVC	TLC L (% predicted)	DLCO (% predicted)

6MWT:

Imaging

HRCT: Y | N Results:

Biopsy

Biopsy performed: Y | N Specify type of biopy and location(s):
Results:

Bronchoscopy

Performed: Y | N
Results:

Serologies

ANA by IFA:
RF:
CCP:
Other serologies:

* If signicant exposure present, describe timing, extent and nature of exposure.

† Standard questioning for connective tissue disease symptoms may include: dry eyes, dry mouth, myalgia, arthralgia, morning stiness, Raynaud's phenomena, rash, skin changes, dysphagia, paresthesia and weakness. Additional questioning at discretion of treating physician.

‡ Comment if medication has temporal association with clinical presentation, include details on dosing, duration of use of medication when appropriate.

Figure 5.1 ILD history template. Initial consultation with a patient with suspected interstitial lung disease (ILD) requires a detailed history to explore possible aetiologies of his or her lung disease.

seen in respiratory-bronchiolitis-associated ILD (RB-ILD) or bronchiolitis obliterans. Patients frequently report their disease being mislabelled as 'asthma', 'emphysema', 'chronic obstructive pulmonary disease' or 'bronchitis' before ultimately being diagnosed with ILD (10). As symptoms progress, patients often experience constitutional symptoms such as fatigue and weight loss.

While most ILDs have primarily respiratory-related symptoms, those with an underlying connective tissue disease (CTD) can have several extra-pulmonary manifestations of disease (see section below). In addition, patients with hypersensitivity pneumonitis (HP) can also present with symptoms of fevers, chills and a flu-like illness, which are seen more commonly with the acute form of HP.

MEDICATION HISTORY

A detailed medication history is helpful to identify potential culprit medications. Key factors include the duration of time the patient used the medication, temporal relationship with clinical symptoms and dosages. In addition, herbal supplements, over-the-counter medications and substances of abuse must also be considered as potential causes of a patient's underlying ILD. While numerous medications have been associated with ILD, more commonly encountered medications associated with ILD include nitrofurantoin, amiodarone, statins, methotrexate and chemotherapy agents such as bleomycin, paclitaxel and chlorambucil. The website http://www.pneumotox.com provides a useful and easily accessible reference tool for reviewing medications and their link to ILD. This resource is frequently updated and includes 23,150 references in their database as of May 18, 2015 (19).

Additional consideration must be given to radiation history. Radiation pneumonitis may present subacutely in the following 4–12 weeks post-therapy, while other patients may experience a more insidious onset of symptoms months to years following radiation treatment. In a systematic review of lung cancer patients, the prevalence of radiation pneumonitis ranged from 13% to 37% (20). The risk for radiation pneumonitis increases when given with concurrent chemotherapy or in those with pre-existing lung problems. The total dose of radiation, number of fractions and radiation dose per fraction are associated with an increased risk of radiation pneumonitis (21). The total volume of lung exposed to radiation is another consideration when assessing a patient with suspected radiation pneumonitis.

OCCUPATIONAL AND EXPOSURE HISTORY

Smoking history should be obtained on all patients. Smoking is an identified risk factor for several ILDs including IPF, desquamative interstitial pneumonia (DIP), RB-ILD, and pulmonary Langerhans cell histiocytosis. Smoking is also linked to several comorbidities prevalent among patients with IPF including lung cancer, gastroesophageal reflux, coronary artery disease and emphysema.

A detailed review of the patient's work history, home environment and hobbies should be performed to elicit potential exposures. Questions should centre on the nature and duration of the exposure and if protective gear, such as masks, was used. Specifically, clinicians need to inquire about the precise tasks and duties individuals performed at their jobs or while participating in hobbies to have a clear understanding of the nature of the exposure. Given the latency period of certain exposures, such as asbestos, the clinical history should be comprehensive and include a chronological occupational history.

Numerous examples of occupational ILD appear in the literature; however, identification often requires a high index of suspicion. Identifying occupational lung disease, such as asbestosis, may have important implications to patients and their families regarding work compensation and disability applications. Inhalation of dusts, minerals and inorganic materials such as coal, silica and asbestos may lead to pneumoconiosis. Silicosis remains among the most common occupational lung diseases globally (22). Silica is found in glass, ceramics, abrasives and numerous other manufacturing products. Metals such as beryllium, used in the manufacturing industry, and cobalt, used to make machine parts or tools for drilling, grinding and cutting, have been linked to granulomatous responses in the lung and hard metal pneumoconiosis (23,24).

'Outbreaks' of occupational lung disease have also been reported (25,26). For example, HP presentations were reported among metal grinding machinists who worked with water-based metal working fluids known to harbour *Mycobacterium*. This led investigators to identify a specific myco-bacterial genotype across 10 industrial centres in Canada and the United States where these HP cases had been reported (27). Identifying patterns of disease related to place of work or geography may assist clinicians with earlier disease detection and prevention.

Exposures associated with HP vary by geography. Possible exposures include non-tuberculous mycobacterial organisms, bacteria such as thermophilic actinomycete species, fungi such as *Aspergillus* species, chemicals and high/low molecular weight protein from avian proteins in feces, serum and feathers. While classically described among bird owners (bird fancier's disease) who own pigeons, parakeets and other domesticated house birds, HP may also be seen with exposure to feather/down products found in pillows, comforters, furniture and coats. Another potential antigenic source includes indoor hot tubs where non-tuberculous mycobacteria thrive in the warm environment (28,29). In a retrospective series of 85 HP cases, approximately half confirmed by surgical lung biopsy, bird antigens and hot tub lung in the setting of *Mycobacterium avium-intracellulare* (MAI) exposure were the two most commonly identified causes (30). Another study cited birds and mould as common HP culprits (31). Interestingly, only a small subset of individuals, less than 10%, who are in close proximity with birds, develop bird fancier's disease (32).

The use of a checklist describing commonly encountered HP exposures that are specific to the practicing clinician's area, may be useful to assist patients with reviewing their home and work environment to identify potential exposures. Checklists should reflect regional clinical experience, such as swamp coolers in warmer climates or specific practices in agricultural areas. In addition, reviewing exposures at follow-up appointments may be helpful. Additional measures such as site visits or home assessments by a trained industrial hygienist may be warranted. Despite these efforts, a clearly identifiable antigen is only found in 37%–75% of cases (30,31,33). Cases in which a causative antigen cannot be identified are associated with poorer survival (31).

FAMILY HISTORY AND GENETICS

Up to 20% of IIPs are familial (34–36). Numerous genes have been associated with sporadic and familial forms of pulmonary fibrosis (Table 5.1) (37). For example, genetic studies of IPF patients and their families demonstrate that 18% of kindreds are genetic carriers of TERT mutations (38), while 3% of sporadic cases have a TERT mutation (39). It is important to recognize that family members may present with various forms of fibrotic lung disease including unclassifiable ILD, HP and non-specific interstitial pneumonia (NSIP), although IPF remains the most common (39–41). In addition, patients with familial fibrosis tend to be younger than their counterparts with sporadic pulmonary fibrosis (35,41).

Dyskeratosis congenita is a disease manifesting from telomere dysfunction. Inheritance may be autosomal dominant, X-linked, autosomal recessive and sporadic (42). Clinically, patients develop nail dystrophy, skin abnormalities and oral leucoplakia. Dyskeratosis congenita is also associated with bone marrow failure, malignancy and pulmonary fibrosis, and patients may present at any age.

Several other genetic disorders may have clinical manifestations that include pulmonary fibrosis. Patients with neurofibromatosis, an autosomal dominant disease, present with café au lait spots, axillary and inguinal freckling and cutaneous neurofibromas. When present, ILD is most commonly found to have lower lobe predominant reticulations and fibrosis on thoracic high-resolution computed tomography (HRCT) imaging (43). Lymphangioleiomyomatosis (LAM) may be seen in isolation or in the setting of tuberous sclerosis (TS). TS is an autosomal dominant inherited disease, although it may also present sporadically, characterized by hamartomas and angiomyolipomas, which develop in multiple organs including brain, kidneys and skin. Burt–Hogg–Dubé (BHD), which arises from a mutation in the folliculin gene, is another autosomal dominant disease associated with benign fibrofolliculomas of the skin, renal malignancies and lung cysts (44). Hermansky-Pudlak syndrome presents with albinism, platelet dysfunction leading to bleeding disorders and pulmonary fibrosis, in addition to other organ involvement. Diseases due to metabolic errors, such as Gaucher disease (type 1) and Niemann–Pick

Table 5.1 Genes associated with familial and/or sporadic pulmonary fibrosis

	Implicated gene	Physiologic role
Alveolar epithelial genes	Surfactant protein C (SFTPC) Surfactant protein A2 (SFTPA2) ATP-binding cassette member A3 (ABCA3)	Alveolar surfactant proteins associated with maintaining stability of the alveolar epithelium
Genes associated with maintaining telomere length	Telomerase reverse transcriptase (TERT)	Catalytic component of the enzyme telomerase; participates in maintaining telomere length
	Telomerase RNA component (TERC)	Component of telomerase complex that is responsible for maintenance of telomere length by encoding nucleotide repeats (TTAGGG) to the ends of chromosomes
	Dyskeratosis congenital 1, Dyskerin (DKC1)	Encodes a component of the telomerase complex; maintains telomere repeats at chromosome ends
	Regulator of telomere elongation helicase 1 (RTEL1)	Component of DNA helicases implicated in telomere length maintenance
Mucin production	Mucin B5 (MUC5B)	Encodes an airway mucin glycoprotein
Genes associated with immune pathways	Toll interacting protein (TOLLIP)	Ubiquitin binding protein that inhibits toll-like receptor pathways; regulates innate immune responses, including the TGF-ß signalling pathway

Source: Zhou W, Wang Y. Appl Clin Genet. 2016;9:5–13.

(type B) may also present with manifestations of pulmonary fibrosis.

While guidelines on how to manage screening and risk of developing ILD in the setting of familial fibrosis are presently lacking, and access to genetic testing is not yet widely available, identification of familial patterns of fibrotic lung disease is an important area to explore due to its impact on counselling of patients, their families and their children.

SIGNS AND SYMPTOMS OF CONNECTIVE TISSUE DISEASE

The prevalence of ILD among patients with rheumatoid arthritis (RA), systemic sclerosis (SSc), idiopathic inflammatory myopathy (IIM), mixed connective tissue disease (MCTD), and Sjögren syndrome ranges from 4% to 90% (45). Patients may present with an established diagnosis of an underlying CTD; however, in others, the ILD may be the initial manifestation of their CTD. Thus clinicians must maintain a high level of suspicion.

Patients with an established diagnosis of CTD who develop indolent symptoms of dyspnoea, cough and fatigue should be evaluated for the presence of ILD. Patients who present with a rapidly progressive ILD over weeks to months should be considered for an IIM diagnosis. Diagnosis can be challenging if the onset of ILD precedes the appearance of myositis symptoms (46). Additionally, IIM consists of a heterogeneous group of diseases ranging from classical dermatomyositis (DM) with proximal muscle weakness, heliotropic rash and inflammatory myositis with elevated CK and aldolase to clinical amyopathic dermatomyositis (CADM), also known as DM siné myositis. Specific consideration for CADM may be important as it is associated with severe ILD, yet lacks evidence of inflammatory myositis and the clinical symptoms of muscle weakness (47).

All patients presenting with ILD should be evaluated for clinical features that may suggest an underlying autoimmune process. Patient reports of small joint swelling (e.g. hands, wrists, ankles), morning stiffness or joint deformities suggest a diagnosis of RA. Additional suggestive symptoms of a CTD include Raynaud phenomenon, digital swelling, nail changes, digital ulceration, skin changes, rash, sicca symptoms, dysphagia and muscle weakness. Consultation with a rheumatologist to confirm a diagnosis of CTD is recommended.

EXPLORE POSSIBLE COMORBIDITIES

Patients with ILD may experience a number of comorbidities (48,49). Whether this is due to shared risk factors, such as smoking, or a consequence of the disease itself remains unknown. The importance of recognizing and identifying associated comorbidities is underlined by their impact on morbidity, mortality and overall quality of life. Common comorbidities include gastroesophageal reflux, obstructive sleep apnoea, lung cancer, emphysema, pulmonary hypertension, depression and anxiety. Additional prospective studies are needed to better understand how these comorbidities present in the context of ILD and how they should be managed.

PHYSICAL EXAMINATION

The physical exam in a patient with suspected ILD aims to confirm the presence of ILD, but also provides clues to the underlying aetiology of the lung disease and any associated comorbidities.

Findings that suggest a diagnosis of ILD include resting or exertional hypoxemia. Velcro-like bilateral inspiratory crackles on examination of the chest further support the diagnosis. A lack of crackles makes a diagnosis of IPF less likely; however, crackles may be absent in non-IPF ILD subtypes. Patients with chronic hypoxemia may develop clubbing of the nail beds; however, digital clubbing is often a late finding. In addition, clubbing may be seen with other pulmonary and systemic diseases such cystic fibrosis and cyanotic heart disease. Evidence of premature grey hair, particularly in those with a family history of ILD, may raise the clinical suspicion of an underlying telomeropathy.

Careful review of the skin, joints, muscles and nails may provide evidence of an undiagnosed CTD.

Specific features that should alert the clinician to an underlying CTD include puffy hands, sclerodactyly, periungal erythema, telangiectasias, Raynaud phenomena, fissuring of the digits (mechanic hands), digital ulceration, calcinosis, Gottron's papules, rashes, skin thickening, abnormalities in the capillary nail folds, evidence of active synovitis, joint deformity and muscle weakness.

Several inherited disorders, which may manifest with ILD, have specific clinical findings that should alert the clinician to suspect an underlying genetic disease. Notable examples include albinism in dyskeratosis congenita, hypopigmented ash leaf spots and shagreen patches in tuberous sclerosis, and fibrofolliculomas in Bert–Hogg–Dubé.

Finally, as discussed above, patients with ILD have an increased risk of several comorbidities. An assessment for pulmonary hypertension should be performed by looking for evidence of raised right-sided heart pressures in the form of an elevated jugular venous pulse, a right-sided heave, a loud pulmonic valve closure sound (P_2) or a tricuspid regurgitation murmur. In addition, patients with primary or secondary pulmonary hypertension may demonstrate evidence of a pulsatile liver, ascites and lower leg oedema.

NON-INVASIVE DIAGNOSTIC TESTING

SEROLOGIES

ILD may be the heralding clinical manifestation for a patient with an undiagnosed CTD. As part of the evaluation of a patient with suspected ILD, a basic serologic screen including anti-nuclear antibody (ANA), rheumatoid factor (RF) and anti-cyclic citrullinated peptide (CCP) is recommended (13). ANA by immunofluorescence is preferred, as it is more specific compared to ANAs obtained by enzyme-linked immunosorbent assay (ELISA). Serologic results must be interpreted within the individual patient's clinical context. Approximately 20% of patients with IPF are found to have positive autoantibodies, and similar rates are found in healthy controls (50). Positive but low ANA titres may be seen in up to 30% of healthy volunteers (51,52). Thus the presence of autoantibodies alone is insufficient to confirm a diagnosis of a CTD. The diagnosis of a specific CTD must be established on the basis of the integration of clinical, physical and serologic manifestations in consultation with a rheumatology consultant.

RF is positive in 70%–80% of patients with RA. It is a moderately specific autoantibody with specificity improving with higher titres, but can be an insensitive test in the setting of a suspected ILD. CCP is more specific for RA with a specificity of 95%–98% (53–56). Co-positivity is helpful for determining a diagnosis of RA in the appropriate clinical setting, with one meta-analysis reporting a diagnostic odds ratio (DOR) of 33.02 (CI, 23.89–45.64) when both are positive (57).

A more extended panel of serologies should be obtained depending on the clinical scenario. Sjögren's syndrome, most commonly associated with clinical symptoms of dry eyes and dry mouth, may be associated with SSA and SSB antibodies. In the setting of clinical suspicion for SSc, additional serologies include anti-centromere antibodies, Scl-70, anti-topoisomerase antibody and polymerase III antibodies. Patients may also demonstrate overlap with myositis and other CTDs, such as SSc. Serologic markers in this setting include AntiRo-60/SSA, AntiRo-52/TRIM21, AntiLa/SSB, AntiU1RNP, PM/Scl and AntiKu (58–61).

Clinicians should maintain a high index of suspicion for IIM, as these patients may present with negative ANA and normal to mildly elevated CK and aldolase levels, or they may fail to demonstrate clinical evidence of myositis and are thus vulnerable to being under-recognized as having an IIM (62,63). Additionally, the ILD may precede development of other supportive features of antisynthetase syndrome (64). Of the myositis-associated autoantibodies, anti-Jo-1 is the most commonly encountered autoantibody in patients with DM and polymyositis (PM). Other prominent anti-tRNA synthetase antibodies include PL-7 and PL-12, which are associated with the presence of ILD (64,65) and less commonly associated with myositis compared to those with anti-Jo-1 positivity (46). Additional anti-tRNA synthetase autoantibodies include KS, OJ, EJ, SC, JS, YRS and ZO, although these are considered rare (66–69). Availability for testing may vary by institution.

Another commonly encountered scenario is an ILD patient who exhibits features of CTD but has insufficient evidence to meet criteria for a CTD diagnosis. The recently coined term 'interstitial pneumonia with autoimmune features' (IPAF) aims to identify this subgroup of patients with ILD by incorporating clinical, serological and /or morphological features that support the presence of an underlying autoimmune process (70). For patients with a 'flavour' of autoimmune disease on initial presentation, it is reasonable to re-evaluate periodically for evidence of additional clinical or serologic evidence to support the development of a defined CTD.

The importance of identifying CTD-associated ILD relates to improved prognosis (71,72) and variation in pharmacologic therapy, as compared to the treatment of IPF. While all new ILD patients should undergo a basic serologic screen, clinicians may consider ordering a more extensive serologic panel in several settings:

1. History or physical examination suggestive of CTD
2. Younger patient
3. Female sex
4. Rapidly progressive ILD
5. High-resolution computed tomography (HRCT) pattern of non-specific interstitial pneumonia (NSIP), organizing pneumonia (OP) or mixed picture of NSIP-OP overlap

Individuals with ILD and clinical evidence suggestive of an underlying CTD benefit from early consultation with a rheumatologist, even in the setting of negative serologies.

PULMONARY FUNCTION TESTING

The role of pulmonary function testing is to document baseline status, monitor for disease progression, predict prognosis and provide objective evidence of response to therapy. Full pulmonary function testing, including spirometry, lung volumes and diffusion capacity, is performed at baseline. Spirometry alone is insufficient, as a reduction in vital capacity should be confirmed with concomitant reduction in total lung capacity (73). Once a disease pattern is confirmed, spirometry and diffusion capacity are sufficient in follow-up. Physiologic testing is preferred for longitudinal monitoring of disease, as it is more sensitive than CT and minimizes unnecessary radiation.

The most commonly encountered physiologic pattern in ILD is restriction, although additional physiologic patterns may be seen in certain ILD subtypes (Table 5.2). Physiologic patterns observed in ILD include obstruction, normal or pseudo-normal lung volumes, isolated reduction in diffusion capacity, pure restriction and reduced diffusion capacity out of proportion to the disease.

Changes in lung function over time offer important prognostic information, aiding clinicians with determining the appropriate timing for starting/stopping therapy and/or referral for lung transplantation assessment. In a multivariate analysis of patients with IPF and fibrotic NSIP, baseline diffusion capacity (DLCO) and change of forced vital capacity (FVC) of >10% over 6 months

were found to be independent risk factors for death (74). Additional studies demonstrate a decline in FVC (75–79) and diffusion capacity over 6–12 months are associated with decreased survival (75,77–79). However, previous physiologic decline does not appear to predict future clinical course in patients with IPF (77).

6-MINUTE WALK TEST

The 6-minute walk test (6MWT) provides information on the patient's functional status and disease progression over time, and it provides a measure to assess response to therapy over time. Reduced baseline 6-minute walk distances are independently associated with increased mortality

Table 5.2 Physiologic patterns of disease in interstitial lung disease

Restrictive Pattern

$\Downarrow$FVC, $\Downarrow$FEV$_1$, N/$\Uparrow$FEV$_1$/FVC ratio, $\Downarrow$TLC, $\Downarrow$DLCO

- Idiopathic pulmonary fibrosis
- Non-specific interstitial pneumonia
- Connective tissue disease-associated interstitial lung disease
- Hypersensitivity pneumonitis
- Sarcoidosis
- Organizing pneumonia
- Desquamative interstitial pneumonia
- Lymphoid interstitial pneumonia
- Pulmonary Langerhans cell histiocytosis

Mixed Obstructive and Restrictive Pattern

$\Downarrow$FVC, $\Downarrow$FEV$_1$, $\Downarrow$FEV$_1$/FVC ratio, N/$\Downarrow$TLC, $\Downarrow$DLCO

- Respiratory bronchiolitis-associated interstitial lung disease
- Chronic obstructive lung disease with pulmonary fibrosis

Obstructive Pattern

N FVC, $\Downarrow$FEV$_1$, $\Downarrow$FEV$_1$/FVC ratio, N/$\Uparrow$TLC, $\Downarrow$DLCO (may demonstrate air trapping)

- Bronchiolitis obliterans
- Lymphangioleiomyomatosis
- Endobronchial sarcoidosis

Normal with Isolated Diffusion Capacity

N FVC, N FEV$_1$, N FEV$_1$/FVC ratio, N TLC, $\Downarrow$DLCO

- Chronic obstructive lung disease with pulmonary fibrosis (pseudonormalization of lung volumes)
- Early ILD with associated pulmonary hypertension
- Lymphangioleiomyomatosis
- Pulmonary Langerhans cell histiocytosis

Normal

N FVC, N FEV$_1$, N FEV$_1$/FVC ratio, N TLC, N DLCO

- Any ILD in early disease

Abbreviations: DLCO = diffusion capacity; FEV$_1$ = forced volume in 1 second; FVC = forced vital capacity; N = normal; TLC = total lung capacity.

(80,81). In addition, a change in 6MWT provides prognostic information. In an analysis of patients enrolled in the gamma interferon trial, a decline of 50 meters or more at 24 weeks was associated with a fourfold increase in mortality (HR 4.27; 95% CI 2.57–7.10, $p < 0.001$) (82).

HIGH-RESOLUTION COMPUTED TOMOGRAPHY SCAN

As outlined in the American Thoracic Society/European Respiratory Society/Japanese Respiratory Society/Latin American Thoracic Association (ATS/ERS/JRS/ALAT) statement for diagnosis and management of IPF, all patients require a non-contrast, high-resolution computed tomography (HRCT) scan at baseline for diagnosis. Reconstructed slice collimation ≤2 mm is recommended, with ≤1.25 mm slice thickness preferred and reconstructed images spaced at ≤2 cm. Images should be captured at full inspiration to minimize respiratory motion artefact. For the initial evaluation of a patient with suspected ILD, expiratory images are also performed to allow for the assessment of air trapping. Prone images should be collected as these help discern true disease from atelectasis (13). Honeycombing may also be more evident on these views. Follow-up imaging may be required for monitoring of suspicious pulmonary nodules or if there is evidence of clinical deterioration.

The radiographic patterns of specific forms of ILD are discussed in detail in a separate chapter. However, careful attention should be made to features of the UIP pattern, including basal distribution, honeycombing, reticulations, traction bronchiectasis and the absence of inconsistent features such as extensive ground glass, centrilobular nodules or air trapping (13). The presence of the UIP pattern is strongly associated with a diagnosis of IPF (83,84), mitigating the need for surgical lung biopsy in the appropriate clinical scenario.

especially eosinophil counts, are useful when considering a diagnosis such as eosinophilic pneumonia. Transbronchial biopsies are of limited utility in many forms of ILD but may be particularly helpful when considering infection or sarcoidosis.

A surgical lung biopsy may be required for definitive diagnosis in cases of ILD where clinical data and radiographic imaging fail to provide a clear diagnosis. The surgical approach is most commonly via video-assisted thoracoscopic surgery (VATS). Review of histopathologic specimens by an experienced lung pathologist with integration of clinical and radiological data in a multidisciplinary format is recommended (13,15). The addition of histopathologic data offers important clinical implications, changing diagnosis in 42%–90% of cases in one systematic review of the literature (85). Diagnostic yield is high, ranging between 74% and 96% across studies (86–88).

Relative contraindications to surgical lung biopsy include patient preference, advanced age, reduced DLCO (<35%), reduced FVC (<55%), mechanical ventilation, preoperative resting hypoxemia, pulmonary hypertension, concurrent acute exacerbation, immunosuppression and significant underlying comorbidities. The surgical risks and diagnostic benefits associated with pursuing a surgical lung biopsy should be reviewed and individualized to the patient. A surgical lung biopsy is associated with a 30-day postoperative mortality range between 1.8% and 4.5% (86,87,89–92).

For patients proceeding to surgical lung biopsy, samples from two or more lobes are recommended (93). Sampling is guided by HRCT appearance, with surgical samples selected from areas with normal parenchyma adjacent to honeycomb lung or abnormal parenchyma whenever possible, while avoiding areas of dense fibrosis (94). When discordance in histologic pattern is present, for example NSIP and UIP, disease behaviour models that of UIP (95).

INVASIVE DIAGNOSTIC TESTING

Bronchoscopy is a useful tool in the evaluation of patients with ILD when there is concern for underlying infection, which is frequently a complication of immunosuppressive therapy. Further, bronchoalveolar lavage differential cell counts,

ROLE OF MULTIDISCIPLINARY DISCUSSION

International guidelines stress the importance of multidisciplinary discussion (MDD) for establishing a diagnosis of ILD (13,15). Given the complexities in establishing a diagnosis (particularly when

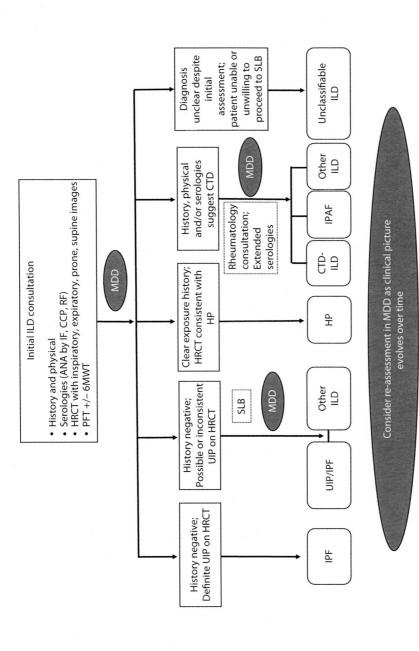

Figure 5.2 Application of multidisciplinary discussion in an iterative format to achieve a consensus diagnosis for patients with ILD. Multidisciplinary discussion (MDD) among clinicians, thoracic radiologists and lung pathologists improves diagnostic agreement and confidence (96). However, despite a thorough initial assessment, establishing a specific ILD diagnosis may be challenging. Iterative multidisciplinary discussion may assist in management of cases, allowing for integration of new data, as it becomes available. (Abbreviations: 6MWT = 6-minute walk test; ANA = anti-nuclear antibody; CCP = anti-cyclic citrullinated peptide; CTD = connective tissue disease; HP = hypersensitivity pneumonitis; HRCT = high-resolution computed tomography; IF = immunofluorescence; ILD = interstitial lung disease; IPAF = interstitial pneumonia with autoimmune features; IPF = idiopathic pulmonary fibrosis; MDD = multidisciplinary discussion; NSIP = non-specific interstitial pneumonia; PFT = pulmonary function testing; RF = rheumatoid factor; SLB = surgical lung biopsy; UIP = usual interstitial pneumonia.)

HRCT scans are not diagnostic, surgical lung biopsies are unavailable due to patient wishes or severity of disease or the pathology is non-diagnostic), MDD among individuals with expertise in ILD (from the disciplines of clinical pulmonary medicine, thoracic radiology and lung pathology) is imperative. The use of iterative and integrated MDD improves inter-observer agreement and diagnostic confidence (96). The importance applies beyond the IIPs to CTD and other forms of ILD (63).

MDD itself may be an imperfect process, subject to bias of the participating individuals, their degree of expertise and the data presented in case format. While consensus diagnosis is considered the gold standard, this should not necessarily be a corollary for accuracy. It is important to recognize the iterative nature of an MDD, with cases being presented when additional diagnostic data are available, such as serologies, follow-up HRCT imaging or histopathology. A suggested approach to ILD diagnosis using MDD is outlined in Figure 5.2. This approach emphasizes returning to cases as additional data become available and as clinicians gather information on the individual patient's disease behaviour. For example, cases deemed unclassifiable may benefit from periodic review in MDD, as their disease behaviour over time may help establish a firm diagnosis. While MDDs are charged with establishing a diagnosis, survey data from a purposeful sample of 10 centres from Australia, United States, Canada, United Kingdom and France on the use of MDD, report that 80% of MDDs also establish management plans and 60% establish treatment recommendations, although the organization of MDDs differs widely (97).

MDD can be used to distinguish between idiopathic NSIP and other non-idiopathic ILDs such as HP and drug toxicity. In one series of multidisciplinary workshops, an alternative diagnosis to idiopathic NSIP was determined in more than a third of cases (98). In cases where a clear exposure is lacking, HP may be difficult to diagnose, again placing emphasis on the importance of an integrated MDD review whenever possible. Finally, with widespread availability of anti-fibrotic therapy, use of MDD to establish a consensus diagnosis of IPF may be increasingly important to ensure application of these costly drugs to the appropriate patient population.

In summary, ILDs comprise a heterogeneous group of lung diseases that can be challenging to diagnose. The clinical evaluation of a patient with a suspected ILD is an essential component to the diagnostic evaluation, and it includes a careful history, drug and work history, relevant exposure history, family history and identification of signs/symptoms to suggest an underlying CTD. The clinical evaluation along with the physiologic, radiologic and, when available, histopathologic data should be discussed in a MDD format in order to establish an accurate and confident ILD diagnosis.

REFERENCES

1. Kornum JB, Christensen S, Grijota M, Pedersen L, Wogelius P, Beiderbeck A et al. The incidence of interstitial lung disease 1995–2005: A Danish nationwide population-based study. *BMC Pulmon Med.* 2008;8:24.

2. Gribbin J, Hubbard RB, Le Jeune I, Smith CJ, West J, Tata LJ. Incidence and mortality of idiopathic pulmonary fibrosis and sarcoidosis in the UK. *Thorax.* 2006;61(11):980–5.

3. Raghu G, Chen SY, Yeh WS, Maroni B, Li Q, Lee YC et al. Idiopathic pulmonary fibrosis in US Medicare beneficiaries aged 65 years and older: Incidence, prevalence, and survival, 2001–11. *Lancet Respir Med.* 2014;2(7):566–72.

4. Harari S, Madotto F, Caminati A, Conti S, Cesana G. Epidemiology of idiopathic pulmonary fibrosis in Northern Italy. *PloS One.* 2016;11(2):e0147072.

5. Noble PW, Albera C, Bradford WZ, Costabel U, Glassberg MK, Kardatzke D et al. Pirfenidone in patients with idiopathic pulmonary fibrosis (CAPACITY): Two randomised trials. *Lancet.* 2011;377(9779):1760–9.

6. Richeldi L, du Bois RM, Raghu G, Azuma A, Brown KK, Costabel U et al. Efficacy and safety of nintedanib in idiopathic pulmonary fibrosis. *New Engl J Med.* 2014;370(22):2071–82.

7. King TE, Jr, Bradford WZ, Castro-Bernardini S, Fagan EA, Glaspole I, Glassberg MK et al. A phase 3 trial of pirfenidone in patients with idiopathic pulmonary fibrosis. *New Engl J Med.* 2014;370(22):2083–92.

8. Jin GY, Lynch D, Chawla A, Garg K, Tammemagi MC, Sahin H et al. Interstitial lung abnormalities in a CT lung cancer screening population: Prevalence and progression rate. *Radiology.* 2013;268(2):563–71.

9. Salvatore M, Henschke CI, Yip R, Jacobi A, Eber C, Padilla M et al. JOURNAL CLUB: Evidence of interstitial lung disease on low-dose chest CT images: Prevalence, patterns, and progression. *AJR Am J Roentgenol.* 2016;206(3):487–94.

10. Collard HR, Tino G, Noble PW, Shreve MA, Michaels M, Carlson B et al. Patient experiences with pulmonary fibrosis. *Respir Med.* 2007;101(6):1350–4.

11. ten Klooster L, Nossent GD, Kwakkel-van Erp JM, van Kessel DA, Oudijk EJ, van de Graaf EA et al. Ten-year survival in patients with idiopathic pulmonary fibrosis after lung transplantation. *Lung.* 2015;193(6):919–26.

12. Christie JD, Edwards LB, Kucheryavaya AY, Benden C, Dipchand AI, Dobbels F et al. The Registry of the International Society for Heart and Lung Transplantation: 29th Adult Lung and Heart-Lung Transplant Report-2012. *J Heart Lung Transplant.* 2012;31(10):1073–86.

13. Raghu G, Collard HR, Egan JJ, Martinez FJ, Behr J, Brown KK et al. An official ATS/ERS/JRS/ALAT statement: Idiopathic pulmonary fibrosis: Evidence-based guidelines for diagnosis and management. *Am J Respir Crit Care Med.* 2011;183(6):788–824.

14. Travis WD, Costabel U, Hansell DM, King TE, Jr., Lynch DA, Nicholson AG et al. An official American Thoracic Society/European Respiratory Society statement: Update of the international multidisciplinary classification of the idiopathic interstitial pneumonias. *Am J Respir Crit Care Med.* 2013;188(6):733–48.

15. Raghu G, Rochwerg B, Zhang Y, Garcia CA, Azuma A, Behr J et al. An official ATS/ERS/JRS/ALAT clinical practice guideline: Treatment of idiopathic pulmonary fibrosis. An update of the 2011 clinical practice guideline. *Am J Respir Crit Care Med.* 2015;192(2):e3–19.

16. Papiris SA, Daniil ZD, Malagari K, Kapotsis GE, Sotiropoulou C, Milic-Emili J et al. The Medical Research Council dyspnea scale in the estimation of disease severity in idiopathic pulmonary fibrosis. *Respir Med.* 2005;99(6):755–61.

17. Manali ED, Stathopoulos GT, Kollintza A, Kalomenidis I, Emili JM, Sotiropoulou C et al. The Medical Research Council chronic dyspnea score predicts the survival of patients with idiopathic pulmonary fibrosis. *Respir Med.* 2008;102(4):586–92.

18. Holland AE, Fiore JF, Jr., Bell EC, Goh N, Westall G, Symons K et al. Dyspnoea and comorbidity contribute to anxiety and depression in interstitial lung disease. *Respirology (Carlton, Vic).* 2014;19(8):1215–21.

19. The Drug-Induced Respiratory Disease Website, Dijon, France. http://www.pneumotox.com/ (Accessed 1 May 2016).

20. Rodrigues G, Lock M, D'Souza D, Yu E, Van Dyk J. Prediction of radiation pneumonitis by dose-volume histogram parameters in lung cancer—A systematic review. *Radiother Oncol.* 2004;71(2):127–38.

21. Roach M 3rd, Gandara DR, Yuo HS, Swift PS, Kroll S, Shrieve DC et al. Radiation pneumonitis following combined modality therapy for lung cancer: Analysis of prognostic factors. *J Clin Oncol.* 1995;13(10):2606–12.

22. Rosenman KD, Reilly MJ, Henneberger PK. Estimating the total number of newly-recognized silicosis cases in the United States. *Am J Ind Med.* 2003;44(2):141–7.

23. Nemery B, Verbeken EK, Demedts M. Giant cell interstitial pneumonia (hard metal lung disease, cobalt lung). *Semin Respir Crit Care Med.* 2001;22(4):435–48.

24. Fontenot AP, Amicosante M. Metal-induced diffuse lung disease. *Semin Respir Crit Care Med.* 2008;29(6):662–9.

25. Fox J, Anderson H, Moen T, Gruetzmacher G, Hanrahan L, Fink J. Metal working fluid-associated hypersensitivity pneumonitis: An outbreak investigation and case-control study. *Am J Ind Med.* 1999;35(1):58–67.

26. Lougheed MD, Roos JO, Waddell WR, Munt PW. Desquamative interstitial pneumonitis and diffuse alveolar damage in textile workers. Potential role of mycotoxins. *Chest.* 1995;108(5):1196–200.

27. Wallace RJ, Jr., Zhang Y, Wilson RW, Mann L, Rossmoore H. Presence of a single genotype of the newly described species *Mycobacterium immunogenum* in industrial metalworking fluids associated with hypersensitivity pneumonitis. *Appl Environ Microbiol.* 2002;68(11):5580–4.

28. Sood A, Sreedhar R, Kulkarni P, Nawoor AR. Hypersensitivity pneumonitis-like granulomatous lung disease with nontuberculous mycobacteria from exposure to hot water aerosols. *Environ Health Perspect.* 2007;115(2):262–6.

29. Glazer CS, Martyny JW, Lee B, Sanchez TL, Sells TM, Newman LS et al. Nontuberculous mycobacteria in aerosol droplets and bulk water samples from therapy pools and hot tubs. *J Occup Environ Hyg.* 2007;4(11):831–40.

30. Hanak V, Golbin JM, Ryu JH. Causes and presenting features in 85 consecutive patients with hypersensitivity pneumonitis. *Mayo Clin Proc.* 2007;82(7):812–6.

31. Fernandez Perez ER, Swigris JJ, Forssen AV, Tourin O, Solomon JJ, Huie TJ et al. Identifying an inciting antigen is associated with improved survival in patients with chronic hypersensitivity pneumonitis. *Chest.* 2013;144(5):1644–51.

32. Rodriguez de Castro F, Carrillo T, Castillo R, Blanco C, Diaz F, Cuevas M. Relationships between characteristics of exposure to pigeon antigens. Clinical manifestations and humoral immune response. *Chest.* 1993;103(4):1059–63.

33. Mooney JJ, Elicker BM, Urbania TH, Agarwal MR, Ryerson CJ, Nguyen ML et al. Radiographic fibrosis score predicts survival in hypersensitivity pneumonitis. *Chest.* 2013;144(2):586–92.

34. Marshall RP, Puddicombe A, Cookson WO, Laurent GJ. Adult familial cryptogenic fibrosing alveolitis in the United Kingdom. *Thorax.* 2000;55(2):143–6.

35. Garcia-Sancho C, Buendia-Roldan I, Fernandez-Plata MR, Navarro C, Perez-Padilla R, Vargas MH et al. Familial pulmonary fibrosis is the strongest risk factor for idiopathic pulmonary fibrosis. *Respir Med.* 2011;105(12):1902–7.

36. Coghlan MA, Shifren A, Huang HJ, Russell TD, Mitra RD, Zhang Q et al. Sequencing of idiopathic pulmonary fibrosis-related genes reveals independent single gene associations. *BMJ Open Respir Res.* 2014;1(1):e000057.

37. Zhou W, Wang Y. Candidate genes of idiopathic pulmonary fibrosis: Current evidence and research. *Appl Clin Genet.* 2016;9:5–13.

38. Diaz de Leon A, Cronkhite JT, Katzenstein AL, Godwin JD, Raghu G, Glazer CS et al. Telomere lengths, pulmonary fibrosis and telomerase (TERT) mutations. *PloS One.* 2010;5(5):e10680.

39. Cronkhite JT, Xing C, Raghu G, Chin KM, Torres F, Rosenblatt RL et al. Telomere shortening in familial and sporadic pulmonary fibrosis. *Am J Respir Crit Care Med.* 2008;178(7):729–37.

40. George G, Rosas IO, Cui Y, McKane C, Hunninghake GM, Camp PC et al. Short telomeres, telomeropathy, and subclinical extrapulmonary organ damage in patients with interstitial lung disease. *Chest.* 2015;147(6):1549–57.

41. Fernandez BA, Fox G, Bhatia R, Sala E, Noble B, Denic N et al. A Newfoundland cohort of familial and sporadic idiopathic pulmonary fibrosis patients: Clinical and genetic features. *Respir Res.* 2012; 13:64.

42. Savage SA, Alter BP. Dyskeratosis congenita. *Hematol Oncol Clin North Am.* 2009;23(2):215–31.

43. Devine MS, Garcia CK. Genetic interstitial lung disease. *Clin Chest Med.* 2012;33(1):95–110.

44. Nickerson ML, Warren MB, Toro JR, Matrosova V, Glenn G, Turner ML et al. Mutations in a novel gene lead to kidney tumors, lung wall defects, and benign tumors of the hair follicle in patients with the Birt-Hogg-Dube syndrome. *Cancer Cell.* 2002;2(2):157–64.

45. Wallace B, Vummidi D, Khanna D. Management of connective tissue diseases associated interstitial lung disease: A review of the published literature. *Curr Opin Rheumatol.* 2016;28(3):236–45.

46. Hervier B, Devilliers H, Stanciu R, Meyer A, Uzunhan Y, Masseau A et al. Hierarchical cluster and survival analyses of antisynthetase syndrome: Phenotype and outcome are correlated with anti-tRNA synthetase antibody specificity. *Autoimmun Rev.* 2012;12(2):210–7.

47. Gerami P, Schope JM, McDonald L, Walling HW, Sontheimer RD. A systematic review of adult-onset clinically amyopathic dermatomyositis (dermatomyositis sine myositis): A missing link within the spectrum of the idiopathic inflammatory myopathies. *J Am Acad Dermatol.* 2006;54(4):597–613.

48. Collard HR, Ward AJ, Lanes S, Cortney Hayflinger D, Rosenberg DM, Hunsche E. Burden of illness in idiopathic pulmonary fibrosis. *J Med Econ.* 2012;15(5):829–35.

49. de Boer K, Lee JS. Under-recognised co-morbidities in idiopathic pulmonary fibrosis: A review. *Respirology (Carlton, Vic).* 2016;21(6):995–1004.

50. Lee JS, Kim EJ, Lynch KL, Elicker B, Ryerson CJ, Katsumoto TR et al. Prevalence and clinical significance of circulating autoantibodies in idiopathic pulmonary fibrosis. *Respir Med.* 2013;107(2):249–55.

51. Tan EM, Feltkamp TE, Smolen JS, Butcher B, Dawkins R, Fritzler MJ et al. Range of antinuclear antibodies in 'healthy' individuals. *Arthritis Rheum.* 1997;40(9):1601–11.

52. Solomon DH, Kavanaugh AJ, Schur PH. Evidence-based guidelines for the use of immunologic tests: Antinuclear antibody testing. *Arthritis Rheum.* 2002;47(4):434–44.

53. Jansen AL, van der Horst-Bruinsma I, van Schaardenburg D, van de Stadt RJ, de Koning MH, Dijkmans BA. Rheumatoid factor and antibodies to cyclic citrullinated peptide differentiate rheumatoid arthritis from undifferentiated polyarthritis in patients with early arthritis. *J Rheumatol.* 2002;29(10):2074–6.

54. Nishimura K, Sugiyama D, Kogata Y, Tsuji G, Nakazawa T, Kawano S et al. Meta-analysis: Diagnostic accuracy of anti-cyclic citrullinated peptide antibody and rheumatoid factor for rheumatoid arthritis. *Ann Intern Med.* 2007;146(11):797–808.

55. Ates A, Karaaslan Y, Aksaray S. Predictive value of antibodies to cyclic citrullinated peptide in patients with early arthritis. *Clin Rheumatol.* 2007;26(4):499–504.

56. Whiting PF, Smidt N, Sterne JA, Harbord R, Burton A, Burke M et al. Systematic review: Accuracy of anti-citrullinated peptide antibodies for diagnosing rheumatoid arthritis. *Ann Intern Med.* 2010;152(7):456–64; w155–66.

57. Sun J, Zhang Y, Liu L, Liu G. Diagnostic accuracy of combined tests of anticyclic citrullinated peptide antibody and rheumatoid factor for rheumatoid arthritis: A meta-analysis. *Clin Exper Rheumatol.* 2014;32(1):11–21.

58. Vancsa A, Gergely L, Ponyi A, Lakos G, Nemeth J, Szodoray P et al. Myositis-specific and myositis-associated antibodies in overlap myositis in comparison to primary dermatopolymyositis: Relevance for clinical classification: Retrospective study of 169 patients. *Joint Bone Spine.* 2010;77(2):125–30.

59. Ghirardello A, Borella E, Beggio M, Franceschini F, Fredi M, Doria A. Myositis autoantibodies and clinical phenotypes. *Auto Immun Highlights.* 2014;5(3):69–75.

60. Menendez A, Gomez J, Escanlar E, Caminal-Montero L, Mozo L. Clinical associations of anti-SSA/Ro60 and anti-Ro52/TRIM21 antibodies: Diagnostic utility of their separate detection. *Autoimmunity.* 2013;46(1):32–9.

61. D'Aoust J, Hudson M, Tatibouet S, Wick J, Mahler M, Baron M et al. Clinical and serologic correlates of anti-PM/Scl antibodies in systemic sclerosis: A multicenter study of 763 patients. *Arthritis Rheumatol.* 2014;66(6):1608–15.

62. Mittoo S, Gelber AC, Christopher-Stine L, Horton MR, Lechtzin N, Danoff SK. Ascertainment of collagen vascular disease in patients presenting with interstitial lung disease. *Respir Med.* 2009;103(8):1152–8.

63. Chartrand S, Swigris JJ, Peykova L, Chung J, Fischer A. A multidisciplinary evaluation helps identify the antisynthetase syndrome in patients presenting as idiopathic interstitial pneumonia. *J Rheumatol.* 2016;43(5):887–92.

64. Kalluri M, Sahn SA, Oddis CV, Gharib SL, Christopher-Stine L, Danoff SK et al. Clinical profile of anti-PL-12 autoantibody. Cohort study and review of the literature. *Chest.* 2009;135(6):1550–6.

65. Yamasaki Y, Yamada H, Nozaki T, Akaogi J, Nichols C, Lyons R et al. Unusually high frequency of autoantibodies to PL-7 associated with milder muscle disease in Japanese patients with polymyositis/dermatomyositis. *Arthritis Rheum.* 2006;54(6):2004–9.

66. Lega JC, Reynaud Q, Belot A, Fabien N, Durieu I, Cottin V. Idiopathic inflammatory myopathies and the lung. *Eur Respir Rev.* 2015;24(136):216–38.

67. Hamaguchi Y, Fujimoto M, Matsushita T, Kaji K, Komura K, Hasegawa M et al. Common and distinct clinical features in adult patients with anti-aminoacyl-tRNA synthetase antibodies: Heterogeneity within the syndrome. *PloS One.* 2013;8(4): e60442.

68. Mahler M, Miller FW, Fritzler MJ. Idiopathic inflammatory myopathies and the anti-synthetase syndrome: A comprehensive review. *Autoimmun Rev.* 2014;13(4–5):367–71.

69. Watanabe K, Handa T, Tanizawa K, Hosono Y, Taguchi Y, Noma S et al. Detection of antisynthetase syndrome in patients with idiopathic interstitial pneumonias. *Respir Med.* 2011;105(8):1238–47.

70. Fischer A, Antoniou KM, Brown KK, Cadranel J, Corte TJ, du Bois RM et al. An official European Respiratory Society/ American Thoracic Society research statement: Interstitial pneumonia with autoimmune features. *Eur Respir J.* 2015;46(4):976–87.

71. Park JH, Kim DS, Park IN, Jang SJ, Kitaichi M, Nicholson AG et al. Prognosis of fibrotic interstitial pneumonia: Idiopathic versus collagen vascular disease-related subtypes. *Am J Respir Crit Care Med.* 2007;175(7):705–11.

72. Suda T, Kono M, Nakamura Y, Enomoto N, Kaida Y, Fujisawa T et al. Distinct prognosis of idiopathic nonspecific interstitial pneumonia (NSIP) fulfilling criteria for undifferentiated connective tissue disease (UCTD). *Respir Med.* 2010;104(10):1527–34.

73. Pellegrino R, Viegi G, Brusasco V, Crapo RO, Burgos F, Casaburi R et al. Interpretative strategies for lung function tests. *Eur Respir J.* 2005;26(5):948–68.

74. Jegal Y, Kim DS, Shim TS, Lim CM, Do Lee S, Koh Y et al. Physiology is a stronger predictor of survival than pathology in fibrotic interstitial pneumonia. *Am J Respir Crit Care Med.* 2005;171(6):639–44.

75. Collard HR, King TE, Jr., Bartelson BB, Vourlekis JS, Schwarz MI, Brown KK. Changes in clinical and physiologic variables predict survival in idiopathic pulmonary fibrosis. *Am J Respir Crit Care Med.* 2003;168(5):538–42.

76. Flaherty KR, Mumford JA, Murray S, Kazerooni EA, Gross BH, Colby TV et al. Prognostic implications of physiologic and radiographic changes in idiopathic interstitial pneumonia. *Am J Respir Crit Care Med.* 2003;168(5):543–8.

77. Schmidt SL, Tayob N, Han MK, Zappala C, Kervitsky D, Murray S et al. Predicting pulmonary fibrosis disease course from past trends in pulmonary function. *Chest.* 2014;145(3):579–85.

78. du Bois RM, Weycker D, Albera C, Bradford WZ, Costabel U, Kartashov A et al. Ascertainment of individual risk of mortality for patients with idiopathic pulmonary fibrosis. *Am J Respir Crit Care Med.* 2011;184(4):459–66.

79. Latsi PI, du Bois RM, Nicholson AG, Colby TV, Bisirtzoglou D, Nikolakopoulou A et al. Fibrotic idiopathic interstitial pneumonia: The prognostic value of longitudinal functional trends. *Am J Respir Crit Care Med.* 2003;168(5):531–7.

80. Lederer DJ, Arcasoy SM, Wilt JS, D'Ovidio F, Sonett JR, Kawut SM. Six-minute-walk distance predicts waiting list survival in idiopathic pulmonary fibrosis. *Am J Respir Crit Care Med.* 2006;174(6):659–64.

81. Caminati A, Bianchi A, Cassandro R, Mirenda MR, Harari S. Walking distance on 6-MWT is a prognostic factor in idiopathic pulmonary fibrosis. *Respir Med.* 2009;103(1):117–23.

82. du Bois RM, Weycker D, Albera C, Bradford WZ, Costabel U, Kartashov A et al. Six-minute-walk test in idiopathic pulmonary

fibrosis: Test validation and minimal clinically important difference. *Am J Respir Crit Care Med.* 2011;183(9):1231–7.

83. Raghu G, Mageto YN, Lockhart D, Schmidt RA, Wood DE, Godwin JD. The accuracy of the clinical diagnosis of new-onset idiopathic pulmonary fibrosis and other interstitial lung disease: A prospective study. *Chest.* 1999;116(5):1168–74.

84. Hunninghake GW, Zimmerman MB, Schwartz DA, King TE, Jr., Lynch J, Hegele R et al. Utility of a lung biopsy for the diagnosis of idiopathic pulmonary fibrosis. *Am J Respir Crit Care Med.* 2001;164(2):193–6.

85. Han Q, Luo Q, Xie JX, Wu LL, Liao LY, Zhang XX et al. Diagnostic yield and postoperative mortality associated with surgical lung biopsy for evaluation of interstitial lung diseases: A systematic review and meta-analysis. *J Thorac Cardiovasc Surg.* 2015;149(5):1394–401.e1.

86. Rotolo N, Imperatori A, Dominioni L, Facchini A, Conti V, Castiglioni M et al. Efficacy and safety of surgical lung biopsy for interstitial disease. Experience of 161 consecutive patients from a single institution in Italy. *Sarcoidosis Vasc Diffuse Lung Dis.* 2015;32(3):251–8.

87. Morris D, Zamvar V. The efficacy of video-assisted thoracoscopic surgery lung biopsies in patients with Interstitial Lung Disease: A retrospective study of 66 patients. *J Cardiothorac Surg.* 2014;9:45.

88. Sigurdsson MI, Isaksson HJ, Gudmundsson G, Gudbjartsson T. Diagnostic surgical lung biopsies for suspected interstitial lung diseases: A retrospective study. *Ann Thorac Surg.* 2009;88(1):227–32.

89. Bando M, Ohno S, Hosono T, Yanase K, Sato Y, Sohara Y et al. Risk of acute exacerbation after video-assisted thoracoscopic lung biopsy for interstitial lung disease. *J Bronchology Interv Pulmonol.* 2009;16(4):229–35.

90. Park JH, Kim DK, Kim DS, Koh Y, Lee SD, Kim WS et al. Mortality and risk factors for surgical lung biopsy in patients with idiopathic interstitial pneumonia. *Eur J Cardiothorac Surg.* 2007;31(6): 1115–9.

91. Kreider ME, Hansen-Flaschen J, Ahmad NN, Rossman MD, Kaiser LR, Kucharczuk JC et al. Complications of video-assisted thoracoscopic lung biopsy in patients with interstitial lung disease. *Ann Thorac Surg.* 2007;83(3):1140–4.

92. Lettieri CJ, Veerappan GR, Helman DL, Mulligan CR, Shorr AF. Outcomes and safety of surgical lung biopsy for interstitial lung disease. *Chest.* 2005;127(5):1600–5.

93. American Thoracic Society/European Respiratory Society International Multidisciplinary Consensus Classification of the Idiopathic Interstitial Pneumonias. This joint statement of the American Thoracic Society (ATS), and the European Respiratory Society (ERS) was adopted by the ATS board of directors, June 2001 and by the ERS executive committee, June 2001. *Am J Respir Crit Care Med.* 2002;165(2):277–304.

94. Bradley B, Branley HM, Egan JJ, Greaves MS, Hansell DM, Harrison NK et al. Interstitial lung disease guideline: The British Thoracic Society in collaboration with the Thoracic Society of Australia and New Zealand and the Irish Thoracic Society. *Thorax.* 2008;63 (Suppl 5):v1–58.

95. Flaherty KR, Travis WD, Colby TV, Toews GB, Kazerooni EA, Gross BH et al. Histopathologic variability in usual and nonspecific interstitial pneumonias. *Am J Respir Crit Care Med.* 2001;164(9):1722–7.

96. Flaherty KR, King TE, Jr., Raghu G, Lynch JP 3rd, Colby TV, Travis WD et al. Idiopathic interstitial pneumonia: What is the effect of a multidisciplinary approach to diagnosis? *Am J Respir Crit Care Med.* 2004;170(8):904–10.

97. Jo HE, Corte TJ, Moodley Y, Levin K, Westall G, Hopkins P et al. Evaluating the interstitial lung disease multidisciplinary meeting: A survey of expert centres. *BMC Pulm Med.* 2016;16:22.

98. Travis WD, Hunninghake G, King TE, Jr, Lynch DA, Colby TV, Galvin JR et al. Idiopathic nonspecific interstitial pneumonia: Report of an American Thoracic Society project. *Am J Respir Crit Care Med.* 2008;177(12):1338–47.

6

Role of invasive testing in ILD diagnosis

J SCOTT FERGUSON AND KEITH C MEYER

INTRODUCTION

Optimal management of patients with interstitial lung disease (ILD) is dependent on establishing an accurate, specific ILD diagnosis that allows clinicians to recommend appropriate therapeutic interventions that are likely to help and not harm patients (1,2). Because patients with different forms of ILD frequently have similar symptoms, signs and findings on routine chest radiographs as well as inconclusive laboratory test results, some form of invasive testing is often required to make or confirm a specific diagnosis. In many instances a high-resolution computed tomography (HRCT) scan of the thorax can reveal a pattern that is pathognomonic for a specific form of ILD (thereby obviating the need for invasive procedures) or reveals a pattern that narrows the differential diagnosis considerably (3–5). However, if the diagnosis remains unclear, clinicians can utilize a number of invasive procedures to identify and diagnose specific forms of ILD (Figures 6.1 and 6.2). Flexible bronchoscopy (FB) has been used for more than three decades to

evaluate patients with ILD, and surgical lung biopsy (SLB) has been used for over half a century. With the development of advanced surgical techniques, the flexible bronchoscope, an improved ability to interpret diagnostic patterns in histopathologic specimens and the advent of pharmacologic therapies that can induce remission or significantly slow the tempo of disease progression for many types of ILD, invasive testing has become more commonplace and accepted in the evaluation of these patients (1,6–8).

INDICATIONS AND TECHNIQUES FOR BRONCHOSCOPIC PROCEDURES

BRONCHOSCOPY

FB has been used in the clinical setting for over 40 years and can be performed with a high degree of safety by appropriately trained clinicians and support personnel. Bronchoscopy is generally well-tolerated and can be performed under

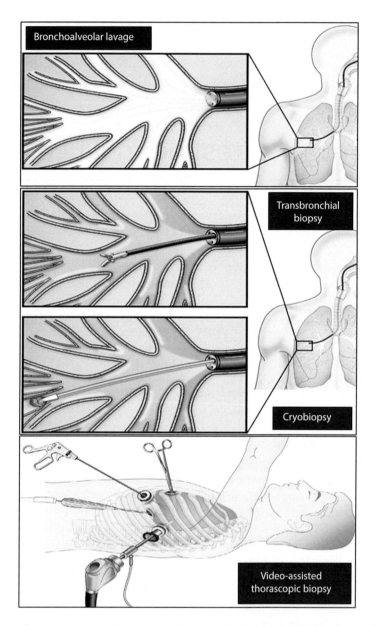

Figure 6.1 Invasive diagnostic procedures. BAL is best performed with the distal end of the broncho-scope wedged in a segmental bronchus. TBLB is best performed by passing a forceps to within 2–3 centimeters of the pleura under fluoroscopic guidance to obtain specimens. Similarly, a cryoprobe is passed in a similar location to obtain specimens via TBLCB. Finally, surgical lung biopsies are best performed with video-assistance, and procedures are typically performed with a maximum of three or four puncture sites.

moderate sedation with topical anaesthesia. Key safety aspects include adequate subject monitoring (heart rate, electrocardiogram tracing, blood pressure, continuous pulse oximetry), pre-procedure assessment of risk factors (significant cardiopulmonary compromise, recent ischaemic cardiac events, bleeding diatheses, unstable medical conditions), adequate training in bronchoscopic procedures, and the ability to promptly respond to complications that may occur during or following the procedure. The upper and lower airways should be completely inspected to detect any mucosal abnormalities. Pre-procedure HRCT scanning can be very useful to target areas of the lung that are most likely to yield diagnostic specimens when performing lavage or lung biopsy (9,10).

BRONCHOALVEOLAR LAVAGE

Bronchoalveolar lavage (BAL) (Figure 6.1) allows the retrieval of distal airspace cells, infectious agents (if present) and acellular components of airspace surface liquid (e.g. cytokines, other glycoproteins, surfactant components, markers consistent with gastroesophageal reflux and microaspiration). BAL can detect or exclude infection, and immune cell patterns can point to or strongly support specific ILD diagnoses (9). However, smoking can affect cell numbers and subsets as well as acellular components, and BAL must be performed properly to obtain an adequate specimen that accurately reflects components of airspace surface liquid from peripheral bronchoalveolar areas (Table 6.1). A total of at least 100 mL in divided aliquots should be used in a given segment when performing the lavage, and at least 30% of the total lavage fluid should be retrieved to ensure that adequate sampling of distal airspace cells and epithelial surface liquid has been accomplished. Additionally, a clinical laboratory must be available that can process and examine BAL fluids according to specific published guidelines so that an accurate interpretation can be made from the data that are obtained.

BAL as a stand-alone procedure is unlikely to provide a definitive ILD diagnosis, but it can provide valuable information that when combined with HRCT imaging and other clinical data may make or strongly implicate a specific diagnosis (Table 6.2). The ATS Task Force Report on BAL for

Table 6.1 Key aspects of performing bronchoalveolar lavage

Procedure	• Use pre-procedure HRCT to choose target site(s) • Right middle lobe or lingula give best return and can be used as target site if involvement of parenchyma on HRCT is diffuse • Place distal end of bronchoscope in wedge position (segmental or subsegmental bronchus) • Total instilled volume of isotonic saline should be 100–300 mL in three to five sequentially instilled and aspirated aliquots; total volume of retrieved fluid should be ≥30% of total instilled volume • Minimize aliquot dwell time (immediately aspirate after aliquot instillation is complete) • Avoid overloading target area with excessive fluid instillation (excessive distention can cause inflammatory mediator release) • Optimal volume for pooled BAL sample for cellular analysis is 10–20 mL
Specimen transport, processing and analysis	• Rapid transport to the clinical laboratory for processing and analysis is optimal • Cell counts can be obtained via haemocytometer or automated analyzer • Prepare slides via cytospin method and stain for nucleated immune cell identification and determination of differential cell count • Subject BAL aliquots to appropriate staining, molecular probes and culture if infection is a consideration (e.g. bacteria, mycobacteria, fungi, viruses as appropriate) • Perform lymphocyte subset determination only if such is considered useful for diagnosis (e.g. suspicion of sarcoidosis) • Ensure proper training of laboratory personnel for recognizing and identifying BAL cell types • Examine ≥300 nucleated BAL cell randomly per slide to obtain differential cell counts; average counts from multiple slides • Note presence of bronchial and squamous epithelial cells • Clinicians familiar with BAL cell patterns and ILD should interpret BAL cell patterns and other findings

Table 6.2 Interpretation of BAL findings

Observation	Suggested/consistent diagnosis
Lymphocytosis (>15%)	Sarcoidosis, HP, NSIP, CTD-ILD, IPAF, OP, drug reaction, CBD, LIP, lymphoproliferative disorder, infection (mycobacterial, viral)
Lymphocytes ≥25%	Sarcoidosis, HP, cellular NSIP, drug reaction, CBD, LIP, lymphoproliferative disorder, CTD-ILD, IPAF
Lymphocytosis with CD4/CD8 lymphocyte subset ratio >4	Highly specific for sarcoidosis (especially if other inflammatory cell types are not increased)
Eosinophilia (>1%)	Eosinophilic pneumonia, drug reaction, eosinophilic granulomatosis with polyangiitis, infection (*Pneumocystis*, helminths, fungal, bacterial), asthma, bronchiolitis, OP, ABPA, UIP/IPF
Eosinophils ≥25%	Eosinophilic pneumonia
Neutrophilia (>3%)	Infection, UIP/IPF, aspiration pneumonia, CTD-ILD, IPAF, ARDS, DAD, OP, pneumoconiosis, AIP, AEIPF, fibrotic HP, airway disorders (asthma, COPD, inhalation injury, bronchitis, bronchiolitis)
Neutrophils ≥50%	AIP, DAD, AEIPF, pulmonary infection
Milky BAL fluid with PAS-positive amorphous debris	PAP
Bloody fluid with increasing RBC content of sequential aliquots	DAH, pulmonary haemorrhage
High haemosiderin score	DAH, DAD
In vitro lymphocyte proliferative response to specific beryllium antigen	CBD
Expanded macrophage population containing smoking-related inclusions with no or minor increases in other cell types	DIP, RBILD
Prominent foamy macrophages	Amiodarone toxicity (also seen with amiodarone exposure without toxicity)
Monotypic lymphocytes	Pulmonary lymphoma
Malignant cells	Carcinoma
Squamous epithelial cells >5%	Aspiration of upper airway secretions; sample may be unsuitable for BAL analysis
Bronchial epithelial cells >5%	Sample may be unsuitable for BAL analysis
CD1a+ cells (Langerhans cells) ≥5% (immunohistochemistry on slide preparations much more reliable than flow cytometry)	PLCH

Abbreviations: AEIPF = acute exacerbation of idiopathic pulmonary fibrosis; AIP = acute interstitial pneumonia; ARDS = acute respiratory distress syndrome; CBD = chronic beryllium disease; COPD = chronic obstructive pulmonary disease; CPFE = combined pulmonary fibrosis and emphysema; CTD-ILD = connective tissue disease-associated interstitial lung disease; DAD = diffuse alveolar damage; DAH = diffuse alveolar haemorrhage; DIP = desquamative interstitial pneumonia; EP = eosinophilic pneumonia; HP = hypersensitivity pneumonitis; IIP = idiopathic interstitial pneumonia; IPAF = interstitial pneumonia with autoimmune features; IPF = idiopathic pulmonary fibrosis; LAM = lymphangioleiomyomatosis; LIP = lymphoid interstitial pneumonia; NSIP = non-specific interstitial pneumonia; OP = organizing pneumonia; PAP = pulmonary alveolar proteinosis; PLCH = pulmonary Langerhans cell histiocytosis; PPFE = pleuro-parenchymal fibroelastosis; RBILD = respiratory bronchiolitis interstitial lung disease; UIP = usual interstitial pneumonia.

the diagnosis of ILD recommends using recently obtained HRCT imaging to choose an appropriate segment of the lung and performing the lavage from a wedge position in a segmental bronchus (9). The right middle lobe or the lingula of the left upper lobe are likely the best regions to perform lavage when diffuse disease is present (fluid retrieval will usually be optimal in these locations), and areas with ground-glass opacification or profuse nodular change are more likely to provide useful diagnostic information rather than areas with extensive fibrosis. In addition to total and differential cell counts of nucleated immune cells, BAL fluid and sediment can be analysed for infection or the presence of malignant cells. The gross appearance of freshly retrieved BAL fluid may provide useful diagnostic information; progressively increasing amounts of blood in sequential aliquots are consistent with diffuse alveolar haemorrhage, and white-tan discoloration of BAL fluid with rapidly settling tan sediment due to the effects of gravity implicates pulmonary alveolar proteinosis as a diagnosis. Significant BAL lymphocytosis or eosinophilia may provide strong support for a specific diagnosis when combined with imaging and clinical data. However, routine determination of BAL lymphocyte subsets is unlikely to provide useful diagnostic information.

BAL is a very safe procedure, but complications may still occur. Over-distending a lung segment with excessive amounts of instilled saline should be avoided; this can increase the risk of complications such as post-bronchoscopy fever or more serious adverse events. BAL has also been reported to trigger acute exacerbations of idiopathic pulmonary fibrosis (IPF), but this is a rare complication of BAL.

ENDOSCOPIC LUNG BIOPSY

Transbronchial lung biopsy (TBLB) has been used to obtain lung tissue for histopathologic analysis for over 50 years (Figure 6.1). While such biopsies were originally obtained through a rigid bronchoscope, which allowed only the middle and lower lobes to be biopsied, development of the flexible bronchoscope also allowed sampling from upper lobe regions. Endobronchial biopsies may provide useful tissue sampling, especially if mucosal abnormalities such as superficial nodules (e.g. sarcoidosis) or ulceration (e.g. vasculitis, infection) are present. As is the

case for performing BAL, TBLB is best performed away from areas of advanced fibrosis (to avoid areas where it is difficult to pinch off tissue from the surrounding parenchyma) and target areas of ground-glass opacities or more profuse nodules. Multiple biopsies, when performed with an adequately sized forceps (e.g. 2.2 mm alligator forceps) while using fluoroscopic guidance to place the forceps in an appropriate distal biopsy site, can provide good tissue sampling for some forms of ILD such as sarcoidosis or organizing pneumonia. However, TBLB is likely to be non-diagnostic if areas of extensive and/or advanced fibrotic disease are targeted, especially if HRCT imaging shows features consistent with a form of IIP. Additionally, due to the small size of the biopsy specimens, crush artefact may obscure features that could be otherwise diagnostic. TBLB can be especially useful when granulomatous inflammation consistent with a diagnosis of sarcoidosis is present (8), and TBLB can be combined with endobronchial ultrasound (EBUS)-guided transbronchial needle aspiration of enlarged mediastinal and hilar lymph nodes (if such are found to present on HRCT) to increase the likelihood of obtaining diagnostic tissue (11,12). Finally, combining BAL data with TBLB may narrow a differential diagnosis or increase confidence in making a final diagnosis without having to resort to more invasive procedures (Table 6.3).

Transbronchial lung cryobiopsy (TBLCB), which uses compressed gas to freeze lung tissue at the site where a cryoprobe is placed (which is then retracted to retrieve an attached tissue specimen) is a method (Figure 6.1) that was first reported in 2009 for the diagnosis of diffuse lung disease (13). TBLCB can retrieve much larger tissue specimens with better preserved tissue architecture than TBLB allows, and it can substantially increase the utility of bronchoscopy when attempting to make a confident diagnosis of IPF in patients who lack a typical UIP pattern on HRCT (14,15). When properly performed, results can approach that of surgical lung biopsy (SLB); specimen size is considerably larger than that obtained via TBLB, distortion of tissue due to crush artefacts is substantially less, and diagnostic yield ranges up to 80%. However, some studies have reported a significant incidence of haemorrhage or pneumothorax with TBLCB (15).

Histopathologic patterns in specimens obtained via TBLCB or TBLB could be integrated with other analytic techniques such as genomic analysis

Table 6.3 Utility of endoscopic lung biopsy and/or bronchoalveolar lavage in ILD diagnosis

ILD diagnosis	BAL potentially useful?	TBLB potentially diagnostic/ useful?	Confidence potentially improved by combining TBLB with BAL
Sarcoidosis	Yes	Yes	+++
HP (acute)	Yes	Yes	+++
Organizing pneumonia	Yes	Yes	+++
Drug reaction	Yes	Yes	+++
Eosinophilic pneumonia	Yes	Yes	+++
IPF	Lymphocytosis suggests alternative diagnosis	±	±
NSIP	Lymphocytosis supports cellular NSIP	Yes (cellular NSIP)	+
DIP/RBILD	±	±	+
PAP	Yes	Yes	++
CTD-ILD or IPAF	Lymphocytosis	Yes	++
DAH	Yes	±	+
Pulmonary capillaritis	±	Yes	+
Granulomatosis with polyangiitis	±	Yes	+
LIP	±	Yes	+
Pulmonary lymphoma	Yes	Yes	+
Lymphangitic carcinomatosis	Yes	Yes	+
Multifocal lung adenocarcinoma	±	Yes	+
PLCH	±	Yes	+
CBD	Yes	Yes	+++
LAM	Yes	Yes	+
Amyloidosis	No	Yes	±
AIP or AEIPF	Yes	No	No

Abbreviations: AEIPF = acute exacerbation of idiopathic pulmonary fibrosis; AIP = acute interstitial pneumonia; BAL = bronchoalveolar lavage; CBD = chronic beryllium disease; CTD-ILD = connective tissue disease-associated interstitial lung disease; DAD = diffuse alveolar damage; DAH = diffuse alveolar haemorrhage; DIP = desquamative interstitial pneumonia; EP = eosinophilic pneumonia; HP = hypersensitivity pneumonitis; IPAF = interstitial pneumonia with autoimmune features; IPF = idiopathic pulmonary fibrosis; LAM = lymphangioleiomyomatosis; LIP = lymphoid interstitial pneumonia; NSIP = non-specific interstitial pneumonia; OP = organizing pneumonia; PAP = pulmonary alveolar proteinosis; PLCH = pulmonary Langerhans cell histiocytosis; RBILD = respiratory bronchiolitis interstitial lung disease; TBLB = transbronchial lung biopsy; UIP = usual interstitial pneumonia.

to yield a more precise diagnosis and profiling of specific forms of ILD at the time of diagnosis. Newer approaches that use molecular-based methods that allow transcriptomic profiling that can detect gene signatures that are specific for an ILD entity such as UIP may allow accurate differentiation of UIP from non-UIP forms of ILD (16), and these methods may be adaptable to specimens retrieved via TBLB or TBLCB.

ENDOSCOPIC ULTRASOUND AND NEEDLE ASPIRATION

Transbronchial needle aspiration (TBNA) of mediastinal lesions was first reported in the 1940s, and the advent of endobronchial ultrasound (EBUS) has allowed EBUS-TBNA to be readily performed on enlarged hilar or mediastinal lymph nodes, which can be especially helpful in diagnosing and staging neoplasms (17). The yield for finding non-caseating granulomas via EBUS-TBNA has been reported to range up to 94% when sampling mediastinal nodes in patients with suspected sarcoidosis. EBUS-TBNA can also be used to diagnose tuberculosis, lymphoma or histoplasmosis in the appropriate clinical setting (17).

SURGICAL LUNG BIOPSY

A confident diagnosis of IPF can be made without proceeding to invasive procedures if HRCT shows a definite usual interstitial pneumonia (UIP) pattern and there is no evidence of an alternative cause such as the presence of a connective tissue disease (CTD) (18). However, if a definite UIP pattern is lacking, making a definitive diagnosis requires proceeding to an invasive procedure if risks to the patient do not outweigh the potential benefit of undergoing an invasive procedure (19). If the ultimate diagnosis is a form of IIP, especially IPF, a bronchoscopic approach (especially if TBLCB is not available and only BAL and/or TBLB can be performed) is less likely to facilitate establishing a definitive diagnosis, and SLB may be a better approach (20,21). A SLB specimen obtained via video-assisted thoracic surgery (VATS) or open biopsy is, if properly performed, likely to provide an excellent specimen that preserves tissue architecture and shows a histopathologic pattern that can usually be interpreted as definitively diagnostic of a specific disease entity. However, although SLB has been considered the gold standard (particularly when combined with multidisciplinary discussion of all clinical data by experts to attain diagnostic agreement), one must weigh risks and benefits when considering a SLB, especially when patients are elderly and/or frail, have ventilatory compromise, are known to have moderate-to-severe pulmonary hypertension or have multiple co-morbidities (19,21). A VATS biopsy (Figure 6.1) has a significantly lower risk of mortality than open lung biopsy, although the reported risk of 30-day mortality with a VATS biopsy ranges from 1% to 3%, and other significant complications such as prolonged air leak, broncho-pleural fistula, trapped lung, infection or persistent chest pain may occur (19). Additionally, the mortality risk for patients whose ultimate diagnosis is IPF may be even higher, especially if an open lung biopsy is performed rather than a VATS

biopsy. SLB (or thoracic surgery for other indications such as malignancy) has been associated with triggering acute exacerbations of IPF. However, confirming the diagnosis of UIP/IPF and differentiating among specific forms of IIP may not be possible without performing a SLB.

OTHER PROCEDURES THAT MAY PROVIDE USEFUL DIAGNOSTIC INFORMATION

Evaluation of pleural abnormalities

Pleural abnormalities may occur with various types of ILD, such as CTD-ILD, EP, sarcoidosis, pleuro-parenchymal fibroelastosis (PPFE), drug pneumotoxicity, pneumoconiosis (asbestosis, CWP, silicosis) and amyloidosis. Therefore, pleural thickening or fluid may need to be evaluated to determine the nature of pleural changes and to rule out infection. Thoracentesis, closed pleural biopsy or thoracoscopy can all be useful in specific settings to determine the cause of pleural disease or accumulation of pleural fluid that occurs in the setting of suspected or established ILD.

Detection of pathologic gastroesophageal reflux

An excessive degree of gastroesophageal reflux (GER) combined with subclinical aspiration episodes may play a significant role in the pathogenesis of some forms of ILD (22), and GER disease (GERD) has been highly associated with IPF and with other forms of fibrotic ILD, such as systemic sclerosis (scleroderma). It has been suggested that aspiration may play a role in triggering and/or driving lung inflammation and fibrosis in IPF and scleroderma and may be a cause of AEIPF events. Additionally, oesophageal dysmotility, which is highly prevalent in patients with scleroderma and may be found in other forms of CTD, may especially predispose such patients to aspiration of gastric contents that can trigger lung injury, inflammation, and a fibrotic response. Therefore, using diagnostic techniques, such as oesophageal manometry to detect oesophageal functional abnormalities plus impedance/pH testing to detect and characterize GER, may detect abnormalities that could potentially play an important role in initiating, driving and/or exacerbating some forms of ILD.

Table 6.4 Advantages, disadvantages, and risks of invasive diagnostic procedures

Procedure	Advantages	Disadvantages	Risks
BAL	• High degree of safety • Easily performed • Can detect infection • Can provide airspace nucleated immune cell profile (e.g. lymphocytosis) • Can be very useful with acute onset ILD (e.g. EP)	• Usually non-diagnostic as stand-alone test • Clinical lab must be able to process and analyse cells and fluid adequately	• Post-bronchoscopy fever • May trigger AEIPF episode • Infection
Endoscopic biopsy	• Safe if performed by adequately trained individuals • Can target multiple sites • Can retrieve diagnostic tissue for many forms of ILD	• Relatively small specimen size • Unable to adequately sample tissue in areas of significant fibrosis (limited sensitivity for IIP) • Tissue crush artefact is common • Fluoroscopy is required to visualize forceps positioning	• Haemorrhage • Pneumothorax • Infection • May trigger AEIPF episode
EBUS with needle aspiration	• Can diagnose sarcoidosis • Useful to diagnose malignancy, tuberculosis, histoplasmosis	• Equipment and laboratory support availability • Limited utility (useful only if adenopathy is present)	• Haemorrhage • Infection
Bronchoscopic cryobiopsy	• Larger tissue specimens with preserved architecture • Can provide tissue that is diagnostic of IIP (up to 80% yield)	• May have excessive bleeding • Not available at many centres	• Haemorrhage • Pneumothorax • Infection • May trigger AEIPF episode
Surgical lung biopsy (VATS)	• Controlled setting • Can visualize pleural surface • Larger size lung tissue specimens can be sampled • Multiple lung geographic regions can be biopsied • Optimal specimens for histopathologic analysis	• Requires general anaesthesia • Pleural catheter must be placed and maintained post-op • Requires pain control post-op • May not be readily available at smaller centers	• Infection • Prolonged air leak • Bronchopleural fistula • Trapped lung • Persistent/refractory incision site pain • 1%–3% 30-day mortality • May trigger AEIPF episode

Abbreviations: AEIPF = acute exacerbation of IPF; BAL = bronchoalveolar lavage; EBUS = endobronchial ultrasound; EP = eosinophilic pneumonia; ILD = interstitial lung disease; VATS = video-assisted thoracoscopic surgery.

SUMMARY

Many tools are available that clinicians can use to attain an accurate diagnosis of ILD. Less invasive testing, such as bronchoscopy with BAL, has an excellent safety profile and may suffice to reach a confident diagnosis, but more invasive testing may be required. The various advantages, disadvantages and potential risks of the various invasive procedures that clinicians can use to diagnose specific forms of ILD should be carefully considered when clinical decision making is undertaken to reach an ultimate diagnosis (Table 6.4). A key component of the diagnostic approach is having clinicians, radiologists and pathologists with expertise in ILD participating in a multidisciplinary discussion (Figure 6.2), whenever needed, to optimize the validity of a

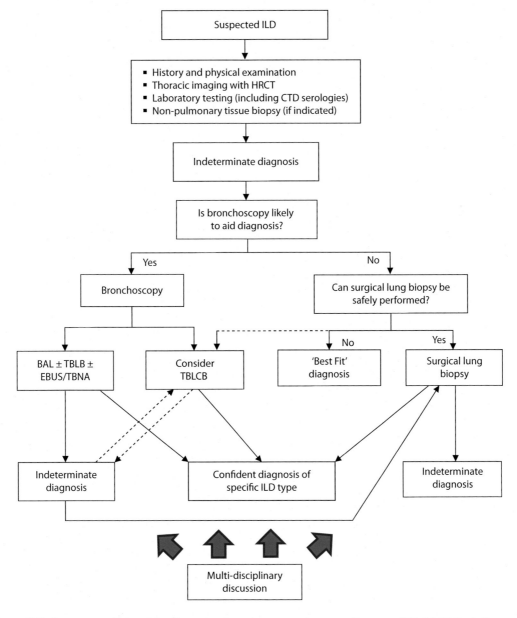

Figure 6.2 A suggested algorithm for using invasive procedures to diagnose ILD. Multidisciplinary discussions among specialists enhance the accuracy and confidence of specific diagnoses.

final diagnosis (23). Advances in diagnostic instruments and techniques in the coming decades, such as using a machine-learning approach to obtain a genomic signature via high-dimensional transcriptional data obtained from biopsy tissue (16), will hopefully lead to the ability to use procedures that are less invasive than SLB to obtain specimens from which specific forms of ILD can be confidently diagnosed. As such approaches become refined and enter the clinical arena, a crucial step toward providing personalized medicine for patients with ILD will undoubtedly be enhanced.

REFERENCES

1. Meyer KC. Diagnosis and management of interstitial lung disease. *Translat Respir Med.* 2014;2:4. doi: 10.1186/2213-0802-2-4. eCollection 2014.
2. Collard HR, King TE Jr. Diffuse lung disease: Classification and evaluation. In: Baughman RP, du Bois RM, eds. *Diffuse Lung Disease: A Practical Approach.* 2nd ed. New York, NY: Springer; 2012:85–100.
3. Walsh SL, Hansell DM. High-resolution CT of interstitial lung disease: A continuous evolution. *Semin Respir Crit Care Med.* 2014;35(1):129–44.
4. Sverzellati N, Lynch DA, Hansell DM, Johkoh T, King TE Jr, Travis WD. American Thoracic Society-European Respiratory Society Classification of the Idiopathic Interstitial Pneumonias: Advances in Knowledge since 2002. *Radiographics.* 2015;35(7): 1849–71.
5. Oikonomou A. Role of imaging in the diagnosis of diffuse and interstitial lung diseases. *Curr Opin Pulm Med.* 2014;20(5):517–24.
6. Leslie KO. My approach to interstitial lung disease using clinical, radiological and histopathological patterns. *J Clin Pathol.* 2009;62:387–401.
7. Poletti V, Chilosi M, Olivieri D. Diagnostic invasive procedures in diffuse infiltrative lung diseases. *Respiration.* 2004;71(2): 107–19.
8. Chapman JT, Mehta AC. Bronchoscopy in sarcoidosis: Diagnostic and therapeutic interventions. *Curr Opin Pulm Med.* 2003; 9(5):402–7.
9. Meyer KC, Raghu G, Baughman RP Brown KK, Costabel U, du Bois RM et al. An official American Thoracic Society clinical practice guideline: The clinical utility of bronchoalveolar lavage cellular analysis in interstitial lung disease. *Am J Respir Crit Care Med.* 2012;185(9):1004–14.
10. Meyer KC, Raghu G. Bronchoalveolar lavage for the evaluation of interstitial lung disease: Is it clinically useful? *Eur Respir J.* 2011;38(4):761–9.
11. Gupta D, Dadhwal DS, Agarwal R, Gupta N, Bal A, Aggarwal AN. Endobronchial ultrasound-guided transbronchial needle aspiration vs conventional transbronchial needle aspiration in the diagnosis of sarcoidosis. *Chest.* 2014;146(3):547–56.
12. Trisolini R, Lazzari Agli L, Tinelli C, De Silvestri A, Scotti V, Patelli M. Endobronchial ultrasound-guided transbronchial needle aspiration for diagnosis of sarcoidosis in clinically unselected study populations. *Respirology.* 2015;20(2):226–34.
13. Babiak A, Hetzel J, Krishna G, Fritz P, Moeller P, Balli T et al. Transbronchial cryobiopsy: A new tool for lung biopsies. *Respiration.* 2009;78(2):203–8.
14. Ravaglia C, Bonifazi M, Wells AU, Tomassetti S, Gurioli C, Piciucchi S et al. Safety and diagnostic yield of transbronchial lung cryobiopsy in diffuse parenchymal lung diseases: A comparative study versus video-assisted thoracoscopic lung biopsy and a systematic review of the literature. *Respiration.* 2016;91(3):215–27.
15. Johannson KA, Marcoux VS, Ronksley PE, Ryerson CJ. Diagnostic yield and complications of transbronchial lung cryobiopsy for interstitial lung disease. A systematic review and Metaanalysis. *Ann Am Thorac Soc.* 2016;13(10):1828–38.
16. Kim SY, Diggans J, Pankratz D, Huang J, Pagan M, Sindy N et al. Classification of usual interstitial pneumonia in patients with interstitial lung disease: Assessment of a machine learning approach using high-dimensional transcriptional data. *Lancet Respir Med.* 2015;3(6):473–82.
17. Wahidi MM, Herth F, Yasufuku K, Shepherd RW, Yarmus L, Chawla M Technical aspects of endobronchial ultrasound-guided

transbronchial needle aspiration: CHEST guideline and expert panel report. *Chest.* 2016;149(3):816–35.

18. Raghu G, Collard HR, Egan JJ, Martinez FJ, Behr J, Brown KK et al. An official ATS/ERS/JRS/ALAT statement: Idiopathic pulmonary fibrosis: Evidence-based guidelines for diagnosis and management. *Am J Respir Crit Care Med.* 2011;183(6):788–824.

19. Nguyen W, Meyer KC. Surgical lung biopsy for the diagnosis of interstitial lung disease: A review of the literature and recommendations for optimizing safety and efficacy. *Sarcoidosis Vasc Diffuse Lung Dis.* 2013; 30(1):3–16.

20. Sheth JS, Belperio JA, Fishbein MC, Kazerooni EA, Lagstein A, Murray S et al. Utility of transbronchial vs surgical lung biopsy in the diagnosis of suspected fibrotic interstitial lung disease. *Chest.* 2017;151(2):389–99.

21. Raj R, Raparia K, Lynch DA, Brown KK. Surgical lung biopsy for interstitial lung diseases. *Chest.* 2017;151(5):1131–40.

22. Raghu G, Meyer KC. Silent gastro-oesophageal reflux and microaspiration in IPF: Mounting evidence for anti-reflux therapy? *Eur Respir J.* 2012;39(2):242–45.

23. Flaherty KR, King TE Jr, Raghu G, Lynch JP 3rd, Colby TV, Travis WD et al. Idiopathic interstitial pneumonia: What is the effect of a multidisciplinary approach to diagnosis? *Am J Respir Crit Care Med.* 2004;170(8):904–10.

7

General principles of ILD diagnosis and management

MELISSA WICKREMASINGHE, RICHARD J HEWITT AND ATHOL WELLS

INTRODUCTION

Interstitial lung diseases (ILDs) are a heterogenous group of over 300 diseases with a limited repertoire of treatment options. Diagnosis can present a considerable challenge to the clinician. ILDs can be classified into disorders of known cause, granulomatous diseases, other causes and idiopathic interstitial pneumonias (IIPs) (Figure 7.1), with the latter group updated in 2013 to include major, minor IIPs and unclassifiable disease (Table 7.1) (1,2). Classifications can be justified for a number of reasons including the identification of important distinctions in the natural history and treated course. This applies to the IIP classification, which consists of the definition of clinical entities built on histopathologic and high-resolution computed tomography (HRCT) features. The IIP classification can be used as a template for the formulation of an optimal management plan. By contrast, an aetiologic classification of ILD is useful for diseases that are managed by removing the underlying cause or treating the underlying cause directly. However, it does not discriminate between important idiopathic ILD entities and fails to address emergent phenotypes that are diagnostically challenging (3).

Placing an individual patient in a discrete IIP category is not always straightforward. Overlapping pathological and radiological patterns, discrepancies between the two modalities, inter-observer disagreement and incomplete data

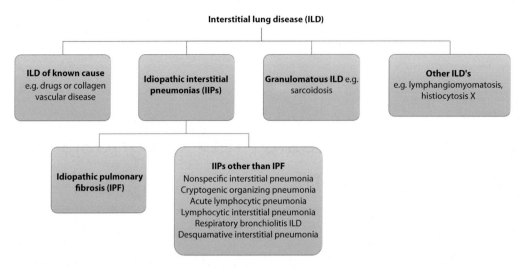

Figure 7.1 Classification of interstitial lung disease (ILD). (Adapted from Thomeer M et al. *Eur Respir J.* 2008;31(3):585–91.)

in individual patients contribute to diagnostic uncertainty. Dependence upon a single diagnostic modality such as surgical lung biopsy (SLB) does not address these problems and can be misleading. Since the millennium, it has become generally accepted that histologic findings should no longer be viewed as a diagnostic reference standard. Indeed, no diagnostic reference standard currently exists in ILD. Multidisciplinary diagnosis (MDD), a process that consists of the integration and reconciliation of clinical, HRCT and histologic data,

is now the preferred diagnostic approach in ILD and is the only means of reaching a broad diagnostic consensus. MDD has yet to be validated against an external standard, in part because any theoretical reference standard would itself be integrated within a MDD.

In the majority of ILD patients, an established diagnosis can be made from diagnostic criteria defined by expert groups. However, in many patients, a confident diagnosis cannot be made by this means, leading to therapeutic paralysis. A 'working diagnosis' must instead be constructed, based on a combination of suggestive diagnostic features and clinical reasoning, often including observation of serial disease behaviour. In this way, it is usually possible to make useful statements on likely outcome and to formulate a logical management plan. Reliance solely on inflexible diagnostic criteria, built on an incomplete evidence base (especially with regard to rare disorders and emerging entities) often results in major diagnostic and management uncertainty which is stressful for patients and for clinicians alike. A broad approach based on clinical reasoning allows the clinician to overcome difficulties related to the striking variability in quantity, quality and interpretation of data which is ever-present in routine clinical practice. Recognized diagnostic criteria are an essential starting point in the construction of an ILD diagnosis. However, criteria applied at a single point in time are often inconclusive and in many cases, accurate diagnosis requires the

Table 7.1 Revised classification of idiopathic interstitial pneumonias

Revised classification of idiopathic interstitial pneumonias: Multidisciplinary diagnoses
Major Idiopathic Interstitial Pneumonias
Idiopathic pulmonary fibrosis
Idiopathic non-specific interstitial pneumonia
Respiratory bronchiolitis–interstitial lung disease
Desquamative interstitial lung disease
Cryptogenic organizing pneumonia
Acute interstitial pneumonia
Rare Idiopathic Interstitial Pneumonias
Idiopathic lymphoid interstitial pneumonia
Idiopathic pleuroparenchymal
Unclassifiable Idiopathic Interstitial Pneumonias

Source: Adapted from Travis WD et al. *Am J Respir Crit Care Med.* 2013;188(6):733–48.

integration of responsiveness to therapy and disease progression over time.

Thus, major diagnostic uncertainty is an ever-present reality for ILD clinicians. Experienced ILD practitioners have generally developed personal diagnostic and management algorithms with skill sets to deal with areas of disease that are less well researched or protocolized. The art of ILD management, when the diagnosis is uncertain, lies in the distillation of information that identifies (a) logical treatment goals and (b) the optimal method of monitoring disease in order to evaluate whether treatment goals are met. It is often possible to be decisive in this regard when the disease is unclassifiable.

The disease behaviour classification (DBC), first put forward in 2003 was refined and formally proposed for use in unclassifiable disease in the updated IIP classification of 2013 (2,4). In this approach, patterns of disease behaviour can be broadly subdivided into 'reversible and self-limited'; 'reversible with risk of progression'; 'stable with residual disease'; 'progressive, irreversible disease with potential for stabilization'; and 'progressive, irreversible disease despite therapy' (exemplified by IPF) (Table 7.2). This pragmatic approach can be used as a basis for confident management in unclassifiable disease with the logic of management immediately apparent. Confidence on likely outcome and optimal management often greatly reduces patient stress: with that in mind, disease behaviour 'diagnoses' can usefully be stated in lieu of a histospecific diagnosis, when one cannot be made. Indeed, even when a specific diagnosis is attainable, the definition of goals and optimal management and monitoring using the disease behaviour classification is a useful tool in ensuring good communication with the patient.

However, the disease behaviour classification should not be regarded as a substitute for exact diagnosis but rather a powerful complementary approach. Knowledge of the exact diagnosis establishes what patterns of disease behaviour are possible in an individual patient. Thus, the formal classification of the IIPs and the broad classification of disease behaviour both address the essential goal of diagnosis: to identify the likely future natural history and treated course of disease.

It is possible that in the future, greater management precision than is currently possible will be achieved with the integration of biomarkers and genetic data in a mechanism-based classification (3).

Table 7.2 Characterization of different disease patterns as a guide to treatment approach and monitoring strategy

Pattern of disease	Broad treatment approach	Monitoring strategy
Self-limited inflammation	Remove cause/observe or treat (usually with steroid therapy) in short term	Short-term monitoring to confirm disease regression
Major inflammation with risk of progression to fibrosis	Anti-inflammatory therapy (eventually high dose) for a response, then rationalize lower-dose therapy to maintain response	Monitor in short term to quantify the response to high-dose treatment; monitor less frequently in long term to ensure that gains are preserved
Stable fibrosis	Observation alone (in treatment-naïve patients, a treatment trial may be considered)	Long-term monitoring to ensure ongoing stability
Progressive fibrosis with stabilization realistic	Treat with steroid or immunosuppressive therapy, high dose if necessary to stabilize; consider anti-fibrotic drugs	Long-term monitoring to confirm absence of progression
Inexorably progressive fibrosis	Consider therapy to slow progression but avoid toxic agents	Long-term monitoring to quantify rapidity of progression with a view to transplant or for effective palliation

Source: Adapted from Wells A. In: Spiro SG, Silvestri GA, Agustí ABT, eds. *Clinical Respiratory Medicine.* 4th ed. Philadelphia: WB Saunders; 2012:588–98.

The ultimate goal of this approach is 'personalized medicine' with optimal treatment regimens based on core pathogenetic pathways that vary greatly in disorders that we currently regard as single disease entities. However, it is entirely uncertain whether this approach will hold the key to future diagnostic evaluation.

In this chapter, the fundamentals of ILD diagnosis are discussed, including (a) an algorithm-based approach and key strategic questions; (b) review of the role of and evidence for MDT approach; and (c) discussion of the most difficult diagnostic challenges faced by ILD clinicians. The core principles of ILD management are discussed with reference both to management when the diagnosis is established and the problem of unclassifiable disease.

GENERAL PRINCIPLES OF ILD DIAGNOSIS

A diagnostic algorithm is shown in Figure 7.2. In a case of suspected ILD a full history, examination and investigations are laid out in detail in Chapter 5. This includes HRCT, lung function tests and detailed blood tests. In a minority, a diagnostic radiological pattern and clinical context may be

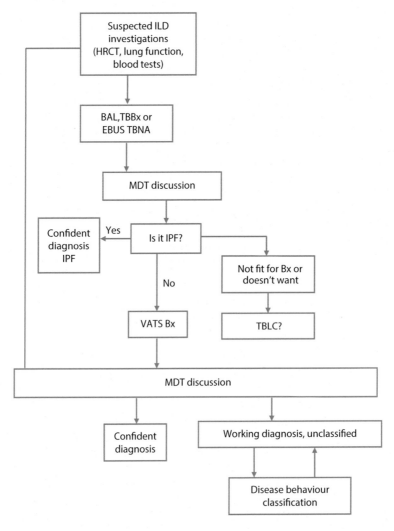

Figure 7.2 Diagnostic algorithm for interstitial lung disease (ILD) (Abbreviations: BAL = bronchoalveolar lavage; EBUS TBNA = endobronchial ultrasound-guided transbronchial needle aspirate; TBBx = transbronchial lung biopsy; TBLC = transbronchial lung cryobiopsy; VATS Bx = video-assisted thoracoscopic surgery lung biopsy). (Adapted from Behr J. *Clin Chest Med.* 2012;33(1):1–10.)

immediately evident, e.g. classical UIP (usual interstitial pneumonia) or lymphangioleiomyomatosis (LAM). However the majority will be considered for further investigation such as bronchoalveolar lavage (BAL), transbronchial biopsy, transbronchial lung cryobiopsy or endobronchial ultrasound-guided transbronchial needle aspirate (EBUS TBNA).

BAL is discussed in detail elsewhere in this book. There is considerable variation in the use of BAL in ILD diagnostic algorithms, ranging from the routine performance of BAL in some European cohorts to the non-performance of BAL in the United States (6). However, a balanced approach can be justified, in which BAL is used in selected patients to answer specific clinical questions (7). The value added by BAL in patients with suspected IPF has not been definitively quantified, apart from a single under-powered study in which 8% of patients presenting with clinical and HRCT features compatible with IPF were found to have a BAL lymphocytosis of >30% and were ultimately diagnosed with chronic hypersensitivity pneumonitis (CHP) or non-specific interstitial pneumonia (NSIP) (8). In many patients with CHP, clinical and HRCT features overlap with IPF and the major utility of BAL in suspected IPF is in the identification of a significant lymphocytosis, often leading to a MDD of CHP. In occasional cases, a high profusion of asbestos bodies in BAL fluid may provide support for a diagnosis of asbestosis.

There is a growing international consensus that clinical, HRCT, BAL and other data (including serologic features suggesting the existence of an underlying connective tissue disease [CTD]) should be integrated in multidisciplinary team (MDT) discussion, before a decision is made to proceed to a diagnostic surgical biopsy. Surgical lung biopsy (SLB), once viewed as a diagnostic reference standard in ILD, has significant risks in elderly patients, especially if there are major co-morbidities, moderate-to-severe pulmonary function impairment, or an underlying diagnosis of IPF (9). The 2%–4% mortality associated with SLB is largely due to acute exacerbations occurring post-operatively and is associated with a high in-hospital mortality. However, it should not be forgotten that failure to make an accurate ILD diagnosis is associated with inaccurate management. Thus, SLB remains justified in ILD when the risks of the procedure are judged to be lower than the risks resulting from incomplete information.

Although histologic information is the most important diagnostic determinant in patients undergoing SLB, careful MDT review is required. In some cases, histological findings are discrepant with HRCT and clinical information. Occasionally, histologic patterns are difficult to classify, accounting for significant inter-observer variation between pathologists (10). The possibility of 'sampling error' should not be overlooked. In some patients with IPF, the cardinal histologic pattern of UIP may be admixed with areas of NSIP. For this reason, it is now standard practice to take biopsies from at least two sites, preferably from separate lobes.

The recent development of transbronchial lung cryobiopsy (TBLC) offers a less invasive approach with an acceptable diagnostic yield. In a recent meta-analysis, encompassing 16 series, the yield from cryobiopsy was 81%, applying equally to the definition of a histologic pattern and the formulation of a multidisciplinary diagnosis (11). TBLC may have particular utility in the confident identification of a UIP pattern in patients with suspected IPF (12). At the time of writing, TBLC is increasingly used as a routine diagnostic modality in European centres but has yet to be adopted elsewhere. Critical scrutiny is likely to centre on the risks of pneumothorax and bleeding and safety and diagnostic yield in less experienced hands.

THE MULTIDISCIPLINARY PROCESS

The concept of a consensus MDD was first described in 2002, although practiced in some referral centres in earlier decades. Previously, a histologic diagnosis had been regarded as the diagnostic reference standard. The aim of the MDT is to reach a working diagnosis in insufficiently characterized patients by consensus, with a minimum core group of a pathologist, radiologist and clinician. All potentially important clinical information for each patient is discussed, with reconciliation of clinical, imaging and histologic data.

It should be stressed at the outset that MDD in ILD is not a diagnostic reference standard. In part, this reflects difficulties in its validation: any test against which MDT diagnosis might be validated is, in reality, integrated into diagnosis. The multidisciplinary process exists because it is now acknowledged that there is no diagnostic reference standard in ILD: clinical, HRCT and histologic evaluation all have significant diagnostic limitations when used in isolation. Put simply, MDD is now the preferred diagnostic approach in ILD because it allows the integration of the evidence base with the act of clinical reasoning.

The value of the ILD MDT lies in dynamic interactive discussion, leading to higher inter-observer agreement and greater diagnostic confidence (13,14). MDT improves diagnostic agreement in ILDs within both community and academic centres (15). In a recent study, MDT discussion resulted in a change from the histological diagnosis in 30% and increased diagnostic confidence from 'probable' to 'confident' in a further 17% of cases (16). In another series, the MDT discussion led to a change in the ILD diagnosis in 48/90 (53%) patients (17).

With particular reference to IPF, the American Thoracic Society/European Respiratory Society/Japanese Respiratory Society/Latin American Thoracic Association (ATS/ERS/JRS/ALAT) 2011 guideline highlights the importance of MDD (18). However, it should be stressed that the formulaic approach to MDD in that document, consisting of the tabulated integration of histologic and HRCT data, is very different from the interactive discussion between clinicians, radiologists and pathologists which is the true essence of the MDT approach. This discrepancy largely reflects the fact that guideline statements are driven by the existing evidence base and a desire to formulate strict diagnostic criteria. The value of MDD lies in the fact that many patients do not meet current diagnostic criteria. In such cases, a diagnosis can be made only with the integration of data and clinical reasoning, in which all potentially relevant diagnostic information is considered in each patient. This includes non-standardized data (such as observed disease behaviour) which is highly informative in some cases but inconclusive or lacking in others. It can be argued that in evidence-based guideline statements, the diagnostic primacy of standardized diagnostic tools is over-emphasized and the important art of diagnosis by means of clinical reasoning is under-valued (19,20).

Despite its advantages, the MDT approach has significant limitations. Broadly parallel expertise in the three sub-specialties is required, and there is a danger that diagnostic decisions will be driven by the most experienced or most vocal group member. When formal diagnostic criteria are not met, the process is highly subjective. The end product consists of the formulation of a 'working diagnosis', made with variable confidence, with no immediate means of evaluating diagnostic accuracy.

In this regard, reassuring information comes from a recent study in which MDT diagnoses were made at seven expert centres from the same patient data (21). Although agreement on diagnosis was only moderately good overall, there was good agreement on a diagnosis of IPF, probably as a result of the widespread discussion of this problem in recent years. MDTs made the diagnosis of IPF more frequently and with greater confidence than clinicians and radiologists in isolation. Agreement on a diagnosis of CTD-ILD was also good, but there was poor agreement on CHP highlighting the need for the development of more robust diagnostic criteria for this disease.

THE MULTIDISCIPLINARY DIAGNOSIS OF IPF

The distinction between IPF and other ILDs is the most important task accomplished in multidisciplinary diagnosis (MDD). IPF is the most prevalent idiopathic ILD, has the worst outcome, and is now managed with anti-fibrotic therapy, with aggressive immunomodulation associated with a poor outcome. By contrast, other ILDs (with the exception of a handful of rare disorders) can be broadly conceptualized as forms of immune dysregulation. If this key distinction cannot be made with use of non-invasive tests, a decision must be made on whether to proceed to SLB or TBLC.

In the ATS/ERS/JRS/ALAT 2011 IPF guideline algorithm, diagnosis is deceptively straightforward. The assumption is made that if HRCT appearances are not classical for UIP in the correct clinical context, IPF can only be diagnosed by SLB: no alternative approach is suggested. However, as discussed earlier, SLB is impracticable in a major proportion of patients with suspected IPF for a number of reasons. In up to half of IPF patients, 2011 guideline diagnostic criteria are not satisfied, a SLB cannot be performed and disease must be viewed as unclassifiable, a scenario occurring most frequently with an HRCT appearance of 'possible UIP' in patients not undergoing surgical lung biopsy.

It should be acknowledged that the 2011 IPF guideline was developed when no proven treatment existed in IPF and it appeared reasonable to treat IPF and major differential diagnoses (HP, NSIP) with immunomodulation (generally triple therapy with low dose prednisolone, azathioprine and anti-oxidant therapy). At that time, patient management was not compromised by diagnostic uncertainty if IPF was suspected and rigorous IPF diagnostic criteria had advantages for study design. However, this is no longer the case. The large sub-group of IPF patients with non-classical HRCT appearances are, in effect, disenfranchised by current guideline criteria. Without a diagnosis of IPF, anti-fibrotic therapy will not be approved by regulatory bodies.

Pending guideline revision, MDTs can only act to reach 'working diagnoses' of IPF in this patient subset. Based on demographic data, absence of support for HP (exposure history, BAL findings) or CTD-ILD with a high likelihood of NSIP (clinical history, serologic findings) and, in some cases, observed deterioration despite immunomodulatory therapy, a diagnosis of IPF can and should often be made. A 'working diagnosis', made when formal criteria are not satisfied, is often highly confident and should serve as a basis for confident management. In other cases, when an alternative tentative diagnosis of HP or NSIP is made initially, subsequent review in a MDT meeting is appropriate if there is progression of disease despite treatment. Repetition of HRCT is useful as progression to a UIP-like appearance, compatible with IPF, is sometimes disclosed.

OTHER DIAGNOSTIC CHALLENGES FOR THE ILD CLINICIAN

Although specific diseases are discussed individually in other chapters, it is worth pulling together some challenging subtypes and emerging phenotypes in ILD that need further consideration of the general principles for their diagnosis and management. These include unclassifiable disease, interstitial pneumonia with autoimmune features (IPAF), sub-clinical disease, unrecognized CHP with a

UIP pattern, smoking-related ILD, an acute presentation and finally possible UIP.

SUB-CLINICAL DISEASE, INTERSTITIAL LUNG ABNORMALITIES AND EARLY DISEASE

With the advent of lung cancer screening programmes, limited interstitial abnormalities, termed 'interstitial lung abnormalities' (ILAs) are increasingly identified (22). In recent studies, the prevalence of ILAs has been 6%–7% in elderly cohorts, increasing in current or former heavy smokers, with the majority of ILAs consisting of limited sub-pleural reticulation (with a minority having an overtly fibrotic HRCT pattern). Recently, annual loss of forced vital capacity (FVC) of over 60 mL/year has been documented in subjects with progressive ILAs on serial HRCT (23). Importantly, FVC decline was found to be predictive of mortality. Thus it appears likely that ILAs represent early IPF in an important sub-group although, in the absence of biomarker or histologic information no immediate diagnosis of IPF can be made.

Given these observations, it is appropriate to monitor ILAs with annual PFT and HRCT. It should be expected that this recommendation will generate considerable patient concern, especially in patients who have a family history of lung fibrosis. However, a routine algorithm is required, given the desirability of early treatment in IPF and the increasing use of HRCT screening programs to detect lung cancer in current and former smokers.

ILAs should not be treated with anti-fibrotic agents but the sub-group with serial progression poses a particular difficulty for clinicians. In asymptomatic patients, the concept of 'sub-clinical IPF' is attractive but diagnostic SLB or TCLB should be considered before treatment is instituted. In established IPF, emerging data show that disease progression and treatment effects are virtually identical, irrespective of the initial FVC value (24,25). However, even when FVC values are well preserved in pharmaceutical trials, a large proportion of patients have symptoms or demonstrate desaturation during a 6-minute walk test. The role of anti-fibrotic therapy in sub-clinical asymptomatic IPF, in the absence of abnormal minute walk data, is not known.

INTERSTITIAL PNEUMONIA WITH AUTOIMMUNE FEATURES

Some patients with ILD have non-specific clinical features and serological evidence of an underlying autoimmune condition but these do not meet formal rheumatologic criteria for a CTD (26) This clinical scenario variously termed 'undifferentiated CTD-related ILD' and 'lung dominant CTD' is encountered both in NSIP and in patients with UIP on HRCT or biopsy. In the latter case, the differential diagnosis lies between ILD due to an occult CTD and IPF. The distinction is important as management differs radically between the two entities. It is known that in a handful of patients with typical clinical and HRCT features of IPF, anti-CCP antibody positivity can precede the clinical picture of rheumatoid arthritis by many years. A UIP pattern on HRCT or biopsy is also present in a minority of ILD patients with systemic sclerosis and, less frequently, in other CTDs.

The difficulty for clinicians is that until recently, no consensus has existed in published series as to the definition of this patient sub-group. An ERS/ATS research statement has now been published, outlining diagnostic criteria for 'interstitial pneumonia with autoimmune features' (IPAF) (27). The new term signifies the importance of standardizing diagnostic criteria in the hope that the prognostic significance and optimal management of IPAF will be clarified.

Diagnostic criteria for IPAF are shown in Table 7.3. It should be stressed that IPAF is not an established entity – it is likely that with further studies, diagnostic criteria will be modified. However, the IPAF designation does at least justify the empirical use of cautious immunomodulation as initial therapy in this patient sub-group (e.g. low-dose corticosteroid therapy, mycophenolate mofetil at a dose of 650 mg b.d.). Aggressive immunomodulation is less appropriate when the differential diagnosis is IPF, given the poor outcome with immune-modulation in the PANTHER IPF treatment trial (28).

UNCLASSIFIABLE DISEASE

Unclassifiable disease was introduced as a concept in the 2002 IIP consensus classification document and was formally recognized in the IIP classification in the 2013 updated document (2). The term 'unclassifiable disease' applies when a first-choice diagnosis cannot be stated with at least a 50% likelihood. Most commonly, disease is unclassifiable due to the absence of key data (most frequently, the non-performance of a biopsy), or discrepancies between clinical, imaging and histologic data.

Previous studies suggest that unclassifiable disease accounts for 9%–15% of all ILD cases (29–31). Many cases are deemed unclassifiable because a biopsy is contraindicated due to patient co-morbidity, age or patient preference. In the current era, fewer cases than previously have biopsies performed and so the frequency of unclassifiable ILD may be now higher than 10%. Although an experienced MDT group may reduce the proportion of patients that are considered unclassifiable, it is clear that a significant proportion of patients will remain unclassified. The most frequent differential diagnoses for unclassifiable cases are HP, IPF and NSIP (31).

In the study by Ryerson et al. 2013, cases with histopathologic features of 'end-stage' fibrotic disease were likely to be unclassifiable (31). Seventeen percent of patients with unclassifiable disease demonstrated a UIP pattern on HRCT, as judged by 2011 IPF guidelines definitions, whereas 50% of patients had a possible UIP pattern. With the planned revision of the IPF diagnostic guidelines in 2017/2018, it is likely that in many elderly patients with 'possible UIP' on HRCT, IPF diagnostic criteria will be met, reducing the prevalence of unclassifiable disease.

However, management of unclassifiable disease is likely to remain problematic. The disease behaviour classification (DBC) was endorsed for use in unclassifiable disease in the 2013 IIP classification update and serves to identify logical treatment goals and monitoring strategies (2). In a recent study the DBC and the previously validated ILD-gender age physiology (GAP) prognostic system were compared in a cohort of patients with unclassifiable ILD (32). The two systems were found to be complementary, providing independent prognostic guidance. In unclassifiable disease, the prognosis is intermediate between IPF and other ILDs, suggesting that IPF is, in reality, the diagnosis in a major sub-group (31,32). It appears likely that if TCLB is increasingly used internationally, the prevalence of unclassifiable disease will be reduced.

Table 7.3 Classification criteria for IPAF

Classification criteria for 'interstitial pneumonia with autoimmune features'

1. Presence of an interstitial pneumonia (by HRCT or surgical lung biopsy) *and*,
2. Exclusion of alternative aetiologies *and*,
3. Does not meet criteria of a defined connective tissue disease *and*,
4. At least one feature from at least two of these domains:

1. Clinical domain
   a. Distal digital fissuring (i.e. 'mechanic hands')
   b. Distal digital tip ulceration
   c. Inflammatory arthritis *or* polyarticular morning joint stiffness ≥60 min
   d. Palmar telangiectasia
   e. Raynaud phenomenon
   f. Unexplained digital oedema
   g. Unexplained fixed rash on the digital extensor surfaces (Gottron sign)
2. Serological domain
   a. ANA ≥1:320 titre, diffuse, speckled, homogenous patterns *or*
      i. ANA nucloelar pattern (any titre) *or*
      ii. ANA centromere pattern (any titre)
   b. Rheumatoid factor ≥2× upper limit of normal
   c. Anti-CCP
   d. Anti-dsDNA
   e. Anti-Ro (SS-A)
   f. Anti-La (SS-B)
   g. Anti-ribonucleoprotein
   h. Anti-Smith
   i. Anti-topoisomerase (Scl-70)
   j. Anti-tRNA synthetase (e.g. Jo-1, PL-7, PL-12; others are: EJ, OJ, KS, Zo, tRS)
   k. Anti-PM-Scl
   l. Anti-MDA-5
3. Morphological domain
   a. Suggestive radiology patterns by HRCT:
      i. NSIP
      ii. OP
      iii. NSIP with OP overlap
      iv. LIP
   b. Histopathology patterns or features by surgical lung biopsy:
      i. NSIP
      ii. OP
      iii. NSIP with OP overlap
      iv. LIP
      v. Interstitial lymphoid aggregates with germinal centres
      vi. Diffuse lymphoplasmacytic infiltration (with or without lymphoid follicles)
   c. Multi-compartment involvement (in addition to interstitial pneumonia):
      i. Unexplained pleural effusion or thickening
      ii. Unexplained pericardial effusion or thickening
      iii. Unexplained intrinsic airways disease[a] (by PFT, imaging or pathology)
      iv. Unexplained pulmonary vasculopathy

Source: Adapted from Fischer A et al. *Eur Respir J.* 2015;46(4):976–87.
Abbreviations: ANA = antinuclear antibody; HRCT = high-resolution computed tomography; LIP = lymphoid interstitial pneumonia; NSIP = non-specific interstitial pneumonia; OP = organizing pneumonia; PFT = pulmonary function testing.
[a] Includes airflow obstruction, bronchiolitis or bronchiectasis.

THE RECOGNITION OF UNDERLYING UIP AND ITS DIAGNOSTIC SIGNIFICANCE

Honeycombing, the cardinal HRCT feature of UIP, is not always easy to identify. Differentiating honeycombing from traction bronchiectasis or paraseptal emphysema can be challenging, even for experts (33). In an early study, interobserver agreement for honeycombing between expert thoracic radiologists was not clinically acceptable, with a weighted kappa coefficient of only 0.31 (34). In a later study of expert evaluation, higher kappa values (0.40–0.58) were achieved for the distinction between traction bronchiectasis, emphysema and honeycombing (33). In a recent study in which less experienced radiologists were included, acceptable agreement was achieved in designating HRCT appearances as UIP, possible UIP and 'inconsistent with UIP' (weighted kappa = 0.47) (35). However, the fact that agreement was, at best, moderate in all the above studies highlights the difficulty in identifying UIP on HRCT in many cases.

An important second problem is that UIP occurs in disorders other than IPF, especially in HP and CTD-ILD (Table 7.4). The need for a detailed exposure history and meticulous assessment for possible connective tissue disease has been highlighted earlier in this chapter and is especially important when UIP is present and a diagnosis other than IPF needs to be excluded. Many patients with features of IPF have exposures compatible with HP or asbestosis. In a recent study, the careful elicitation of occult environmental triggers led to the reclassification of IPF in many cases (36). Clinical signs suggestive of secondary UIP include inspiratory squeaks/squawks favouring HP and evidence of systemic connective tissue disorders.

In many cases, UIP is present on HRCT but there are ancillary features suggestive of diagnoses other than IPF (e.g. stand-alone bronchiectasis in

Table 7.4 Secondary UIP: Different contexts

Causes of secondary UIP pattern
Asbestosis
Chronic hypersensitivity pneumonitis
Rheumatoid arthritis-ILD
Other CTD
Fibrotic sarcoid

CTD, an upper zone predominance or the presence of areas of mosaic attenuation in HP). The presence of pleural thickening raises the possibility of CTD or asbestosis, with the latter more likely when there is pleural calcification. However, many patients with moderate asbestos exposure have related pleural abnormalities on HRCT, without the exposure threshold required to make a diagnosis of asbestosis.

The need for evaluation of ancillary features applies equally to histologic findings. HP should be suspected when UIP is associated with bronchocentric inflammation, bridging of fibrosis between airways, a significant component of organizing pneumonia or loosely formed granulomas. In CTD, UIP may be characterized by bronchocentric inflammation or enlarged lymphoid follicles. The diagnosis of asbestosis is suggested by a high profusion of asbestos bodies and a lower profusion of fibroblastic foci than generally seen in IPF.

Given the complexity of ancillary information in all three disciplines, the cut and thrust of MDT discussion is diagnostically crucial, with the need for interactive debate and the reconciliation of conflicting data. The considerable diagnostic difficulties are illustrated by the poor agreement between expert MDTs for diagnoses of HP and NSIP, when the same patient data are considered (21). In the same study, agreement on ancillary features of CTD was poor both for radiologists and pathologists. These data can be misinterpreted as a failure of MDD but in reality, MDT discussion serves an essential role in establishing that in some cases, diagnosis is genuinely uncertain and must be revisited with the integration of subsequent observed disease behaviour.

SMOKING-RELATED ILD

Smoking-related ILD (SRILD) encompasses a spectrum of lung disease associated with cigarette smoking, including cases of desquamative interstitial pneumonia (DIP), RBILD and a small subgroup of patients with smoking-related NSIP. IPF is not regarded as a SRILD, although associated with an increased prevalence of smoking.

The most difficult diagnostic challenge in SRILD is the interpretation of interstitial abnormalities on HRCT when there is concurrent emphysema. Agreement between radiologists on the presence or absence of honeycombing, a cardinal feature of IPF, is only moderate (33). In part, discrepant calls on honeycombing are due to the presence of emphysema: the combination of fine intralobular fibrosis and emphysema can simulate a UIP pattern. The integration of clinical information, including longitudinal disease behaviour, is required in such cases if a robust multidisciplinary diagnosis of IPF is to be achieved.

Combined pulmonary fibrosis and emphysema (CPFE), a distinct phenotype, is associated with a particularly high mortality in some reports, in part due to pulmonary hypertension (37). CPFE is characterized by paradoxical preservation of lung volumes, including FVC, but a severe reduction in measures of gas transfer. It is likely that the adverse outcomes and high prevalence of pulmonary hypertension in CPFE reflect the fact that lung disease is more severe when emphysema and pulmonary fibrosis co-exist than in patients with isolated pulmonary fibrosis.

ACUTE ILD

Acute ILD may occur *de novo* (not discussed in the current chapter) or as an acute exacerbation of a known ILD (most commonly IPF).

Acute exacerbations of IPF (AEIPF) have recently been redefined by consensus as an episode of worsening shortness of breath within the previous 30 days and the presence of ground-glass opacification (representing diffuse alveolar damage) on HRCT superimposed on a background of fibrosis, not explained by heart failure (38). The existence of known triggers such as infection or reflux with microaspiration is no longer considered to be an exclusion criterion. AEIPF have a notoriously poor outcome with the majority of patients dying during the cardinal hospital admission. In IPF the 3-month mortality was 81% in patients with more extensive disease (abnormal lung >50% on HRCT) and 55% in those with less extensive disease (HRCT abnormal lung <50%) (39). It is estimated that AEIPF occur in 10% of IPF patients per year. Acute exacerbations are seen less frequently in other fibrosing lung diseases including HP, RA (in which the outcome is as poor as in IPF) and other CTDs (in which the outcome is better). The unifying feature is the presence of diffuse alveolar damage.

In diseases other than IPF, there is a wide differential for clinical and HRCT features of an acute exacerbation and this applies especially to patients with CTD. The lack of specific imaging characteristics (essentially the rapid development of ground-glass opacification on a background of pre-existing ILD) means that the differential diagnosis should include cardiac failure, pulmonary embolism, worsening interstitial disease other than diffuse alveolar damage and, in patients on immunosuppressive therapy, opportunistic infection or drug-induced lung disease (e.g. methotrexate). In CTD, both drug-induced disease and intrinsic worsening of ILD are treated with aggressive immunosuppression and thus the key diagnostic test is BAL to exclude infection.

FAMILIAL DISEASE

A family history of ILD is evident in up to 20% of patients with ILD with genetic mutations increasingly being identified, some of which may have prognostic value (39). Patients with familial disease can present at a younger age, have atypical radiology and be difficult to classify (40).

GENERAL PRINCIPLES OF MANAGEMENT

Possible scenarios after the completion of diagnostic evaluation are

- An established MDD (likelihood >90%), based either on satisfaction of formal diagnostic criteria or on a highly confident 'working diagnosis' made by clinical reasoning
- A provisional diagnosis, made either with high confidence (likelihood 70%–90%) or low confidence (likelihood 50%–70%)
- Unclassifiable disease (diagnostic likelihood of first choice diagnosis, if any, <50%).

Optimal management consists of

- The designation of logical treatment goals and appropriate monitoring to ensure that goals are achieved
- Treatment of complications and co-morbidities
- Palliation of symptoms and optimization of quality of life
- End of life planning

Accurate management requires that doctors and patients work in partnership with clear communication of treatment goals and patient needs. The emergence of charters to benchmark standards of care expected by patients (e.g. IPF charter UK, European charter) is a much needed development. There is an increasing focus on patient-reported outcomes (formalizing patient views on the value of an intervention) and patient-reported experiences (documenting the patient journey and the quality of management pathways from the patient's perspective).

Good communication is essential. In many cases, confident prognostic evaluation and management, discussed for individual ILDs in other chapters, are based on a confident diagnosis. However, when the diagnosis is uncertain, the clear delineation of diagnostic uncertainties and the designation of logical treatment goals is required. In this regard, the disease behaviour classification is often helpful for its lack of medical jargon and clear statement of realistic treatment aims. It is also important to stress the ways in which observed disease behaviour may modify the management plan with time.

A key part of the doctor-patient dynamic is to introduce the concept of risk/benefit thinking, with an emphasis of the trade-off between treatment benefits and adverse effects from therapy. If this dialogue is not undertaken, the emergence of significant side effects is likely to seriously undermine confidence in medical advice. Moreover, if the patient is informed of likely side effects, it is often possible to continue therapies with temporary dose reductions or a period of treatment cessation followed by careful reintroduction or a change to alternative treatment.

A diagnosis of IPF can be viewed as a 'special case' as many patients are acutely aware of the prognostic implications. Communication of the diagnosis must be handled in a similar way to a diagnosis of malignancy, given the similarities in life expectancy between IPF and the more aggressive cancers. Nurse specialists have a pivotal role in ensuring that a management plan addresses not only treatment for the disease to improve life expectancy but also symptoms and quality of life in a holistic fashion.

A statement on likely outcomes is valued by most patients and this requires accurate prognostic evaluation. To a certain extent, the formulation of a confident diagnosis allows reported disease-specific outcomes to be discussed with the patient. In individual ILDs, the severity of disease at presentation is a key consideration – it is often helpful to indicate the impact of the disease using a simple scale of severity (e.g. a simple five-point scale, ranging from sub-clinical to end-stage disease). In some diseases, more nuanced staging systems exist (e.g. the GAP index in IPF [41], limited/extensive staging in lung disease in systemic sclerosis) but the challenge is to interpret the stage of disease in language readily understood by patients. In the future, molecular and genetic markers and signatures may be an important part of this process.

Even when the prognosis is likely to be good, it is necessary to stress that there is a wide range of possible outcomes. It is often helpful to indicate that even with expert evaluation, the clinician is required to make statements that capture the scenarios of 'good luck', 'average luck' and 'bad luck'. The importance of reviewing disease behaviour with time, as a guide to long-term outcome, can be emphasized to the patient.

If an ILD is difficult to classify and worsens significantly despite therapy in the next 6–12 months, the likelihood of IPF with atypical HRCT features increases substantially (hence the maxim 'if it behaves like IPF it probably is IPF'). In this scenario, further MDT evaluation should be undertaken, in order to make a working diagnosis of IPF which may be highly confident or provisional.

TREATMENT OPTIONS

Current therapies addressed at improving life expectancy and improving symptoms or delaying loss of quality of life can be broadly sub-divided into anti-fibrotic therapies (for IPF) and treatments of immune dysregulation, broadly appropriate in most non-IPF disorders. Specific therapies are addressed in detail in other chapters covering individual ILDs.

In general, treatment should be instituted early in the course of disease if there is major inflammation, especially when there is supervening fibrosis, or if progression of fibrotic disease can be expected. In some patients with HP, sarcoidosis or CTD-ILD, disease may be limited in extent or there is reason to believe that there is intrinsic stability. In these cases, careful observation without immediate intervention can be justified. However, in IPF, progression is the rule. The current ruling by the National Institute for Health and Care Excellence (NICE), the UK regulatory body, that anti-fibrotic therapy cannot be funded in IPF until the FVC level is less than 80% is not justified by existing evidence (which indicates that earlier treatment is effective) and is clearly driven by considerations other than the existing evidence base.

In relation to the disease behaviour classification, the following treatment strategies are appropriate:

- Careful observation
  - This applies to diseases in which there is self-limited inflammation, including cases with a known trigger which can be avoided (e.g. mild HP or drug-induced disease).
  - This also applies to the scenario of 'burnt out disease' in which there is limited lung fibrosis and it is reasonable to delay intervention in the hope that it will not be needed.
- Initial high-dose therapy
  - This approach is appropriate when there is major inflammation, requiring treatment in its own right, especially if there is supervening fibrosis. High-dose corticosteroid therapy to achieve a response is often sufficient (except in systemic sclerosis, in which there is a risk of steroid-induced renal crisis), but in many cases early immunosuppressive therapy is required.
  - Once a short-term response has been achieved and it is clear that additional improvement is not a realistic goal, it is important to identify the minimal dose of longer-term treatment required to preserve gains. It is often necessary to continue treatment for many years, in the hope that treatment cessation will eventually be achieved.
- Treatment to stabilize irreversible disease
  - It is often obvious at presentation that disease is progressive and irreversible but in non-IPF disorders such as other IIPs, HP, CTD-ILD and sarcoidosis, the prevention of disease progression is the cardinal treatment goal. In this scenario, high-dose initial treatment may achieve little but should always be undertaken if significant coexistent inflammation cannot be excluded.
  - As long-term therapy will usually be required, side effects are a key consideration. In some cases, low-dose corticosteroid therapy may suffice but when disease is already extensive, an immunosuppressive agent may also be needed.
- Treatment to slow the progression of irreversible disease
  - This aim applies to those patients in whom the initial goal is long-term stabilization of disease but there is inexorable disease progression despite treatment. Retardation of disease progression is a worthwhile goal, provided that side effects are not prohibitive.
  - In IPF, this treatment goal can be articulated from the outset. There is now convincing evidence that anti-fibrotic therapy retards disease progression in IPF but no suggestion that long-term stabilization is achievable.
  - In patients with inexorably progressive fibrotic disease, other treatment options include lung transplantation and enrolment in trials of novel agents. Timely referral to a transplant unit before disease is pre-terminal is essential. If there are no overt contraindications to transplantation, progression to a DLCO level of <40% should prompt consideration of referral.

The above schema applies to treatments used in an attempt to improve life expectancy (with the important second goal of improving symptoms and quality of life). Other interventions are wholly symptomatic and this includes pulmonary rehabilitation and the optimal use of oxygen therapy, not addressed further in this chapter.

In advanced disease, early palliative care involvement is appropriate. Palliative care physicians are essentially specialists in maximizing quality of life and their involvement long before disease is pre-terminal is often highly fruitful. It is necessary to confront the misconception that palliative care input is useful only in the last weeks of life. Planning for end-stage care is a difficult art in which palliative care expertise is pivotal and is discussed elsewhere.

CO-MORBID CONDITIONS

The detection and management of co-morbid conditions and complications in ILD are essential and are covered thoroughly in Chapter 25 and elsewhere. Briefly, one must investigate for or address a number of co-morbidities or complications.

PULMONARY HYPERTENSION

Pulmonary hypertension (PH) is a common finding in advanced ILD and denotes a poor prognosis when severe. Specialist evaluation may be necessary, both to confirm the diagnosis and for consideration of targeted pulmonary hypertension therapies in carefully selected cases.

SLEEP-DISORDERED BREATHING

This should be identified, if necessary with polysomnography, and symptomatic obstructive sleep apnoea (OSA) treated on quality-of-life grounds and importantly to prevent significant hypoxia worsening any pulmonary hypertension particularly in those under consideration for transplantation.

IMMUNITY AGAINST INFLUENZA AND PNEUMOCOCCAL INFECTIONS

Vaccination, prompt treatment of infection with antibiotics and avoidance of infectious contacts are advised. Infections can be a driver of disease and trigger acute exacerbations.

GASTRO-EOSOPHAGEAL REFLUX DISEASE

The reported prevalence of gastro-eosophageal reflux disease (GORD) in IPF is variable (42). In some diseases such as scleroderma GORD is a prominent feature and requires treatment. The role of GORD in IPF disease pathogenesis is contentious, and data regarding the role for routine antacid therapy in limiting disease progression are conflicting so further prospective studies are required (43).

LUNG CANCER

The prevalence of lung cancer in patients with IPF is increased (prevalence reported as 15% in one study), and it clearly influences survival (44) and a high index of suspicion of this should be maintained.

CARDIAC DISEASE

Coronary artery disease (CAD) is a co-morbidity seen in over 60% of IPF patients (45). Direct cardiac involvement is an important disease-specific consideration in sarcoidosis and CTDs particularly scleroderma and idiopathic inflammatory myopathies.

SUMMARY

The diagnostic process in ILD can be challenging with major diagnostic uncertainty a reality for today's ILD clinician. The MDT allows integration of evidence base, patient data and clinical reasoning in these challenging cases to achieve a consensus. The disease behaviour classification can be used as a powerful complementary approach to diagnosis as a basis for a confident management plan in challenging cases with unclassifiable disease. In the future greater diagnostic and management precision may become available by integration of biomarker and genetic data in a mechanism-based classification system but until then the general principles for diagnosis and management laid out in this chapter will need to be used.

REFERENCES

1. Demedts M, Costabel U. ATS/ERS international multidisciplinary consensus classification of the idiopathic interstitial pneumonias. *Eur Respir J.* 2002;19(5):794–6.
2. Travis WD, Costabel U, Hansell DM, King TE, Lynch DA, Nicholson AG et al. An official American Thoracic Society/European Respiratory Society statement: Update of the international multidisciplinary classification of the idiopathic interstitial pneumonias. *Am J Respir Crit Care Med.* 2013;188(6):733–48.
3. Ryerson CJ, Collard HR. Update on the diagnosis and classification of ILD. *Curr Opin Pulm Med.* 2013;19(5):453–9.
4. Wells A. Chapter 46 – Approach to diagnosis of diffuse lung disease. In: Spiro

SG, Silvestri GA, Agustí ABT, eds. *Clinical Respiratory Medicine*. 4th ed. Philadelphia, PA: WB Saunders; 2012:588–98.

5. Behr J. Approach to the diagnosis of interstitial lung disease. *Clin Chest Med*. 2012;33(1):1–10.

6. Behr J, Kreuter M, Hoeper MM, Wirtz H, Klotsche J, Kosche D et al. Management of patients with idiopathic pulmonary fibrosis in clinical practice: The INSIGHTS-IPF registry. *Eur Respir J*. 2015;46(1):186–96.

7. Wells AU. Managing diagnostic procedures in idiopathic pulmonary fibrosis. *Eur Respir Rev*. 2013;22(128):158–62.

8. Ohshimo S, Bonella F, Cui A, Beume M, Kohno N, Guzman J et al. Significance of bronchoalveolar lavage for the diagnosis of idiopathic pulmonary fibrosis. *Am J Crit Care Med*. 2009;179(11):1043–7.

9. Hutchinson JP, Fogarty AW, McKeever TM, Hubbard RB. In-hospital mortality following surgical lung biopsy for interstitial lung disease in the USA: 2000–2011. *Am J Respir Crit Care Med*. 2015;193:1161–7.

10. Thomeer M, Demedts M, Behr J, Buhl R, Costabel U, Flower CDR et al. Multidisciplinary interobserver agreement in the diagnosis of idiopathic pulmonary fibrosis. *Eur Respir J*. 2008;31(3):585–91.

11. Ravaglia C, Bonifazi M, Wells AU, Tomassetti S, Gurioli C, Piciucchi S et al. Safety and diagnostic yield of transbronchial lung cryobiopsy in diffuse parenchymal lung diseases: A comparative study versus video-assisted thoracoscopic lung biopsy and a systematic review of the literature. *Respiration*. 2016;91(3):215–27.

12. Tomassetti S, Wells AU, Costabel U, Cavazza A, Colby T V, Rossi G et al. Bronchoscopic lung cryobiopsy increases diagnostic confidence in the multidisciplinary diagnosis of idiopathic pulmonary fibrosis. *Am J Respir Crit Care Med*. 2016;193(7):745–52.

13. Tomassetti S, Piciucchi S, Tantalocco P, Dubini A, Poletti V. The multidisciplinary approach in the diagnosis of idiopathic pulmonary fibrosis: A patient case-based review. *Eur Respir Rev*. 2015;24(135):69–77.

14. Flaherty KR, King TE, Raghu G, Lynch JP, Colby T V, Travis WD et al. Idiopathic

interstitial pneumonia: What is the effect of a multidisciplinary approach to diagnosis? *Am J Respir Crit Care Med*. 2004;170(8):904–10.

15. Flaherty KR, Andrei AC, King TE, Raghu G, Colby T V, Wells A et al. Idiopathic interstitial pneumonia: Do community and academic physicians agree on diagnosis? *Am J Respir Crit Care Med*. 2007;175(10):1054–60.

16. Burge P, Reynolds J, Trotter S, Burge G, Walters G. Histologist's original opinion compared with multidisciplinary team in determining diagnosis in interstitial lung disease. *Thorax*. 2016;72(3):280–1.

17. Jo HE, Glaspole IN, Levin KC, McCormack SR, Mahar AM, Cooper WA et al. Clinical impact of the interstitial lung disease multidisciplinary service. *Respirology*. 2016;21(8):1438–44.

18. Raghu G, Collard HR, Egan JJ, Martinez FJ, Behr J, Brown KK et al. An Official ATS/ERS/JRS/ALAT Statement: Idiopathic pulmonary fibrosis: Evidence-based guidelines for diagnosis and management. *Am J Respir Crit Care Med*. 2011;183(6):788–824.

19. Wells AU. Any fool can make a rule and any fool will mind it. *BMC Med*. 2016;14(1):23.

20. Behr J. Guidelines or guidance for better idiopathic pulmonary fibrosis management? *BMC Med*. 2016;14(1):24.

21. Walsh SLF, Wells AU, Desai SR, Poletti V, Piciucchi S, Dubini A et al. Multicentre evaluation of multidisciplinary team meeting agreement on diagnosis in diffuse parenchymal lung disease: A case-cohort study. *Lancet Respir Med*. 2016;4(7):557–65.

22. Jin GY, Lynch D, Chawla A, Garg K, Tammemagi MC, Sahin H et al. Interstitial lung abnormalities in a CT lung cancer screening population: Prevalence and progression rate. *Radiology*. 2013;268(2):563–71.

23. Araki T, Putman RK, Hatabu H, Gao W, Dupuis J, Latourelle JC et al. Development and progression of interstitial lung abnormalities in the Framingham heart study. *Am J Respir Crit Care Med*. 2016;194(12):1514–22.

24. Kolb M, Richeldi L, Behr J, Maher TM, Tang W, Stowasser S et al. Nintedanib in patients with idiopathic pulmonary fibrosis and preserved lung volume. *Thorax*. 2017;72:340–6.

25. Noble PW, Albera C, Bradford WZ, Costabel U, Du Bois RM, Fagan EA et al. Pirfenidone for idiopathic pulmonary fibrosis: Analysis of pooled data from three multinational phase 3 trials. *Eur Respir J.* 2016;47(1):243–53.

26. Kinder BW, Collard HR, Koth L, Daikh DI, Wolters PJ, Elicker B et al. Idiopathic nonspecific interstitial pneumonia: Lung manifestation of undifferentiated connective tissue disease? *Am J Respir Crit Care Med.* 2007;176(7):691–7.

27. Fischer A, Antoniou KM, Brown KK, Cadranel J, Corte TJ, Du Bois RM et al. An official European Respiratory Society/ American Thoracic Society research statement: Interstitial pneumonia with autoimmune features. *Eur Respir J.* 2015;46(4):976–87.

28. Idiopathic Pulmonary Fibrosis Clinical Research Network, Raghu G, Anstrom KJ, King TE, Lasky JA, Martinez FJ. Prednisone, azathioprine, and N-acetylcysteine for pulmonary fibrosis. *N Engl J Med.* 2012;366(21):1968–77.

29. Karakatsani A, Papakosta D, Rapti A, Antoniou KM, Dimadi M, Markopoulou A et al. Epidemiology of interstitial lung diseases in Greece. *Respir Med.* 2009;103(8):1122–9.

30. Thomeer MJ, Vansteenkiste J, Verbeken EK, Demedts M. Interstitial lung diseases: Characteristics at diagnosis and mortality risk assessment. *Respir Med.* 2004;98(6):567–73.

31. Ryerson CJ, Urbania TH, Richeldi L, Mooney JJ, Lee JS, Jones KD et al. Prevalence and prognosis of unclassifiable interstitial lung disease. *Eur Respir J.* 2013;42(3):750–7.

32. Hyldgaard C, Bendstrup E, Wells AU, Hilberg O. Unclassifiable interstitial lung diseases: Clinical characteristics and survival. *Respirology.* 2017;22(3):494–500.

33. Watadani T, Sakai F, Johkoh T, Noma S, Akira M, Fujimoto K et al. Interobserver variability in the CT assessment of honeycombing in the lungs. *Radiology.* 2013;266(3):936–44.

34. Lynch DA, Godwin JD, Safrin S, Starko KM, Hormel P, Brown KK et al. High-resolution computed tomography in idiopathic pulmonary fibrosis: Diagnosis and prognosis. *Am J Respir Crit Care Med.* 2005;172(4): 488–93.

35. Walsh SLF, Calandriello L, Sverzellati N, Wells AU, Hansell DM, Observer UIP. Interobserver agreement for the ATS/ERS/ JRS/ALAT criteria for a UIP pattern on CT. *Thorax.* 2016;71(1):45–51.

36. Morell F, Villar A, Montero M-Á, Muñoz X, Colby T V, Pipvath S et al. Chronic hypersensitivity pneumonitis in patients diagnosed with idiopathic pulmonary fibrosis: A prospective case-cohort study. *Lancet Respir Med.* 2013;1(9):685–94.

37. Cottin V, Cordier JF. Combined pulmonary fibrosis and emphysema: An experimental and clinically relevant phenotype. *Am J Respir Crit Care Med.* 2005;172(12):1605; author reply 1605-6.

38. Collard HR, Ryerson CJ, Corte TJ, Jenkins G, Kondoh Y, Lederer DJ et al. Acute exacerbation of idiopathic pulmonary fibrosis an international working group report. *Am J Respir Crit Care Med.* 2016;194(3):265–75.

39. García-Sancho C, Buendía-Roldán I, Fernández-Plata MR, Navarro C, Pérez-Padilla R, Vargas MH et al. Familial pulmonary fibrosis is the strongest risk factor for idiopathic pulmonary fibrosis. *Respir Med.* 2011;105(12):1902–7.

40. Lee HY, Seo JB, Steele MP, Schwarz MI, Brown KK, Loyd JE et al. High-resolution CT scan findings in familial interstitial pneumonia do not conform to those of idiopathic interstitial pneumonia. *Chest.* 2012;142(6):1577–83.

41. Ley B, Ryerson CJ, Vittinghoff E, Ryu JH, Tomassetti S, Lee JS et al. A multidimensional index and staging system for idiopathic pulmonary fibrosis. *Ann Intern Med.* 2012;156(10):684–91.

42. Raghu G, Amatto VC, Behr J, Stowasser S. Comorbidities in idiopathic pulmonary fibrosis patients: A systematic literature review. *Eur Respir J.* 2015;46(4):1113–30.

43. Margaritopoulos GA, Antoniou KM, Wells AU. Comorbidities in interstitial lung diseases. *Eur Respir Rev.* 2017;26(143).

44. Kreuter M, Ehlers-Tenenbaum S, Palmowski K, Bruhwyler J, Oltmanns U, Muley T et al. Impact of comorbidities on mortality in patients with idiopathic pulmonary fibrosis. *PLoS One*. 2016;11(3):1–18.

45. Nathan SD, Basavaraj A, Reichner C, Shlobin OA, Ahmad S, Kiernan J et al. Prevalence and impact of coronary artery disease in idiopathic pulmonary fibrosis. *Respir Med*. 2010;104(7):1035–41.

8

Idiopathic pulmonary fibrosis: Epidemiology, natural history and pathophysiology

ZULMA YUNT, JEFFREY J SWIGRIS AND AMY L OLSON

EPIDEMIOLOGY OF IDIOPATHIC PULMONARY FIBROSIS

BACKGROUND

While idiopathic pulmonary fibrosis (IPF) is the most common of the idiopathic interstitial pneumonias (1), it was once considered a rare, orphan disease. Today, epidemiologic studies suggest that the burden of IPF is considerably greater than previously recognized, and is growing. This highlights the importance of ongoing research into this devastating disease.

In the past, a number of factors have hampered investigators in their conduct of large-scale epidemiologic studies in IPF: (1) the condition was thought to be rare; (2) diagnostic criteria and modalities were evolving (e.g. high-resolution computed tomography); and (3) *International Classification of Diseases* (*ICD*) codes lacked a specific code for IPF. More recently, these limitations have been overcome with the development of large population databases (both national and international) that include healthcare claims information to determine incidence and prevalence, death certificate databases to determine mortality rates and the development of *ICD* codes that allow researchers to specifically identify IPF and fibrotic lung disease (post-inflammatory pulmonary fibrosis [PIPF]).

Unfortunately, there are limitations associated with the use of these large datasets including diagnostic validity (e.g. was the diagnosis of IPF correct?) and under-coding (e.g. in a patient with IPF, was the diagnosis recorded either in the healthcare claims database or on the death certificate?). Smaller population-based studies are likely to have more accurate diagnoses, but it is not clear that local trends represent national trends. Although both of these types of studies have limitations, they allow for a general understanding of the burden and trends in IPF.

INCIDENCE, PREVALENCE AND TRENDS OVER TIME

The incidence of disease is a rate defined as 'the number of new cases of a disease that occur during a specified period of time in a population at risk for developing the disease', while the prevalence of disease is a ratio and is defined as 'the number of affected persons present in the population at a specific time divided by the number of persons in the population at that time' (2).

The United States

In the early 1990s, a National Heart, Lung, and Blood Institute (NHLBI) Workshop summary reported that little data were available on the occurrence of IPF in the general population (3). Following this, in 1994, Coultas and colleagues published the first regional epidemiologic investigation into the incidence and prevalence of interstitial lung diseases – including IPF – in persons over 18 years of age in the United States (4). They established a population-based registry in Bernalillo County, New Mexico, using primary care and pulmonary physician's records, pathology reports, hospital discharge diagnoses, death certificates and autopsies, and collected data from 1988 to 1993. They reported the incidence of IPF as 10.7 per 100,000 person-years in men and 7.4 per 100,000 person-years in women. The prevalence of IPF was 20.2 cases per 100,000 persons in men and 13.2 cases per 100,000 persons overall. When stratified by age and gender, both the incidence and prevalence of IPF were higher in men than in women and increased with increasing age.

Using data from 1996 to 2000, Raghu and colleagues examined the incidence and prevalence of IPF using data from a healthcare claims processing centre (5). This processing centre services a healthcare plan that covers approximately 3 million persons residing in 20 states – mostly in the South Atlantic, South Central, and North Central Regions of the United States. Using these data, they then estimated IPF incidence and prevalence for the entire United States. Using broad case-finding criteria (age >18, one or more medical encounters for IPF (*ICD-9* code 516.3), and no medical encounters with diagnostic codes for any other type of ILD after an IPF encounter, they estimated an incidence rate of 16.3 per 100,000 persons/year and a prevalence of 42.7 per 100,000 persons, respectively. Using narrow case-finding criteria (the broad case definition in addition to at least one medical claim with a procedure code for a surgical lung biopsy, transbronchial biopsy or computed tomography of the thorax), the estimated incidence rate and prevalence were 6.8 per 100,000 persons/year and 14 per 100,000 persons, respectively. Similar to the findings of Coultas and colleagues, both the incidence and prevalence increased with age, and there were higher rates in men than women. From these two studies it appeared that the incidence and prevalence had increased – but definitive evidence was lacking for this trend given the uncertainty that these broad case-finding criteria accurately captured patients with lone IPF.

Using data from patients evaluated at their centre between 1997 and 2005, Fernández-Pérez and colleagues completed a population-based, historical cohort study in Olmsted County, Minnesota (6). These investigators likewise created narrow and broad case-finding criteria. Narrow criteria included a usual interstitial pneumonia (UIP) pattern of surgical lung biopsy or a definite UIP pattern on high-resolution computed tomography (HRCT), while broad criteria included a possible UIP pattern on HRCT scan. The age- and sex-adjusted incidence (for those over the age of 50) was 8.8 cases per 100,000 person-years (95% CI = 5.3–12.4) and 17.4 cases per 100,000 person-years (95% CI = 12.4–22.4) using the narrow and broad definitions, respectively. The age- and sex-adjusted prevalence (for those over the age of 50) was 27.9 cases per 100,000 persons (95% CI = 10.4–45.4) and 63 cases per 100,000 persons (95% CI = 36.4–89.6). These investigators found a decrease in the incidence rate over the last 3 years of the study. Given the small number of incident cases in this study (47 cases based on broad-case finding criteria), it is not clear that these results can be considered representative of national trends during this period of time.

Using a 5% random sample of Medicare beneficiaries (aged 65 years and older) from 2001 to 2011 and using *ICD*-9 codes 516.3 (IPF) and 515 (post-inflammatory pulmonary fibrosis [PIPF]), Raghu and colleagues completed a second large-scale epidemiologic study to determine the annual incidence and cumulative prevalence of IPF (7). Over this time period, the incidence of IPF remained stable with an overall estimate of 93.7 cases per 100,000 person-years (95% CI = 91.9–95.4). However, the annual cumulative prevalence increased from 202.2 cases per 100,000 persons in 2001 to 494.2 cases per 100,000 persons in 2011. These investigators also found that cases diagnosed in 2007 had longer survival times (4 years [95% CI = 3.8–4.5]) than those diagnosed in the earlier years (3.3 years [95% CI = 3–3.8]), explaining – in part – the stable incidence rates, but the increasing cumulative prevalence.

Given the stable incidence, but increasing prevalence, in Medicare beneficiaries from 2001 to 2011, Raghu and colleagues then examined a younger population for comparison (8). Using an administrative patient claims dataset that encompassed more than 45 managed care health plans covering more than 89 million people, they determined the incidence and prevalence of cases aged 18–64 from 2005 to 2010. Using a narrow case-finding definition, the annual incidence decreased from 2.9 to 2.4 new cases per 100,000 person-years and the annual prevalence ranged from 4.6 to 6.7 per 100,000 person-years over this period of time. Using a broad case-finding definition, the annual incidence decreased from 5.1 to 3.6 new cases per 100,000 person-years and the annual prevalence range from 8.4 to 11.3 per 100,000 person-years. Unlike the stable incidence and increasing prevalence noted in the older, Medicare population, in this younger cohort the incidence declined over time while the prevalence plateaued. These trends were mainly driven by younger patients (18–44 years), suggesting that they are the result of more accurate IPF diagnoses in the later time periods.

Recently, using the HealthCore Integrated Research Database, Esposito and colleagues examined the positive predictive value (PPV) of a broad case definition of IPF (*ICD*-9 code 516.3 or 515). The broad definition entailed an IPF diagnosis made by a physician and no alternative diagnosis 6 months prior or after (9). This definition was found to have a PPV of 44.4% (95% CI = 29.6%–60%), suggesting that using a health claims database overestimates both the incidence and the prevalence of IPF. Using this database and the broad case-finding definition, investigators determined an incidence of 14.6 per 100,000 person-years and a prevalence of 125.2 per 100,000 persons over time period from 2006 to 2012 after correcting for the PPV and standardizing the claims cohort to the US population.

Comparison of the two most comparable studies that used national healthcare databases, Raghu (7) and Esposito (9), it appears that the incidence and prevalence of IPF have trended up over time (Table 8.1). Unlike a diagnosis of cancer, which results in mandatory reporting of disease and allows for more precise estimates of incidence, prevalence and mortality rates, there is no mandatory reporting of IPF in the United States or elsewhere (10). However, efforts are underway to start a national IPF patient registry, which may more precisely expand our understanding of the epidemiology of IPF.

The United Kingdom

Large-scale epidemiologic studies from the United Kingdom have reported an increase in the incidence of IPF over time. Using a large longitudinal, general practice database in the United Kingdom and the diagnostic codes for 'cryptogenic fibrosing alveolitis' and 'idiopathic pulmonary fibrosis' (these clinical terms had been used interchangeably), Gribbin and colleagues found that the overall incidence of IPF doubled from 1991 to 2003 (11). The overall crude incidence of IPF was 4.6 cases per 100,000 person-years, and the annual increase in the incidence of IPF was 11% per year (rate ratio 1.11; 95% CI = 1.09–1.13). These investigators could not determine if the increase in incidence was related to an actual increase in disease burden, or was due to other factors such as improved diagnostic accuracy given the expanding use of HRCT over this time period.

Using the same database, Navaratnam and colleagues expanded on this prior work (10). In their

Table 8.1 Incidence and prevalence of IPF in United States

Study	Time period	Incidence in men (per 100,000 persons/year)	Incidence in women (per 100,000 persons/year)	Prevalence in men (per 100,000 population)	Prevalence in women (per 100,000 population)
Coultas et al. (4) (age >18)	1988–1993	10.7 cases	7.4 cases	20.2 cases	13.2 cases
Raghu et al. (5) (age >18)	1996–2000	Incidence in men and women		Prevalence in men and women	
Narrow definition		6.8 cases		14.0 cases	
Broad definition		16.3 cases		42.7 cases	
Fernández-Pérez et al. (6) (age >50)	1997–2005	Incidence in men and women (from 1997 to 2005)		Prevalence in men and women (in 2005)	
Narrow definition		8.8 cases		27.9 cases	
Broad definition		17.4 cases		63 cases	
Raghu et al. (7) (age >65)	2001–2011	Incidence in men and women		Prevalence in men and women	
Broad definition		93.7 cases		202.2 cases (in 2001) 494.5 cases (in 2011)	
Raghu et al. (8) (age 18–64)	2005–2010	Incidence in men and women		Prevalence in men and women	
Narrow definition		2.9 cases (2005) 2.4 cases (2010)		4.6 cases (2005) 6.7 cases (2010 – plateaued)	
Broad definition		5.1 cases (2005) 3.6 cases (2010)		8.4 cases (2005) 11.3 cases (2010 – plateaued)	
Esposito et al. (9) (age 50–100)	2006–2012				
Broad definition		14.6 cases		125.2 cases	

study, the diagnostic codes were expanded to include not only 'cryptogenic fibrosing alveolitis' and 'idiopathic pulmonary fibrosis', but also other fibrotic diagnostic codes including 'diffuse pulmonary fibrosis', 'idiopathic fibrosing alveolitis NOS' and 'Hamman–Rich syndrome', in an attempt to capture all cases of IPF. This group of fibrotic diseases was termed IPF-clinical syndrome (IPF-CS). From 2000 to 2008, the overall crude incidence of IPF-CS was 7.44 per 100,000 person-years – nearly double the incidence rate of the prior decade. Further, the incidence of IPF-CS increased by 5% annually over this time period (rate ratio 1.05; 95% CI = 1.03–1.06) – or at a somewhat slower rate than the prior decade. It remained unclear if these findings represented a true increase in disease burden, or were the result of increased awareness given the then recently published international consensus statement on the diagnosis and treatment of IPF (12) and/or the beginning of multi-centre treatment trials for IPF. (13,14)

Canada

Using two national administrative databases from the Canadian Institute for Health Information, Hopkins and colleagues examined the incidence and prevalence of IPF in Canada from 2007 to 2011 (15). Using broad and narrow case-finding definitions – they reported a broad incidence and prevalence in men of 21.3 per 100,000 person-years and 45.3 per 100,000 persons and a narrow incidence and prevalence of 10.5 per 100,000 person-years and 22.3 per 100,000 persons. In women, the broad incidence and prevalence were of 16.2 per 100,000 persons-years and 38.2 per 100,000 persons, while the incidence and prevalence were 7.4 per 100,000 person-years and 17.7 per 100,000 persons. These estimates were in line with those seen in the United States and the United Kingdom.

Other countries

Although beyond the scope of this chapter, Hutchinson and colleagues recently published a systematic review on the global incidence of IPF. In general, the incidence of IPF appeared to be increasing worldwide and rates seemed to be converging. As more countries begin to collect large-scale data on IPF, a better understanding of the global incidence of IPF will be possible (16).

MORTALITY RATES AND TRENDS OVER TIME

Mortality rates are defined as the total number of deaths from a cause in 1 year divided by the number of people alive within that population at midyear (17). Death certificate data and national census data allow for this calculation. In a disease that is lethal within a relatively short period of time – such as in IPF – mortality rates should parallel incidence rates. Thus, trends in mortality rates may increase our confidence when reviewing trends in incidence rates.

The validity of death certificate data has not been fully investigated. In the new era of *ICD-10* coding, Hutchinson and colleagues recently examined the death certificates from 124 IPF deaths in the United Kingdom. Of these deaths, 82% had a diagnostic code somewhere on the death certificate for IPF (J84.1) or interstitial lung disease unspecified (ILD-U) (J84.9). Most deaths were coded correctly as IPF (92%), and only 8% were coded as ILD-U. This suggests that death certificate data may underestimate mortality rates by ~20% (18). It is unclear if these findings apply to death certificate data from other countries, and more research on the validity of death certificate data is needed.

The United States

Using US death certificate data from 1979 to 1991, Mannino and colleagues reported that the age-adjusted mortality from pulmonary fibrosis (PF) (*ICD-9* codes 516.3 [IPF] and 515 [PIPF]) increased from 48.6 deaths per million to 50.9 deaths per million – or 4.7% – in men, and increased from 21.4 deaths per million to 27.3 deaths per million – or 27.1% – in women. Geographic variation was identified within this study; mortality rates were higher in the West and Southeast, and were lower in the Midwest and Northeast (19).

Expanding on this work, our group examined US death certificate data from 1992 to 2003. PF mortality rates increased from 49.7 deaths per million to 64.3 death per million – or 29.4% – in men, and from 42.3 deaths per million to 58.4 deaths per million – or 38.1% – in women. Similar to Mannino and colleagues, we found mortality rates increased with increasing age, were higher in men than in women, and were increasing at a faster pace in women than in men (20).

Hutchinson and colleagues recently examined US death certificate data from 2000 to 2010. Using the broad *ICD-10* code J84 (other interstitial lung diseases, but includes IPF and ILD-U) and only 'underlying cause of death' on death certificates, mortality rates increased by 1% per year (annual increase 1.01; 95% CI = 1.011–1.014). In 2010, the age-adjusted mortality rate was 7.8 per 100,000 persons (or 78 deaths per million).

Other countries

Hutchinson and colleagues also examined death certificate data from ten other countries including England and Wales, Australia, Canada, Japan, Northern Ireland, New Zealand, Scotland, Spain and Sweden from 2000 to 2010 (18). Using the broad *ICD-10* code J84 and the death certificate 'underlying cause of death' only, these investigators found that mortality rates increased in all countries from 1% to 4% per year, except in Northern Ireland where data years were limited (from 2009 to 2011) and the increase was large (25%). A meta-analysis of rate ratios from all eleven countries (including the United States) showed a 2% annual increase over time (rate ratio, 1.02; 95% CI = 1.01–1.03). For the most recent years available, age-standardized mortality rates showed variation by country; countries with the lowest mortality rates included Sweden (4.68 per 100,000 de) and New Zealand (5.55 per 100,000). Countries with mortality rates similar to the United States included Australia (6.49 per 100,000) and Canada (7.52 per 100,000). Countries with the highest mortality rates included England and Wales (9.84 per 100,000) and Japan (10.26 per 100,000).

RISK FACTORS

Studies examining risk factors for the development of IPF have typically been retrospective, and subject to a number of limitations including recall and misclassification biases (21). Studies that demonstrate a dose–response relationship strengthen the likelihood of identifying a true risk factor. Genetic risk factors are discussed in Chapter 4.

Cigarette smoking

Smoking has been identified as a risk factor for both IPF and familial pulmonary fibrosis (FPF). Baumgartner and colleagues conducted a multicentre case–control study of smoking and the risk of IPF in the United States (22). A total of 248 cases of IPF were identified between 1989 and 1993 from 16 collaborating centres and compared to 491 controls matched on age, sex and geography. A history of ever smoking was associated with a 60% increased risk for the development of IPF (OR = 1.6; 95% CI = 1.1–2.2), while current smoking was not associated with an elevated risk (OR = 1.06; 95% CI = 0.6–1.8). A dose–response relationship was not identified; however, among former smokers, a trend in time since cessation of smoking and risk of IPF was identified. Those who had more recently quit smoking (<2.5 years prior) had the highest risk for the development of IPF (OR = 3.5%; 95% CI = 1.1–11.9) while those who quit smoking in the remote past (>25 years prior) had the lowest risk (OR = 1.3; 95% CI = 0.7–2.3).

Miyake and colleagues examined smoking and risk for the development of IPF in Japan (23). Similar to Baumgartner and colleagues, they did not identify a dose–response relationship. Instead they found that when compared to non-smokers, only those who had a pack-year history between 20 and 39.9 had an increased risk for the development of IPF (OR = 2.26; 95% CI = 1.3–3.8). Those with a lower pack-year history and those with a higher pack-year history did not have an increased risk.

A meta-analysis, which included these two studies and an additional three studies from the United Kingdom and Japan, found ever smoking was associated with a 58% increase in the risk for the development of IPF (summary OR = 1.58; 95% CI = 1.27–1.97) (24). Given the high prevalence of smoking, it was estimated that 49% of IPF cases could be prevented by entirely eliminating smoking in the population.

Similar to IPF, Steele and colleagues found an association between smoking and the development of FPF. In their case–control study, 309 cases of FPF were compared to 360 unaffected family members. After adjustment for age and sex, ever smoking was associated with a greater than threefold odds of developing lung disease (OR = 3.6; 95% CI = 1.3–9.8) (25).

Occupational exposures

A number of studies have found an association between dust and/or dusty environments and IPF.

METAL DUSTS

Taskar and Coultas conducted a meta-analysis of five case-controlled studies published between 1990 and 2005, and found a significant association between metal dust exposure and the development of IPF (summary OR = 2.44, 95% CI = 1.74–3.40) (24). In one, it appeared that this association held true only for those with ≥5 years of exposure and suggests a possible dose–response relationship (26). An additional study, not included in this meta-analysis, found an association between metal dusts and the development of IPF – but only after a prolonged exposure. Hubbard and colleagues analysed data from the pension fund archives of a metal engineering company and found no relationship between metal dust and the development of IPF, until one was exposed for more than 10 years (OR = 1.71; 95% CI = 1.09–2.68) (27). Two additional studies found no relationship between metal dusts and the development of IPF, but did not account for extent or duration of exposure (28,29).

WOOD DUSTS

A meta-analysis of five case–control studies found an association between wood dusts and the development of IPF (summary OR = 1.94; 95% CI = 1.34–2.81) (24). Two of the five studies did not find an association and this may have been the result of the type of wood dust exposure (26,30). One study out of Sweden found an association between birch and hardwood dust and IPF – but not fir dust (28).

LIVESTOCK, FARMING AND AGRICULTURAL CHEMICALS

Two case–control studies suggest an association between exposure to livestock and IPF (summary OR = 2.17; 95% CI = 1.20–2.26) (24). One of the studies found a dose–response relationship – for those with <5 years of exposure to livestock, no association was identified. However, for those with >5 years of exposure an association to the development of IPF was found (OR = 3.3; 95% CI = 1.3–8.3) (26).

Additional studies investigating farming (or residing in an agricultural region) found an association (summary OR = 1.65; 95% CI = 1.20–2.26) with the development of IPF (24,26,31). One of these studies also found an association between exposure to agricultural chemicals and IPF (OR = 3.32; 95% CI = 1.22–9.05) (31).

SAND, STONE AND SILICA

A meta-analysis of four case–control studies found an association between sand, stone and silica dusts and the development of IPF (summary OR = 1.97; 95% CI = 1.09–3.55) (24). Only one of the four studies did not find an association (30).

MISCELLANEOUS EXPOSURES

Hair dressing, raising birds or residing in an urban/polluted area has been associated with the development of IPF and has been reported in case-control studies (26,31).

In summary, it appears that smoking and exposure to certain dusts are associated with the development of IPF; however, the exact role of these exposures in the development of IPF needs to be further elucidated and may further our understanding of the pathophysiology of this disease.

CLINICAL PRESENTATION AND NATURAL HISTORY OF DISEASE

CLINICAL PRESENTATION

IPF occurs more often in men and the incidence of IPF increases with older age – patients are typically over the age of 50. Further, a majority of patients are former smokers. The most recent international guideline for the diagnosis and management of IPF states that 'IPF should be considered in all adult patients with unexplained chronic exertional dyspnoea, and commonly presents with cough, bibasilar inspiratory crackles, and finger clubbing' (1). The clinical evaluation for suspected IPF is discussed in Chapter 5.

NATURAL HISTORY OF DISEASE

The development of dyspnoea in IPF has typically been described as 'insidious' with symptoms preceding the diagnosis by 1–3 years and with a median survival of 2–3 years after diagnosis (1,32–34). However, as multiple clinical trials have been completed, it has now become evident that the natural history of IPF is heterogeneous – and it is difficult to predict the disease course in any given individual (Figure 8.1) (35). Some will have long-term stability, others will have rapid progression

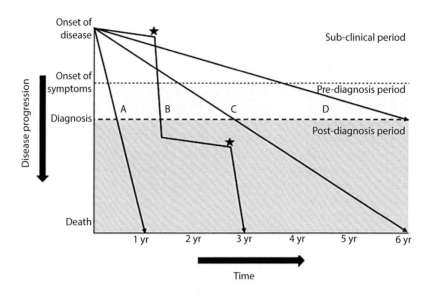

Figure 8.1 Potential clinical courses of idiopathic pulmonary fibrosis (IPF). As disease progresses, there is a subclinical period in which only radiographic findings of disease may be present, followed by a symptomatic period consisting of both pre-diagnosis and post-diagnosis clinical phases. The rate of decline and progression to death may be rapid (line A), slow (lines C and D), or mixed (curve B), with periods of relative stability interposed with periods of acute decline (star). (Reprinted from Ley B et al. Clinical course and prediction of survival in idiopathic pulmonary fibrosis. *Am J Respir Crit Care Med.* 2011;183(4):431–40. Copyright 2011, with permission from American Thoracic Society.)

and others appear to have periods of stability marked by acute exacerbation(s) (see below). At the same time, investigators are discovering a significant population of patients with subclinical disease. The cause of this clinical heterogeneity is unknown, but it has been hypothesized that complex interactions between the host (e.g. genetic variation and ageing) and his or her environment (e.g. smoking, environmental exposures) are at play. Further, co-morbid conditions (e.g. pulmonary hypertension) likely play a role.

Survival predication models

Over the years, a number of prediction models based on one or more clinical variables have been generated, though validation is lacking for most (34,36,37). Recognizing the wide variation in the clinical course of patients with IPF and the limitations of the then available prediction models, Ley and colleagues published a multidimensional index and staging system for IPF in an attempt to predict 1 -, 2-, and 3-year mortality in 2012 (38). Using data from 228 IPF patients, these investigators developed both a complex model and a simple

point-scoring system that included gender, age and two physiologic variables at the time of diagnosis (forced vital capacity [FVC] and diffusion of carbon monoxide [DLCO]) – termed 'GAP'. The complex model and the simple point-scoring system were applied to a second cohort for validation, and the simple point-scoring system was found to have a discriminatory power similar to the more complex model for predicting mortality (Tables 8.2 and 8.3). Further, discrimination was good when used at follow-up time points from 6 to 24 months, although there was some over-prediction of the risk of mortality specifically for the lower risk groups.

Salisbury and colleagues then applied the GAP Index and staging system to 657 IPF patients from three tertiary referral centres to determine whether the GAP stage predicted future pulmonary decline and whether interval pulmonary function decline predicts mortality after accounting for the GAP stage (39). These investigators found that baseline GAP stage predicted death or lung transplantation. However, GAP stage could not predict the rate of future pulmonary function decline – and after accounting for the GAP stage, a decline of

Table 8.2 The GAP (gender, age and physiology) index

	Predictor	Points
	Gender	
G	Female	0
	Male	1
	Age Years	
A	≤60	0
	61–65	1
	>65	2
	Physiology	
	FVC % predicted	
	>75	0
	50–75	1
	<50	2
P	DLCO % predicted	
	>55	0
	36–55	1
	≤35	2
	Cannot perform	3

Source: Kolb M, Collard HR. *Eur Respir Rev.* 2014;23(132):220–4. doi:10.1183/09059180. 00002114.

Note: Maximum possible points = 8. Abbreviations: DLCO = diffusing capacity of the lung for carbon monoxide; FVC = forced vital capacity.

Table 8.3 GAP mortality prediction

Stage	I	II	III
Points	0–3	4–5	6–8
Mortality years			
1	5.6	16.2	39.2
2	10.9	29.9	62.1
3	16.3	42.1	76.8

Source: Kolb M, Collard HR. *Eur Respir Rev.* 2014;23(132):220–4. doi:10.1183/09059180. 00002114.

Note: Individual 1-, 2- and 3-year mortality is shown by stage as determined by GAP score. GAP = gender, age and two lung function variables.

≥10% in FVC or DLCO independently predicted death or transplantation. Thus, (1) GAP stage predicts survival, but not future physiologic decline, and (2) physiologic decline adds prognostic information to baseline stage. These findings highlight the heterogeneity of this disease course in patients with IPF.

Phenotypic subgroups of disease progression

SLOW PROGRESSORS

Studies conducted prior to the development of the 2002 consensus statement on the classification of the idiopathic interstitial pneumonias (IIPs) reported that nearly 30% of subjects with IPF were alive 10 years from diagnosis (40–42). Given that idiopathic non-specific interstitial pneumonia (i-NSIP) was – for the first time – given 'provisional diagnosis' status in this 2002 consensus statement and NSIP has been associated with a longer survival than IPF (the estimated 10-year survival in NSIP is 73.2%), it is likely that many of the long-term survivors referred to in this document had underlying i-NSIP (43).

More recent studies, however, suggest that a cohort of IPF patients do have prolonged survival. Nathan and colleagues identified 357 patients with IPF seen at their centre (transplants excluded) from 2000 to 2009. Patients who were alive at 5 years were more likely to have prolonged survival (Figure 8.2) (44).

RAPID PROGRESSORS

It is now recognized that a subset of patients with IPF present with accelerated disease. Selman and colleagues compared IPF patients presenting with <6 months of symptoms (rapid progressors) to

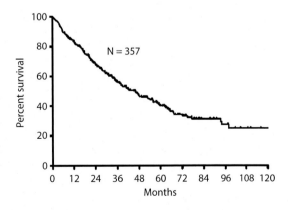

Figure 8.2 Survival of patients with IPF from the time of initial PFT, with transplantation recipients excluded. (Reprinted from *Chest*, 140(1), Nathan SD et al., Long-term course and prognosis of idiopathic pulmonary fibrosis in the new millennium, 221–9, Copyright 2011, with permission from Elsevier.)

those presenting with >24 months of symptoms (slow progressors) (45). While there were no differences between groups at baseline in terms of age, physiology or gas exchange parameters; rapid progressors were more likely to be male (OR = 6.5; 95% CI = 1.4–29.5) and either former or current smokers (OR = 3.04; 95% CI = 1.1–8.3). Further, rapid progressors had a significantly increased risk of death (HR = 9; 95% CI = 4.48–18.3). Rapid progressors also had a unique gene expression pattern with overexpression of genes involved in morphogenesis, oxidative stress and migration and proliferation of fibroblasts and smooth muscle cells. Similarly, Boon and colleagues examined IPF patients with clinically stable or progressive disease, and identified a molecular expression signature of 134 transcripts that sufficiently distinguished stable from progressive IPF (46). The results of these studies underscore the molecular heterogeneity in IPF and likely explain – in part – differences in rates of progression. Given these findings, future prognostic models may need to account for variables at the genetic and/or molecular level in order to accurately predict disease course in an individual patient.

Acute exacerbations of IPF

For over 30 years, it has been recognized that some patients with IPF will experience an acute respiratory decline. When these sudden respiratory declines have no apparent cause, they are termed 'acute exacerbations' of IPF (AE-IPF), and these events have been associated with significant morbidity and mortality.

In 2007, in an attempt to standardize the definition of AE-IPF, Collard and colleagues in the National Institutes of Health–sponsored IPF Clinical Trials Network (IPFNet), published a proposed diagnostic criteria for an AE-IPF: (1) a previous or concurrent diagnosis of IPF; (2) unexplained development of dyspnoea or worsening within 30 days; (3) high-resolution computed tomography (HRCT) with new bilateral ground-glass abnormality and/or consolidation superimposed on a background pattern consistent with IPF; (4) no evidence of pulmonary infection by endotracheal aspirate or bronchoalveolar lavage (BAL); and (5) exclusion of alternative causes including left heart failure, pulmonary embolism and identifiable causes of acute lung injury (47).

These criteria have been widely adopted over the past decade and have led to a better understanding of the current state of knowledge regarding AE-IPF. With this in mind, in 2016, an international working group proposed a revised definition of AE-IPF as 'an acute, clinically significant respiratory deterioration characterized by evidence of new widespread alveolar abnormality'. The group proposed revised diagnostic criteria: (1) previous or concurrent diagnosis of IPF; (2) acute worsening or development of dyspnoea typically <1 month duration; (3) computed tomography with new bilateral ground-glass and/or consolidation superimposed on a background pattern consistent with usual interstitial pneumonia; and (4) deterioration not fully explained by cardiac failure or fluid overload (48).

The incidence of AE-IPF varies in the literature and likely reflects differences in the population studied (e.g. disease severity), how these events were defined and how monitoring for these events was conducted. For example, using the placebo arms of previously conducted randomized controlled trials may have missing data and underestimate the incidence, whereas cohort studies may overestimate the incidence depending on the criteria used to define an exacerbation.

In a recent meta-analysis that included the placebo arms of six randomized controlled trials, the overall weighted average of AE-IPF was 4.1 per 100 patient-years. Further, rates were lower in studies that excluded severe disease when compared to those studies that did not (2.8 versus 12.3 AE-IPF per 100 patient-years, $p < 0.0001$) (49). In a small US cohort study, the incidence of AE-IPF was found to be 13 per 100 patient-years (6).

A Korean retrospective cohort study, conducted by Song and colleagues, identified 461 patients with IPF with a median follow-up time of 22.9 months and found that 96 patients (20.8%) had a definite AE-IPF (as defined by the Collard criteria) or a suspected AE-IPF (when an endotracheal aspirate or BAL was not performed) (50). The 1-, 2- and 3-year incidence of AE-IPF was 14.2%, 18.8% and 20.7%, respectively. After an AE-IPF, immediate outcomes were poor; 50% of the patients died during the hospitalization and the median survival was 2.2 months from the onset of the AE-IPF. Of those who were admitted to an intensive care unit (~50% of the AE-IPF cohort) outcomes were even worse, with an 80% mortality rate.

While the precise aetiology for AE-IPF is not known, it has been hypothesized that unrecognized external insults that could lead to acute lung injury (ALI) in a normal host (e.g. infection, microaspiration) may lead to ALI in IPF. Further, it has also been hypothesized that intrinsic biological dysfunction of an IPF lung may be more susceptible not only to these external insults but also mechanical stresses – as AE-IPF have been reported after both thoracic and extrathoracic surgeries as well as bronchoscopies (48).

Several risk factors for AE-IPF have been identified; low FVC has been the most consistent risk factor among studies (48). Other physiologic and clinical parameters including low diffusing capacity for carbon monoxide, short 6-minute-walk distance, increased dyspnoea, pulmonary hypertension, comorbid coronary artery disease, younger age and obesity have also been associated with an increased risk (48,49).

Thus, AE-IPF are common, are associated with clinical and physiologic risk factors, significantly shorten survival – and are, unfortunately, part of the natural history of disease. Given this, investigators are actively trying to determine the precise aetiology, pathobiology and optimal management of these devastating events.

Subclinical disease

Over the past decade, subclinical interstitial lung disease, defined by the presence of interstitial lung abnormalities (ILAs) on HRCT, has gained significant interest for a number of reasons: (1) though not universally a precursor to the development of IPF, ILAs are clinically significant – their presence is associated with increased mortality; (2) in both familial IPF (FIPF) cohorts and in non-familial cohorts these findings are relatively common; (3) ILAs may represent a very early stage of disease that would allow for early intervention; and (4) ILAs may provide an opportunity to better understand inciting events that allow for progression to clinical disease.

Studies of family members of patients with FIPF have shed light on the significance of subclinical disease/ILAs. Rosas and colleagues identified 143 asymptomatic subjects from 18 kindreds with FIPF. Of these asymptomatic subjects, HRCT imaging identified abnormalities consistent with ILD in 31 (22%) subjects. Compared to affected family members, those with asymptomatic changes were younger (46 years versus 67 years, $p < 0.001$), and both groups had significantly more smokers than compared to related subjects without disease. These findings suggest that progression from asymptomatic to symptomatic disease may occur over decades and that smoking appears to be a risk factor, but it is still not known what proportion of these asymptomatic patients will develop clinically overt disease (51).

The hypothesis that disease characterized by radiographic changes alone (subclinical disease) identifies patients at risk for the development of clinically apparent IPF is supported by studies of patients with ILA on HRCT and lung cancer who undergo lobectomy and develop AE-IPF. Chida and colleagues examined 1,148 patients with primary lung cancer who underwent thoracotomy and identified 15 patients who developed postoperative acute respiratory distress syndrome (ARDS) (52). Of these cases, 11 patients (73%) had both ILA on preoperative computed tomography (CT) and a histologic UIP pattern of fibrosis in resected lung tissue. In a separate study, Araya and colleagues reviewed 14 autopsy cases of acute interstitial pneumonia (AIP) and found that 50% of cases had evidence of subpleural fibrosis – suggesting that at least some cases of AIP may actually represent an acute exacerbation of subclinical fibrosis (53).

Recently, investigators from four large prospective studies came together to study the significance of ILAs (51). The Framingham Heart Study found that ILAs were present in 177 (7%) of 2,633 participants, the AGES-Reykjavik (Age Gene/Environment Susceptibility) Study found ILAs were present in 378 (7%) of 5,320 participants, the COPDGene Study found ILAs were present in 156 (8%) of 2,068 participants, and the ECLIPSE (Evaluation of COPD Longitudinally to Identify Predictive Surrogate Endpoints) Study found ILAs were present in 157 (9%) of 1,670 participants. Recently, Putman and colleagues reported all-cause mortality over an approximate 3- to 9-year median follow-up time, and found that after adjustment for a number of covariates, ILAs were associated with a higher risk of death in all four of these prospective cohort studies (Table 8.4) (54). Further, in the AGES-Reykjavik cohort, these investigators were able to determine that the higher mortality rate could be explained by a higher rate of death

Table 8.4 Hazard ratio (HR) for death with interstitial lung abnormalities (ILAs)

Prospective cohort study	HR	95% CI	p Value
Framingham Health Study	2.7	95% CI = 1.1–6.6	$p = 0.03$
AGES-Reykjavik	1.3	95% CI = 1.2–1.4	$p < 0.001$
COPDGene	1.8	95% CI = 1.1–2.8	$p = 0.01$
ECLIPSE	1.4	95% CI = 1.1–2.0	$p = 0.02$

due to respiratory disease – specifically pulmonary fibrosis. Thus, ILA appears to be associated with an increased risk of death, but the current data have not identified specific risk factors for progression to clinical respiratory disease – which likely occurs in only a minority of cases given the percentage of ILAs identified and the relatively low prevalence of IPF (~0.002%–0.04%) (54). Additional longitudinal studies of large cohorts are needed to address these questions.

Specific clinical phenotypes that appear to impact the natural history of disease

IPF AND PULMONARY HYPERTENSION

The presence of pulmonary arterial hypertension in patients with IPF is recognized to shorten survival (63,64). Initially, IPF-related pulmonary hypertension was thought to be due to loss of lung volume and vascular destruction. However, there is not a clear association between physiologic impairment and the presence or degree of pulmonary hypertension, suggesting that additional pathophysiologic abnormalities are involved (55,56).

IPF AND EMPHYSEMA (COMBINED PULMONARY FIBROSIS AND EMPHYSEMA [CPFE])

It is unclear if emphysema and pulmonary fibrosis is a distinct clinically entity, or the result of two smoking-related diseases. CPFE does have suggestive pulmonary function testing typically revealing relatively preserved static and forced lung volumes, but with a disproportionately low diffusion capacity. Pulmonary hypertension is the most important complication of this condition, affecting 47%–90% of patients and shortening survival (57). Mejía and colleagues found that patients with CPFE exhibited higher mortality compared to IPF alone; a Cox regression model showed that the two

most important variables associated with mortality were a FVC of <50% predicted (HR, 2.6; 95% CI = 1.19–4.54, $p = 0.016$) and an estimated systolic pulmonary artery pressure of ≥75 mm Hg (HR, 2.25; 95% CI = 1.12–4.54, $p = 0.022$) suggesting that the worse outcome was in part driven by severe pulmonary hypertension (58).

PATHOPHYSIOLOGY OF IPF

IPF is characterized by excess collagen and matrix deposition within interstitial spaces resulting in airspace obliteration and loss of normal alveolar physiology. While progress has been made in understanding the pathogenesis of IPF, much remains unknown. In particular, the inciting mechanisms and pathways that drive excessive fibrosis formation in this disease remain elusive. Generally speaking, IPF is thought by many to be the result of abnormal wound healing responses that lead to exaggerated collagen deposition and scar formation. This scar formation has been likened to cancer with propagation of invasive collagen-producing fibroblasts that behave more aggressively than normal fibroblasts (59–61). It is now understood that genetic predisposition plays a role in many cases of IPF. It is possible that underlying genetic factors in conjunction with environmental exposures together lead to the disease. The link between genetics, environment and the observed pathophysiologic disease mechanisms in IPF is an area of significant interest and active investigation. An overview of current understanding regarding the pathophysiology of IPF is provided in Figure 8.3 (62).

ROLE OF GENETICS

Clues to the importance of a genetic component in the development of pulmonary fibrosis came from

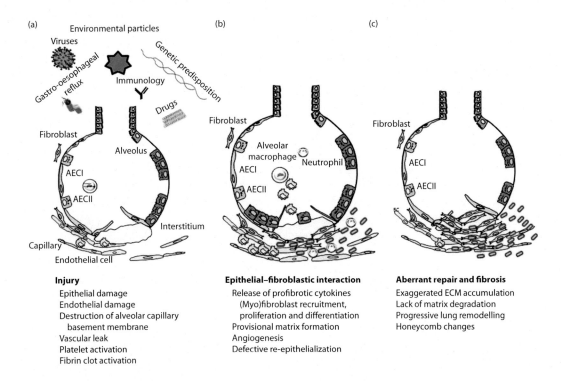

Figure 8.3 The major elements involved in induction and progression of fibrosis. **(a)** The onset of fibrosis is characterized by both injury and susceptibility to the formation of progressive fibrosis. Many different injurious agents have been identified that lead to epithelial and endothelial damage, vascular leak and fibrin clot formation. **(b)** This is followed by an abnormal repair process characterized by an abnormal re-epithelialization, abundance of myofibroblasts and the formation of a collagen matrix. **(c)** The process proceeds to excessive matrix formation leading to architectural distortion and finally death. (Abbreviations: AEC = alveolar epithelial cell; ECM = extracellular matrix.) (Reproduced from Wuyts WA et al. The pathogenesis of pulmonary fibrosis: A moving target. *Eur Respir J.* 2013;41(5):1207–18, with permission of the European Respiratory Society.)

the recognition of familial disease and from specific known genetic disorders including dyskeratosis congenita and Hermansky–Pudlak syndrome. Dyskeratosis congenita is a rare, heritable condition characterized by bone marrow failure and mucocutaneous features, and is commonly complicated by pulmonary fibrosis (63,64). The disease is caused by genetic mutations in genes responsible for telomerase maintenance. This observation led to an examination of telomerase genes in familial forms of lung fibrosis not associated with dyskeratosis congenita. This identified an association between familial pulmonary fibrosis (FPF) and mutations in *TERT* and *TERC* (65,66). Similarly, other studies identified variants in genes encoding surfactant protein C (SFTPC), surfactant protein A2 (SFTPA2) (67–69). Together however, these mutations account for only a minority of cases of pulmonary fibrosis.

Until recently, an association between genetics and sporadic IPF remained less certain. Within the past decade, however, large genome-wide linkage and association studies have identified several gene loci clearly associated with increased IPF risk (70–72). Most notable is the single-nucleotide polymorphism (SNP) within the promoter region of the gene encoding Mucin 5B (*MUC5B*). This variant, identified in 2011, was found to occur in 34% of FPF cases, 38% of IPF cases and 9% of healthy controls (71). Its association with IPF risk has been confirmed by various studies though the variant occurs only rarely in certain Asian populations (70,72–75). The *MUC5B* mutation correlates with increased *MUC5B* mRNA expression in the lung and distal airways; however, the biologic link between this finding and development of lung fibrosis is unknown. The role of genetics in IPF is reviewed in greater detail in a separate chapter.

While recent studies have confirmed an important genetic component to IPF disease risk, environmental risk factors are also recognized (see above) (1). While neither genetics nor environmental exposures alone fully account for the development of IPF, the combination of both factors is important for development of disease. To this end, epigenetic mechanisms have recently received attention as a possible link between genes and environment in IPF. Epigenetics refers to the study of cellular and physiologic changes caused by post-translational modification of gene expression without change in the genetic code itself. Several studies have now demonstrated that epigenetic modifications can regulate gene expression in genes associated with IPF disease pathogenesis including α-SMA, cyclooxygenase-2, chemokine IP-10, Thy-1 and miR17~92 (76–81). Epigenomic studies examining global DNA methylation profiles in large IPF cohorts have identified differential profiles in IPF versus healthy controls and have identified similarities between profiles in IPF and lung cancer (82,83). Further investigations are needed to understand the relevance of these epigenetic findings and IPF disease pathogenesis.

EPITHELIAL DYSFUNCTION IN IPF

Alveolar epithelial cell (AEC) abnormalities constitute a well-established feature of IPF. Early reports found that AECs in IPF demonstrated abnormal apoptotic cell death, atypical proliferation and hyperplasia and development of bronchiolar features (84–88). Today, repeated epithelial injury and abnormal repair is considered central to disease pathogenesis in IPF. This aberrant repair compromises epithelial reconstitution and impairs normal epithelial–mesenchymal ultrastructure and cell–cell interaction. The full spectrum of epithelial dysfunction in IPF remains unknown but recent reports have provided more detail as to the molecular and functional abnormalities of AECs that contribute to lung fibrosis.

Repeated micro-injury to the epithelium from viruses, aspiration, cigarette smoke or other inhalants is hypothesized to result in aberrant activation of epithelial cells. This then leads to epithelial cell apoptosis and capillary leak of coagulation factor-rich fluid creating a provisional matrix within

alveolar and interstitial spaces (89,90). The matrix includes a variety of proteins and clotting factors including fibrin, fibronectin, tissue factor, factor VII and factor Xa. Studies in animal models of lung fibrosis have demonstrated a role for coagulation factors, particularly thrombin and factor Xa in the activation of myofibroblasts via transforming growth factor-β (TGF-β) (91,92). It is thought that impaired fibronolytic action by dysfunctional AECs plays a role in propagation of this procoagulant matrix IPF.

In the setting of IPF, AECs exhibit signs of endoplasmic reticulum (ER) stress (93,94). ER stress occurs when cellular demand for proteins exceeds the ER's capacity for production resulting in a buildup of unfolded proteins within the ER. This triggers an 'unfolded protein response' (UPR) that ultimately leads to cell death through apoptosis if left unchecked. UPR has been implicated as an important source of AEC apoptosis in IPF and may also play a role in promoting epithelial–mesenchymal transition (EMT) in AECs (95,96).

EMT refers to a process by which mature epithelial cells transform into cells with mesenchymal phenotypes in response to tissue remodelling or injury (97). EMT occurs normally during embryogenesis. However, in adults, EMT has been implicated as a source of tissue fibroblasts in various forms of pathologic organ fibrosis including IPF (97,98). It also plays a critical role in malignant tumour progression (99). Among the most important inducers of EMT in the lung is activation by transforming growth factor beta (TGF-β) (100,101). While EMT has been intermittently observed in IPF, its precise role in disease pathogenesis remains unclear.

FIBROBLASTS IN IPF

Fibroblasts are the hallmark cell of lung fibrosis in IPF. Fibroblasts are present in normal lungs; however in the setting of IPF, an exaggerated expansion of this population occurs and fibroblasts differentiate into abnormal collagen-producing myofibroblasts. The origin of fibroblasts in IPF remains a topic of debate and active investigation. Historically it was believed that resident lung mesenchymal cells alone gave rise to IPF fibroblasts, however, evidence increasingly points to alternate origins for these cells. Circulating bone marrow–derived progenitor cells called fibrocytes are one important source (102,103). These cells increase in number during acute exacerbation and appear to correlate with disease activity and prognosis in IPF (104). EMT and possibly endothelial–mesenchymal transition (EndoMT) also contribute to the fibroblast population expansion in IPF (100,105,106). Lung pericytes constitute another postulated source (107). Once present, IPF fibroblast populations are furthered augmented by a heightened proliferative capacity and development of apoptotic resistance (61,108–110). Biologic mechanisms that regulate proliferation and apoptosis in resolving injury and normal wound healing appear to be lost in the setting of IPF (111).

Fibroblasts in IPF adopt a matrix-producing (myofibroblast) phenotype via a variety of mechanisms, many characterized by abnormal epithelial-mesenchymal signalling or crosstalk. Epithelial cells directly signal fibroblasts through release of growth factors, including TGF-β, which trigger conversion of fibroblasts to myofibroblasts. AECs also signal to fibroblasts through release of proteins associated programmes of embryonic development including Wnt glycoproteins and sonic hedgehog (112–114). Overexpression of these proteins in lung fibrosis suggests that re-activation of developmental pathways is a feature of IPF disease pathogenesis. Recent evidence also points to the role of impaired autophagy and mitophagy in activation myofibroblast differentiation (115).

Mechanical properties of the extracellular matrix itself may drive myofibroblast differentiation. Extracellular matrix deposition in IPF results in increased lung rigidity or stiffness, and studies have demonstrated differential fibroblast behavior and programming in responses to growth on stiff matrix (116). Stiffness activates mechanotransduction pathways that regulate myofibroblast differentiation, possibly through actin cytoskeletal remodelling (117,118). Precise mechanosensing mechanisms and signalling pathways are not fully known but offer hope as a new target for therapy in IPF.

Once activated, myofibroblasts express alpha-smooth muscle actin (α-SMA) conferring a more contractile phenotype than normal fibroblasts. These cells secrete large amounts of collagen-1-rich extracellular matrix and have invasive properties that contribute to the expansion of fibrosis in IPF (59,60,119). Fibroblast foci are considered the leading edge of fibrosis and are composed of polyclonal highly active, collagen-secreting myofibroblasts (120). Currently little is known regarding the mechanisms that drive to relentless propagation of myofibroblasts in IPF. In addition, the mechanisms responsible for observed periods of progression versus stability in patients with IPF are unknown.

CONCLUSION

While IPF was once considered an orphan disease, epidemiologic studies suggest that mortality rates are similar to some common malignancies. The natural history is not one of 'insidious' progression, but may progress rapidly, intermittently or even very slowly. The current pathophysiologic evidence now suggests that IPF is due to a combination of genetic and environmental factors that incite abnormal activation of epithelial cells and fibroblast. Inflammation is no longer thought to play a significant role in IPF disease pathogenesis, and anti-inflammatory therapies have demonstrated lack of efficacy and even harm in patients in IPF (121). Although we have gained important insight into this disease over the past two decades, only a greater understanding of the underlying pathophysiology will lead to new, targeted therapy.

REFERENCES

1. Raghu G, Collard HR, Egan JJ, Martinez FJ, Behr J, Brown KK et al. An official ATS/ERS/JRS/ALAT statement: Idiopathic pulmonary fibrosis: Evidence-based guidelines for diagnosis and management. *Am J Respir Crit Care Med*. 2011;183(6):788–824.

2. Gordis L, Measuring the occurrence of disease: 1. morbidity. In: Leon GO, ed. *Epidemiology*. 3rd ed. Philadelphia, PA: Elsevier Saunders; 2004:32–47.

3. Cherniack RM, Crystal RG, Kalica AR. NHLBI Workshop summary. Current concepts in idiopathic pulmonary fibrosis: A road map for the future. *Am Rev Respir Dis*. 1991;143(3):680–3.

4. Coultas DB, Zumwalt RE, Black WC, Sobonya RE. The epidemiology of interstitial lung diseases. *Am J Respir Crit Care Med*. 1994;150(4):967–72.

5. Raghu G, Weycker D, Edelsberg J, Bradford WZ, Oster G. Incidence and prevalence of idiopathic pulmonary fibrosis. *Am J Respir Crit Care Med.* 2006;174(7):810–6.

6. Fernandez Perez ER, Daniels CE, Schroeder DR, St Sauver J, Hartman TE, Bartholmai BJ et al. Incidence, prevalence, and clinical course of idiopathic pulmonary fibrosis: A population-based study. *Chest.* 2010; 137(1):129–37.

7. Raghu G, Chen SY, Yeh WS, Maroni B, Li Q, Lee YC et al. Idiopathic pulmonary fibrosis in US Medicare beneficiaries aged 65 years and older: Incidence, prevalence, and survival, 2001–11. *Lancet Respir Med.* 2014;2(7):566–72.

8. Raghu G, Chen SY, Hou Q, Yeh WS, Collard HR. Incidence and prevalence of idiopathic pulmonary fibrosis in US adults 18–64 years old. *Eur Respir J.* 2016;48(1):179–86.

9. Esposito DB, Lanes S, Donneyong M, Holick CN, Lasky JA, Lederer D et al. Idiopathic pulmonary fibrosis in United States Automated Claims. Incidence, prevalence, and algorithm validation. *Am J Respir Crit Care Med.* 2015;192(10):1200–7.

10. Navaratnam V, Fleming KM, West J, Smith CJ, Jenkins RG, Fogarty A et al. The rising incidence of idiopathic pulmonary fibrosis in the U.K. *Thorax.* 2011;66(6):462–7.

11. Gribbin J, Hubbard RB, Le Jeune I, Smith CJ, West J, Tata LJ. Incidence and mortality of idiopathic pulmonary fibrosis and sarcoidosis in the UK. *Thorax.* 2006;61(11):980–5.

12. American Thoracic Society. Idiopathic pulmonary fibrosis: Diagnosis and treatment. International consensus statement. American Thoracic Society (ATS), and the European Respiratory Society (ERS). *Am J Respir Crit Care Med.* 2000;161(2 Pt 1):646–64.

13. Ziesche R, Hofbauer E, Wittmann K, Petkov V, Block LH. A preliminary study of long-term treatment with interferon gamma-1b and low-dose prednisolone in patients with idiopathic pulmonary fibrosis. *N Engl J Med.* 1999;341(17):1264–9.

14. Raghu G, Brown KK, Bradford WZ, Starko K, Noble PW, Schwartz DA et al. A placebo-controlled trial of interferon gamma-1b in patients with idiopathic pulmonary fibrosis. *N Engl J Med.* 2004;350(2):125–33.

15. Hopkins RB, Burke N, Fell C, Dion G, Kolb M. Epidemiology and survival of idiopathic pulmonary fibrosis from national data in Canada. *Eur Respir J.* 2016;48(1):187–95.

16. Hutchinson J, Fogarty A, Hubbard R, McKeever T. Global incidence and mortality of idiopathic pulmonary fibrosis: A systematic review. *Eur Respir J.* 2015;46(3): 795–806.

17. Gordis L. More on causal inferences: Bias, confounding, and interaction. In: Leon G, ed. *Epidemiology.* 3rd ed. Philadelphia, PA: Elsevier Saunders; 2004:224–39.

18. Hutchinson JP, McKeever TM, Fogarty AW, Navaratnam V, Hubbard RB. Increasing global mortality from idiopathic pulmonary fibrosis in the twenty-first century. *Ann Am Thorac Soc.* 2014;11(8):1176–85.

19. Mannino DM, Etzel RA, Parrish RG. Pulmonary fibrosis deaths in the United States, 1979–1991. An analysis of multiple-cause mortality data. *Am J Respir Crit Care Med.* 1996;153(5):1548–52.

20. Olson AL, Swigris JJ, Lezotte DC, Norris JM, Wilson CG, Brown KK. Mortality from pulmonary fibrosis increased in the United States from 1992 to 2003. *Am J Respir Crit Care Med.* 2007;176(3):277–84.

21. Raphael K. Recall bias: A proposal for assessment and control. *Int J Epidemiol.* 1987;16(2):167–70.

22. Baumgartner KB, Samet JM, Stidley CA, Colby TV, Waldron JA. Cigarette smoking: A risk factor for idiopathic pulmonary fibrosis. *Am J Respir Crit Care Med.* 1997;155(1):242–8.

23. Miyake Y, Sasaki S, Yokoyama T, Chida K, Azuma A, Suda T et al. Occupational and environmental factors and idiopathic pulmonary fibrosis in Japan. *Ann Occup Hyg.* 2005;49(3):259–65.

24. Taskar VS, Coultas DB. Is idiopathic pulmonary fibrosis an environmental disease? *Proc Am Thorac Soc.* 2006;3(4):293–8.

25. Steele MP, Speer MC, Loyd JE, Brown KK, Herron A, Slifer SH et al. Clinical and pathologic features of familial interstitial

pneumonia. *Am J Respir Crit Care Med.* 2005;172(9):1146–52.

26. Baumgartner KB, Samet JM, Coultas DB, Stidley CA, Hunt WC, Colby TV et al. Occupational and environmental risk factors for idiopathic pulmonary fibrosis: A multicenter case-control study. Collaborating centers. *Am J Epidemiol.* 2000;152(4):307–15.

27. Hubbard R, Cooper M, Antoniak M, Venn A, Khan S, Johnston I et al. Risk of cryptogenic fibrosing alveolitis in metal workers. *Lancet.* 2000;355(9202):466–7.

28. Gustafson T, Dahlman-Hoglund A, Nilsson K, Strom K, Tornling G, Toren K. Occupational exposure and severe pulmonary fibrosis. *Respir Med.* 2007;101(10):2207–12.

29. Harris JM, Cullinan P, McDonald JC. Occupational distribution and geographic clustering of deaths certified to be cryptogenic fibrosing alveolitis in England and Wales. *Chest.* 2001;119(2):428–33.

30. Scott J, Johnston I, Britton J. What causes cryptogenic fibrosing alveolitis? A case-control study of environmental exposure to dust. *BMJ.* 1990;301(6759):1015–7.

31. Iwai K, Mori T, Yamada N, Yamaguchi M, Hosoda Y. Idiopathic pulmonary fibrosis. Epidemiologic approaches to occupational exposure. *Am J Respir Crit Care Med.* 1994;150(3):670–5.

32. Nicholson AG, Colby TV, du Bois RM, Hansell DM, Wells AU. The prognostic significance of the histologic pattern of interstitial pneumonia in patients presenting with the clinical entity of cryptogenic fibrosing alveolitis. *Am J Respir Crit Care Med.* 2000;162(6):2213–7.

33. King TE, Jr., Schwarz MI, Brown K, Tooze JA, Colby TV, Waldron JA, Jr. et al. Idiopathic pulmonary fibrosis: Relationship between histopathologic features and mortality. *Am J Respir Crit Care Med.* 2001;164(6):1025–32.

34. King TE, Jr., Tooze JA, Schwarz MI, Brown KR, Cherniack RM. Predicting survival in idiopathic pulmonary fibrosis: Scoring system and survival model. *Am J Respir Crit Care Med.* 2001;164(7):1171–81.

35. Ley B, Collard HR, King TE, Jr. Clinical course and prediction of survival in idiopathic pulmonary fibrosis. *Am J Respir Crit Care Med.* 2011;183(4):431–40.

36. Wells AU, Desai SR, Rubens MB, Goh NS, Cramer D, Nicholson AG et al. Idiopathic pulmonary fibrosis: A composite physiologic index derived from disease extent observed by computed tomography. *Am J Respir Crit Care Med.* 2003;167(7):962–9.

37. du Bois RM, Weycker D, Albera C, Bradford WZ, Costabel U, Kartashov A et al. Ascertainment of individual risk of mortality for patients with idiopathic pulmonary fibrosis. *Am J Respir Crit Care Med.* 2011;184(4):459–66.

38. Ley B, Ryerson CJ, Vittinghoff E, Ryu JH, Tomassetti S, Lee JS et al. A multidimensional index and staging system for idiopathic pulmonary fibrosis. *Ann Intern Med.* 2012;156(10):684–91.

39. Salisbury ML, Xia M, Zhou Y, Murray S, Tayob N, Brown KK et al. Idiopathic pulmonary fibrosis: Gender-age-physiology index stage for predicting future lung function decline. *Chest.* 2016;149(2):491–8.

40. Turner-Warwick M, Burrows B, Johnson A. Cryptogenic fibrosing alveolitis: Clinical features and their influence on survival. *Thorax.* 1980;35(3):171–80.

41. Carrington CB, Gaensler EA, Coutu RE, FitzGerald MX, Gupta RG. Natural history and treated course of usual and desquamative interstitial pneumonia. *N Engl J Med.* 1978;298(15):801–9.

42. American Thoracic S, European Respiratory S. American Thoracic Society/European Respiratory Society International Multidisciplinary Consensus Classification of the Idiopathic Interstitial Pneumonias. This joint statement of the American Thoracic Society (ATS), and the European Respiratory Society (ERS) was adopted by the ATS board of directors, June 2001 and by the ERS Executive Committee, June 2001. *Am J Respir Crit Care Med.* 2002;165(2):277–304.

43. Travis WD, Hunninghake G, King TE, Jr., Lynch DA, Colby TV, Galvin JR et al. Idiopathic nonspecific interstitial pneumonia: Report of an American Thoracic Society project. *Am J Respir Crit Care Med.* 2008;177(12):1338–47.

44. Nathan SD, Shlobin OA, Weir N, Ahmad S, Kaldjob JM, Battle E et al. Long-term course and prognosis of idiopathic pulmonary fibrosis in the new millennium. *Chest.* 2011;140(1):221–9.

45. Selman M, Carrillo G, Estrada A, Mejia M, Becerril C, Cisneros J et al. Accelerated variant of idiopathic pulmonary fibrosis: Clinical behavior and gene expression pattern. *PLoS One.* 2007;2(5):e482.

46. Boon K, Bailey NW, Yang J, Steel MP, Groshong S, Kervitsky D et al. Molecular phenotypes distinguish patients with relatively stable from progressive idiopathic pulmonary fibrosis (IPF). *PLoS One.* 2009;4(4):e5134.

47. Collard HR, Moore BB, Flaherty KR, Brown KK, Kaner RJ, King TE, Jr. et al. Acute exacerbations of idiopathic pulmonary fibrosis. *Am J Respir Crit Care Med.* 2007;176(7):636–43.

48. Collard HR, Ryerson CJ, Corte TJ, Jenkins G, Kondoh Y, Lederer DJ et al. Acute exacerbation of idiopathic pulmonary fibrosis. An international working group report. *Am J Respir Crit Care Med.* 2016;194(3):265–75.

49. Atkins CP, Loke YK, Wilson AM. Outcomes in idiopathic pulmonary fibrosis: A meta-analysis from placebo controlled trials. *Respir Med.* 2014;108(2):376–87.

50. Song JW, Hong SB, Lim CM, Koh Y, Kim DS. Acute exacerbation of idiopathic pulmonary fibrosis: Incidence, risk factors and outcome. *Eur Respir J.* 2011;37(2):356–63.

51. Rosas IO, Ren P, Avila NA, Chow CK, Franks TJ, Travis WD et al. Early interstitial lung disease in familial pulmonary fibrosis. *Am J Respir Crit Care Med.* 2007;176(7):698–705.

52. Chida M, Ono S, Hoshikawa Y, Kondo T. Subclinical idiopathic pulmonary fibrosis is also a risk factor of postoperative acute respiratory distress syndrome following thoracic surgery. *Eur J Cardiothorac Surg.* 2008;34(4):878–81.

53. Araya J, Kawabata Y, Jinho P, Uchiyama T, Ogata H, Sugita Y. Clinically occult subpleural fibrosis and acute interstitial pneumonia a precursor to idiopathic pulmonary fibrosis? *Respirology.* 2008;13(3):408–12.

54. Putman RK, Hatabu H, Araki T, Gudmundsson G, Gao W, Nishino M et al. Association between interstitial lung abnormalities and all-cause mortality. *JAMA.* 2016;315(7):672–81.

55. Nathan SD, Noble PW, Tuder RM. Idiopathic pulmonary fibrosis and pulmonary hypertension: Connecting the dots. *Am J Respir Crit Care Med.* 2007;175(9):875–80.

56. Nathan SD, Shlobin OA, Ahmad S, Urbanek S, Barnett SD. Pulmonary hypertension and pulmonary function testing in idiopathic pulmonary fibrosis. *Chest.* 2007;131(3):657–63.

57. Lin H, Jiang S. Combined pulmonary fibrosis and emphysema (CPFE): An entity different from emphysema or pulmonary fibrosis alone. *J Thorac Dis.* 2015;7(4):767–79.

58. Mejia M, Carrillo G, Rojas-Serrano J, Estrada A, Suarez T, Alonso D et al. Idiopathic pulmonary fibrosis and emphysema: Decreased survival associated with severe pulmonary arterial hypertension. *Chest.* 2009;136(1):10–5.

59. White ES, Thannickal VJ, Carskadon SL, Dickie EG, Livant DL, Markwart S et al. Integrin $\alpha4\beta1$ regulates migration across basement membranes by lung fibroblasts: A role for phosphatase and tensin homologue deleted on chromosome 10. *Am J Respir Crit Care Med.* 2003;168(4):436–42.

60. Li Y, Jiang D, Liang J, Meltzer EB, Gray A, Miura R et al. Severe lung fibrosis requires an invasive fibroblast phenotype regulated by hyaluronan and CD44. *J Exp Med.* 2011;208(7):1459–71.

61. Ramos C, Montano M, Garcia-Alvarez J, Ruiz V, Uhal BD, Selman M et al. Fibroblasts from idiopathic pulmonary fibrosis and normal lungs differ in growth rate, apoptosis, and tissue inhibitor of metalloproteinases expression. *Am J Respir Cell Mol Biol.* 2001;24(5):591–8.

62. Wuyts WA, Agostini C, Antoniou KM, Bouros D, Chambers RC, Cottin V et al. The pathogenesis of pulmonary fibrosis: A moving target. *Eur Respir J.* 2013;41(5):1207–18.

63. Vulliamy TJ, Marrone A, Knight SW, Walne A, Mason PJ, Dokal I. Mutations in

dyskeratosis congenita: Their impact on telomere length and the diversity of clinical presentation. *Blood.* 2006;107(7):2680–5.

64. Ballew BJ, Savage SA. Updates on the biology and management of dyskeratosis congenita and related telomere biology disorders. *Expert Rev Hematol.* 2013;6(3):327–37.

65. Armanios MY, Chen JJ, Cogan JD, Alder JK, Ingersoll RG, Markin C et al. Telomerase mutations in families with idiopathic pulmonary fibrosis. *N Engl J Med.* 2007;356(13):1317–26.

66. Tsakiri KD, Cronkhite JT, Kuan PJ, Xing C, Raghu G, Weissler JC et al. Adult-onset pulmonary fibrosis caused by mutations in telomerase. *Proc Natl Acad Sci U S A.* 2007;104(18):7552–7.

67. Nogee LM, Dunbar AE, 3rd, Wert SE, Askin F, Hamvas A, Whitsett JA. A mutation in the surfactant protein C gene associated with familial interstitial lung disease. *N Engl J Med.* 2001;344(8):573–9.

68. Thomas AQ, Lane K, Phillips J, 3rd, Prince M, Markin C, Speer M et al. Heterozygosity for a surfactant protein C gene mutation associated with usual interstitial pneumonitis and cellular nonspecific interstitial pneumonitis in one kindred. *Am J Respir Crit Care Med.* 2002;165(9):1322–8.

69. Wang Y, Kuan PJ, Xing C, Cronkhite JT, Torres F, Rosenblatt RL et al. Genetic defects in surfactant protein A2 are associated with pulmonary fibrosis and lung cancer. *Am J Hum Genet.* 2009;84(1):52–9.

70. Fingerlin TE, Murphy E, Zhang W, Peljto AL, Brown KK, Steele MP et al. Genome-wide association study identifies multiple susceptibility loci for pulmonary fibrosis. *Nat Genet.* 2013;45(6):613–20.

71. Seibold MA, Wise AL, Speer MC, Steele MP, Brown KK, Loyd JE et al. A common MUC5B promoter polymorphism and pulmonary fibrosis. *N Engl J Med.* 2011;364(16):1503–12.

72. Noth I, Zhang Y, Ma SF, Flores C, Barber M, Huang Y et al. Genetic variants associated with idiopathic pulmonary fibrosis susceptibility and mortality: A genome-wide association study. *Lancet Respir Med.* 2013;1(4):309–17.

73. Borie R, Crestani B, Dieude P, Nunes H, Allanore Y, Kannengiesser C et al. The MUC5B variant is associated with idiopathic pulmonary fibrosis but not with systemic sclerosis interstitial lung disease in the European Caucasian population. *PLoS One.* 2013;8(8):e70621.

74. Horimasu Y, Ohshimo S, Bonella F, Tanaka S, Ishikawa N, Hattori N et al. MUC5B promoter polymorphism in Japanese patients with idiopathic pulmonary fibrosis. *Respirology.* 2015;20(3):439–44.

75. Wei R, Li C, Zhang M, Jones-Hall YL, Myers JL, Noth I et al. Association between MUC5B and TERT polymorphisms and different interstitial lung disease phenotypes. *Transl Res.* 2014;163(5):494–502.

76. Hu B, Gharaee-Kermani M, Wu Z, Phan SH. Epigenetic regulation of myofibroblast differentiation by DNA methylation. *Am J Pathol.* 2010;177(1):21–8.

77. Hu B, Gharaee-Kermani M, Wu Z, Phan SH. Essential role of MeCP2 in the regulation of myofibroblast differentiation during pulmonary fibrosis. *Am J Pathol.* 2011;178(4):1500–8.

78. Coward WR, Watts K, Feghali-Bostwick CA, Knox A, Pang L. Defective histone acetylation is responsible for the diminished expression of cyclooxygenase 2 in idiopathic pulmonary fibrosis. *Mol Cell Biol.* 2009;29(15):4325–39.

79. Coward WR, Watts K, Feghali-Bostwick CA, Jenkins G, Pang L. Repression of IP-10 by interactions between histone deacetylation and hypermethylation in idiopathic pulmonary fibrosis. *Mol Cell Biol.* 2010;30(12):2874–86.

80. Sanders YY, Pardo A, Selman M, Nuovo GJ, Tollefsbol TO, Siegal GP et al. Thy-1 promoter hypermethylation: A novel epigenetic pathogenic mechanism in pulmonary fibrosis. *Am J Respir Cell Mol Biol.* 2008;39(5):610–8.

81. Dakhlallah D, Batte K, Wang Y, Cantemir-Stone CZ, Yan P, Nuovo G et al. Epigenetic regulation of miR-17~92 contributes to the pathogenesis of pulmonary fibrosis. *Am J Respir Crit Care Med.* 2013;187(4):397–405.

82. Sanders YY, Ambalavanan N, Halloran B, Zhang X, Liu H, Crossman DK et al. Altered

DNA methylation profile in idiopathic pulmonary fibrosis. *Am J Respir Crit Care Med.* 2012;186(6):525–35.

83. Rabinovich EI, Kapetanaki MG, Steinfeld I, Gibson KF, Pandit KV, Yu G et al. Global methylation patterns in idiopathic pulmonary fibrosis. *PLoS One.* 2012;7(4):e33770.

84. Kuwano K, Kunitake R, Kawasaki M, Nomoto Y, Hagimoto N, Nakanishi Y et al. P21Waf1/Cip1/Sdi1 and p53 expression in association with DNA strand breaks in idiopathic pulmonary fibrosis. *Am J Respir Crit Care Med.* 1996;154(2 Pt 1):477–83.

85. Maeyama T, Kuwano K, Kawasaki M, Kunitake R, Hagimoto N, Matsuba T et al. Upregulation of Fas-signalling molecules in lung epithelial cells from patients with idiopathic pulmonary fibrosis. *Eur Respir J.* 2001;17(2):180–9.

86. Coalson JJ. The ultrastructure of human fibrosing alveolitis. *Virchows Arch A Pathol Anat Histol.* 1982;395(2):181–99.

87. Katzenstein AL. Pathogenesis of 'fibrosis' in interstitial pneumonia: An electron microscopic study. *Hum Pathol.* 1985;16(10):1015–24.

88. Kawanami O, Ferrans VJ, Crystal RG. Structure of alveolar epithelial cells in patients with fibrotic lung disorders. *Lab Invest.* 1982;46(1):39–53.

89. Ahluwalia N, Shea BS, Tager AM. New therapeutic targets in idiopathic pulmonary fibrosis. Aiming to rein in runaway wound-healing responses. *Am J Respir Crit Care Med.* 2014;190(8):867–78.

90. King TE, Jr., Pardo A, Selman M. Idiopathic pulmonary fibrosis. *Lancet.* 2011;378(9807):1949–61.

91. Scotton CJ, Krupiczojc MA, Konigshoff M, Mercer PF, Lee YC, Kaminski N et al. Increased local expression of coagulation factor X contributes to the fibrotic response in human and murine lung injury. *J Clin Invest.* 2009;119(9):2550–63.

92. Bogatkevich GS, Tourkina E, Silver RM, Ludwicka-Bradley A. Thrombin differentiates normal lung fibroblasts to a myofibroblast phenotype via the proteolytically activated receptor-1 and a protein kinase C-dependent pathway. *J Biol Chem.* 2001;276(48):45184–92.

93. Korfei M, Ruppert C, Mahavadi P, Henneke I, Markart P, Koch M et al. Epithelial endoplasmic reticulum stress and apoptosis in sporadic idiopathic pulmonary fibrosis. *Am J Respir Crit Care Med.* 2008;178(8):838–46.

94. Tanjore H, Blackwell TS, Lawson WE. Emerging evidence for endoplasmic reticulum stress in the pathogenesis of idiopathic pulmonary fibrosis. *Am J Physiol Lung Cell Mol Physiol.* 2012;302(8):L721–9.

95. Zhong Q, Zhou B, Ann DK, Minoo P, Liu Y, Banfalvi A et al. Role of endoplasmic reticulum stress in epithelial-mesenchymal transition of alveolar epithelial cells: Effects of misfolded surfactant protein. *Am J Respir Cell Mol Biol.* 2011;45(3):498–509.

96. Tanjore H, Cheng DS, Degryse AL, Zoz DF, Abdolrasulnia R, Lawson WE et al. Alveolar epithelial cells undergo epithelial-to-mesenchymal transition in response to endoplasmic reticulum stress. *J Biol Chem.* 2011;286(35):30972–80.

97. Kalluri R, Neilson EG. Epithelial-mesenchymal transition and its implications for fibrosis. *J Clin Invest.* 2003;112(12):1776–84.

98. Iwano M, Plieth D, Danoff TM, Xue C, Okada H, Neilson EG. Evidence that fibroblasts derive from epithelium during tissue fibrosis. *J Clin Invest.* 2002;110(3):341–50.

99. Guarino M, Rubino B, Ballabio G. The role of epithelial-mesenchymal transition in cancer pathology. *Pathology.* 2007;39(3):305–18.

100. Kim KK, Kugler MC, Wolters PJ, Robillard L, Galvez MG, Brumwell AN et al. Alveolar epithelial cell mesenchymal transition develops *in vivo* during pulmonary fibrosis and is regulated by the extracellular matrix. *Proc Natl Acad Sci U S A.* 2006;103(35):13180–5.

101. Jayachandran A, Konigshoff M, Yu H, Rupniewska E, Hecker M, Klepetko W et al. SNAI transcription factors mediate epithelial-mesenchymal transition in lung fibrosis. *Thorax.* 2009;64(12):1053–61.

102. Hashimoto N, Jin H, Liu T, Chensue SW, Phan SH. Bone marrow-derived progenitor cells in pulmonary fibrosis. *J Clin Invest.* 2004;113(2):243–52.

103. Andersson-Sjoland A, de Alba CG, Nihlberg K, Becerril C, Ramirez R, Pardo

A et al. Fibrocytes are a potential source of lung fibroblasts in idiopathic pulmonary fibrosis. *Int J Biochem Cell Biol.* 2008;40(10):2129–40.

104. Moeller A, Gilpin SE, Ask K, Cox G, Cook D, Gauldie J et al. Circulating fibrocytes are an indicator of poor prognosis in idiopathic pulmonary fibrosis. *Am J Respir Crit Care Med.* 2009;179(7):588–94.

105. Hashimoto N, Phan SH, Imaizumi K, Matsuo M, Nakashima H, Kawabe T et al. Endothelial-mesenchymal transition in bleomycin-induced pulmonary fibrosis. *Am J Respir Cell Mol Biol.* 2010;43(2):161–72.

106. Willis BC, Borok Z. TGF-beta-induced EMT: Mechanisms and implications for fibrotic lung disease. *Am J Physiol Lung Cell Mol Physiol.* 2007;293(3):L525–34.

107. Hung C, Linn G, Chow YH, Kobayashi A, Mittelsteadt K, Altemeier WA et al. Role of lung pericytes and resident fibroblasts in the pathogenesis of pulmonary fibrosis. *Am J Respir Crit Care Med.* 2013;188(7):820–30.

108. Chang W, Wei K, Jacobs SS, Upadhyay D, Weill D, Rosen GD. SPARC suppresses apoptosis of idiopathic pulmonary fibrosis fibroblasts through constitutive activation of beta-catenin. *J Biol Chem.* 2010;285(11):8196–206.

109. Maher TM, Evans IC, Bottoms SE, Mercer PF, Thorley AJ, Nicholson AG et al. Diminished prostaglandin E2 contributes to the apoptosis paradox in idiopathic pulmonary fibrosis. *Am J Respir Crit Care Med.* 2010;182(1):73–82.

110. Nho RS, Hergert P, Kahm J, Jessurun J, Henke C. Pathological alteration of FoxO3a activity promotes idiopathic pulmonary fibrosis fibroblast proliferation on type i collagen matrix. *Am J Pathol.* 2011;179(5):2420–30.

111. Desmouliere A, Redard M, Darby I, Gabbiani G. Apoptosis mediates the decrease in cellularity during the transition between granulation tissue and scar. *Am J Pathol.* 1995;146(1):56–66.

112. Coon DR, Roberts DJ, Loscertales M, Kradin R. Differential epithelial expression of SHH and FOXF1 in usual and nonspecific interstitial pneumonia. *Exp Mol Pathol.* 2006;80(2):119–23.

113. Vuga LJ, Ben-Yehudah A, Kovkarova-Naumovski E, Oriss T, Gibson KF, Feghali-Bostwick C et al. WNT5A is a regulator of fibroblast proliferation and resistance to apoptosis. *Am J Respir Cell Mol Biol.* 2009;41(5):583–9.

114. Konigshoff M, Kramer M, Balsara N, Wilhelm J, Amarie OV, Jahn A et al. WNT1-inducible signaling protein-1 mediates pulmonary fibrosis in mice and is upregulated in humans with idiopathic pulmonary fibrosis. *J Clin Invest.* 2009;119(4):772–87.

115. Kobayashi K, Araya J, Minagawa S, Hara H, Saito N, Kadota T et al. Involvement of PARK2-mediated mitophagy in idiopathic pulmonary fibrosis pathogenesis. *J Immunol.* 2016;197(2):504–16.

116. Booth AJ, Hadley R, Cornett AM, Dreffs AA, Matthes SA, Tsui JL et al. Acellular normal and fibrotic human lung matrices as a culture system for *in vitro* investigation. *Am J Respir Crit Care Med.* 2012;186(9):866–76.

117. Huang X, Yang N, Fiore VF, Barker TH, Sun Y, Morris SW et al. Matrix stiffness-induced myofibroblast differentiation is mediated by intrinsic mechanotransduction. *Am J Respir Cell Mol Biol.* 2012;47(3):340–8.

118. Zhou Y, Huang X, Hecker L, Kurundkar D, Kurundkar A, Liu H et al. Inhibition of mechanosensitive signaling in myofibroblasts ameliorates experimental pulmonary fibrosis. *J Clin Invest.* 2013;123(3):1096–108.

119. Klingberg F, Hinz B, White ES. The myofibroblast matrix: Implications for tissue repair and fibrosis. *J Pathol.* 2013;229(2):298–309.

120. Cool CD, Groshong SD, Rai PR, Henson PM, Stewart JS, Brown KK. Fibroblast foci are not discrete sites of lung injury or repair: The fibroblast reticulum. *Am J Respir Crit Care Med.* 2006;174(6):654–8.

121. Idiopathic Pulmonary Fibrosis Clinical Research N, Raghu G, Anstrom KJ, King TE, Jr., Lasky JA, Martinez FJ. Prednisone, azathioprine, and N-acetylcysteine for pulmonary fibrosis. *N Engl J Med.* 2012;366(21):1968–77.

122. Kolb M, Collard HR. *Eur Respir Rev.* 2014;23(132):220–4.

9

Idiopathic pulmonary fibrosis: How should a confident diagnosis be made?

BRIDGET F COLLINS AND GANESH RAGHU

OVERVIEW

While the 2011 evidence-based idiopathic pulmonary fibrosis (IPF) guidelines established criteria for the diagnosis of IPF, making the diagnosis can still be challenging in clinical practice (1). The IPF guidelines outlined the following diagnostic criteria for IPF: (1) exclusion of other known causes of interstitial lung disease (ILD) such as connective tissue disease-associated ILD (CTD-ILD), domestic/occupational exposures known to be associated with pulmonary fibrosis, non-IPF forms of idiopathic interstitial pneumonia (IIP) and hypersensitivity pneumonitis (HP); (2) the presence of a usual interstitial pneumonia (UIP) pattern on high-resolution computed tomography (HRCT) of the chest in patients who have not undergone a surgical lung biopsy (SLB); and (3) specific combinations of HRCT and SLB histopathologic patterns in patients who undergo SLB (1). Although new evidence has accumulated since the 2011 guidelines were published, the 2011 diagnostic criteria remain the gold standard until the diagnostic guidelines are updated.

HISTORY, PHYSICAL EXAM AND LABORATORY TESTING

As described in the previous chapter, the most common presenting symptoms among patients with IPF are cough and dyspnoea (1). Symptom onset may be insidious and may precede diagnosis by 1–2 years, and radiographic abnormalities may occur before symptom onset (2–4). In a recent, small qualitative study of European patients with IPF, 87% of patients reported that it took over 1 year from symptom onset until they were given a diagnosis of IPF (5).

A detailed current and past medical history that includes family medical history is absolutely necessary to rule out potential alternate aetiologies of ILD such as CTD-ILD or HP. Elicitation of a detailed exposure history is particularly important; Morell et al. found that when 46 patients diagnosed with IPF in one region using the 2011 guideline criteria were re-evaluated using a prompted, detailed exposure history accompanied by additional testing (lung biopsy, bronchial challenge, etc.) at a centre with special expertise in diagnosing HP, 43% of the patients were subsequently diagnosed with chronic HP (6). CTD-ILD should also be eliminated as a possibility prior to making a diagnosis of IPF. A detailed history of CTD signs and symptoms should be taken, and multidisciplinary discussion (MDD), particularly with input from rheumatology consultants, can be helpful in recognizing cases of suspected CTD-ILD. Clinicians should also obtain a history of current and prior medication use and chemotherapy treatment, as drug toxicity can rarely manifest as UIP (7,8).

The physical exam most often reveals bibasilar crackles, and fingernail clubbing is present in up to 50% of patients (1,9). Patients should also be thoroughly evaluated for extra-pulmonary symptoms and signs of CTD, such as skin rashes, sclerodactyly and musculoskeletal abnormalities; these can raise suspicion of a specific and an alternative diagnosis for the presence of ILD, rather than concluding that the aetiology is idiopathic.

Regarding laboratory testing, a serum precipitin panel for antigens associated with HP may be considered, but it is important to note that the detection of positive antibodies only provides evidence of exposure; the results do not confirm or refute a diagnosis of chronic HP. Also, standardized panels are not used across all laboratories. CTD serologies, in particular antinuclear antibody (ANA) and rheumatoid factor (RF) titres, should be obtained in all patients regardless of symptoms, as ILD may be the initial manifestation of the presence of a CTD in some patients (10,11). However, ANA and RF have low specificity and may be seen in a substantial subset of the healthy elderly population (11–13). Indeed, patients with low titre autoantibodies who do not have signs or symptoms that suggest the presence of a CTD can still be considered to have IPF. Pulmonary function testing among patients with IPF most often shows restriction and a reduced diffusion capacity for carbon monoxide (1).

ROLE OF THORACIC IMAGING

All patients suspected to have ILD/IPF should undergo a HRCT, which is more sensitive than chest radiograph for detecting interstitial abnormalities (14). The HRCT technique is important; the HRCT protocol should include thin (1–2 mm) contiguous sections, and inspiratory/expiratory as well as prone/supine views should be considered (1,15). A HRCT diagnosis of definite UIP has a positive predictive value of 90%–100% for histopathologic UIP on SLB, and in the appropriate clinical setting, an IPF diagnosis can be made in the absence of lung biopsy when a definite UIP pattern on HRCT is observed (1,16,17). Radiographic criteria for UIP are shown in Table 9.1, and examples of HRCT images are shown in Figure 9.1. HRCT criteria for UIP include subpleural, basilar predominance of reticular abnormalities and honeycombing with or without traction bronchiectasis in the absence of features inconsistent with UIP (e.g. extent of ground-glass opacities greater

Table 9.1 High-resolution computed tomography criteria for usual interstitial pneumonia (UIP) pattern

UIP pattern (all four)	Possible UIP (all three)	Inconsistent with UIP
1. Subpleural, basilar predominance	1. Subpleural, basilar predominance	1. Upper or mid-lung predominance
2. Reticulation	2. Reticulation	2. Peribronchovascular predominance
3. Honeycombing +/– traction bronchiectasis	3. Absence features inconsistent with UIP (column 3)	3. Extensive ground-glass abnormalities (extent > reticular abnormality)
4. Absence of features inconsistent with UIP (column 3)		4. Profuse micronodules (bilateral, predominantly upper lobe)
		5. Discrete cysts (multiple, bilateral, not in areas of honeycombing)
		6. Diffuse air trapping (bilateral, in ≥3 lobes
		7. Consolidation in bronchopulmonary segment(s)

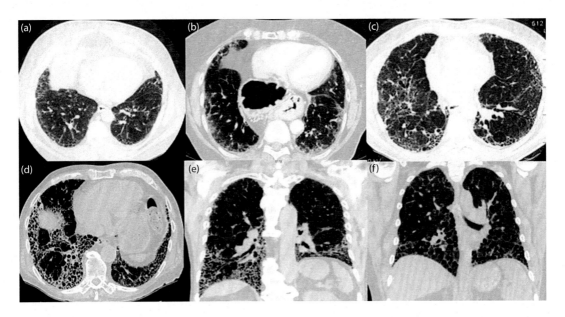

Figure 9.1 UIP on HRCT. **(a)** 61-year-old man with IPF, **(b)** 77-year-old woman with IPF and large hiatal hernia, **(c,d)** 81-year-old man with IPF, and **(e,f)** 60-year-old man with IPF.

than reticulation) (1). Honeycombing on HRCT is defined as clustered cystic airspaces, which are usually of comparable diameter (3–10 mm generally, but up to 2.5 cm possible) and are subpleural with well-defined walls (1,18). However, a UIP pattern on HRCT is not synonymous with a diagnosis of IPF and may be seen in other diseases such as CTD-ILD or chronic HP.

When HRCT features meet diagnostic criteria for UIP but honeycombing is absent, the pattern is classified as possible UIP (1). In patients with a possible UIP pattern, surgical lung biopsy should be considered. Among patients with IPF referred by pulmonologists for participation in the ARTEMIS-IPF study, 94% with possible UIP had histopathological UIP on SLB and were diagnosed with IPF, suggesting that a possible UIP pattern on HRCT in the appropriate clinical setting with the diagnosis made at a tertiary referral center by ILD experts may be sufficient to establish a diagnosis of IPF (19). However, patients referred for the ARTEMIS-IPF study were a select group; therefore, this result may not apply uniformly to all patients with possible UIP. SLB may be helpful in distinguishing between IPF, chronic HP and CTD-ILD in patients with a possible UIP pattern on HRCT. Some investigators have modified the criteria of the possible UIP pattern to include traction bronchiectasis without honeycombing, and

patients who have not undergone a SLB to show evidence of UIP have been enrolled in IPF clinical trials. Use of the pattern/term 'probable UIP' for such patients, which was shown in one study to more closely correlate with histopathologic UIP than other forms of what is currently described as possible UIP ('indeterminate UIP' in that study), has been proposed (20–22). Undoubtedly such accumulating evidence from a variety of investigations will be reviewed in the anticipated update to the evidence-based guidelines for the diagnosis of IPF.

ROLE OF OBTAINING PATHOLOGIC TISSUE SPECIMENS (WHEN REQUIRED) AND TECHNIQUES

Histopathologically, a pattern of UIP demonstrates spatial and temporal heterogeneity wherein areas of normal lung alternate with areas of interstitial fibrosis (with fibrosis dominating over inflammation) along with honeycomb change (Figure 9.2) (23,24). The subpleural and paraseptal regions are most often affected. Fibroblastic foci, which are areas of proliferating fibroblasts and myofibroblasts that are not specific for UIP, are present

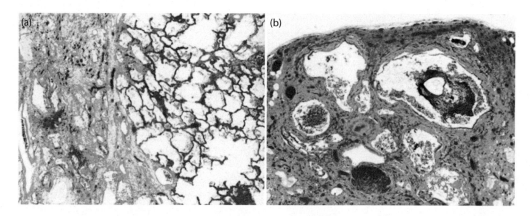

Figure 9.2 UIP histopathology from surgical lung biopsy. **(a)** UIP with abrupt transitions between fibrotic and non-fibrotic lung. **(b)** Microcystic honeycombing.

(1,23,24). Notably, the UIP pattern can also be found in asbestosis, chronic HP, CTD-ILD and ILD due to drug toxicity. Histopathology demonstrating a UIP pattern is not synonymous with a diagnosis of IPF, and individual cases should be evaluated via MDD (see below) that considers the clinical context as well as radiographic features (Table 9.2).

In the appropriate clinical setting, the histopathology pattern of UIP on SLB substantiates a diagnosis of IPF. While bronchoalveolar lavage (BAL) and transbronchial lung biopsies may be helpful in excluding other causes of respiratory symptoms or non-IPF ILD such as sarcoidosis, transbronchial biopsies are unlikely to yield an adequate amount of tissue to make a diagnosis of

Table 9.2 Integration of HRCT and surgical lung biopsy patterns in IPF diagnosis; final diagnosis requires multidisciplinary discussion

HRCT pattern	Surgical lung biopsy pattern	IPF diagnosis?
UIP	• UIP	IPF
	• Probable UIP	
	• Possible UIP	
	• Non-classifiable fibrosis	
	• Not UIP	Not IPF
Possible UIP	• UIP	IPF
	• Probable UIP	
	• Possible UIP	Probable IPF
	• Non-classifiable fibrosis	
	• Not UIP	Not IPF
Inconsistent with UIP	• UIP	Possible IPF
	• Probable UIP	Not IPF
	• Possible UIP	
	• Non-classifiable fibrosis	
	• Not UIP	

Source: Reprinted from Raghu G et al. An official ATS/ERS/JRS/ALAT statement: Idiopathic pulmonary fibrosis: Evidence-based guidelines for diagnosis and management. *Am J Respir Crit Care Med.* 2011;183(6):788–824. Copyright 2017, with permission from American Thoracic Society.

UIP. Therefore, SLB performed by video-assisted thoracoscopy (VATS) or thoracotomy is needed to make a confident diagnosis of UIP (1,25). With the recent advent of transbronchial lung cryobiopsy (TLC), some centres report adequate diagnostic yield in lung biopsy specimens obtained via TLC techniques (26). Regardless of whether SLB or TLC is performed to retrieve diagnostic tissue, lung biopsy specimens from at least two to three different bronchopulmonary segments/lobes must be obtained in patients suspected to have IIP/IPF (27). Histopathology from SLB specimens may demonstrate UIP in one segment and NSIP in a different biopsied segment, and such cases are classified as discordant UIP (1,27,28). Clinical behaviour in patients with discordant biopsies is similar to that of patients with concordant UIP (UIP in all biopsy segments) (27,28).

Concerns about the need to obtain a SLB include the risk of precipitating an acute exacerbation of ILD as well as risks of mortality and other complications. Patients with IPF seem particularly vulnerable to stress incurred with thoracic as well as non-thoracic surgery; rates of acute respiratory decline among patients with IPF undergoing thoracic surgical cancer resection range from 7% to 32% (29,30). Additionally, acute exacerbations of IPF have been reported following SLB and even following BAL (31,32). Among patients with ILD, mortality rates of SLB have generally ranged from 1% to 5% in various case series, although some series report higher rates (33–36). While the diagnostic yield is similar between VATS biopsy and open lung biopsy, morbidity and mortality are lower with VATS than with open lung biopsy (33,37,38). A study of 2,820 patients with ILD in the United Kingdom found that in-hospital, 30-day and 90-day mortality rates with SLB were 1.7%, 2.4% and 3.9%, respectively; increasing age, open thoracotomy and the number of patient comorbidities were associated with poorer outcomes (39). Other studies have found pre-operative oxygen dependence and pulmonary hypertension to be associated with greater mortality for VATS (34). Whether SLB is elective also affects mortality risk. In a US study, elective SLB had a lower in-hospital mortality than non-elective procedures (1.7% versus 16%); additional risk factors for increased mortality included male sex, increasing age, increasing number of comorbidities,

open biopsy approach and a provisional diagnosis of IPF or CTD-ILD (40).

Yield and safety of TLC in IPF deserve further mention. One small trial compared TLC to SLB in patients with ILD and demonstrated that in 72% of cases, findings from TLC were congruent with other clinical data and facilitated reaching a definitive diagnosis (41). Complications following TLC included pneumothorax (19%) and severe endobronchial bleeding (53%), although only 2 of 17 patients with severe bleeding required rigid bronchoscopy for clot extraction (41). A study of 69 patients with fibrotic ILD reported adequate TLC specimens in 99% of cases (median number of tissue pieces obtained was three), and pathologists reported high confidence in their ability to identify a specific pattern from TLC samples in 76% of patients including 77% with UIP (42). Complications included pneumothorax in 28%, death from acute exacerbation in 1.4% and prolonged bleeding in 1.4% (42). When compared to SLB, peri-operative mortality was 1.7% (one patient) with TLC versus 3.4% (two patients) with SLB among patients with fibrotic ILD, and all deaths were attributed to acute exacerbation of IPF (26). Hospitalization time was on average 3 days with TLC compared to 6 days with SLB, and pneumothorax occurred in 33% of patients who underwent TLC (26). The authors found that both TLC and SLB similarly affected multidisciplinary diagnosis of IPF with similar changes in diagnostic impression, confidence and interobserver agreement (26).

KEYS TO RECOGNIZING NON-IPF FIBROTIC ILD: MIMICS OF IPF AND CONFOUNDING CO-MORBID CONDITIONS

Diagnosis of IPF requires exclusion of other causes of fibrotic lung disease. Chronic HP is a very important consideration, and nearly half of a cohort of patients diagnosed with IPF by 2011 criteria were recognized as actually having chronic HP following additional exposure history and testing (6). Chronic HP may demonstrate a UIP pattern on histopathology that is indistinguishable from that seen in IPF (23,43). In the absence of poorly formed granulomas, there may be some additional clues on SLB such as peribronchiolar inflammation and/or fibrosis to suggest a diagnosis of HP, and biopsy from more than one lobe may also be helpful (23,43). In addition to a thorough exposure history, BAL may be helpful; BAL lymphocytosis of >30%, typically with CD8T cell predominance, is highly suggestive of chronic HP (44,45).

CTD-ILD may also mimic IPF, particularly in patients with rheumatoid arthritis (RA), where the most common pattern of ILD is UIP (46,47). Suspicion for possible CTD-ILD should be particularly high in women and in patients less than 50 years of age (1,45). Patients should undergo a thorough history and physical exam to elicit symptoms and signs of CTD such as Raynaud phenomenon, arthritis, muscle weakness, skin changes and oesophageal motility problems. As described above, a CTD panel should be sent in most patients suspected to have IPF (1). ILD

may be the initial manifestation of CTD in some patients, and high titres of antibodies such as RF and anti-CCP or positive antibodies for inflammatory myositis or systemic sclerosis should raise this possibility (10,48,49).

Asbestosis can also mimic IPF. In addition to a significant exposure history, findings on HRCT such as pleural thickening or plaques may provide clues to a diagnosis of asbestosis, although pleural findings are not universal in patients exposed to asbestos, and pleural abnormalities may be due to other causes (45,50). HRCT findings of coarser fibrosis, parenchymal bands and subpleural curvilinear lines are more common in asbestosis than in patients with IPF (50,51). Histopathologic microscopic diagnosis of asbestosis requires interstitial fibrosis and the presence of asbestos bodies (52). Fibrosis in asbestosis is often accompanied

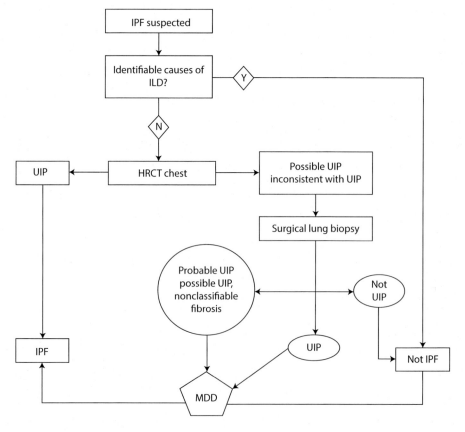

Figure 9.3 Diagnostic algorithm for IPF based on 2011 guidelines. (Reprinted from Raghu G et al. An official ATS/ERS/JRS/ALAT statement: Idiopathic pulmonary fibrosis: Evidence-based guidelines for diagnosis and management. *Am J Respir Crit Care Med.* 2011;183[6]:788–824. Copyright 2017, with permission from American Thoracic Society.)

Clinical cases

CASE 1

A 75-year-old man presents with 1 year of nonproductive cough and shortness of breath. One year ago at this time he was able to walk his dog 2 miles per day, but now he is only able to walk ½ mile before he must stop and catch his breath. He is a former smoker (1 pack per day for 15 years) and quit 35 years ago. HRCT images are shown here.

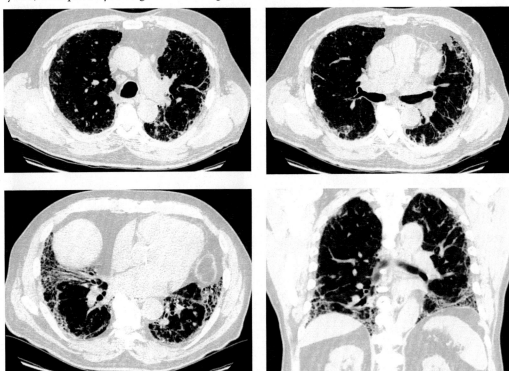

Question: What is the next best step in evaluation and management?

1. Perform bronchoscopy with bronchoalveolar lavage and transbronchial biopsies.
2. Obtain an occupational and domestic exposure history.
3. Initiate daily prednisone.
4. Initiate anti-fibrotic therapy.

The next best step is to obtain additional occupational and domestic exposure history. The HRCT scan shows a UIP pattern of pulmonary fibrosis with peripheral basilar predominant subpleural reticulation and traction bronchiectasis. There is also honeycombing. While the UIP pattern on HRCT is sufficient to diagnose IPF in the right clinical setting, the provider must first eliminate potential exposures that may be associated with hypersensitivity pneumonitis (HP) as well as signs and symptoms of connective tissue disease (CTD), as the UIP pattern may be seen in chronic HP, asbestosis, as well as in CTD-associated ILD (especially in rheumatoid arthritis).

The patient had a parakeet as a child, but he has not owned birds since the age of 15. He has no concerning occupational or domestic exposures. He does not have signs or symptoms of CTD, and a full panel of CTD serologies including anti-nuclear antibody, rheumatoid factor, anti-cyclic-citrullinated peptide antibody and a myositis panel are negative. Based on this information (in addition to the HRCT demonstrating a UIP pattern) the patient is diagnosed with IPF.

CASE 2

A 70-year-old man presents with 4 years of progressive exertional dyspnoea. He has never smoked, and while he and his wife live on 25 acres of land, the area is wooded. They have no pets (including birds). Past medical history is notable for obstructive sleep apnoea for which he uses a continuous positive airway pressure (CPAP) apparatus. HRCT images are shown below. Connective tissue disease serologies were obtained and were unremarkable. Pulmonary function testing (PFT) is unremarkable other than a reduced DLCO value (adjusted for peripheral blood haemoglobin content) at 71% of the predicted normal value.

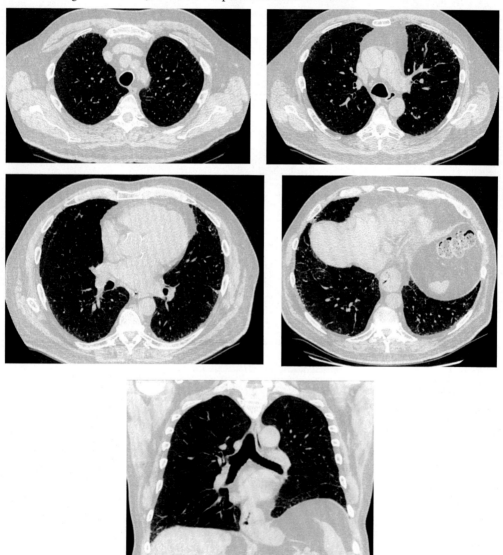

Question: What is the next best step in evaluation and management of this patient?

1. Perform bronchoscopy with transbronchial lung biopsies only.
2. Diagnose the patient with IPF and discuss anti-fibrotic therapy.
3. Refer for surgical lung biopsy.
4. Ask the patient to return in 12 months with repeat pulmonary function tests.

The next best step would be to refer the patient for surgical lung biopsy (SLB). While bronchoalveolar lavage (BAL) may be helpful in distinguishing among some forms of ILD (for instance sarcoidosis and chronic HP tend to exhibit BAL differential cell count lymphocytosis), transbronchial lung biopsies alone are typically not helpful for a patient with a possible UIP pattern on HRCT such as is the case for this patient. While a possible UIP pattern in a patient without a history of exposures that could lead to HP or signs or symptoms of CTD is considered by some to be adequate to diagnose IPF in the appropriate clinical setting, other possibilities such as chronic HP in response to occult antigen exposure remain on the list of potential diagnoses. Given the patient's mild disease on HRCT and only mildly impaired DLCO on PFTs, it may be reasonable to observe the patient and have him return with PFTs and then intervene if he has a significant decline in PFT values – 12 months would be too long of a period to wait to see if the lung disease progresses.

The patient underwent SLB, and findings were consistent with chronic HP. The patient had been planning to move to another home, and when he did so, his symptoms improved. However, an offending antigen was never identified.

by mild pleural fibrosis, and fibroblastic foci are rare (in contrast to IPF) (52). Sarcoidosis is another fibrotic lung disease that could mimic IPF, although fibrosis in advanced pulmonary sarcoidosis is typically mid- to upper lobe predominant in a peri-bronchovascular distribution, and advanced pulmonary sarcoidosis and UIP differ histopathologically (53,54).

Patients with IPF are at increased risk of multiple co-morbid conditions, and mortality is actually attributable to non-IPF conditions in a significant proportion of patients with IPF (2,55–57). Co-morbid conditions and associated symptoms may make the diagnosis of IPF more complex. Rates of venous thromboembolism, gastro-oesphageal reflux, pulmonary hypertension, coronary artery disease, chronic obstructive pulmonary disease, emphysema, lung cancer, sleep apnoea, anxiety and depression are increased among patients with IPF compared to that in age- and sex-matched controls (56,58–60).

MULTIDISCIPLINARY DISCUSSION

Multidisciplinary discussion (MDD) among pulmonologists with experience in ILD, chest radiologists and lung pathologists experienced in histopathologic patterns of IIP/ILD has been shown to improve diagnostic confidence and accuracy in the diagnosis of IIPs including IPF (1,61–63). MDD is especially helpful in cases where radiologic and histopathologic patterns are discordant, and MDD is recommended by the IPF evidence-based guidelines (1). While the IPF guidelines recommend MDD, commonly utilized at centres with expertise in ILD diagnosis, differences in how MDD is conducted exist (e.g. attendee specialties, amount and type of data presented and approach to diagnosis), even among specialized centres (64). There may be a role for additional evidence-based guidelines on composition and conduct of MDDs in the future. Figure 9.3 shows a diagnostic algorithm for IPF (including the incorporation of MDD), based on the 2011 evidence-based guidelines.

REFERENCES

1. Raghu G, Collard HR, Egan JJ. An official ATS/ERS/JRS/ALAT statement: Idiopathic pulmonary fibrosis: Evidence-based guidelines for diagnosis and management. *Am J Respir Crit Care Med.* 2011;183(6):788–824.

2. Ley B, Collard HR, King Jr TE. Clinical course and prediction of survival in idiopathic pulmonary fibrosis. *Am J Respir Crit Care Med.* 2011;183:10.

3. Kim DS, Collard HR, King Jr TE. Classification and natural history of the idiopathic interstitial pneumonias. *Proc Am Thorac Soc.* 2006;3:8.

4. Nagai S, Kitaichi M, Itoh H, Nishimura K, Izumi T, Colby TV. Idiopathic non-specific interstitial pneumonia/fibrosis: Comparison with idiopathic pulmonary fibrosis and BOOP. *Eur Respir J.* 1998;12:10.

5. Russell AM, Ripamonti E, Vancheri C. Qualitative European survey of patients with idiopathic pulmonary fibrosis: Patients' perspectives of disease and treatment. *BMC Pulm Med.* 2016;16(10):7.

6. Morell F, Villar A, Montero MA, Munoz X, Colby TV, Pipvath S et al. Chronic hypersensitivity pneumonitis in patients diagnosed with idiopathic pulmonary fibrosis: A prospective case-cohort study. *Lancet Respir Med.* 2013;1(9):10.

7. Wuyts WA, Cavazza A, Rossi G, Bonella F, Sverzellati N, Spagnolo P. Differential diagnosis of usual interstitial pneumonia: When is it truly idiopathic? *Eur Respir Rev.* 2014;23:12.

8. Myers JL, Limper AH, Swenson SJ. Drug-induced lung disease: A pragmatic classification incorporating HRCT appearances. *Semin Respir Crit Care Med.* 2003;24(4):10.

9. Meltzer EB, Noble PW. Idiopathic pulmonary fibrosis. *Orphanet J Rare Dis.* 2008;3(8):15.

10. Hu Y, Wang LS, Wei YR, Du SS, Du YK, He X et al. Clinical characteristics of connective tissue disease-associated interstitial lung disease in 1,044 Chinese patients. *Chest.* 2016;149(1):9.

11. Fischer A, Lee JS, Cottin V. Interstitial lung disease evaluation: Detecting connective tissue disease. *Respiration.* 2015;90:8.

12. Goodwin JS, Searles RP, Tung KS. Immunological responses of healthy elderly population. *Clin Exp Immunol.* 1982;48(2):8.

13. Manoussakis MN, Tziofas AG, Silis MP, Pange PJ, Goudevenos J, Moutsopoulos HM. High prevalence of anti-cardiolipin and other autoantibodies in a healthy elderly population. *Clin Exp Immunol.* 1987;69(3):9.

14. Mathieson JR, Mayo JR, Staples CA, Muller NL. Chronic diffuse infiltrative lung disease: Comparison of diagnostic accuracy of CT and chest radiography. *Radiology.* 1989;171(1):6.

15. Mayo JR. CT evaluation of diffuse infiltrative lung disease: Dose considerations and optimal technique. *J Thorac Imaging.* 2009;24(4):8.

16. Raghu G, Mageto YN, Lockhart D, Schmidt RA, Wood DE, Godwin JD. The accuracy of the clinical diagnosis of new-onset idiopathic pulmonary fibrosis and other interstitial lung disease: A prospective study. *Chest.* 1999;116(5):7.

17. Swenson SJ, Aughenbaugh GL, Myers JL. Diffuse lung disease: Diagnostic accuracy of CT in patients undergoing surgical biopsy of the lung. *Radiology.* 1997;205(1):6.

18. Hansell DM, Bankier A, Macmahon H, McLoud TC, Muller NL, Remy J. Fleischner society: Glossary of terms for thoracic imaging. *Radiology.* 2008;246:25.

19. Raghu G, Lynch D, Godwin JD, Webb R, Colby TV, Leslie KO et al. Diagnosis of idiopathic pulmonary fibrosis with high-resolution CT in patients with little or no radiological evidence of honeycombing: Secondary analysis of a randomised trial. *Lancet Respir Med.* 2014;2(4):8.

20. Raghu G, Wells AU, Nicholson AG, Richeldi L, Flaherty KR, Le Maulf F et al. Effect of nintedanib in subgroups of idiopathic pulmonary fibrosis by diagnostic criteria. *Am J Respir Crit Care Med.* 2017;195(1):78–85.

21. Richeldi L, du Bois RM, Raghu G, Azuma A, Brown KK, Costabel U et al. Efficacy and safety of nintedanib in idiopathic pulmonary fibrosis. *NEJM.* 2014;370(22):12.

22. Chung JH, Chawla A, Peljito AL, Cool CD, Groshong SD, Talbert JL et al. CT scan findings of probable usual interstitial pneumonitis have a high predictive value for histologic usual interstitial pneumonitis. *Chest.* 2015;147(2):10.

23. Visscher DW, Myers JL. Histologic spectrum of idiopathic interstitial pneumonias. *Proc Am Thorac Soc.* 2006;3:8.

24. Katzenstein AA, Myers JL. Idiopathic pulmonary fibrosis. Clinical relevance of pathologic classification. *Am J Respir Crit Care Med.* 1998;157:15.

25. Meyer KC, Raghu G, Baughman RP, Brown KK, Costabel U, du Bois RM et al. An official American Thoracic Society clinical practice guideline: The clinical utility of bronchoalveolar lavage cellular analysis in interstitial lung disease. *Am J Respir Crit Care Med.* 2012;185(9):11.

26. Tomassetti S, Wells AU, Costabel U, Cavazza A, Colby TV, Rossi G et al. Bronchoscopic lung cryobiopsy increases diagnostic confidence in the multidisciplinary diagnosis of idiopathic pulmonary fibrosis. *Am J Respir Crit Care Med.* 2016;193(7):8.

27. Monaghan H, Wells AU, Colby TV, du Bois RM, Hansell DM, Nicholson AG. Prognostic implications of histologic patterns in multiple surgical lung biopsies from patients with idiopathic interstitial pneumonias. *Chest.* 2004;125:5.

28. Flaherty KR, Travis WD, Colby TV, Toews GB, Kazerooni EA, Gross BH et al. Histopathologic variability in usual and non-specific interstitial pneumonias. *Am J Respir Crit Care Med.* 2001;164(9):6.

29. Collard HR, Ryerson CJ, Corte TJ, Jenkins G, Kondoh Y, Lederer DJ et al. Acute exacerbation of idiopathic pulmonary fibrosis. An international working group report. *AJRCCM.* 2016;194(3):11.

30. Ghatol A, Ruhl AP, Danoff SK. Exacerbations in idiopathic pulmonary fibrosis triggered by pulmonary and nonpulmonary surgery: A case series and comprehensive review of the literature. *Lung.* 2012;190(4):8.

31. Samejima S, Tajiri M, Ogura T, Baba T, Omori T, Tsuboi M et al. Thoracoscopic lung biopsy in 285 patients wth diffuse pulmonary disease. *Asian Cardiovasc Thorac Ann.* 2015;23(2):7.

32. Sakamoto K, Taniguchi H, Kondoh Y, Wakai K, Kimura T, Kataoka K et al. Acute exacerbation of IPF following diagnostic bronchoalveolar lavage procedures. *Respir Med.* 2012;106(3):7.

33. Nguyen W, Meyer KC. Surgical lung biopsy for the diagnosis of interstitial lung disease: A review of the literature and recommendations for optimizing safety and efficacy. *Sarcoidosis Vasc Diffuse Lung Dis.* 2013;30(1):14.

34. Kreider ME, Hansen-Flaschen J, Ahmad NN, Rossman MD, Kaiser LR, Kucharczuk JC et al. Complications of video-assisted thoracoscopic lung biopsy in patients with interstitial lung disease. *Ann Thorac Surg.* 2007;83(3):5.

35. Blackhall V, Asif M, Renieri A, Civitelli S, Kirk A, Jilaihawi A et al. The role of surgical lung biopsy in the management of interstitial lung disease: Experience from a single institution in the UK. *Interact Cardiovasc Thorac Surg.* 2013;17(2):5.

36. Lettieri CJ, Veerappan GR, Helman DL, Mulligan CR, Shorr AF. Outcomes and safety of surgical lung biopsy for interstitial lung disease. *Chest.* 2005;127:6.

37. Bensard DD, McIntyre Jr RC, Waring BJ, Simon JS. Comparison of video thoracoscopic lung biopsy to open lung biopsy in the diagnosis of interstitial lung disease. *Chest.* 2003;103(3):6.

38. Miller JD, Urschel JD, Cox G, Olak J, Young JE, Kay JM et al. A randomized, controlled trial comparing thoracoscopy and limited thoracotomy for lung biopsy in interstitial lung disease. *Ann Thorac Surg.* 2000;70(5):4.

39. Hutchinson JP, McKeever TM, Fogarty AW, Navaratnam V, Hubbard RB. Surgical lung biopsy for the diagnosis of interstitial lung disease in England: 1997–2008. *Eur Respir J.* 2016;48(5):1453–61.

40. Hutchinson JP, Fogarty AW, McKeever TM, Hubbard RB. In-hospital mortality after surgical lung biopsy for interstitial lung disease in the United States. 2000–2011. *Am J Respir Crit Care Med.* 2016;193(10):7.

41. Hagmeyer L, Theegarten D, Wohlschlager J, Treml M, Matthes S, Priegnitz C et al. The role of transbronchial cryobiopsy and surgical lung biopsy in the diagnostic algorithm of interstitial lung disease. *Clin Respir J.* 2016;10(5):7.

42. Luca Casoni G, Tomassetti S, Cavazza A, Colby TV, Dubini A, Ryu JH et al.

Transbronchial lung cryobiopsy in the diagnosis of fibrotic interstitial lung disease. *PLOS One.* 2014;9(2):7.

43. Trahan S, Hanak V, Ryu JH, Myers JL. Role of surgical lung biopsy in separating chronic hypersensitivity pneumonia from usual interstitial pneumonia/idiopathic pulmonary fibrosis. *Chest.* 2008;134:7.

44. Ohshimo S, Bonella F, Cui A, Beume M, Kohno N, Guzman J et al. Significance of bronchoalveolar lavage for the diagnosis of idiopathic pulmonary fibrosis. *Am J Respir Crit Care Med.* 2009;179(11):5.

45. Spagnolo P, Tonelli R, Cocconcelli E, Stefani A, Richeldi L. Idiopathic pulmonary fibrosis; Diagnostic pitfalls and therapeutic challenges. *Multidiscip Respir Med.* 2012;7(1):42.

46. Lee HK, Kim DS, Yoo B, Seo JB, Rho JY, Colby TV, Kitaichi M. Histopathologic pattern and clinical features of rheumatoid arthritis-associated interstitial lung disease. *Chest.* 2005;127(6):9.

47. Tanaka N, Kim JS, Newell JD, Brown KK, Cool CD, Meehan R et al. Rheumatoid arthritis-related lung diseases: CT findings. *Radiology.* 2004;232(1):11.

48. Homma Y, Ohtsuka Y, Tanimura K, Kusaka H, Munakata M, Kawakami Y et al. Can interstitial pneumonia as the sole presentation of collagen vascular diseases be differentiated from idiopathic interstitial pneumonia. *Respiration.* 1995;62(5):4.

49. Saketkoo LA, Ascherman DP, Cottin V, Christopher-Stine L, Danoff SK, Oddis CV. Interstitial lung disease in idiopathic inflammatory myopathy. *Curr Rheumatol Rev.* 2010;6(2):12.

50. Akira M, Yamamoto S, Inoue Y, Sakatani M. High resolution CT of asbestosis and idiopathic pulmonary fibrosis. *Am J Radiol.* 2003;181:7.

51. Misumi S, Lynch DA. Idiopathic pulmonary fibrosis/usual interstitial pneumonia. Imaging diagnosis, spectrum of abnormalities, and temporal progression. *Proc Am Thorac Soc.* 2006;3(4):8.

52. Roggli V, Gibbs AR, Attanoos R, Churg A, Popper H, Cagle P et al. Pathology of asbestosis – An update of the diagnostic criteria. *Arch Pathol Lab Med.* 2010;134:19.

53. Zhang C, Chan KM, Schmidt LA, Myers JL. Histopathology of explanted lungs from patients with a diagnosis of pulmonary sarcoidosis. *Chest.* 2016;149(2):499–507.

54. Nunes H, Brillet PY, Valeyre D, Brauner MW, Wells AU. Imaging in sarcoidosis. *Semin Respir Crit Care Med.* 2007;28(1):18.

55. Panos RJ, Mortenson RL, Niccoli SA, King Jr TE. Clinical deterioration in patients with idiopathic pulmonary fibrosis; Causes and assessment. *Am J Med.* 1990;88(4):9.

56. King CS, Nathan SD. Idiopathic pulmonary fibrosis: Effects and optimal management of comorbidities. *Lancet Respir Med.* 2017;5(1):72–84.

57. Kreuter M, Ehlers-Tenenbaum S, Palmowski K, Bruhwyler J, Oltmanns U, Muley T et al. Impact of comorbidities on mortality in patients with idiopathic pulmonary fibrosis. *PloS One.* 2016;11(3):18.

58. Raghu G, Amatto VC, Behr J, Stowasser S. Comorbidities in idiopathic pulmonary fibrosis patients: A systematic literature review. *Eur Resp J.* 2015;46(4):18.

59. Collard HR, Ward AJ, Lanes S, Cortney Hayflinger D, Rosenberg DM, Hunsche E. Burden of illness in idiopathic pulmonary fibrosis. *J Med Econ.* 2012;15(5):7.

60. Lancaster LH, Mason WR, Parnell JA, Rice TW, Loyd JE, Milstone AP et al. Obstructive sleep apnea is common in idiopathic pulmonary fibrosis. *Chest.* 2009;136(3):7.

61. Flaherty KR, King Jr TE, Raghu G, Lynch JP, Colby TV, Travis WD et al. Idiopathic interstitial pneumonia: What is the effect of a multidisciplinary approach to diagnosis? *Am J Respir Crit Care Med.* 2004;170(8):7.

62. Tomassetti S, Piciucchi S, Tantalocco P, Dubini A, Poletti V. The multidisciplinary approach in the diagnosis of idiopathic pulmonary fibrosis: A patient case-based review. *Eur Respir Rev.* 2015;24:9.

63. Flaherty KR, Andrei AC, King Jr TE, Raghu G, Colby TV, Wells A et al. Idiopathic interstitial pneumonia: Do community and academic physicians agree on diagnosis? *Am J Respir Crit Care Med.* 2007;175(10):7.

64. Jo HE, Corte TJ, Moodley Y, Levin K, Westall G, Hopkins P et al. Evaluating the interstitial lung diseases multidisciplinary meeting: A survey of expert centers. *BMC Pulm Med.* 2016;16:6.

10

Management of idiopathic pulmonary fibrosis

DAMIAN AD BRUCE-HICKMAN, HELEN GARTHWAITE,
MELISSA HEIGHTMAN, AND BIBEK GOOPTU

INTRODUCTION

Idiopathic pulmonary fibrosis (IPF) is possibly the most rapidly progressive, chronic fibrosing condition in any organ. It is associated with a median survival of 3 years from diagnosis. The overall incidence of diagnosed IPF is increasing, in part as awareness of the diagnosis increases. Indeed, recent epidemiologic findings from the Respiratory Health of the Nation study in the United Kingdom indicate that IPF is twice as common as previously believed, with around 0.5 cases diagnosed per 1,000 of the UK population (1). Moreover, although it is considered a rare disease, IPF is strongly associated with ageing. In patients ≥70 years in age, its incidence is estimated between 1 and 4 per 1,000, and it is responsible for 1% of deaths in the United Kingdom (1–3). Clinical need remains under-served in terms of its diagnosis and effective treatment. Nevertheless, the direction of travel over recent years in both these aspects is encouraging. The evolution of guidelines and algorithms for multidisciplinary diagnosis of IPF (4) has been associated with increased consistency between specialist centres internationally (5). This appears to be accompanied by good identification of cases in which typically 'IPF-like' disease behaviour – progressive decline despite therapeutic intervention – is predicted, allowing proactive management planning. Within this 'typical' picture of disease progression, heterogeneity is increasingly recognized at both clinical and molecular levels, allowing the possibility of more personalized care in the future (6).

In recent years the first treatments proven to reduce disease progression have come to market and been licensed for use in IPF. Moreover, a range of new therapeutic approaches are in development based upon improved understanding of disease mechanisms. Indeed, in IPF there is a feedback loop between these processes. The response to a treatment approach, or its lack, can provide new insights into the pathologic relevance of different processes *in vivo*. The clinical definition of IPF and of underlying cellular and molecular processes relative to other interstitial lung diseases (ILDs) has therefore improved in step with differentiation of effective from ineffective or even harmful therapies. The therapeutic approach has moved from nihilism, via attempts to control disease progression with steroid and immunosuppressive treatments now deemed harmful, to focus upon more directly anti-fibrotic treatments (7). In parallel, the model of pathogenesis has developed (8) from one in which cell-mediated inflammation might cause fibrosis in IPF to one in which an inappropriately triggered wound healing response could lead to scarring without immune cell involvement (9). In this chapter we consider the current approach to diagnosing IPF, emerging sub-phenotyping possibilities, current and emerging therapeutic options and contexts of care. We also discuss complications

associated with the disease and highlight areas of current uncertainty.

EVALUATION AND DIAGNOSIS

The diagnosis of IPF may be aided by the presence of characteristic features. However, these are not entirely specific, and so the possibility of other non-IPF ILDs must be assessed and excluded. In addition, IPF may ultimately be considered the most likely diagnosis even in the context of some atypical features or confounding factors. Last, the diagnosis of IPF should be coupled with some assessment of modifiable co-factors and risk stratification. A detailed clinical assessment is therefore required together with a range of investigations, and findings should be integrated with the benefit of a specialist multidisciplinary team meeting. Subsequently, repeated assessments of key elements in the history, examination and diagnostic investigations can help monitor disease progression.

RELEVANT FEATURES OF PRESENTATION AND HISTORY

IPF typically develops with an insidious clinical onset. A gradual increase in exertional dyspnoea is the most common initial symptom, and this is often accompanied by a non-productive cough. There is a median 1- to 2-year lag between initial presentation and the diagnosis of IPF (10). Initial presentations are often attributed to common causes of dyspnoea such as chronic obstructive pulmonary disease (COPD), heart failure or chest infection (acute bronchitis or pneumonia). This may occur due to genuine co-morbidity with these conditions or due to misdiagnosis. Conversely, patients may present as a result of radiologic investigations undertaken as part of the management of a co-morbidity, often at a pre-symptomatic stage of disease. IPF is more common in men than women (1,4,11), and increasing age is associated with worsened prognosis. Smoking, while not considered 'causative' is a well-defined risk factor (12). Gastro-(o)esophageal reflux disease (GER, GERD, GORD) has been implicated in driving progression of IPF (13) as have infective exacerbations (14,15). Potentially relevant exposures to other pneumotoxic stimuli should also be assessed. These include drugs (16), invasive ventilation, heavy and sustained contact with asbestos or silica dust or triggers of hypersensitivity pneumonitis (e.g. avian antigens, moulds, paraben-containing hair dyes). Endogenous drivers of ILD should also be considered by screening for features in the history suggesting rheumatoid or connective tissue disease, vasculitis or sarcoidosis.

EXAMINATION

On examination the presence of clubbing is far more common in IPF than other ILDs (17,18), while the presence of clinical features suggestive of rheumatoid or other connective tissue disease (CTD) should be noted for evaluation of differential diagnoses. Low body mass index (BMI) is associated with worse outcome. Hypoxaemia and cyanosis may already be apparent upon initial evaluation, as may signs of secondary pulmonary hypertension and right heart failure. On auscultation of the chest, end-inspiratory crackles are a typical finding, and these are characteristically most evident in lower zones. Auscultation of squawks indicates a bronchiolitic process that is not characteristic of IPF, and this finding may prompt consideration of alternative ILDs (hypersensitivity pneumonitis, respiratory bronchiolitis ILD) or infection. In the abdomen, hepatomegaly or splenomegaly could support an alternative diagnosis of sarcoidosis.

PULMONARY FUNCTION TESTING

Pulmonary function tests are highly informative in assessing disease severity and are the most sensitive objective measure of progression. Typically in IPF the spirometry is restrictive with reductions in forced expiratory volume in 1 second (FEV_1) and forced vital capacity (FVC) that do not lead to a forced expiratory ratio <0.7 in the absence of a co-existent obstructive lung disease. Lung volumes are generally reduced, as is gas transfer as measured by the transfer factor indicating the diffusion capacity for carbon monoxide (DLCO, TLCO). The transfer coefficient for carbon monoxide (KCO, equal to DLCO/alveolar volume) is relatively preserved in IPF, as the underlying process of interstitial fibrosis concomitantly reduces alveolar volume and gas transfer by similar factors. Therefore, if the KCO is not relatively preserved this should prompt

consideration of other pathologies and complications (e.g. co-existent emphysema, pulmonary hypertension, pulmonary thromboembolic disease or vasculopathy). In general, FVC is a less sensitive indicator of the extent of IPF than DLCO (19,20). Patients with a DLCO of ≥40% predicted at diagnosis have better median survival than patients whose DLCO is <40% predicted (21). However FVC is more readily assessable and has better reproducibility than DLCO; therefore, it can be useful in monitoring disease progression once the diagnosis is established. In the United Kingdom, the National Institute for Health and Care Excellence (NICE) have established FVC criteria that are currently used to stratify access to anti-fibrotic treatment in IPF in the National Health Service (NHS) (22,23). Six-minute walk testing can be used to screen for a hypoxaemic response, with desaturations <88% at diagnosis indicating worse prognosis (24).

Many patients with IPF have coexistent emphysema. This can contribute to worsening DLCO while tending to preserve lung volumes against the reductions associated with IPF progression. These factors likely explain why a composite physiologic index (CPI) that incorporates both spirometric and gas transfer indices is a better predictor of CT-defined extent of IPF than the most sensitive single test (DLCO) and also predicts prognosis (25). CPI relates DLCO, FVC and FEV_1 to extent of disease (% of affected tissue as assessed by CT) by the following formula:

$$91.0 - (0.65 \times DLCO \, (\% \, predicted))$$
$$- (0.53 \times FVC \, (\% \, predicted))$$
$$+ (0.34 \times FEV_1 \, (\% \, predicted))$$

SEROLOGY

Serologic investigations are indicated to screen for auto-immune, hypersensitivity or sarcoid drivers of fibrosing ILD. Auto-immune conditions of particular relevance that may be associated with IPF-like appearances on computed tomography (CT) scanning are rheumatoid disease and microscopic polyangiitis. Rheumatoid disease tendencies can be screened by rheumatoid factor and anti-citrullinated cyclic peptide (anti-CCP) assays and microscopic polyangiitis by assessing for perinuclear anti-neutrophil cytoplasmic antibody (pANCA) and/or anti-myeloperoxidase (anti-MPO) positivity. In addition, a common differential for radiologic findings in IPF in the absence of honeycombing is non-specific interstitial pneumonia (NSIP). Evidence suggests that this differential diagnosis is often associated with an underlying CTD process, even when the initial presentation seems idiopathic (26,27). A wider auto-immune screen is therefore helpful in screening for CTDs associated with NSIP. This would include screening for antinuclear antibodies (ANAs) and extractable nuclear antigen antibodies (ENAs). Hypersensitivity pneumonitis can mimic IPF in terms of radiology and clinical course. Testing for specific precipitin antibodies supporting the immune recognition of relevant triggers may be undertaken. However, the results are frequently non-definitive (28). Positive findings indicate exposure rather than a pathogenic mechanism, while negative findings do not exclude immunologic recognition of an epitope not included in the assay. In approximately 50% of hypersensitivity pneumonitis diagnoses a trigger is not identified despite both detailed history taking and precipitin screening. Last, angiotensin-converting enzyme (ACE) may be used to screen for a sarcoidosis tendency. However, this is not highly sensitive, and screening may be confounded by the common use of ACE inhibitors as anti-hypertensive agents in the population at risk of IPF.

RADIOLOGY

The characteristic changes of IPF give rise to reticulonodular opacities with bibasal predominance on plane chest radiographs. On high-resolution (HR) computed tomographic (CT) chest imaging they are seen as subpleural reticulations with or without honeycomb changes. The predominant distribution of these findings, in addition to being bibasilar, may be seen to follow a postero-anterior shift from caudal to cranial images, the so-called 'propeller blade' distribution. The fibrotic nature of the process is demonstrated by architectural distortion within the lung parenchyma with tractional dilatation of airways (often described as traction bronchiectasis) and retraction of the oblique fissure. Widespread ground-glass opacification (particularly away from the areas of fibrotic change), areas of consolidation or mosaic attenuation are not typical features of IPF and should prompt consideration of alternative or superimposed pulmonary processes. Such considerations currently lead to an interpretive approach to CT scans in cases where IPF is a diagnostic possibility according to international consensus guidelines (4). Radiologic conclusions that appearances indicate 'definite', 'possible' or are 'inconsistent with' a usual interstitial pneumonia (UIP) pattern are advised. UIP was originally defined in terms of the histologic correlate of IPF that can also be seen in other conditions, e.g. rheumatoid-related ILD and chronic hypersensitivity pneumonitis, similar to the experience with the characteristic CT appearances. Use of the term UIP permits integration with findings from clinical assessment and other investigations to arrive at an overall consensus diagnosis of IPF or an alternative diagnosis. It is therefore often now used to describe CT changes typical of IPF, where biopsy would be overwhelmingly likely to show UIP histopathology.

Historically, HRCT and volumetric CT chest acquisition protocols were distinct. The former collected high-resolution cross-sectional imaging data in a discontinuous thin section (interspaced) manner. The latter collected lower-resolution imaging data that combined cross-sectional signals within broader sections in a continuous distribution, thereby involving a much higher radiation dose to the patient. In recent years, the introduction of more advanced CT scanners and lower radiation dose protocols means that there is far less difference in the radiation dose between discontinuous HRCT and volumetric acquisitions. Moreover the volumetric data are recorded in a way that allows high-resolution images to be reconstructed in a continuous sequence rather than interspaced. The increased information from this technique has advantages in IPF. It allows more reliable comparison of equivalent cross sections in serial imaging and improves discrimination between honeycombing and tractional dilatation of crowded airways subpleurally.

In addition to supporting a diagnosis of IPF, CT scanning screens for relevant complications and co-morbidities (29). Pulmonary hypertension may be indicated by enlargement of the pulmonary artery diameter >29 mm and/or relative to the aortic diameter or by other signs including oedema in the mediastinal recess between the aorta and pulmonary artery (30). Coronary artery calcification indicates increased risk of ischaemic heart disease. IPF confers an increased risk of lung cancer, a cause of 10%–17% of IPF deaths in a range of studies (31–33); therefore, CT chest imaging may also identify nodules requiring further investigation.

Serial imaging may be helpful in assessing rate of disease progression. However, it is often not necessary for this alone, especially if lung function tests and clinical course are consistent. However, repeated CT scanning may distinguish between deterioration due to IPF progression and other causes, and it may be required to investigate unexpected findings on serial pulmonary function testing.

HIGH-VOLUME BRONCHOALVEOLAR LAVAGE

Interstitial lung disease workup may include a high-volume bronchoalveolar lavage (BAL) for differential cell count analysis. Current guidelines recommend instillation of 100–300 mL normal saline through a flexible bronchoscope wedged in a bronchus. Where possible, the targeted site should be defined as affected by activity of the disease process under investigation by CT appearances (34). BAL contributes to the diagnosis of IPF largely where the diagnosis is not definitive following clinical and radiologic evaluation, and BAL may help exclude more auto-inflammatory ILDs from the differential. In IPF the BAL is characterized by alveolar macrophage predominance, and neutrophilia (>3% of total count) is often present. Increased neutrophil numbers and proportions have been correlated to the extensiveness of disease observed on CT (35). The presence of a lymphocytosis (>25%) suggests an alternative diagnosis with chronic hypersensitivity pneumonitis, rheumatoid-related UIP and NSIP important in this context. BAL sample culture can also be useful to screen for active bacterial infection. However, the significance of bacterial presence below the threshold for detection by standard culture and/or viral factors for IPF progression is an area of active interest. Such possibilities are being considered following the observation that antibiotic treatment with co-trimoxazole was associated with reduced mortality in IPF patients who received immunomodulatory medication (36). An increased burden of bacteria is seen in IPF BAL compared with controls (healthy smokers) that was predictive of both decline in lung function and death (37). Moreover, the IPF microbiome appears particularly enriched for certain species. While further studies are required to elucidate the clinical significance of these findings, they raise the possibility that more powerful microbiological characterization of BAL samples may become relevant in future stratification of IPF.

HISTOPATHOLOGY

International guidelines have taken account of the high accuracy of multidisciplinary teams to diagnose IPF based upon clinical, serologic and radiologic data and the risk of harm with surgical lung biopsy in the patient population at most risk of IPF. Surgical biopsy is therefore far less common in the diagnosis of IPF than previously. Generally it is reserved for cases where the diagnosis is unclear, BAL analysis is deemed unlikely (or has proven unable) to provide a conclusive answer, and there are major implications for clinical management. UIP histopathology is the microscopic correlate of IPF, and UIP is characterized by fibroblastic foci, which are clusters of fibroblasts and myofibroblasts with surrounding collagen deposition. In two-dimensional tissue sections these are juxtaposed with normal lung and cystic honeycomb change, corresponding to changes visible on CT and microcystic changes below the current resolution limit of this modality in clinical practice. In three dimensions the fibroblastic foci connect to form a 'fibroblastic reticulum' (38).

MULTIDISCIPLINARY MEETING

Joint statements by the American Thoracic Society (ATS) and the European Respiratory Society (ERS) and others on classification of IPF and other ILDs over the past 15 years have advocated a multidisciplinary approach to diagnosis (4,39–41). Multidisciplinary discussion allows clinical, radiologic and, where relevant, cytologic and lung biopsy findings to be integrated to arrive at the most appropriate consensus diagnosis. A recent international, multi-centre study showed this approach leads to excellent agreement on IPF diagnosis among multidisciplinary teams at ILD centres in different countries (5).

In an appropriate clinical context the presence of 'possible' as well as 'definite' UIP patterns may be sufficient to support a diagnosis of IPF at discussion in the multidisciplinary team (MDT) meeting. The increasing incidence of IPF relative to alternative

ILDs with increasing age overwhelmingly favours this diagnosis in the presence of either 'definite' or 'possible' UIP patterns in individuals over 70, absent inconsistent clinical features (42). The concern that a small proportion of patients will be assigned an inappropriate diagnosis of IPF leading to ineffective treatment is somewhat assuaged by findings from *post hoc* analysis of patients treated with the anti-fibrotic agent nintedanib. Beneficial effects of treatment upon lung function decline were no different between patients with radiologic findings of 'possible' or 'definite' UIP, or indeed those with a histopathologic diagnosis of UIP (43).

Where the diagnosis is uncertain pre-biopsy, histopathologic findings may remain one of several factors considered in reaching a diagnosis, rather than the conclusive 'gold standard'. For example, fibroblastic foci are a hallmark lesion of UIP histopathology but may be observed in other ILDs including chronic hypersensitivity pneumonitis or fibrosing organizing pneumonia (44,45). But even where alternative diagnoses are strongly favoured over IPF on radiologic grounds, histopathologic findings may be so consistent with IPF that this is adopted as the final diagnosis. In a study of 55 cases where IPF was diagnosed following biopsy, an alternative diagnosis was favoured in 62% of cases based upon thin-section CT appearances, often with high confidence (46). In these cases the assignment of IPF diagnoses appeared supported by subsequent 'IPF-like' clinical course (i.e. progressive decline in lung function). Alternative diagnoses included NSIP and chronic hypersensitivity pneumonitis. It is now well established that when NSIP appearances are accompanied by 'discordant' UIP histology, the disease progression does indeed match that of IPF (47,48). Similar findings have been reported in chronic hypersensitivity pneumonitis cases with histopathologic patterns of UIP (49). More generally, the most useful approach to define cases in which radiologic, cytologic and/or histopathologic features of IPF and other ILDs do not coincide remains to be fully clarified. The extent to which such conditions behave clinically as IPF in terms of natural history and response to anti-fibrotic versus immunomodulatory therapies is clearly important.

CLINICAL REVIEW

Clinical assessment is an essential component of a multidisciplinary team discussion where diagnoses of IPF and other ILDs are under consideration. Ideally, the discussion should directly involve a clinician who has personally assessed the patient. As CT scanning and invasive sampling are not routinely used as serial measures of disease behaviour in individual patients, regular clinical review is key to the integrity of the diagnostic process. Heterogeneity of clinical course is well known in IPF. Study data indicate that 20%–30% of patients with IPF substantially outperform the median survival, such that they survive to 5 years. However, in some cases the clinical behaviour of a patient diagnosed with IPF may lead to a review of the diagnosis. Examples include spontaneous improvement, long-term stability, steroid responsiveness, development of connective tissue disease features or delayed identification of exposure to a relevant drug or trigger of hypersensitivity pneumonitis. Alternatively, a patient given a different ILD diagnosis may progress unexpectedly in an IPF-like manner. Ongoing clinical review provides the opportunity for re-evaluation of the MDT diagnosis, and this should be pursued where necessary. In the absence of sufficiently fine-grained algorithms to negate potential diagnostic and management dilemmas mentioned in the previous section, the clinician's role in ongoing evaluation of patients following the MDT process remains crucial.

DISCRIMINATING ASBESTOSIS AND IPF

Asbestosis and IPF are generally considered distinct entities. The ATS/ERS statement of 2011 highlights the need to distinguish asbestosis from IPF. However, this can be challenging as the appearances of the two conditions cannot be reliably distinguished by radiologic imaging. The presence of other indicators of asbestos exposure (e.g. pleural plaques, pleuroparenchymal reactions ['crow's feet']) are neither sufficiently sensitive nor specific. Making the distinction has become more important with the advent of anti-fibrotic therapy, which is currently only evidence based and licensed for treatment in IPF. Disease progression is typically much slower in asbestosis than IPF, but there can be overlap between the two time courses. The quantification of asbestos exposure from an occupational history is a critical criterion to aid diagnosis, as very high exposure is required for asbestosis to develop. High-risk exposure histories include construction and shipyard workers, power industry and heating engineers and plumbers active for multiple years in the 1960s–1970s. This was a period during which asbestos use was peaking prior to the introduction of protective regulations on the use of asbestos and personal protective equipment. A threshold of 25 fibre/mL years (equivalent to 25 years at 1 fibre/mL with fibres per millilitre estimated according to activity) is believed necessary to cause parenchymal asbestosis (50). A very high risk exposure such as spraying asbestos pulp without respiratory protection is estimated to cause 1.67 fibre/mL years each day (i.e. 25 fibre/mL year threshold reached in 2–3 weeks), whereas a roofer or car mechanic would accumulate 21 fibre/mL years over 18 years exposure (51). Consistent with this, car mechanics appear to experience low levels of cumulative asbestos exposure and a low incidence of asbestosis (52). Histologic confirmation requires the presence of two or more asbestos bodies in a 1 cm² section or a count of uncoated asbestos bodies within a certain range (determined by local laboratories) (53). Asbestosis is characterized by more collagen deposition and far fewer fibroblastic foci than in IPF (54). However, biopsy may not be necessary to confirm the diagnosis in the context of appropriate imaging appearances if occupational exposure is deemed sufficient.

Asbestos exposure has been proposed as a potential causative agent in IPF. However, a recent study of lung tissue from four multiple asbestos-exposed cohorts (workforces totaling ~25,000, post-mortem tissue reviewed from all 233 appropriate subjects) did not support this (55). The data strongly supported the conclusion that a histopathologic UIP pattern indicated the presence of a coincident ILD such as IPF rather than a process caused by asbestos exposure, regardless of exposure history.

PHARMACOLOGIC THERAPY IN IDIOPATHIC PULMONARY FIBROSIS

Recent years have seen a major shift in the pharmacologic management of IPF. The PANTHER-IPF study demonstrated a clear mortality signal with anti-inflammatory/immunomodulatory strategies with the combination of oral prednisolone and azathioprine specifically studied. Subsequently, the development of novel anti-fibrotic agents, pirfenidone and nintedanib, has provided new treatment strategies supported by an evidence base that is far more robust in its powering and its alignment with current disease classification.

PIRFENIDONE

Pirfenidone is an orally available pyridone derivative that exhibits anti-inflammatory, anti-oxidant and anti-fibrotic properties. Its precise mechanism of action is unclear, but it has been shown to inhibit fibroblast recruitment and expression, resulting in attenuated extracellular matrix synthesis. In animal models it regulates the pro-fibrotic cytokine, transforming growth factor (TGF)-β, reduces production of collagen proteins and reduces the synthesis of the pro-inflammatory cytokine, tumour necrosis factor (TNF)-α (56–58).

Initial open-label and small placebo-controlled trials suggested a treatment effect (59–62) and so paved the way for two pivotal international, multi-centre, randomized, controlled trials, CAPACITY 004 and CAPACITY 006 (63), which compared pirfenidone with placebo in IPF. These studies shared near identical design to enable pooling of the data. They recruited patients with mild-to-moderate disease (defined as an FVC of >50% predicted and DLCO of >35% predicted). Patients received either high- or low-dose pirfenidone or placebo for 72 weeks, and the primary endpoint was change in FVC decline. Taken together the studies suggested a benefit with high-dose (2403 mg/d) treatment, but the individual results were somewhat mixed. This may relate to a better than expected clinical course in the control group of CAPACITY 006 (9% decline from baseline FVC in treatment group compared with 9.6% in control). However the FVC data from CAPACITY 004 (8% decline in treated group versus 12.4% in control, $p = 0.001$) and pooled analysis (8.5% versus 11%, $p = 0.005$) supported a treatment benefit. FVC decline correlates with mortality (64). Consistent with this, a trend to decreased mortality was observed in the treated groups.

On the basis of these results the European Medicines Agency (EMA) approved pirfenidone in 2011, while in the United States, the Food and Drug Administration (FDA) specifically requested a further multinational, placebo-controlled study,

ASCEND ($n = 555$) (65). This trial had a similar design (specifically to permit pooling of data including mortality) with patients receiving either pirfenidone (2403 mg per day) or placebo for 52 weeks. The proportion of patients who had a decline of 10% or more in predicted FVC or who died (the composite primary endpoint) was relatively reduced by 47.9% in the pirfenidone group (16.5% versus 31.8% in the placebo group, number needed to treat = 7). The proportion of subjects with no decline in percent predicted FVC increased by more than twofold (22.7% in the pirfenidone arm versus 9.7% in placebo arm). In the pooled data from ASCEND and the CAPACITY studies, pirfenidone reduced the risk of death from all-cause mortality at 1 year by 48% and reduced IPF deaths by 68%. This was further supported by a Cochrane meta-analysis, which demonstrated that pirfenidone reduced the risk of disease progression or death by 30% (66).

The consequent adoption of pirfenidone for IPF across ILD centres internationally has led to the accumulation of real-world data. In cohorts from multiple centres (67,68), retrospective analyses have demonstrated that the annual slope of decline in FVC decreases with pirfenidone treatment in a fashion similar to the clinical trial observations. This treatment effect does, however, appear to vary among patients with the most pronounced effect seen in patients with the steepest decline prior to treatment initiation.

Pirfenidone has been reasonably well tolerated in studies to date. The major side effects have been gastrointestinal upset (nausea, dyspepsia, vomiting or anorexia), photosensitivity rashes and (usually minor) disturbance of liver enzymes (Table 10.1).

Table 10.1 Frequency of adverse events in CAPACITY studies

Adverse event	Frequency in pirfenidone group ($n = 623$)	Frequency in placebo group ($n = 624$)
Nausea	32.4%	12.2%
Diarrhoea	18.8%	14.4%
Dyspepsia	16.1%	5%
Anorexia	11.4%	3.5%
Rash	26.2%	7.7%
Photosensitivity	9.3%	1.1%

In the CAPACITY studies 15% of subjects discontinued treatment as a consequence of these adverse events compared to a discontinuation rate of 9% in the placebo arm.

Interim data from RECAP, an open-label extension study of the CAPACITY patients, demonstrated a similar number of adverse events with no new safety concerns raised. In addition, at 5 years approximately half of the cohort remained alive and on treatment (69,70). Most frequent adverse events appear to occur in the first 3 months of treatment (71). Taking pirfenidone with food and spacing the tablets out over a meal can minimize gastrointestinal side effects. Skin reactions can be limited by avoiding exposure to strong sunlight and ultraviolet radiation with regular application of high sun protection factor sun block (72).

NINTEDANIB

Nintedanib is a small molecule, intracellular tyrosine kinase inhibitor that targets multiple growth factor receptors involved in the activation of signalling pathways implicated in IPF. These include vascular endothelial growth factor receptors (VEGFr 1, 2 and 3), fibroblast growth factor receptors (FGFr 1, 2 and 3) and platelet-derived growth factor receptors (PDGFr α and β). Its anti-fibrotic and anti-inflammatory activity has been demonstrated in bleomycin animal models and in human lung fibroblasts (73).

On the basis of the TOMORROW study (74), which suggested a 68% reduction in annual FVC decline with the highest dose of nintedanib, two replicate trials, INPULSIS I and II (75), compared the effect of nintedanib 150 mg twice daily with placebo (randomized 3:2) in 1,066 patients over 52 weeks. In both trials there was a significant reduction in the rate of FVC decline. The pooled data demonstrated a relative reduction in FVC decline of 49.2% in favour of the drug. There was a positive treatment effect on quality of life in one trial, and a significant reduction in the time to adjudicated first exacerbation in the pooled data was also demonstrated.

Post hoc subgroup analysis of nintedanib treatment in patients in the INPULSIS studies who did not have a radiologic diagnosis of definite UIP or a tissue biopsy, indicated such patients derived comparable treatment benefits to those who did (43). This observation is clinically valuable. IPF may be diagnosed in this setting despite a greater level of uncertainty than where radiologic or histologic observations definitively support UIP. These findings indicate that the potential for specialists to mislabel an alternative fibrosing ILD (most likely fibrosing NSIP) as IPF is not associated with any clear diminution of the efficacy of nintedanib. It is hoped that data from further studies will also be interpretable in these terms to assess the robustness of this conclusion.

Serious adverse events were observed at similar levels with nintedanib and placebo. The most frequent side effect reported in the treatment arm was diarrhoea, affecting 62% of participants. However, this led to discontinuation of the drug in just 4%, with nearly 80% of cases resolving without the need for a dose reduction. Elevation of liver enzymes was also observed in the INPULSIS studies, affecting approximately 10.8% of patients taking nintedanib (versus 1.2% with placebo), but this rarely led to discontinuation of the drug (1.6% stopped treatment).

TREATING PATIENTS WITH ANTI-FIBROTICS

Both pirfenidone and nintedanib are approved for use in IPF in multiple territories around the world. In the United Kingdom this has been overseen by the NICE, who have issued identical treatment recommendations for both agents (22,76). They can be prescribed by an ILD specialist in patients with FVC of 50%–80% predicted. A decline in FVC of 10% or more over 12 months is considered a treatment failure and should trigger stopping treatment. Treatment may be equally beneficial with FVC >80% (77) or >90% predicted (78) as below these cut-offs, but such patients may not currently meet reimbursement criteria. Moreover, work by Nathan et al. (79) suggests that stopping treatment based on one lung function test demonstrating decline may not be appropriate. Thirty-four (5.5%) and 68 (10.9%) patients, respectively, in pirfenidone and placebo-treated groups experienced a greater than 10% absolute decline in FVC between baseline and at 6 months. Treatment was continued, and in the subsequent 6-month period, significantly fewer patients in the pirfenidone group experienced a second >10% FVC decline compared to the placebo group (5.9% versus 27.9%).

Both anti-fibrotic drugs have a similar effect on FVC, and while pirfenidone has been shown to have a positive effect on mortality (based on pooled data from three randomized controlled trials), nintedanib has demonstrated a favourable effect on exacerbations. Adherence and side-effect profiles are likely to be deciding factors in drug choice. Tablet burden (nine pirfenidone capsules versus two nintedanib daily), the need for sun cream application and the possibility of diarrhoea will probably influence individual patient choice of drug. Nintedanib is used with caution in patients on anti-coagulation or who have had recent haemorrhage, due to a theoretical risk of bleeding. Managing patient expectation of treatment is vital; treating clinicians should convey the aim of slowing decline rather than being able to have an impact on current levels of dyspnoea. In the future, there may also be scope for combining therapies, a particularly attractive prospect given that multiple pathogenic pathways are implicated in propagating disease activity.

The successful development of two anti-fibrotic drugs represents a major advance in IPF management. Together with the increased recognition of IPF and its clinical burden, they have greatly stimulated academic and industry efforts to develop new therapeutic agents. However, significant challenges remain in drug development, including imperfect understanding of pathogenic pathways and lack of consensus on ideal clinical trial design and appropriate study endpoints. A reduction in mortality might be considered the ultimate goal and thus the best measure. However, the number of patients and duration of follow-up required to detect such an effect are often not realistic for a disease that remains relatively rare. In addition, diagnosing and managing ILD in its entirety is a rapidly evolving sub-specialty with classification and diagnostic criteria undergoing continuous critical appraisal and adjustment. As such, accurately phenotyping patients and enrolling a 'pure' cohort can be a challenge.

Prognosis in IPF is variable with ~20% of patients living beyond 5 years. Differing rates of decline in placebo arms of different studies have led to inconsistent results. Some of this heterogeneity may be explained by the existence of distinct IPF sub-phenotypes (also referred to as endotypes). These may vary according to pathogenic mutations and, hence, responses to therapy. Identifying these groups through the use of genetic and molecular biomarker-based research is likely to be important to future treatment trials. Unless novel approaches are developed to reverse fibrosis and restore normal lung architecture, the goal of treatment seems likely to be limited to halting disease progression or performing lung transplantation.

OTHER THERAPIES CURRENTLY USED IN IPF

TREATMENT OF GASTRO-OESOPHAGEAL REFLUX DISEASE

Prevalence of gastro-oesopphageal reflux disease (GERD) is high in IPF patients (87%–94%) compared to the general population (10%–19%) (80,81). GERD in IPF is frequently symptomatically silent and often predates the IPF diagnosis (80,82). In theory, each condition may mechanistically predispose to the other. GERD may result from reduced lung compliance causing increased swings in intrathoracic pressure and oesophageal sphincter dysfunction in IPF. Alternatively, microaspiration due to GERD may be a co-factor in causing epithelial injury during IPF pathogenesis. There is evidence that exposure of human alveolar epithelial cells to components of bile acids stimulates production of transforming growth factor (TGF)-β (83) and expression of connective tissue growth factor (84). Other mechanisms implicated include uptake of pepsin by airway epithelial cells with consequent cytotoxicity (84), and aspiration of endotoxin from bacterial lysis in gastric juice (85). *In vitro* and animal model studies suggest proton pump inhibitors (PPIs) may directly moderate cellular processes implicated in fibrogenesis (reduction in expression of inflammatory cytokines and MMPs and inhibition of lung fibroblast proliferation) (86).

ATS/ERS IPF guidelines conditionally recommend PPIs in IPF regardless of the patient's symptoms of GERD. This recommendation is supported by a number of case series (13,87) but lacks evidence from randomized controlled trials (RCTs). Indeed there is a need for further evidence to better clarify the role of GERD treatment in IPF. Evidence of linear correlation between the severity of GERD and lung function deficit in IPF is lacking (40,80). There also remains some doubt regarding the efficacy of PPIs to prevent lung injury with persistent

levels of reflux found in IPF patients taking them and variable effectiveness on reducing pH of gastric fluid (80). Moreover, gastric fluid from patients on PPIs can still stimulate inflammatory responses from pulmonary epithelial cells (88), which indicates the potential for non-acidic gastro-oesophageal reflux to induce injury.

Conversely, recent *post hoc* analysis of the INPULSIS study demonstrated that patients treated with an anti-acid treatment at baseline had worse outcomes than those who did not receive such treatment (89). Similarly, *post hoc* analyses of antacid use in IPF patients randomized to placebo arms of pirfenidone treatment trials (CAPACITY, ASCEND) showed no benefit and signals of increased overall and pulmonary infection rates in patients with severe IPF (90). A possible explanation for this observation is that PPI use is simply a marker for the extent of pre-existing GERD. Alternately, PPIs alter the gastro-intestinal microbiome (91,92), and their side effects include an increased risk of community-acquired pneumonia (though this is not reflected in increased risk of hospitalization) (93). Robust RCTs of the role of PPIs and other anti-GERD therapies in IPF are therefore indicated.

Other strategies to manage GERD beyond use of anti-acid therapies remain important, such as lifestyle modifications and smoking cessation. The role of prokinetics, such as domperidone and metoclopramide, is unclear. Surgical intervention, such as Nissen fundoplication, is effective in treating GERD and has shown benefits in retrospective analysis in IPF patients (94). Further studies are ongoing to assess the role of such surgery.

PULMONARY REHABILITATION

Recent international regulatory approvals of antifibrotic therapy bring expectations of reduced disease progression rates and of increased survival in IPF. Maximizing functional capability and quality of life alongside the novel anti-fibrotic pharmacotherapies therefore becomes an even more important goal. Reduced exercise tolerance is a central feature of IPF, and limitations to exercise capacity are due to impaired gas exchange, altered breathing mechanics, circulatory impairment due to pulmonary hypertension and respiratory and skeletal muscle dysfunction (95). Desaturation on exercise is a hallmark of the disease due to V/Q mismatching, impaired oxygen diffusion, low mixed venous oxygen content (95) and increased dead space ventilation (96,97).

To date, significant short-term improvements following exercise training have been demonstrated (98,99), and pulmonary rehabilitation is recommended in ATS/ERS (100) and NICE (22,76) guidelines for IPF patients. However, the evidence grade is weak with few studies having been conducted as randomized controlled trials. Increases in 6-minute walk distance (6MWD) between 18 and 81 m have been reported (minimal clinical important difference in 6MWD 24–45 m) (101). Consequent improvements in functional status and quality of life have also been demonstrated (98). Access to pulmonary rehabilitation may not be universal even in ostensibly common healthcare systems where local service commissioning occurs. Patients are typically enrolled in programmes designed to meet the needs of COPD patients, and there is scope to design more targeted programmes to meet the needs of IPF patients, particularly in terms of disease-specific education. The optimal forms of exercise frequency and type in IPF also require further RCT investigation. Studies of the longer-term benefits of pulmonary rehabilitation have yielded mixed results. In two studies some benefits were not sustained beyond 6 or 11 months, but quality of life improvements were more sustained (102). A further study indicated that improvements in walk distance were maintained at 6 months (103) with the change in 6MWD rather than dyspnoea being the strongest correlate of change in quality of life. The role of oxygen supplementation during exercise to optimize activity requires further study (e.g. whether exertional SaO_2 thresholds of 88% [98] or 85% [104] are most appropriate).

SMOKING CESSATION

By definition IPF is considered idiopathic. Conversely, other more inflammatory cell-associated ILD sub-types (e.g. conditions on the respiratory-bronchiolitis-associated ILD [RBILD]/desquamative interstitial pneumonia [DIP] spectrum, Langerhans cell histiocytosis) are regarded as driven by cigarette smoking. Nevertheless, IPF is associated with cigarette smoking, and this has been defined as a risk factor (105). Large, case-control studies in different populations (105–107) have shown that patients with IPF are more likely

to have smoked previously than controls. The UK Million Women Study also found current smokers had 1.5 times the mortality rate from IPF compared to non-smokers (108,109). Conversely other observations supported the contention that current smokers had a longer median survival compared to never or former smokers (109). This could reflect a self-selecting 'healthy smoker' effect whereby people with disease that is mild at presentation or progresses less rapidly are more likely to continue smoking than those who decline (110). A study to explore this found that once baseline disease severity was taken into account, the difference in survival between current and former smokers was lost, and never-smokers survived longer than current or former smokers (111). Given the clear detrimental general effects of smoking on lung health, cessation treatment should be central to all services caring for patients with IPF (as with any respiratory disease). Smoking status of patients or caregivers may prevent safe prescription of long-term oxygen or ambulatory oxygen due to fire risk.

ADDRESSING BREATHLESSNESS IN IPF

Breathlessness is a complex perception (and the reaction to that perception) that is influenced by physiological, psychological and environmental factors and has a tendency to be self-perpetuating (112,113). It is not, *per se*, identical to hypoxaemia. The physiological mechanism of breathlessness in IPF is likely due to a combination of impaired gas exchange, increased ventilatory demand, respiratory and peripheral muscle dysfunction and neural feedback. The restrictive spirometry defect associated with IPF means that the mechanistic details may differ from those more widely studied in obstructive conditions such as COPD.

Non-pharmacologic management can include encouraging airflow over the face (open window, use of a fan) and distraction (reading, relaxation, company, music). Energy conservation with pacing of exertion, controlled breathing exercises and psychological support can also be beneficial (112). Pharmacologic management is typically with oramorph 2.5 mg as needed to 4 hourly. While there are no studies to confirm benefit of this particular regimen in IPF, a small study of low-dose subcutaneous diamorphine indicated that low-dose opiate approaches were safe and effective for this indication (114). If anxiety contributes to breathlessness, anxiolytics such as low-dose benzodiazepine (in the United Kingdom typically lorazepam 0.5 mg) are often prescribed (115).

ROLE OF OXYGEN THERAPY

Most guidelines relating to use of supplemental oxygen in chronic lung disease are drawn from evidence from patients with COPD (116,117), with uncertainty about their applicability to patients with ILD. Long-term oxygen therapy (LTOT) assessment is recommended if resting oxygen saturations are less than 92% and pO_2 <7.3 kPa, or <8 kPa in the presence of pulmonary hypertension (PH). Ambulatory oxygen can be prescribed if there is exertional desaturation below 90% and clear evidence of benefit from its use. Assessing this benefit depends on evidence of increased quality in life as a result of increased walk distance. One retrospective study in 70 patients with IPF showed an increased walk distance of 81.2 m with optimal ambulatory oxygen titration to reach saturations of 90%, although quality of life was not assessed (117). A second placebo-controlled study (4 L/min air versus 4 L/min oxygen) in IPF patients desaturating on walking did not demonstrate increased walk distance (118). More studies may be useful, as there are potential disadvantages of using oxygen treatment (e.g. anxiety regarding equipment failure, increased airway dryness and cough, confined mobility or reinforcement of illness roles). Oxygen prescription may be prohibited in households where ongoing smoking habits increase the risk of fire.

TREATING COUGH

Cough in IPF is common and can occur through IPF-specific mechanisms such as activation of mechanical cough receptors due to anatomical distortion by fibrosis (119). Other causes such as GERD, asthma, post-nasal drip or drug induced (e.g. ACE inhibitors) should be considered. It can be a major cause of symptom burden and impact very negatively on quality of life (120). Additionally, it may predict poor prognosis (121). An association between cough severity and the MUC5B polymorphism has been reported, which may inform future mechanistic research (122).

Current treatment options for cough due to IPF are limited and with minimal evidence base.

Codeine has historically been widely used as a cough suppressant but has not been evaluated in IPF. Thalidomide was shown to improve cough and respiratory quality of life scores significantly in IPF, though with a relatively high rate of associated non-respiratory side effects, and more studies are required to evaluate its overall benefit (123). Gabapentin has been used successfully in refractory chronic cough and is attractive as a non-opiate agent with relatively favourable side effect and interaction profiles (124). It is, therefore, a logical agent for use in IPF but has not yet been specifically validated in this condition. The P2X3 airway vagal afferent nerve receptor has been successfully targeted by an oral antagonist (AF-219) in phase 2 studies (125). A study of its use in IPF cough has recently been completed (ClinicalTrials.gov NCT02502097). Clinical studies evaluating the effect of pirfenidone on cough in IPF are ongoing (ClinicalTrials.gov NCT02009293).

PATIENT-CENTRED CARE AND PALLIATION OF SYMPTOMS

Despite the advent of anti-fibrotic therapies with significant impact on disease progression, IPF remains a difficult condition that is associated with heavy symptom burdens and poor outcomes. While there is an understandable push to institute such therapies, patient-centred care aiming to improve quality of life must remain a priority. The British Lung Foundation has produced an IPF patients' charter in response to poor patient experience of care (126).

The development of specialist ILD centres concentrates diagnostic expertise but leaves a need to ensure local patient-centred support. In such a system it is, therefore, important for specialist centres to build relationships with referring units, primary care and community services to improve referral pathways and patient experience. In the United Kingdom, NICE guidelines require that an ILD nurse specialist forms part of the service and that palliative care needs are assessed and appropriate referral considered (22,23). Under times of financial pressures within healthcare systems, it can be challenging to develop such roles to effectively treat a sizeable patient group in whom comorbidities and frailty are common issues. There is also geographical variation in the extent to which community/integrated respiratory services cater to the needs of IPF patients while residing in their homes. However, in many areas programmes have been developed for chronic respiratory disease in the context of COPD patient care, and it may be most efficient to embed IPF community care within such teams.

The evolving role of integrated care respiratory physicians providing clinical support for these services can allow this to be safely developed. Particular needs in the community relate to safe and effective oxygen prescribing and access to pulmonary rehabilitation (with programmes designed to meet the needs of IPF patients). Partnership of these caregivers with palliative care practitioners may optimize provision of appropriate symptom relief and support in achieving preferred place of death. There is evidence in support of case conferencing to establish palliative care needs and delivery in severe IPF (120), and a new tool (127,128) is being validated to assess palliative care needs of patients and their caregivers for use in an outpatient setting. Establishing evidence-based standards of such collaborative practice may enable more consistent, high-quality care. The St George's Respiratory Questionnaire and more focused quality of life questionnaires have been validated in ILDs as a whole (129,130). They may provide a means to measure service provision against patient-centred, performance-related outcome measures. Understanding and assessing patients' needs can be labour-intensive. Service providers must, therefore, address challenges in balancing this against service pressures associated with increasing incidence and awareness of IPF.

DRUGS UNDERGOING RE-EVALUATION IN IPF: CO-TRIMOXAZOLE

A pilot study of co-trimoxazole in idiopathic ILD demonstrated improvements in FVC, shuttle walk test and Medical Research Council (MRC) dyspnoea score after 3 months (131). Subsequently a multicentre, double-blind RCT studied the effects of co-trimoxazole treatment in a larger IPF cohort (Treating Idiopathic Pulmonary fibrosis with the Addition of Co-trimoxazole, TIPAC) (36). There was no significant difference between the groups in terms of pulmonary function tests including the primary endpoint (FVC change after 12 months) and 6MWD. However, significant improvements were observed in the symptom domain of the St George's Respiratory Questionnaire, reduced need for increased oxygen therapy and reduced rates of infections. Most strikingly, patients who adhered to the treatment protocol had a marked reduction in mortality on co-trimoxazole (hazard ratio of 0.21). However, the study was undertaken before the findings of PANTHER-IPF were known. It is possible that benefit may have accrued from beneficial effects of co-trimoxazole counteracting adverse consequences of immunosuppression (e.g. with azathioprine treatment and/or high-dose prednisolone). With the advent of the anti-fibrotic era in IPF, a 'TIPAC-2' study (EME-TIPAC, ISRCTN registry, ISRCTN17464641) is currently recruiting to establish whether there may be a role for co-trimoxazole in IPF in combination with such treatment.

DRUGS UNDERGOING RE-EVALUATION IN IPF: ANTIOXIDANT THERAPY – N-ACETYL CYSTEINE

N-acetyl cysteine (NAC) can serve as a prodrug to L-cysteine, which can serve as a precursor of the endogenous antioxidant, glutathione, and thereby replenish glutathione levels. Interest in NAC supplementation as a treatment for IPF is based on the rationale that oxidative stress is involved in disease pathogenesis and that glutathione levels are low in the lungs of IPF patients. The IFIGENIA (132) study was the first multicentre, randomized controlled trial in IPF that achieved its primary endpoint. Treatment with NAC, azathioprine and prednisolone (triple therapy) led to a slowing in VC and DLCO decline when compared to placebo plus azathioprine and prednisolone. The study was, however, small, with a high drop-out rate, and since NAC was given in combination, conclusions about how much it alone contributed to such effects in IPF *per se* could not be drawn. PANTHER-IPF (133) was thus designed to address these issues, comparing triple therapy with NAC alone and a third, true placebo arm. The triple therapy arm was stopped early due to an interim review that detected an increase in mortality, hospitalization and adverse events in this group without any detectable treatment benefit to offset such serious harm. The NAC and placebo arms continued. However, no overall treatment benefit was found, and NAC was thus deemed an ineffective therapy for IPF (134).

A *post hoc* genetic analysis of patients who took part in the PANTHER-IPF study suggested that genetic stratification might identify a subgroup of patients benefiting from NAC treatment, although the numbers in the different subgroups were small. The genes studied were related by proximity on chromosome 11p15.5 and encode proteins with immune (Toll interacting protein, TollIP and mucin-5B, Muc5B), anti-oxidant defence and airway mucus properties (Muc5B). Homozygotes for a single-nucleotide polymorphism (SNP) in the *TOLLIP* gene (T allele rs3750920 SNP site, TT genotype subgroup: $n = 17$ treated versus $n = 16$ NAC-treated) appeared to derive a treatment advantage associated with NAC treatment. This reached significance ($p = 0.03$) for a composite endpoint of death, transplant or FVC decline, and the only one of these events observed in this subgroup was FVC decline ($p = 0.06$ for FVC decline alone) (135). This genotype is estimated to be present in ~25% of IPF patients. The same analysis indicated there might be a different subgroup (CC genotype at the same site) in whom treatment was deleterious to survival, with heterozygosity having no discernible effect. There was also a signal for improved outcome in the same composite event for NAC treatment in patients carrying the T polymorphism in the *MUC5B* gene at the rs3750920 site ($n = 34$ placebo versus $n = 46$ NAC-treated, $p = 0.04$). Despite the limitations of this type of study (*post hoc*, with composite endpoints defined retrospectively), this finding has biological plausibility since this allele, while a risk factor for IPF, has been associated with improved survival (136). These findings, therefore, define hypotheses of translational interest. They would require confirmation with data from prospective, genotype-stratified studies with ready availability of appropriate genotyping services before genotype-based decisions about NAC therapy could be recommended in clinical practice.

EMERGING THERAPEUTIC STRATEGIES TARGETING UNDERLYING MECHANISMS OF IPF

The recently approved therapies for the treatment of IPF, pirfenidone and nintedanib, reduce progression of fibrosis as reported by lung function decline, but they were not initially developed for this primary purpose. As a consequence the dominant mechanism(s) of therapeutic action are not entirely clear beyond generally anti-fibroproliferative effects. This is particularly the case for pirfenidone, which appears to be highly pleiotropic with multiple effects upon cytokines, growth factors and collagen secretion *in vitro* (137). Nintedanib was developed as a triple tyrosine kinase inhibitor capable of targeting PDGF, FGF and VEGF signalling and may be a more targeted therapy. However, it may also have independent anti-fibrotic effects, such as modulating IPF fibroblast behaviour (138).

Therefore, the development of pirfenidone and nintedanib therapies for IPF does not perfectly fit a 'rational' model of therapeutic advances growing out of elucidation of disease-specific mechanisms. Nevertheless, studies that define specific pathways in the molecular pathogenesis of IPF open the prospect of more highly targeted therapies. Currently, these may be viewed in the general context of the aberrant wound response model of IPF pathogenesis that is consistent with its histopathologic characteristics and lack of response to anti-inflammatory therapies. A wide range of novel therapeutic approaches currently in development, therefore, target molecules involved in crosstalk between epithelial cells and mesenchymal cells and in mesenchymal cell recruitment and potentiation.

Transforming growth factor (TGF)-β1 signalling is one of the best-characterized pathways in lung fibrosis (139). It is implicated in epithelial cell apoptosis, fibroblast activation, transition of epithelial cells to those with characteristics of mesenchymal cells and differentiation of fibroblasts into myofibroblasts. TGF-β1 is stored in a latent form in the extracellular matrix and can be activated by cleavage and release via the actions of matrix metalloproteinases (MMPs), integrins and by stretch (140,141). Studies of TGF-β1 inhibitors are ongoing. However, the pleiotropic effects of this pathway mean that this approach risks side effects that may underlie its lack of success to date (142,143).

The heterodimer of αv and β6 integrins (αvβ6 integrin) is an attractive target (144). It can both bind and facilitate activation of TGF-β1, has been proposed as a prognostic biomarker of IPF (145) and is found at sites of epithelial injury where there is underlying fibrotic change. Targeting its actions, therefore, provides the potential to modulate the most disease-relevant, pro-fibrotic effects of TGF-β1 signalling in a relatively selective manner. At least two agents have been developed to explore this possibility. An anti-αvβ6 monoclonal antibody is currently being studied in a phase 2 trial (BG00011, previously STX-100, ClinicalTrials.gov NCT01371305). In addition an αvβ6 inhibitor small molecule therapy, GSK3008348, has been completed for the first time in human studies (healthy volunteer and IPF patients, ClinicalTrials.gov NCT02612051).

Galectin-3 is found at the cell surface in alveolar epithelial cells and lung fibroblasts (146). Increased amounts are found in fibroblastic foci relative to normal lung tissue. It stabilizes cell surface TGF-β receptor II and has potential to bind other important cell surface proteins that can mediate fibrosis. Galectin-3 knockout mice are protected from fibrosis in response to lung TGF-β1 overexpression or intratracheal bleomycin, and protection in response to insults in other organs is also observed. Circulating galectin-3 has been identified as a biomarker that correlates with subclinical interstitial lung abnormalities on CT with associated restrictive spirometry in the large Framingham cohort (147) and with IPF and AE-IPF in a smaller study (146). Synthetic galectin-3 ligands can protect lung tissue from fibrotic responses to bleomycin. One such compound, TD-139, is currently completing phase 2 studies (ClinicalTrials.gov: NCT02257177).

The enzyme, lysyl oxidase-like (LOXL)2, contributes to fibrosis by catalysing the cross-linking of fibrillar collagen, thereby reducing compliance. It may also have further profibrotic actions, as cross-linking appears to result in reduced TGF-β1 signalling and reduced fibroblast recruitment (148). LOXL2 levels in patients from recent clinical trials correlated with disease progression and with mortality risk (149). Simtuzumab is a monoclonal antibody that inhibits LOXL2, but a phase 2 trial (ClinicalTrials.gov NCT01769196) of this drug was recently halted after failure to show treatment benefit at a mid-stage data analysis.

The cytokine, IL-13, correlates inversely with FVC in IPF patients (150) and may be important in those who experience rapid progression (151). Inhibition of IL-13 in humanized models of IPF results in reduced extracellular matrix deposition and reduced epithelial cell apoptosis. Monoclonal antibodies directed against IL-13 (lebrikizumab,

tralokinumab) have been used in phase 2 trials. The trial of tralokinumab for IPF (ClinicalTrials.gov NCT01629667) was halted early due to lack of efficacy. The lebrikizumab trial will assess the effects of the drug compared with placebo, both alone and in combination with pirfenidone (ClinicalTrials.gov NCT01872689). An additional agent, SAR156597, that targets both IL-4 and IL-13 is also in phase 2 studies (ESTAIR, ClinicalTrials.gov NCT02345070).

Lysophosphatidic acid (LPA) may represent a key link between alveolar damage and mesenchymal change. LPA concentrations are increased in BAL after lung injury, and it serves as a chemoattractant for fibroblasts (152). LPA signalling increases epithelial cell apoptosis (153), but it promotes resistance to apoptosis in fibroblasts. Mice lacking the LPA1 receptor are protected from fibrotic injury (152). Administration of an LPA1 receptor antagonist ameliorates fibrosis in the mouse bleomycin-induced fibrosis model (154). A clinical trial of an LPA1 receptor antagonist (BMS-986020) has recently been completed (ClinicalTrials.gov NCT01766817).

NADPH-oxidase 4 (Nox4) is an enzyme whose activity generates reactive oxygen species (ROS) in the lung. These effects are regulated by the induction of NFE2-related factor 2 (Nrf2) antioxidant responses. Nox4:Nrf2 imbalance has been identified in IPF fibroblastic foci, and it is implicated in maintenance of pathological senescent myofibroblast phenotypes in IPF (155,156). Moreover, the lungs of aged Nox4 knockout mice retain the ability to recover from a fibrotic insult with resolution of fibrosis; this ability to recover from such injury is characteristic of young mice and is lost in aged wild-type mice. Oral Nox4 inhibitors have been developed (157). Nox4 inhibition with a combined Nox4/Nox1 inhibitor (158) or by metformin treatment (159) limits bleomycin-induced fibrosis in rodent models and inhibits fibroblast transdifferentiation into myofibroblasts. Phase 2 studies of a Nox4/Nox1 inhibitor in diabetic nephropathy were completed in 2015 (ClinicalTrials.gov NCT02010242), and plans for similar studies in IPF have been announced.

Connective tissue growth factor (CTGF) is a matricellular protein that can play roles in epithelial–mesenchymal transition, activation of myofibroblasts, remodelling of extracellular matrix and stimulation of TGF-β release (160).

In mouse models, inhibition of CTGF not only reduced, but could even reverse the fibrotic effects of radiation (161). FG-3019, an inhibitor of CTGF, has been trialed in human subjects with IPF in an open-label study (162). Twenty percent of patients experienced reduction in fibrotic load, as measured by CT scanning. Further placebo-controlled RCTs are required to confirm these findings, and, if successful, to identify and validate stratifying factors associated with differences in response (163).

DISEASE MONITORING

The clinical course in IPF can be varied. While mean survival is between 3 and 5 years, some patients demonstrate slow decline in lung function while others rapidly worsen, and 5% of patients show intermittent periods of rapid acute deterioration or acute exacerbation (10). Patients may present at different points in their disease course. Predicting future disease behaviour and response to treatment at presentation is a valuable goal. Currently, the best-validated tool, also employed in studies of anti-fibrotic drugs, requires longitudinal monitoring of FVC. A 5%–10% decline in absolute FVC at 6 months is associated with twofold increased mortality over the following year (164). However, in practice individual FVC decline <10% cannot be considered robust for clinical decision making. Assessing relative rather than absolute change in FVC may allow earlier detection of disease progression (165). Other parameters shown to predict survival include baseline DLCO, baseline 6MWD and change in 6MWD at 6 months (101), baseline radiologic extent of fibrosis, change in dyspnoea over time (166) and development of acute exacerbations of IPF. Dyspnoea scoring systems validated in IPF include the (Medical Research Council) MRC dyspnoea scale (167); the Clinical, Radiographic and Physiologic (CRP) score (109); and the UCSD Shortness of Breath Questionnaire (SOBQ, used more in clinical studies) (168). Dyspnoea may be confounded by co-morbidity/anxiety, but in addition to being an important indicator of disease progression, it affects quality of life and should be carefully assessed at every consultation. Several composite mortality risk prediction models have been validated in IPF incorporating clinical, physiological and radiologic variables (25,109,169–171).

However identified predictors of mortality may only poorly predict other conventional measures of disease progression prior to this (168).

Biological biomarkers to improve disease phenotyping and increase ability to predict future course are certainly required. Transcriptional phenotyping from lung tissue has identified 134 transcripts that are sufficiently up- or downregulated to distinguish stable from progressive disease (172). Changes in miRNA expression in IPF patients may also provide prognostic information (173). Elevated serum levels of several proteins such as MMP-7, SP-A and KL6/MUC1 (174,175) and of the products of matrix metalloprotease-mediated proteolysis (176) have been associated with worse prognosis in IPF. The role for incorporating such markers into other composite scoring systems is being assessed (177–179).

ACUTE EXACERBATIONS OF IPF (AE-IPF)

BACKGROUND

Most patients with IPF experience gradual decline and chronic disease progression over the course of their disease. However, there is a clinical consensus that acute exacerbations can cause stepwise decline in the course of disease for many patients, which often occurs in the final months of life (10). Acute exacerbations of IPF (AE-IPF) are defined by episodes of new or worsening breathlessness with onset in the last 30 days accompanied by radiologic findings of new infiltrates that are not specifically accounted for by alternative diagnoses (e.g. thromboembolic disease, cardiac failure) (180–183). Diagnostic criteria have altered subtly over time and continue to be subject to discussion. The main change has been to remove the division between infective causes of acute respiratory deterioration and AE-IPF (184). Variations in criteria may, in part, explain the wide range of incidence reporting (74,185), and achieving consensus should improve the ability to detect significant impact of therapeutics in trial settings. Annual rates of hospitalization with IPF-related clinical presentations have increased approximately 5% every year since 1980 (186). Hospitalization is, therefore, likely to account for a disproportionate amount of the clinical experience with IPF in secondary and tertiary care centres.

RISK FACTORS AND PATHOGENESIS OF AE-IPF

Risk of AE-IPF is highest in patients with poor pre-existing lung health. Increased risk is predicted by poor lung function prior to exacerbation, higher baseline dyspnoea and the presence of PH (187,188). When FVC falls below 70% of the predicted normal value, the risk of exacerbation increases dramatically (189,190). In addition, patients who show significant progression of disease with FVC decline over a short time period are more likely to experience exacerbation (188). Given the possible role of exacerbations in driving accelerated decline, the causative relations underlying such correlations cannot be inferred. The time from diagnosis to first exacerbation is wide ranging with retrospective study estimating a range between 3 and 60 months (191). Patients with higher body mass indices may be more susceptible to exacerbation (188), and never-smokers have increased risk in some studies (190). In post-operative patients with IPF, the extensiveness of fibrosis on HRCT may predict risk of exacerbation (192).

An infective driver of AE-IPF is suggested by presentations with cough, shortness of breath, low-grade fever and malaise (15), its seasonality (193) and evidence that immunosuppressed patients have worse prognosis (190). A study of bronchoscopic washings demonstrated that viral nucleic acid could be detected in a minority of patients with AE-IPF, compared with none in stable IPF patients (194). Unexpectedly, the virus most commonly identified in these studies was tenotorque virus (TTV), which is also commonly detected in other forms of acute lung injury.

Microaspiration of refluxed gastric contents may play a role in a subset of exacerbating patients. High BMI is a significant risk factor for both reflux and for exacerbations, and it is well established that abnormal gastro-oesophageal reflux is over-represented in the IPF cohort (80). In a proportion of exacerbating patients, BAL pepsin levels can be significantly elevated compared with stable controls (195).

In line with other chronic respiratory disease, exposure to air pollution has been correlated with exacerbation risk (196). In a retrospective review of pollution levels, patients who experienced exacerbations had significantly higher exposure to ozone and nitrous oxide compared with non-exacerbating IPF controls in the weeks preceding their exacerbation.

Invasive procedures can trigger AE-IPF (e.g. surgery for lung cancer) (15,197,198), lung biopsy (199) and even bronchoalveolar lavage (200). Where mechanical ventilation is required, this and concomitant hyperoxia are likely to be important factors (201,202) in addition to any direct trauma to a specific region of the lung. Thus, AE-IPF has been associated with extrapulmonary surgical procedures, and in AE-IPF following thoracic surgery, more extensive changes are typically observed on the contralateral side to the surgical stimulus (199). Where mechanical ventilation is required, it may, therefore, be prudent to use relatively low pressures and tidal volumes and to use the lowest FiO_2 required to maintain saturations $\geq$92% (202,203).

Histopathologic findings at post-mortem following exacerbation indicate that the most common correlation is with diffuse alveolar damage (DAD) with occasional hyaline membranes on the background of honeycombing (204). However, other patterns are seen including multiple fibroblastic foci and, interestingly, organizing pneumonia (205). Stratification by distinct radiologic patterns of peripheral, multifocal or diffuse new opacification upon CT scanning may correlate with histopathologic changes. In general, diffuse change on CT scanning results in the histopathologic correlate of DAD. In contrast, more peripheral distribution of new opacifications is more likely to show other histopathologic forms including organizing pneumonia and multiple fibroblastic foci. Together, these findings suggest that heterogeneous tissue responses may underlie the clinical entity of AE-IPF with potentially distinct clinical courses and/or responses to therapeutic interventions.

In the research setting a range of molecules have shown promise as circulating biomarkers of AE-IPF. These include KL-6 (206,207), surfactant protein (SP-)D (207), von Willebrand's factor (207), IL-6 (207), total protein C (207), thrombomodulin (207), plasminogen activator inhibitor (PAI-)1 (207), leptin (208), soluble intercellular adhesion molecule-1 (sICAM-1) (209), serum oxidative stress potential (210), the collagen chaperone heat-shock protein (HSP)-47 (211), IL-7 (as a marker of AE-IPF resolution with polymyxin therapy) (212) and galectin-3 (146). Moreover, increased levels of KL-6, SP-D and total protein C may discriminate AE-IPF from both early and late phases of acute lung injury (207). Serum KL-6 has also been identified as a predictor of a radiation pneumonitis response in pre-existing IPF (213).

CLINICAL IMPLICATIONS AND STRATIFYING FEATURES

Exacerbations are associated with poor prognosis in in-patients (214) and reduced life expectancy in the general IPF population (193,215). Experiencing an exacerbating event increases the risk of subsequent exacerbation (196). Overall, around 40% of patients who suffer with AE-IPF will die as a result of exacerbation (216), a mortality risk approaching three times that reported in COPD exacerbators (217). However, a systematic survey during the preparation of this chapter revealed no longitudinal data on the effect of exacerbation on lung function or symptoms (quality of life, exercise capacity) after discharge from hospital. This indicates a gap in the evidence-base in IPF, given the widespread belief that AE-IPF can act as a ratcheting mechanism of accelerated functional decline in this disease.

Patients with poor lung function pre-exacerbation and patients whose gas exchange deteriorates significantly during exacerbation have higher mortality (193). High LDH and CRP predict mortality, as does the circulating fibrocyte count in the research setting (218). The presence of PH is variably associated with worse outcome from exacerbation (187,219).

Investigators who correlated CT appearances with histologic findings in AE-IPF further assessed how they related to clinical behaviour (205). HRCT patterns correlated with exacerbation outcome. A diffuse pattern was associated the worst outcome; all patients with this pattern on the initial CT scan died. Moreover, in patients who had a multifocal pattern of change on initial scan, mortality was uniformly associated with progression to a diffuse pattern. There was no evidence of progression if baseline CT scanning was classified as a peripheral type, and mortality risk was lower. More diffuse CT changes have been correlated with mortality risk in other studies (220). Similarly, retrospective

analysis of AE-IPF in post-mortem cases indicated that the most common pattern of lung injury was DAD, and none showed organizing pneumonia as the sole histopathologic pattern (221). Given concerns that invasive procedures may worsen outcome, the opportunity for *ex vivo* tissue studies in patients with non-fatal AE-IPF is far more limited. It is, therefore, difficult to ascertain how far such histopathologic characteristics define patients with particularly unfavourable prognosis in the context of a given management strategy or represent AE-IPF as a whole.

MANAGEMENT OF AE-IPF

Expert reviews propose a diversity of management strategies in AE-IPF (182,183,222,223), and some aspects are controversial. The current paucity of evidence-based treatment and the prognostic implications of such events should be borne in mind when formulating potential treatment plans. For optimal patient-centred care, these factors should appropriately inform discussions of the proposed options with the patient. In general, patients are currently often treated with antibiotics to cover for bacterial drivers of exacerbation, even in cases lacking clear evidence of this (182). Supportive care is encouraged, with oxygen supplementation and with medications such as opioids or benzodiazepines at doses to alleviate breathlessness. AE-IPF can present with rapid deterioration of respiratory function. Therefore, early decisions regarding the most appropriate thresholds/ceilings for intensification of intervention or escalation of palliative approaches may helpfully focus care most effectively.

Short-term corticosteroid use in AE-IPF remains supported in recent clinical guidelines on IPF (4). Their use has been supported by a recent consensus document created by expert UK physicians, who suggest that such steroid use should be the rule rather than the exception (182). This opinion is weakly evidence based and not universally supported (224,225). Proponents can point towards the logic of likely steroid responsiveness in exacerbations characterized by organizing pneumonia changes and the high mortality of AE-IPF as providing the potential for clinically meaningful intervention. Others argue that steroids may cause harm in IPF patients who exacerbate. Recently, survival was retrospectively compared in groups of exacerbating patients who had ever been or were never managed with corticosteroid and/or immunosuppressive treatment. The AE-IPF events were managed with withdrawal of any ongoing treatment using these agents, broad-spectrum antibiotics and best supportive care. Survival was significantly higher in those patients who had never been treated previously with corticosteroids or immunosuppressants, despite significantly worse lung function prior to exacerbation (225). Survival at 1 year was also significantly better in the never-treated group. However, this effect was lost once repeated attendances for exacerbation in the same patient were excluded. Moreover, the comparison was between long-term management approaches and outcome in AE-IPF, rather than short-course steroid treatment as currently recommended. While removal of non-steroid immunosuppressants would be consistent with many centres' practice for these patients, the apparent removal of ongoing corticosteroid treatment might also have had deleterious consequences. Nevertheless, these data support a case for larger trials to evaluate the positive or deleterious effects of treating AE-IPF with corticosteroids. Ideally such studies might stratify patients by the radiologic pattern of new infiltrates (focal versus diffuse) to provide data on subgroups pre-defined by criteria that can be used alongside standard clinical care.

The histopathologic finding of organizing pneumonia in AE-IPF biopsy and post-mortem tissue provides some reassurance for the continued use of corticosteroids as a short-term treatment in a condition with a generally poor prognosis. Conversely the use of other immunosuppressant medication in AE-IPF is not widespread internationally. This is likely due to attribution of the mortality findings of the PANTHER-IPF and TIPAC studies to immunosuppression with azathioprine more than to steroid use. Nevertheless, the use of immunosuppressive treatment in AE-IPF has been studied to a limited extent, mainly in small retrospective analyses (reviewed by Juarez et al. [203]). Positive findings have been reported with cyclosporin (226,227), tacrolimus (228) and polymyxin-B (229). Further validation in prospective randomized control trials would be required before their clinical use can be widely advocated, and other non-immunosuppressive strategies are likely to be explored in preference for the foreseeable future.

VENTILATORY SUPPORT STRATEGIES FOR ACUTE RESPIRATORY FAILURE IN IPF

The use of mechanical ventilation in AE-IPF is associated with very poor outcome (230–232), and this is highly consistent with findings for respiratory failure in IPF (230,233). Nevertheless, a diagnosis of AE-IPF may not automatically preclude consideration of admission to an intensive care unit (ICU) for ventilatory support. ICU care and ventilation may permit investigations to exclude reversible causes of respiratory deterioration in IPF (e.g. BAL culture for infection, stabilizing patients for CT scanning). In some situations ICU care may also provide the most appropriate setting for discussing and establishing end-of-life care (232,234). The Acute Physiology and Chronic Health Evaluation (APACHE) (235) and Sequential Organ Failure Assessment (236) (SOFA) critical illness scoring systems may allow some stratification of IPF patients referred to the intensive care services. However, there remains a dearth of information on predictors of ICU survival in IPF patients. Given the concern that ventilator-induced lung damage may contribute to worsened AE-IPF, low tidal volumes are favoured to minimize stretch of lung parenchyma (203), by analogy with the management of acute respiratory distress syndrome (ARDS) (237). In contrast, while high PEEP is favoured in ARDS, concern has been raised about this approach in ILD (including IPF) patients with acute respiratory failure. In one study, both higher PEEP values and APACHE-III scores correlated with worse mortality (238); in another, no such extra mortality was apparent once the APACHE-III score was taken into account (239).

Continuous positive airway pressure (CPAP) delivered non-invasively can support ventilation by counteracting the effects of reduced compliance on pressure–volume relationships in the ventilatory cycle in disease. The rationale for considering its use in type 1 respiratory failure associated with AE-IPF, where both the underlying disease and the effects of an exacerbation will reduce compliance, is, therefore, readily appreciable. Non-invasive ventilation (NIV) is typically used to support patients in type 2 respiratory failure. This can be regarded as a poor prognostic indicator in IPF, as ventilatory clearance of CO_2 is generally preserved until the work of breathing overwhelms functional capacity of the respiratory muscles.

Nevertheless small, retrospective studies suggest that CPAP and even NIV can play a beneficial role in management of AE-IPF. In a review of 11 patients referred to an ICU service for respiratory failure (PaO$_2$:FiO$_2$ ratio <300) over a 6-year period, the use of non-invasive pressure support (CPAP and/or NIV) without subsequent ventilation was associated with survival to 3 months in five cases (240). Exclusion criteria included identification of bacterial pathogens in blood and sputum (and in many cases BAL) cultures. All patients were concurrently managed with high-dose corticosteroid therapy and immunosuppression according to local practice for AE-IPF. However a subsequent paper reported similar findings from a single centre administering NIV to patients with IPF and acute respiratory failure (PaO$_2$:FiO$_2$ ratio <250) from all causes (definable infection 8, cardiac decompensation 4, AE-IPF 4) (241). The results are somewhat more encouraging than those of another study into all-cause respiratory failure in IPF in the ICU setting (233). Respiratory rate and B-type natriuretic peptide levels (above laboratory normal range) may be useful to stratify patients requiring ventilatory support who may be successfully managed by non-invasive means (241). Non-invasive ventilatory support may, therefore, help a subgroup of patients with acute respiratory failure in IPF of intermediate severity with preserved right ventricular function. These conclusions require validation in trials designed to minimize risks of selection bias.

If supported, the fact that use of NIV does not prevent direct communication with the patient has further benefits (242). However in both studies the failure of non-invasive pressure support/ventilation strategies was associated with death in all cases, supporting a role for this mode as a reasonable ceiling of care in AE-IPF cases where clinically appropriate. IPF patients tolerate high-flow nasal oxygenation/insufflation (243), but no evidence exists regarding its effectiveness.

In recent years extracorporeal membrane oxygenation (ECMO) has become increasingly used to support acute respiratory failure. A recent retrospective review of ILD cases referred to an ECMO service was interpreted to support its use as a bridge to lung transplantation (244). Three of the 21 cases

managed with ECMO had a diagnosis of IPF with four other cases defined as idiopathic (two NSIP, two acute interstitial pneumonia), but outcomes were not stratified by ILD sub-type. Overall 8 of the patients were listed for lung transplant with 6 surviving to transplant, while of the remaining 13 patients, only one survived to discharge. Therefore, in carefully selected IPF cases where listing for lung transplant is deemed feasible, it may currently be reasonable to consider ECMO support. However more data are required to provide a better evidence base by ILD subtype, and the likely wait time for an appropriate donor lung in a particular region may affect the chance of benefit. Currently, for patients with IPF and acute respiratory failure this very much remains a decision based upon a clinician's judgment following evaluation of the individual case.

PULMONARY HYPERTENSION IN IPF

BACKGROUND

Secondary PH (pre-capillary, Group 3 [245]) is a well-recognized complication in IPF. It is defined by mean pulmonary artery pressure (mPAP) ≥25 mm Hg or left ventricular end diastolic pressure or pulmonary capillary wedge pressure of ≤15 mm Hg, as measured by right heart catheterization. However, it is difficult to diagnose reliably, and treatment evidence is scarce. The incidence of PH in IPF (IPF-PH) is variably reported. Recent longitudinal data suggest that just under half of patients are affected. The incidence increases with time from diagnosis, and PH is observed in 85% of patients requiring lung transplant (246). IPF-PH carries a fourfold higher risk of death compared with IPF patients without PH (187,247). It is a risk factor for exacerbations of IPF (187), and it impacts severely on patients' exercise tolerance (248). In IPF, mPAP (21,249) and right ventricular systolic pressure (RVSP) (250) are predictors of mortality. In patients with severe fibrosis due to a range of ILDs these particular associations may be lost, although pulmonary vascular resistance still predicts mortality (251). This may reflect reduced right ventricular contractility in severe disease.

ASSESSMENT FOR IPF-PH

The presenting features of PH in IPF are non-specific and overlap with the underlying disease process. Patients may suffer from increases in exertional breathlessness, more rapid fatigue and palpitations. Examination of the patient may reveal a loud pulmonary (P2) component of the second heart sound and a pansystolic murmur if raised pulmonary artery systolic pressure (PASP) causes tricuspid regurgitation. Decompensation of right heart function may be demonstrated by elevated jugular venous pressure, pedal oedema and right ventricular heave.

The earliest objective evidence of secondary PH in an IPF patient may come from pulmonary function testing and exercise testing. Progression of interstitial fibrosis is directly reported by correlated reductions in lung volumes (including alveolar volume) and total gas transfer capacity. This is usually sensitively reported by reductions in both FVC and DLCO with relative preservation of the KCO. IPF-PH causes further reduction in gas transfer in the absence of an effect on lung volumes. The development of IPF-PH is, therefore, indicated by decline in gas transfer measures that are disproportionate to any reduction in FVC. Since DLCO is reduced by both interstitial fibrosis and secondary PH components of IPF-PH, it can be used as a single index to stratify risk of this complication in IPF (249). DLCO is significantly lower in patients with IPF-PH, and DLCO <30% relates to a twofold higher risk of concomitant PH relative to TLCO ≥30% (252). As expected, FVC shows little or no correlation with PH at right heart catheterization.

The 6-minute walk test (6MWT) may be used to identify those at risk of having underlying PH. Patients with underlying IPF-PH perform significantly worse on the 6MWT in terms of distance travelled (6MWD) and the distance-saturation product (253,254). Desaturation to SaO_2 values <85% on exertion and the degree to which baseline heart rate is recovered by 1 minute after test completion are indicators of underlying IPF-PH (255,256).

BNP levels correlate with mortality and have prognostic value when measured serially in the IPF population (257). To our knowledge, there are at present no studies directly comparing right heart catheter results with BNP levels in IPF per se. However, BNP correlates strongly with severity of PH on right heart catheterization in a mixed lung fibrosis cohort where IPF was over-represented in the patient pool (258). CT scan findings of pulmonary artery enlargement and oedema in the aorto-pulmonary bay can raise suspicion of IPF-PH. Although they are not well validated (259) for this purpose, they may predict patient outcome to some extent (260,261).

Currently, there is no specific evidence-based treatment for IPF-PH outside of the usual standard of IPF care. The use of right heart catheterization to formally confirm a diagnosis of IPF-PH and evaluate it in detail is, therefore, not common outside of evaluation of transplant fitness/needs. Echocardiography is a well-tolerated screening investigation for PH and is more commonly used in IPF-PH. In one study it accurately measured RVSP in only 40% of IPF patients studied (255). However, echocardiographic measurements of tricuspid annular plane systolic excursion (TAPSE) and the right-left ventricular diameter ratio predicted mortality in a cohort of IPF patients undergoing right heart catheterization at a transplant centre (262). This study did not report correlations of measurements obtained by echocardiography with pressures observed at right heart catheterization.

TREATMENT

No specific treatments are robustly supported by current evidence for the treatment of secondary PH in IPF. Moreover, trials of agents used to treat idiopathic pulmonary arterial hypertension (IPAH) in IPF populations have generally not targeted an IPF-PH population per se. Anti-coagulation is used in the management of IPAH (263,264), and IPF patients may have a prothrombotic tendency relative to the general population (265). However, the ACE-IPF trial found an excess of mortality when warfarin was combined with prednisolone in treating IPF patients compared with prednisolone alone, resulting in early cessation of the study (266). Novel anti-coagulants have not been studied in this context, and the role of heparin in IPF remains a matter of discussion (267).

Therapies aimed at causing pulmonary vasodilatation are useful in alleviating PAH. However in the presence of interstitial fibrosis, vasodilation to relive secondary pulmonary hypertension carries the potential to concomitantly worsen V/Q mismatch (268). Although sildenafil appears safe to use in patients with IPF, primary outcome efficacy data are lacking. The largest RCT to date for sildenafil in advanced IPF (STEP-IPF) failed to show a significant improvement in its primary outcome measure (6MWD increase) with sildenafil (185). However, the trial data showed efficacy in clinically relevant secondary endpoints. Sildenafil treatment increased PaO_2 and DLCO, and it significantly improved dyspnoea scores and quality of life. *Post hoc* analyses indicated that in patients with RVSD identified on echocardiography, sildenafil resulted in significant preservation of exercise tolerance as assessed by 6MWT (269). In contrast, patients have shown no evidence of improved pulmonary haemodynamics, mortality, improved functional parameters or symptoms with the endothelin receptor antagonist, bosentan, in IPF (270) or in PH associated with fibrotic idiopathic ILD (271). Indeed studies of the use of another member of this drug class, ambrisentan, in IPF were terminated early due to safety concerns (272). Similarly a trial of a soluble guanylate cyclase stimulator approved for use in PAH and CTEPH, riociguat, in PH associated with idiopathic ILD was terminated early due to concern that it was associated with increased mortality risk in this disease group.

Hypoxemia is well established as a driver of secondary PH and tends to worsen during sleep. Moreover, hypoxia-inducible pathways may contribute to fibrosis (273). Support of nocturnal oxygenation in IPF patients is, therefore, of interest as a strategy to limit progression of IPF-PH. IPF patients demonstrate a greater degree of desaturation during sleep than occurs during maximal exercise (274). The maximal difference between SaO_2 while awake and nocturnal saturation correlates with RVSP measured by echocardiography and mortality. Fascinatingly, it has also been correlated with the apnea–hypopnea index. Obstructive sleep apnoea (OSA) is a common comorbidity in IPF cohort, but it differs from non-IPF associated OSA in that traditional risk assessment tools (including questionnaire screening) do not predict likelihood of a diagnostic sleep study (275). Sleep disturbance is a significant predictive factor for poor quality of life outcome in IPF patients and is improved by CPAP when OSA is diagnosed (276). CPAP lowers pulmonary artery pressures in OSA (277), but this has not been explicitly studied in OSA associated with IPF. Not all evidence supports

a role for OSA or hypopnea as the main driver of nocturnal desaturation, and CPAP in IPF patients with OSA is variably tolerated (278). However, when it is tolerated, better functional outcomes are observed (279). LTOT is currently prescribed for IPF by analogy with the evidence-based practice in COPD where it increases survival and can reduce pulmonary artery pressure (280). Indeed, improving right heart function is a major goal of such treatment (281). Oxygen supplementation to support nocturnal oxygenation during sleep in COPD reduces pulmonary artery pressures (282). However there is currently no specific evidence base for its use in IPF either as LTOT or to target nocturnal hypoventilation as a driver of secondary PH in this condition.

In summary, IPF-PH bears grave consequences for the patient, both in terms of increased mortality and functional capacity. Diagnosis requires clinical vigilance, and treatment options remain limited.

LUNG TRANSPLANTATION

Many issues relating to lung transplant in IPF are common to transplantation in other ILDs, and this topic is dealt with more comprehensively elsewhere in this textbook. However appropriate referral for lung transplantation is an important facet of clinical care in IPF, and some general and specific issues are highlighted here. Fewer than 1% of patients with IPF receive lung transplant, although the median life expectancy after lung transplant in this group is currently 4.5 years and improving (283). This is similar to the situation following transplant for other idiopathic interstitial pneumonias (284). It appears worse than for non-ILD indications (α_1-antitrypsin deficiency emphysema, usual COPD, cystic fibrosis), but this comparison does not take into account age of recipients or their co-morbidities, and these characteristics of the IPF recipient population may be less favourable for post-transplant long-term survival. Waiting list mortality is 14%–67% with exercise tolerance an independent risk factor for dying while awaiting transplant (285). A 6MWD threshold of 207 m may define a fourfold increased mortality risk for those walking less than this distance threshold compared with those exceeding it.

As co-morbidities reduce fitness for transplant, younger IPF patients with rapid decline are better candidates for referral. However relatively few patients with IPF are younger than 70 years, and so alternative working diagnoses that are more amenable to stabilization may be investigated before IPF is confirmed. This delay may be associated with pulmonary function decline and, therefore, tend to worsen survival on the waiting list. Close liaison with transplant assessment services is, therefore, helpful to minimize risk of delayed referral without hindering appropriate investigation of alternative diagnoses. The advent of anti-fibrotic therapies may slow rates of decline and thereby reduce mortality before and during assessment and on waiting lists. But some of these anticipated benefits may be somewhat attenuated by increased co-morbidity as age at referral increases.

CONCLUSION: HOW FAR HAVE WE COME?

The understanding of IPF, including its distinction from other types of ILD, has evolved to define a disease entity that is increasingly coherent in its radiologic, histologic and temporal phenotypes. The field was arguably slow to advance from appreciating that such insights provided the justification for rebutting nihilistic views of pulmonary fibrosis as a whole to undertaking therapeutic studies of immunomodulatory treatments recommended on the basis of expert opinion and previous findings in patients diagnosed according to superseded criteria. When such studies were undertaken, however, the validity of the more precise definition of IPF was upheld by the clarity of the results, albeit with mixed implications for managing patients. First, in contrast to more adaptive immune, cell-driven fibrotic processes, such a treatment regimen was associated strongly with increased mortality. Any concern that IPF represented a disease process wholly unamenable to any treatment approach was then rapidly rebutted by findings that anti-fibrotic agents clearly slowed the rate of disease progression. This not only provided a clear evidence base for IPF treatments that are now prescribed in the clinic, but it also showed that pathways of disease progression in IPF could be targeted. Whether these can be reversed, or whether stabilization of decline is the best possible goal in IPF remains to be determined.

IPF phenotyping, therefore, appears to have provided the opportunity to identify such effects. It can be seen as vindication of a 'splitting' approach to the diagnosis and management of ILDs. Further benefits may, therefore, accrue from sub-phenotyping and stratification of what we currently understand as IPF, based upon continued improvements in understanding markers of disease aetiology, co-factors, activity and/or progression. Molecular insights can support such an approach, particularly in diseases whose previous unified definitions have contributed to their apparent intractability. Current areas of interest for sub-phenotyping include stratification according to microbiomics (37), biomarkers (286), microRNA profiles (287) and genotyping. *MUC5B* (135,136) and *TOLLIP* (135) gene polymorphisms have been associated with specific behaviours within IPF. The genetics of non-autoinflammatory familial pulmonary fibrosis may also identify pathways where milder mutations contribute to the pathogenesis of apparently sporadic IPF. Constituents of the telomerase complex may exemplify this (288). There is, therefore, potential for further genes of interest to be identified through studies such as the UK 100,000 Genomes Project where familial pulmonary fibrosis is included as a rare disease of specific interest (289).

Improved understanding can also work in the opposite direction by defining targetable disease mechanisms that are shared between patients diagnosed with different conditions. There may be potential for this in the case of IPF and other fibrosing ILDs with similar features to IPF. The natural history of idiopathic ILD with radiology suggestive of fibrotic NSIP is near-identical to 'typical IPF' if histology demonstrates UIP (47). However, fibrotic NSIP may be diagnosed and treated with immune modulation on radiological grounds without histological correlation, particularly in younger people. This can be rationalized if NSIP is considered a predominantly auto-inflammatory condition, even in the absence of a clear-cut diagnosis of auto-immune disease (26,27). In this case, stabilization or even clinical improvement may be possible with immunomodulatory treatment. In contrast, current anti-fibrotic treatments merely reduce rate of decline, and are not at present evidence based in such situations. Nevertheless, there is a potential overlap between some cases diagnosed as fibrotic NSIP and patients from the INPULSIS trial with 'possible' UIP pattern disease, who derived the same treatment benefit with nintedanib as 'definite' IPF patients (43). Risks of harm contribute to the dilemma. Surgical biopsy carries an increased risk of disease acceleration and death (290–292). However, treatment with immune suppressive approaches might have similar deleterious consequences to those seen in the PANTHER-IPF study if an underlying IPF-like disease process pertains. The risk of inaction is missing the best chance to arrest or slow a disease process and thereby allowing irreversible deterioration to occur to some degree.

Things become even less clear where clinico-radiologic evaluation supports diagnosis of a different non-auto-immune ILD that shows evidence of progressive fibrosis. This can be observed in relatively young patients with CT appearances suggestive of cryptogenic organizing pneumonia or hypersensitivity pneumonitis in the absence of a clearly identified inhalational trigger. Fibroblastic foci are not entirely specific for IPF, and even surgical biopsy may miss characteristic features of a disease process. Therefore, what histologic criteria should constitute 'sufficiently characteristic' UIP histology to switch the consensus diagnosis of a MDT to a diagnosis of IPF? In cases where the radiology is suggestive of chronic HP or COP, how robustly reproducible are such judgments of UIP histology between histopathologists? To what extent does the confidence of identifying a dominant UIP process in these circumstances depend upon the experience of the histopathologist? Do such patients have 'IPF-like' responses to treatment, deriving benefit from anti-fibrotic treatment and harm from immune suppressive treatment? If so, it might make sense to recommend a lower threshold for biopsy, even in non-IPF ILDs where radiology seemed conclusive.

Diagnostic benefits would need to be balanced against risk of harm from biopsy. It has long been recognized that transbronchial lung biopsy with conventional bronchoscopy is insufficient for this purpose. However, it may be possible to reduce the risks of achieving adequate sampling of parenchymal tissue to aid with diagnosis of IPF currently associated with the requirement for surgical lung biopsy. A recent study indicates that transbronchial cryobiopsy may provide similarly diagnostic histopathology to surgical lung biopsy in diagnosing IPF and other fibrosing ILDs (293). Similar increases in

MDT diagnostic certainty were observed following assessment of either cryobiopsy or surgical lung biopsy samples. Direct comparisons have yet to be performed between cryobiopsy and surgical lung biopsy samples in the same patient. Moreover, the safety profile of cryobiopsy in patients with differing co-morbidities and performance status needs to be more fully evaluated to best guide clinical practice (294). Further technological advances may allow the application of even less invasive methods that can define molecular and cellular characteristics of lesions *in situ*. The use of positron emission tomography (PET) using ligands that target lesion-specific (295) biomarkers has potential to do this if findings can be correlated with histopathological findings (296) and/or clinical behaviour.

At present in individual cases, the combination of applying clinical judgment, including a low threshold for BAL studies, monitoring disease progress closely and readiness to adjust strategy depending upon disease progression is valid. In the United Kingdom, an 'MDT diagnosis' of IPF rather than a proscriptive set of 'typical IPF' criteria allow MDTs to apply some judgment in defining an appropriate population to treat as IPF patients. Even 'snapshot' MDT judgment with relatively little input from histopathologic studies has been shown predict a subsequent 'IPF-like' disease course across international centres reviewing a case series representing a wide spectrum of ILDs (5). However, data from prospective studies including RCTs would be of general benefit to the population(s) in whom biopsy may show features that argue against the radiological phenotype.

Conversely, a recent international consensus statement proposed an entity of 'interstitial pneumonitis with auto-immune features' (IPAF) for research purposes (297). The initial aim is to see whether this classification may identify patients with *forme fruste* auto-immune multisystem disease that includes ILD but does not reach criteria for a definitive connective tissue disease diagnosis. These individuals might be expected to benefit from immunomodulatory treatments. For a diagnosis of IPAF, individuals must have radiologic appearances consistent with an ILD and either serologic or clinical features of a connective tissue disease. Although CT appearances of a 'definite UIP' pattern are not included in the qualifying radiologic criteria, they do include appearances that could be associated with UIP histology (e.g. NSIP). Moreover, at least some patients meeting IPAF criteria will likely have serologic markers of auto-immunity merely through coincidence rather than because the ILD is caused by an auto-immune-mediated process. Immunomodulatory treatment might, therefore, cause harm in some patients diagnosed with IPAF. Evaluation of the IPAF group should include studies that are designed to detect signals of adverse effects in patients treated in this way (298–300).

Related questions remain as to whether pathogenic mechanisms of fibrosing auto-immune ILDs sufficiently overlap with those of IPF such that treatment with both anti-fibrotic and immunomodulatory treatments might be beneficial. An obvious starting point for such studies would be rheumatoid-associated UIP. The role of these anti-fibrotics in asbestos-mediated lung disease is also as yet undefined. Finally, studies are currently underway to establish whether use of pirfenidone and nintedanib in combination is more beneficial than either treatment alone (ClinicalTrials.gov NCT02606877).

REFERENCES

1. British Lung Foundation, Respiratory Health of the Nation Study. Idiopathic pulmonary fibrosis statistics, 2016. https://www.blf.org.uk/support-for-you/idiopathic-pulmonary-fibrosis-ipf/statistics. Accessed 17 October 2016.
2. Raghu G, Weycker D, Edelsberg J, Bradford WZ, Oster G. Incidence and prevalence of idiopathic pulmonary fibrosis. *Am J Respir Crit Care Med.* 2006;174(7):810–6.
3. Nalysnyk L, Cid-Ruzafa J, Rotella P, Esser D. Incidence and prevalence of idiopathic pulmonary fibrosis: Review of the literature. *Eur Respir Rev.* 2012;21(126):355–61.
4. Raghu G, Collard HR, Egan JJ, Martinez FJ, Behr J, Brown KK et al. An official ATS/ERS/JRS/ALAT statement: Idiopathic pulmonary fibrosis: Evidence-based guidelines for diagnosis and management. *Am J Respir Crit Care Med.* 2011;183(6):788–824.
5. Walsh SL, Wells AU, Desai SR, Poletti V, Piciucchi S, Dubini A et al. Multicentre evaluation of multidisciplinary team meeting agreement on diagnosis in diffuse parenchymal lung disease: A case-cohort study. *Lancet Respir Med.* 2016;4(7):557–65.
6. Clarke DL, Murray LA, Crestani B, Sleeman MA. Is personalised medicine the key to heterogeneity in idiopathic pulmonary fibrosis? *Pharmacol Ther.* 2017;169:35–46.
7. Spagnolo P, Maher TM, Richeldi L. Idiopathic pulmonary fibrosis: Recent advances on pharmacological therapy. *Pharmacol Ther.* 2015;152:18–27.
8. Selman M, King TE, Pardo A, American Thoracic S, European Respiratory S, American College of Chest P. Idiopathic pulmonary fibrosis: Prevailing and evolving hypotheses about its pathogenesis and implications for therapy. *Ann Intern Med.* 2001;134(2):136–51.
9. Maher TM, Wells AU, Laurent GJ. Idiopathic pulmonary fibrosis: Multiple causes and multiple mechanisms? *Eur Respir J.* 2007;30(5):835–9.
10. Ley B, Collard HR, King TE, Jr. Clinical course and prediction of survival in idiopathic pulmonary fibrosis. *Am J Respir Crit Care Med.* 2011;183(4):431–40.
11. Gribbin J, Hubbard RB, Le Jeune I, Smith CJ, West J, Tata LJ. Incidence and mortality of idiopathic pulmonary fibrosis and sarcoidosis in the UK. *Thorax.* 2006;61(11):980–5.
12. Yang IV, Schwartz DA. Epigenetics of idiopathic pulmonary fibrosis. *Transl Res.* 2015;165(1):48–60.
13. Lee JS, Collard HR, Anstrom KJ, Martinez FJ, Noth I, Roberts RS et al. Anti-acid treatment and disease progression in idiopathic pulmonary fibrosis: An analysis of data from three randomised controlled trials. *Lancet Respir Med.* 2013;1(5):369–76.
14. Johannson K, Collard HR. Acute exacerbation of idiopathic pulmonary fibrosis: A proposal. *Curr Respir Care Rep.* 2013;2(4):233.
15. Moore BB, Moore TA. Viruses in idiopathic pulmonary fibrosis. Etiology and exacerbation. *Ann Am Thorac Soc.* 2015;12(Suppl 2):S186–92.
16. Camus P, Bonniaud P, Baudouin N, Fanton A, Camus C, Favroit N et al. Pneumotox On Line – The Drug-Induced Respiratory Disease Website, 2012. Department of Pulmonary Medicine and Intensive Care, University Hospital, Dijon, France; [v2]. http://www.pneumotox.com/. Accessed 17 October 2016.

17. Kanematsu T, Kitaichi M, Nishimura K, Nagai S, Izumi T. Clubbing of the fingers and smooth-muscle proliferation in fibrotic changes in the lung in patients with idiopathic pulmonary fibrosis. *Chest.* 1994; 105(2):339–42.

18. Turner-Warwick M, Burrows B, Johnson A. Cryptogenic fibrosing alveolitis: Clinical features and their influence on survival. *Thorax.* 1980;35(3):171–80.

19. Staples CA, Muller NL, Vedal S, Abboud R, Ostrow D, Miller RR. Usual interstitial pneumonia: Correlation of CT with clinical, functional, and radiologic findings. *Radiology.* 1987;162(2):377–81.

20. Wells AU, King AD, Rubens MB, Cramer D, du Bois RM, Hansell DM. Lone cryptogenic fibrosing alveolitis: A functional-morphologic correlation based on extent of disease on thin-section computed tomography. *Am J Respir Crit Care Med.* 1997;155(4):1367–75.

21. Hamada K, Nagai S, Tanaka S, Handa T, Shigematsu M, Nagao T et al. Significance of pulmonary arterial pressure and diffusion capacity of the lung as prognosticator in patients with idiopathic pulmonary fibrosis. *Chest.* 2007;131(3):650–6.

22. National Institute for Health and Care Excellence. *Pirfenidone for Treating Idiopathic Pulmonary Fibrosis NICE Technology Appraisal Guidance [TA282]* UK: Department of Health, 2013.

23. National Institute for Health and Care Excellence. *Nintedanib for Treating Idiopathic Pulmonary Fibrosis NICE Technology Appraisal Guidance [TA379]* UK: Department of Health, 2016.

24. Lama VN, Flaherty KR, Toews GB, Colby TV, Travis WD, Long Q et al. Prognostic value of desaturation during a 6-minute walk test in idiopathic interstitial pneumonia. *Am J Respir Crit Care Med.* 2003;168(9):1084–90.

25. Wells AU, Desai SR, Rubens MB, Goh NS, Cramer D, Nicholson AG et al. Idiopathic pulmonary fibrosis: A composite physiologic index derived from disease extent observed by computed tomography. *Am J Respir Crit Care Med.* 2003;167(7):962–9.

26. Kinder BW, Collard HR, Koth L, Daikh DI, Wolters PJ, Elicker B et al. Idiopathic nonspecific interstitial pneumonia: Lung manifestation of undifferentiated connective tissue disease? *Am J Respir Crit Care Med.* 2007;176(7):691–7.

27. Suda T, Kono M, Nakamura Y, Enomoto N, Kaida Y, Fujisawa T et al. Distinct prognosis of idiopathic nonspecific interstitial pneumonia (NSIP) fulfilling criteria for undifferentiated connective tissue disease (UCTD). *Respir Med.* 2010;104(10):1527–34.

28. Mohr LC. Hypersensitivity pneumonitis. *Curr Opin Pulm Med.* 2004;10(5):401–11.

29. Lloyd CR, Walsh SL, Hansell DM. High-resolution CT of complications of idiopathic fibrotic lung disease. *Br J Radiol.* 2011;84(1003):581–92.

30. Devaraj A, Hansell DM. Computed tomography signs of pulmonary hypertension: Old and new observations. *Clin Radiol.* 2009;64(8):751–60.

31. Panos RJ, Mortenson RL, Niccoli SA, King TE, Jr. Clinical deterioration in patients with idiopathic pulmonary fibrosis: Causes and assessment. *Am J Med.* 1990;88(4):396–404.

32. Araki T, Katsura H, Sawabe M, Kida K. A clinical study of idiopathic pulmonary fibrosis based on autopsy studies in elderly patients. *Intern Med.* 2003;42(6):483–9.

33. Rudd RM, Prescott RJ, Chalmers JC, Johnston ID, Fibrosing Alveolitis Subcommittee of the Research Committee of the British Thoracic S. British Thoracic Society Study on cryptogenic fibrosing alveolitis: Response to treatment and survival. *Thorax.* 2007;62(1):62–6.

34. Meyer KC, Raghu G, Baughman RP, Brown KK, Costabel U, du Bois RM et al. An official American Thoracic Society clinical practice guideline: The clinical utility of bronchoalveolar lavage cellular analysis in interstitial lung disease. *Am J Respir Crit Care Med.* 2012;185(9):1004–14.

35. Agusti C, Xaubet A, Luburich P, Ayuso MC, Roca J, Rodriguez-Roisin R. Computed tomography-guided bronchoalveolar lavage in idiopathic pulmonary fibrosis. *Thorax.* 1996;51(8):841–5.

36. Shulgina L, Cahn AP, Chilvers ER, Parfrey H, Clark AB, Wilson EC et al. Treating idiopathic pulmonary fibrosis with the addition

of co-trimoxazole: A randomised controlled trial. *Thorax.* 2013;68(2):155–62.

37. Molyneaux PL, Cox MJ, Willis-Owen SA, Mallia P, Russell KE, Russell AM et al. The role of bacteria in the pathogenesis and progression of idiopathic pulmonary fibrosis. *Am J Respir Crit Care Med.* 2014;190(8):906–13.

38. Cool CD, Groshong SD, Rai PR, Henson PM, Stewart JS, Brown KK. Fibroblast foci are not discrete sites of lung injury or repair: The fibroblast reticulum. *Am J Respir Crit Care Med.* 2006;174(6):654–8.

39. Travis WD, Costabel U, Hansell DM, King TE, Jr., Lynch DA, Nicholson AG et al. An official American Thoracic Society/European Respiratory Society statement: Update of the international multidisciplinary classification of the idiopathic interstitial pneumonias. *Am J Respir Crit Care Med.* 2013;188(6):733–48.

40. Raghu G, Rochwerg B, Zhang Y, Garcia CA, Azuma A, Behr J et al. An Official ATS/ERS/JRS/ALAT Clinical Practice Guideline: Treatment of Idiopathic Pulmonary Fibrosis. An Update of the 2011 Clinical Practice Guideline. *Am J Respir Crit Care Med.* 2015;192(2):e3–19.

41. Demedts M, Costabel U. ATS/ERS international multidisciplinary consensus classification of the idiopathic interstitial pneumonias. *Eur Respir J.* 2002;19(5):794–6.

42. Fell CD, Martinez FJ, Liu LX, Murray S, Han MK, Kazerooni EA et al. Clinical predictors of a diagnosis of idiopathic pulmonary fibrosis. *Am J Respir Crit Care Med.* 2010;181(8):832–7.

43. Raghu G, Wells AU, Nicholson AG, Richeldi L, Flaherty KR, Le Maulf F et al. Effect of nintedanib in subgroups of idiopathic pulmonary fibrosis by diagnostic criteria. *Am J Respir Crit Care Med.* 2017;195(1):78–85.

44. Cordier JF. Cryptogenic organising pneumonia. *Eur Respir J.* 2006;28(2):422–46.

45. Takemura T, Akashi T, Kamiya H, Ikushima S, Ando T, Oritsu M et al. Pathological differentiation of chronic hypersensitivity pneumonitis from idiopathic pulmonary fibrosis/usual interstitial pneumonia. *Histopathology.* 2012;61(6):1026–35.

46. Sverzellati N, Wells AU, Tomassetti S, Desai SR, Copley SJ, Aziz ZA et al. Biopsy-proved idiopathic pulmonary fibrosis: Spectrum of nondiagnostic thin-section CT diagnoses. *Radiology.* 2010;254(3):957–64.

47. Flaherty KR, Travis WD, Colby TV, Toews GB, Kazerooni EA, Gross BH et al. Histopathologic variability in usual and nonspecific interstitial pneumonias. *Am J Respir Crit Care Med.* 2001;164(9):1722–7.

48. Monaghan H, Wells AU, Colby TV, du Bois RM, Hansell DM, Nicholson AG. Prognostic implications of histologic patterns in multiple surgical lung biopsies from patients with idiopathic interstitial pneumonias. *Chest.* 2004;125(2):522–6.

49. Myers JL. Hypersensitivity pneumonia: The role of lung biopsy in diagnosis and management. *Mod Pathol.* 2012;25(Suppl 1):S58–67.

50. Tossvainen A. Asbestos, asbestosis, and cancer: The Helsinki criteria for diagnosis and attribution. *Scand J Work Environ Health.* 1997;23(4):311–6.

51. Felten MK, Knoll L, Eisenhawer C, Ackermann D, Khatab K, Hudepohl J et al. Retrospective exposure assessment to airborne asbestos among power industry workers. *J Occup Med Toxicol.* 2010;5:15.

52. Ameille J, Rosenberg N, Matrat M, Descatha A, Mompoint D, Hamzi L et al. Asbestos-related diseases in automobile mechanics. *Ann Occup Hyg.* 2012;56(1):55–60.

53. Wolff H, Vehmas T, Oksa P, Rantanen J, Vainio H. Asbestos, asbestosis, and cancer, the Helsinki criteria for diagnosis and attribution 2014: Recommendations. *Scand J Work Environ Health.* 2015;41(1):5–15.

54. Roggli VL, Gibbs AR, Attanoos R, Churg A, Popper H, Cagle P et al. Pathology of asbestosis – An update of the diagnostic criteria: Report of the asbestosis committee of the College of American Pathologists and Pulmonary Pathology Society. *Arch Pathol Lab Med.* 2010;134(3):462–80.

55. Attanoos RL, Alchami FS, Pooley FD, Gibbs AR. Usual interstitial pneumonia in asbestos-exposed cohorts – Concurrent idiopathic pulmonary fibrosis or atypical asbestosis? *Histopathology.* 2016;69(3):492–8.

56. Kehrer JP, Margolin SB. Pirfenidone diminishes cyclophosphamide-induced lung fibrosis in mice. *Toxicol Lett.* 1997;90(2–3):125–32.

57. Iyer SN, Gurujeyalakshmi G, Giri SN. Effects of pirfenidone on procollagen gene expression at the transcriptional level in bleomycin hamster model of lung fibrosis. *J Pharmacol Exp Ther.* 1999;289(1):211–8.

58. Iyer SN, Wild JS, Schiedt MJ, Hyde DM, Margolin SB, Giri SN. Dietary intake of pirfenidone ameliorates bleomycin-induced lung fibrosis in hamsters. *J Lab Clin Med.* 1995;125(6):779–85.

59. Nagai S, Hamada K, Shigematsu M, Taniyama M, Yamauchi S, Izumi T. Open-label compassionate use one year-treatment with pirfenidone to patients with chronic pulmonary fibrosis. *Intern Med.* 2002;41(12):1118–23.

60. Raghu G, Johnson WC, Lockhart D, Mageto Y. Treatment of idiopathic pulmonary fibrosis with a new antifibrotic agent, pirfenidone: Results of a prospective, open-label Phase II study. *Am J Respir Crit Care Med.* 1999;159(4 Pt 1):1061–9.

61. Azuma A, Nukiwa T, Tsuboi E, Suga M, Abe S, Nakata K et al. Double-blind, placebo-controlled trial of pirfenidone in patients with idiopathic pulmonary fibrosis. *Am J Respir Crit Care Med.* 2005;171(9):1040–7.

62. Taniguchi H, Ebina M, Kondoh Y, Ogura T, Azuma A, Suga M et al. Pirfenidone in idiopathic pulmonary fibrosis. *Eur Respir J.* 2010;35(4):821–9.

63. Noble PW, Albera C, Bradford WZ, Costabel U, Glassberg MK, Kardatzke D et al. Pirfenidone in patients with idiopathic pulmonary fibrosis (CAPACITY): Two randomised trials. *Lancet.* 2011;377(9779):1760–9.

64. Wells AU. Forced vital capacity as a primary end point in idiopathic pulmonary fibrosis treatment trials: Making a silk purse from a sow's ear. *Thorax.* 2013;68(4):309–10.

65. King TE, Jr., Bradford WZ, Castro-Bernardini S, Fagan EA, Glaspole I, Glassberg MK et al. A phase 3 trial of pirfenidone in patients with idiopathic pulmonary fibrosis. *N Engl J Med.* 2014;370(22):2083–92.

66. Spagnolo P, Del Giovane C, Luppi F, Cerri S, Balduzzi S, Walters EH et al. Non-steroid agents for idiopathic pulmonary fibrosis. *Cochrane Database Syst Rev.* 2010;(9):CD003134.

67. Ravaglia C, Gurioli C, Romagnoli M, Casoni G, Tomassetti S, Gurioli C et al. Pirfenidone treatment in idiopathic pulmonary fibrosis: An Italian case series. *Eur Respir J.* 2013;42(Suppl 57):P3370.

68. Oltmanns U, Kahn N, Palmowski K, Trager A, Wenz H, Heussel CP et al. Pirfenidone in idiopathic pulmonary fibrosis: Real-life experience from a German tertiary referral center for interstitial lung diseases. *Respiration.* 2014;88(3):199–207.

69. Costabel U, Albera C, Fagan E, Bradford W, King TE, Noble P et al. Long-term safety of pirfenidone in RECAP, an open-label extension study in patients with idiopathic pulmonary fibrosis, interim results. *Eur Respir J.* 2014;44(Suppl 58):1903.

70. Costabel U, Albera C, Bradford WZ, Hormel P, King TE, Jr., Noble PW et al. Analysis of lung function and survival in RECAP: An open-label extension study of pirfenidone in patients with idiopathic pulmonary fibrosis. *Sarcoidosis Vasc Diffuse Lung Dis.* 2014;31(3):198–205.

71. Koschel D, Cottin V, Skold M, Tomassetti S, Azuma A, Giot C et al. Pirfenidone post-authorization safety registry (PASSPORT) – Interim analysis of IPF treatment. *Eur Respir J.* 2014;44(Suppl 58):1904.

72. Costabel U, Bendstrup E, Cottin V, Dewint P, Egan JJ, Ferguson J et al. Pirfenidone in idiopathic pulmonary fibrosis: Expert panel discussion on the management of drug-related adverse events. *Adv Ther.* 2014;31(4):375–91.

73. Chaudhary NI, Roth GJ, Hilberg F, Muller-Quernheim J, Prasse A, Zissel G et al. Inhibition of PDGF, VEGF and FGF signalling attenuates fibrosis. *Eur Respir J.* 2007;29(5):976–85.

74. Richeldi L, Costabel U, Selman M, Kim DS, Hansell DM, Nicholson AG et al. Efficacy of a tyrosine kinase inhibitor in idiopathic pulmonary fibrosis. *N Engl J Med.* 2011;365(12):1079–87.

75. Richeldi L, du Raghu G, Azuma A, Brown KK, Costabel U et al. Efficacy and safety of nintedanib in idiopathic pulmonary fibrosis. *N Engl J Med.* 2014;370(22):2071–82.

76. National Institute for Health and Care Excellence (NICE). *Nintedanib for Treating Idiopathic Pulmonary Fibrosis NICE Technology Appraisal Guidance [TA379].* UK: Department of Health, 2016.

77. Kolb M, Richeldi L, Kimura T, Stowasser S, Hallman C, du Bois RM. Effect of baseline FVC on decline in lung function with nintedanib in patients with IPF: Results from the INPULSIS® trials. *Am J Resp Crit Care Med.* 2015;191:A1021.

78. Kolb M, Richeldi L, Behr J, Maher TM, Tang W, Stowasser S et al. Nintedanib in patients with idiopathic pulmonary fibrosis and pre-served lung volume. *Thorax.* 2017;72:340–6.

79. Nathan SD, Albera C, Bradford WZ, Costabel U, du Bois RM, Fagan EA et al. Effect of con-tinued treatment with pirfenidone following clinically meaningful declines in forced vital capacity: Analysis of data from three phase 3 trials in patients with idiopathic pulmonary fibrosis. *Thorax.* 2016;71(5):429–35.

80. Raghu G, Freudenberger TD, Yang S, Curtis JR, Spada C, Hayes J et al. High prevalence of abnormal acid gastro-oesophageal reflux in idiopathic pulmonary fibrosis. *Eur Respir J.* 2006;27(1):136–42.

81. Dent J, El-Serag HB, Wallander MA, Johansson S. Epidemiology of gastro-oesophageal reflux disease: A systematic review. *Gut.* 2005;54(5):710–7.

82. Gribbin J, Hubbard R, Smith C. Role of diabetes mellitus and gastro-oesoph-ageal reflux in the aetiology of idio-pathic pulmonary fibrosis. *Respir Med.* 2009;103(6):927–31.

83. Perng DW, Chang KT, Su KC, Wu YC, Wu MT, Hsu WH et al. Exposure of airway epithelium to bile acids associated with gastroesophageal reflux symptoms: A rela-tion to transforming growth factor-beta1 production and fibroblast proliferation. *Chest.* 2007;132(5):1548–56.

84. Perng DW, Wu YC, Tsai CC, Su KC, Liu LY, Hsu WH et al. Bile acids induce CCN2 pro-duction through p38 MAP kinase activation

in human bronchial epithelial cells: A factor contributing to airway fibrosis. *Respirology.* 2008;13(7):983–9.

85. Bathoorn E, Daly P, Gaiser B, Sternad K, Poland C, Macnee W et al. Cytotoxicity and induction of inflammation by pepsin in acid in bronchial epithelial cells. *Int J Inflam.* 2011;2011:569416.

86. Ghebremariam YT, Cooke JP, Gerhart W, Griego C, Brower JB, Doyle-Eisele M et al. Pleiotropic effect of the proton pump inhibitor esomeprazole leading to suppres-sion of lung inflammation and fibrosis. *J Transl Med.* 2015;13:249.

87. Lee JS, Ryu JH, Elicker BM, Lydell CP, Jones KD, Wolters PJ et al. Gastroesophageal reflux therapy is associated with longer survival in patients with idiopathic pulmo-nary fibrosis. *Am J Respir Crit Care Med.* 2011;184(12):1390–4.

88. Mertens V, Blondeau K, Vanaudenaerde B, Vos R, Farre R, Pauwels A et al. Gastric juice from patients 'on' acid suppressive therapy can still provoke a significant inflammatory reaction by human bronchial epithelial cells. *J Clin Gastroenterol.* 2010;44(10):e230–5.

89. Raghu G, Crestani B, Bailes Z, Schlenker-Herceg R, Costabel U. Effect of anti-acid medication on reduction in FVC decline with nintedanib. *Eur Respir J.* 2015;46(Suppl 59):OA4502.

90. Kreuter M, Wuyts W, Renzoni E, Koschel D, Maher TM, Kolb M et al. Antacid therapy and disease outcomes in idiopathic pul-monary fibrosis: A pooled analysis. *Lancet Respir Med.* 2016;4(5):381–9.

91. Paroni Sterbini F, Palladini A, Masucci L, Cannistraci CV, Pastorino R, Ianiro G et al. Effects of proton pump inhibitors on the gastric mucosa-associated microbiota in dyspeptic patients. *Appl Environ Microbiol.* 2016;82(22):6633–44.

92. Jackson MA, Goodrich JK, Maxan ME, Freedberg DE, Abrams JA, Poole AC et al. Proton pump inhibitors alter the composition of the gut microbiota. *Gut.* 2016;65(5):749–56.

93. Filion KB, Chateau D, Targownik LE, Gershon A, Durand M, Tamim H et al. Proton pump inhibitors and the risk of

hospitalisation for community-acquired pneumonia: Replicated cohort studies with meta-analysis. *Gut.* 2014;63(4):552–8.

94. Linden PA, Gilbert RJ, Yeap BY, Boyle K, Deykin A, Jaklitsch MT et al. Laparoscopic fundoplication in patients with end-stage lung disease awaiting transplantation. *J Thorac Cardiovasc Surg.* 2006;131(2):438–46.

95. Holland AE. Exercise limitation in interstitial lung disease – Mechanisms, significance and therapeutic options. *Chron Respir Dis.* 2010;7(2):101–11.

96. Nishiyama O, Taniguchi H, Kondoh Y, Kimura T, Ogawa T, Watanabe F et al. Quadriceps weakness is related to exercise capacity in idiopathic pulmonary fibrosis. *Chest.* 2005;127(6):2028–33.

97. Jackson RM, Gomez-Marin OW, Ramos CF, Sol CM, Cohen MI, Gaunaurd IA et al. Exercise limitation in IPF patients: A randomized trial of pulmonary rehabilitation. *Lung.* 2014;192(3):367–76.

98. Vainshelboim B, Oliveira J, Yehoshua L, Weiss I, Fox BD, Fruchter O et al. Exercise training-based pulmonary rehabilitation program is clinically beneficial for idiopathic pulmonary fibrosis. *Respiration.* 2014;88(5):378–88.

99. Holland A, Hill C. Physical training for interstitial lung disease. *Cochrane Database Syst Rev.* 2008;(4):CD006322.

100. Spruit MA, Singh SJ, Garvey C, ZuWallack R, Nici L, Rochester C et al. An official American Thoracic Society/European Respiratory Society statement: Key concepts and advances in pulmonary rehabilitation. *Am J Respir Crit Care Med.* 2013;188(8):e13–64.

101. du Bois RM, Weycker D, Albera C, Bradford WZ, Costabel U, Kartashov A et al. Six-minute-walk test in idiopathic pulmonary fibrosis: Test validation and minimal clinically important difference. *Am J Respir Crit Care Med.* 2011;183(9):1231–7.

102. Vainshelboim B, Oliveira J, Fox BD, Soreck Y, Fruchter O, Kramer MR. Long-term effects of a 12-week exercise training program on clinical outcomes in idiopathic pulmonary fibrosis. *Lung.* 2015;193(3):345–54.

103. Ryerson CJ, Cayou C, Topp F, Hilling L, Camp PG, Wilcox PG et al. Pulmonary

rehabilitation improves long-term outcomes in interstitial lung disease: A prospective cohort study. *Respir Med.* 2014;108(1):203–10.

104. Holland AE, Hill CJ, Conron M, Munro P, McDonald CF. Short term improvement in exercise capacity and symptoms following exercise training in interstitial lung disease. *Thorax.* 2008;63(6):549–54.

105. Baumgartner KB, Samet JM, Stidley CA, Colby TV, Waldron JA. Cigarette smoking: A risk factor for idiopathic pulmonary fibrosis. *Am J Respir Crit Care Med.* 1997;155(1):242–8.

106. Iwai K, Mori T, Yamada N, Yamaguchi M, Hosoda Y. Idiopathic pulmonary fibrosis. Epidemiologic approaches to occupational exposure. *Am J Respir Crit Care Med.* 1994;150(3):670–5.

107. Garcia-Sancho Figueroa MC, Carrillo G, Perez-Padilla R, Fernandez-Plata MR, Buendia-Roldan I, Vargas MH et al. Risk factors for idiopathic pulmonary fibrosis in a Mexican population. A case-control study. *Respir Med.* 2010;104(2):305–9.

108. Pirie K, Peto R, Reeves GK, Green J, Beral V, Million Women Study C. The 21st century hazards of smoking and benefits of stopping: A prospective study of one million women in the UK. *Lancet.* 2013;381(9861):133–41.

109. King TE, Jr., Tooze JA, Schwarz MI, Brown KR, Cherniack RM. Predicting survival in idiopathic pulmonary fibrosis: Scoring system and survival model. *Am J Respir Crit Care Med.* 2001;164(7):1171–81.

110. Becklake MR, Lalloo U. The 'healthy smoker': A phenomenon of health selection? *Respiration.* 1990;57(3):137–44.

111. Antoniou KM, Hansell DM, Rubens MB, Marten K, Desai SR, Siafakas NM et al. Idiopathic pulmonary fibrosis: Outcome in relation to smoking status. *Am J Respir Crit Care Med.* 2008;177(2):190–4.

112. Parshall MB, Schwartzstein RM, Adams L, Banzett RB, Manning HL, Bourbeau J et al. An official American Thoracic Society statement: Update on the mechanisms, assessment, and management of dyspnoea. *Am J Respir Crit Care Med.* 2012;185(4):435–52.

113. Dorman S, Jolley C, Abernethy A, Currow D, Johnson M, Farquhar M et al. Researching

breathlessness in palliative care: Consensus statement of the National Cancer Research Institute Palliative Care Breathlessness Subgroup. *Palliat Med.* 2009;23(3):213–27.

114. Allen S, Raut S, Woollard J, Vassallo M. Low dose diamorphine reduces breathlessness without causing a fall in oxygen saturation in elderly patients with end-stage idiopathic pulmonary fibrosis. *Palliat Med.* 2005;19(2):128–30.

115. Simon ST, Higginson IJ, Booth S, Harding R, Bausewein C. Benzodiazepines for the relief of breathlessness in advanced malignant and non-malignant diseases in adults. *Cochrane Database Syst Rev.* 2010;(1):CD007354.

116. Nocturnal Oxygen Therapy Trial Group. Continuous or nocturnal oxygen therapy in hypoxemic chronic obstructive lung disease: A clinical trial. *Ann Intern Med.* 1980;93(3):391–8.

117. Frank RC, Hicks S, Duck AM, Spencer L, Leonard CT, Barnett E. Ambulatory oxygen in idiopathic pulmonary fibrosis: Of what benefit? *Eur Respir J.* 2012;40(1):269–70.

118. Medical Research Council Working Party. Long term domiciliary oxygen therapy in chronic hypoxic cor pulmonale complicating chronic bronchitis and emphysema. *Lancet.* 1981;1(8222):681–6.

119. Jones RM, Hilldrup S, Hope-Gill BD, Eccles R, Harrison NK. Mechanical induction of cough in idiopathic pulmonary fibrosis. *Cough.* 2011;7:2.

120. Bajwah S, Higginson IJ, Ross JR, Wells AU, Birring SS, Riley J et al. The palliative care needs for fibrotic interstitial lung disease: A qualitative study of patients, informal caregivers and health professionals. *Palliat Med.* 2013;27(9):869–76.

121. Ryerson CJ, Abbritti M, Ley B, Elicker BM, Jones KD, Collard HR. Cough predicts prognosis in idiopathic pulmonary fibrosis. *Respirology.* 2011;16(6):969–75.

122. Scholand MB, Wolff R, Crossno PF, Sundar K, Winegar M, Whipple S et al. Severity of cough in idiopathic pulmonary fibrosis is associated with MUC5 B genotype. *Cough.* 2014;10:3.

123. Horton MR, Santopietro V, Mathew L, Horton KM, Polito AJ, Liu MC et al. Thalidomide for the treatment of cough in idiopathic pulmonary fibrosis: A randomized trial. *Ann Intern Med.* 2012;157(6):398–406.

124. Ryan NM, Birring SS, Gibson PG. Gabapentin for refractory chronic cough: A randomised, double-blind, placebo-controlled trial. *Lancet.* 2012;380(9853):1583–9.

125. Abdulqawi R, Dockry R, Holt K, Layton G, McCarthy BG, Ford AP et al. P2X3 receptor antagonist (AF-219) in refractory chronic cough: A randomised, double-blind, placebo-controlled phase 2 study. *Lancet.* 2015;385(9974):1198–205.

126. British Lung Foundation. Our IPF Charter, 2016. https://www.blf.org.uk/support-for-you/idiopathic-pulmonary-fibrosis-ipf/project/our-ipf-charter. Accessed 17 October 2016.

127. Byrne A, Sampson C, Baillie J, Harrison K, Hope-Gill B, Hubbard R et al. A mixed-methods study of the care needs of individuals with idiopathic pulmonary fibrosis and their carers—CaNoPy: A study protocol. *BMJ Open.* 2013;3(8).

128. Sampson C, Gill BH, Harrison NK, Nelson A, Byrne A. The care needs of patients with idiopathic pulmonary fibrosis and their carers (CaNoPy): Results of a qualitative study. *BMC Pulm Med.* 2015;15:155.

129. Lechtzin N, Hilliard ME, Horton MR. Validation of the Cough Quality-of-Life Questionnaire in patients with idiopathic pulmonary fibrosis. *Chest.* 2013;143(6):1745–9.

130. Patel AS, Siegert RJ, Brignall K, Gordon P, Steer S, Desai SR et al. The development and validation of the King's Brief Interstitial Lung Disease (K-BILD) health status questionnaire. *Thorax.* 2012;67(9):804–10.

131. Varney VA, Parnell HM, Salisbury DT, Ratnatheepan S, Tayar RB. A double blind randomised placebo controlled pilot study of oral co-trimoxazole in advanced fibrotic lung disease. *Pulm Pharmacol Ther.* 2008;21(1):178–87.

132. Demedts M, Behr J, Buhl R, Costabel U, Dekhuijzen R, Jansen HM et al. High-dose acetylcysteine in idiopathic pulmonary fibrosis. *N Engl J Med.* 2005;353(21):2229–42.

133. Idiopathic Pulmonary Fibrosis Clinical Research N, Raghu G, Anstrom KJ, King TE, Jr., Lasky JA, Martinez FJ. Prednisone, azathioprine, and N-acetylcysteine for pulmonary fibrosis. *N Engl J Med.* 2012;366(21):1968–77.

134. Idiopathic Pulmonary Fibrosis Clinical Research N, Martinez FJ, de Andrade JA, Anstrom KJ, King TE, Jr., Raghu G. Randomized trial of acetylcysteine in idiopathic pulmonary fibrosis. *N Engl J Med.* 2014;370(22):2093–101.

135. Oldham JM, Ma SF, Martinez FJ, Anstrom KJ, Raghu G, Schwartz DA et al. TOLLIP, MUC5B, and the response to N-acetylcysteine among individuals with idiopathic pulmonary fibrosis. *Am J Respir Crit Care Med.* 2015;192(12):1475–82.

136. Peljto AL, Zhang Y, Fingerlin TE, Ma SF, Garcia JG, Richards TJ et al. Association between the MUC5B promoter polymorphism and survival in patients with idiopathic pulmonary fibrosis. *JAMA.* 2013;309(21):2232–9.

137. Antoniu SA. Pirfenidone for the treatment of idiopathic pulmonary fibrosis. *Expert Opin Investig Drugs.* 2006;15(7):823–8.

138. Rangarajan S, Kurundkar A, Kurundkar D, Bernard K, Sanders YY, Ding Q et al. Novel mechanisms for the antifibrotic action of nintedanib. *Am J Respir Cell Mol Biol.* 2016;54(1):51–9.

139. Fernandez IE, Eickelberg O. The impact of TGF-ß on lung fibrosis: From targeting to biomarkers. *Proc Am Thorac Soc.* 2012;9(3):111–6.

140. Annes JP, Munger JS, Rifkin DB. Making sense of latent TGFß activation. *J Cell Sci.* 2003;116(Pt 2):217–24.

141. Hinz B. The extracellular matrix and transforming growth factor-ß1: Tale of a strained relationship. *Matrix Biol.* 2015;47:54–65.

142. Datta A, Scotton CJ, Chambers RC. Novel therapeutic approaches for pulmonary fibrosis. *Br J Pharmacol.* 2011;163(1):141–72.

143. Akhurst RJ, Hata A. Targeting the TGFß signalling pathway in disease. *Nat Rev Drug Discov.* 2012;11(10):790–811.

144. Goodwin A, Jenkins G. Role of integrin-mediated TGFß activation in the pathogenesis of pulmonary fibrosis. *Biochem Soc Trans.* 2009;37(Pt 4):849–54.

145. Saini G, Porte J, Weinreb PH, Violette SM, Wallace WA, McKeever TM et al. αvß6 integrin may be a potential prognostic biomarker in interstitial lung disease. *Eur Respir J.* 2015;46(2):486–94.

146. Mackinnon AC, Gibbons MA, Farnworth SL, Leffler H, Nilsson UJ, Delaine T et al. Regulation of transforming growth factor-ß1-driven lung fibrosis by galectin-3. *Am J Resp Crit Care Med.* 2012;185:537–46.

147. Ho JE, Gao W, Levy D, Santhanakrishnan R, Araki T, Rosas IO et al. Galectin-3 is associated with restrictive lung disease and interstitial lung abnormalities. *Am J Respir Crit Care Med.* 2016;194(1):77–83.

148. Barry-Hamilton V, Spangler R, Marshall D, McCauley S, Rodriguez HM, Oyasu M et al. Allosteric inhibition of lysyl oxidase-like-2 impedes the development of a pathologic microenvironment. *Nat Med.* 2010;16(9):1009–17.

149. Chien JW, Richards TJ, Gibson KF, Zhang Y, Lindell KO, Shao L et al. Serum lysyl oxidase-like 2 levels and idiopathic pulmonary fibrosis disease progression. *Eur Respir J.* 2014;43(5):1430–8.

150. Park SW, Ahn MH, Jang HK, Jang AS, Kim DJ, Koh ES et al. Interleukin-13 and its receptors in idiopathic interstitial pneumonia: Clinical implications for lung function. *J Korean Med Sci.* 2009;24(4):614–20.

151. Murray LA, Zhang H, Oak SR, Coelho AL, Herath A, Flaherty KR et al. Targeting interleukin-13 with tralokinumab attenuates lung fibrosis and epithelial damage in a humanized SCID idiopathic pulmonary fibrosis model. *Am J Respir Cell Mol Biol.* 2014;50(5):985–94.

152. Tager AM, LaCamera P, Shea BS, Campanella GS, Selman M, Zhao Z et al. The lysophosphatidic acid receptor LPA1 links pulmonary fibrosis to lung injury by mediating fibroblast recruitment and vascular leak. *Nat Med.* 2008;14(1):45–54.

153. Funke M, Zhao Z, Xu Y, Chun J, Tager AM. The lysophosphatidic acid receptor LPA1 promotes epithelial cell apoptosis after lung injury. *Am J Respir Cell Mol Biol.* 2012;46(3):355–64.

154. Swaney JS, Chapman C, Correa LD, Stebbins KJ, Bundey RA, Prodanovich PC et al. A novel, orally active LPA(1) receptor antagonist inhibits lung fibrosis in the mouse bleomycin model. *Br J Pharmacol.* 2010;160(7):1699–713.

155. Amara N, Goven D, Prost F, Muloway R, Crestani B, Boczkowski J. NOX4/NADPH oxidase expression is increased in pulmonary fibroblasts from patients with idiopathic pulmonary fibrosis and mediates TGFß1-induced fibroblast differentiation into myofibroblasts. *Thorax.* 2010;65(8):733–8.

156. Hecker L, Logsdon NJ, Kurundkar D, Kurundkar A, Bernard K, Hock T et al. Reversal of persistent fibrosis in aging by targeting Nox4-Nrf2 redox imbalance. *Sci Transl Med.* 2014;6(231):231ra47.

157. Laleu B, Gaggini F, Orchard M, Fioraso-Cartier L, Cagnon L, Houngninou-Molango S et al. First in class, potent, and orally bioavailable NADPH oxidase isoform 4 (Nox4) inhibitors for the treatment of idiopathic pulmonary fibrosis. *J Med Chem.* 2010;53(21):7715–30.

158. Jarman ER, Khambata VS, Cope C, Jones P, Roger J, Ye LY et al. An inhibitor of NADPH oxidase-4 attenuates established pulmonary fibrosis in a rodent disease model. *Am J Respir Cell Mol Biol.* 2014;50(1):158–69.

159. Sato N, Takasaka N, Yoshida M, Tsubouchi K, Minagawa S, Araya J et al. Metformin attenuates lung fibrosis development via NOX4 suppression. *Respir Res.* 2016;17(1):107.

160. Lipson KE, Wong C, Teng Y, Spong S. CTGF is a central mediator of tissue remodeling and fibrosis and its inhibition can reverse the process of fibrosis. *Fibrogenesis Tissue Repair.* 2012;5(Suppl 1):S24.

161. Lipson K, Wirkner U, Sternlicht M, Seeley T, Bickelhaupt S, Peschke P et al. Rapid reversal of radiation-induced murine pneumonitis by treatment with the anti-CTGF monoclonal antibody FG-3019. *Eur Respir J.* 2011;38(Suppl 55):p668.

162. Raghu G, Scholand MB, de Andrade J, Lancaster L, Mageto Y, Goldin J et al. FG-3019 anti-connective tissue growth factor monoclonal antibody: Results of an open-label clinical trial in idiopathic pulmonary fibrosis. *Eur Respir J.* 2016;47(5):1481–91.

163. Richeldi L. Targeted treatment of idiopathic pulmonary fibrosis: One step at a time. *Eur Respir J.* 2016;47(5):1321–3.

164. du Bois RM, Weycker D, Albera C, Bradford WZ, Costabel U, Kartashov A et al. Forced vital capacity in patients with idiopathic pulmonary fibrosis: Test properties and minimal clinically important difference. *Am J Respir Crit Care Med.* 2011;184(12):1382–9.

165. Richeldi L, Ryerson CJ, Lee JS, Wolters PJ, Koth LL, Ley B et al. Relative versus absolute change in forced vital capacity in idiopathic pulmonary fibrosis. *Thorax.* 2012;67(5):407–11.

166. Collard HR, King TE, Jr., Bartelson BB, Vourlekis JS, Schwarz MI, Brown KK. Changes in clinical and physiologic variables predict survival in idiopathic pulmonary fibrosis. *Am J Respir Crit Care Med.* 2003;168(5):538–42.

167. Manali ED, Stathopoulos GT, Kollintza A, Kalomenidis I, Emili JM, Sotiropoulou C et al. The Medical Research Council chronic dyspnoea score predicts the survival of patients with idiopathic pulmonary fibrosis. *Respir Med.* 2008;102(4):586–92.

168. Ley B, Bradford WZ, Vittinghoff E, Weycker D, du Bois RM, Collard HR. Predictors of mortality poorly predict common measures of disease progression in idiopathic pulmonary fibrosis. *Am J Respir Crit Care Med.* 2016;194(6):711–8.

169. du Bois RM, Weycker D, Albera C, Bradford WZ, Costabel U, Kartashov A et al. Ascertainment of individual risk of mortality for patients with idiopathic pulmonary fibrosis. *Am J Respir Crit Care Med.* 2011;184(4):459–66.

170. Ley B, Ryerson CJ, Vittinghoff E, Ryu JH, Tomassetti S, Lee JS et al. A multidimensional index and staging system for idiopathic pulmonary fibrosis. *Ann Intern Med.* 2012;156(10):684–91.

171. Ley B, Bradford WZ, Weycker D, Vittinghoff E, du Bois RM, Collard HR. Unified baseline and longitudinal mortality prediction in idiopathic pulmonary fibrosis. *Eur Respir J.* 2015;45(5):1374–81.

172. Boon K, Bailey NW, Yang J, Steel MP, Groshong S, Kervitsky D et al. Molecular phenotypes distinguish patients with relatively stable from progressive idiopathic pulmonary fibrosis (IPF). *PLoS One.* 2009;4(4):e5134.

173. Li P, Li J, Chen T, Wang H, Chu H, Chang J et al. Expression analysis of serum microRNAs in idiopathic pulmonary fibrosis. *Int J Mol Med.* 2014;33(6):1554–62.

174. Zhang Y, Kaminski N. Biomarkers in idiopathic pulmonary fibrosis. *Curr Opin Pulm Med.* 2012;18(5):441–6.

175. Hamai K, Iwamoto H, Ishikawa N, Horimasu Y, Masuda T, Miyamoto S et al. Comparative study of circulating MMP-7, CCL18, KL-6, SP-A, and SP-D as disease markers of idiopathic pulmonary fibrosis. *Dis Markers.* 2016;2016:4759040.

176. Jenkins RG, Simpson JK, Saini G, Bentley JH, Russell AM, Braybrooke R et al. Longitudinal change in collagen degradation biomarkers in idiopathic pulmonary fibrosis: An analysis from the prospective, multicentre PROFILE study. *Lancet Respir Med.* 2015;3(6):462–72.

177. Kinder BW, Brown KK, McCormack FX, Ix JH, Kervitsky A, Schwarz MI et al. Serum surfactant protein-A is a strong predictor of early mortality in idiopathic pulmonary fibrosis. *Chest.* 2009;135(6):1557–63.

178. DePianto DJ, Chandriani S, Abbas AR, Jia G, N'Diaye EN, Caplazi P et al. Heterogeneous gene expression signatures correspond to distinct lung pathologies and biomarkers of disease severity in idiopathic pulmonary fibrosis. *Thorax.* 2015;70(1):48–56.

179. Jaffar J, Unger S, Corte TJ, Keller M, Wolters PJ, Richeldi L et al. Fibulin-1 predicts disease progression in patients with idiopathic pulmonary fibrosis. *Chest.* 2014;146(4):1055–63.

180. Kondoh Y, Taniguchi H, Kawabata Y, Yokoi T, Suzuki K, Takagi K. Acute exacerbation in idiopathic pulmonary fibrosis. Analysis of clinical and pathologic findings in three cases. *Chest.* 1993;103(6):1808–12.

181. Collard HR, Moore BB, Flaherty KR, Brown KK, Kaner RJ, King TE, Jr. et al. Acute exacerbations of idiopathic pulmonary fibrosis. *Am J Respir Crit Care Med.* 2007;176(7):636–43.

182. Maher TM, Whyte MK, Hoyles RK, Parfrey H, Ochiai Y, Mathieson N et al. Development of a consensus statement for the definition, diagnosis, and treatment of acute exacerbations of idiopathic pulmonary fibrosis using the Delphi technique. *Adv Ther.* 2015;32(10):929–43.

183. Ryerson CJ, Cottin V, Brown KK, Collard HR. Acute exacerbation of idiopathic pulmonary fibrosis: Shifting the paradigm. *Eur Respir J.* 2015;46(2):512–20.

184. Collard HR, Ryerson CJ, Corte TJ, Jenkins G, Kondoh Y, Lederer DJ et al. Acute exacerbation of idiopathic pulmonary fibrosis. An International Working Group report. *Am J Respir Crit Care Med.* 2016;194(3):265–75.

185. Idiopathic Pulmonary Fibrosis Clinical Research N, Zisman DA, Schwarz M, Anstrom KJ, Collard HR, Flaherty KR et al. A controlled trial of sildenafil in advanced idiopathic pulmonary fibrosis. *N Engl J Med.* 2010;363(7):620–8.

186. Navaratnam V, Fogarty AW, Glendening R, McKeever T, Hubbard RB. The increasing secondary care burden of idiopathic pulmonary fibrosis: Hospital admission trends in England from 1998 to 2010. *Chest.* 2013;143(4):1078–84.

187. Judge EP, Fabre A, Adamali HI, Egan JJ. Acute exacerbations and pulmonary hypertension in advanced idiopathic pulmonary fibrosis. *Eur Respir J.* 2012;40(1):93–100.

188. Kondoh Y, Taniguchi H, Katsuta T, Kataoka K, Kimura T, Nishiyama O et al. Risk factors of acute exacerbation of idiopathic pulmonary fibrosis. *Sarcoidosis Vasc Diffuse Lung Dis.* 2010;27(2):103–10.

189. Costabel U, Inoue Y, Richeldi L, Collard HR, Tschoepe I, Stowasser S et al. Efficacy of nintedanib in idiopathic pulmonary fibrosis across prespecified subgroups in INPULSIS. *Am J Respir Crit Care Med.* 2016;193(2):178–85.

190. Song JW, Hong SB, Lim CM, Koh Y, Kim DS. Acute exacerbation of idiopathic pulmonary fibrosis: Incidence, risk factors and outcome. *Eur Respir J.* 2011;37(2):356–63.

191. Kim DS, Park JH, Park BK, Lee JS, Nicholson AG, Colby T. Acute exacerbation of idiopathic pulmonary fibrosis: Frequency and clinical features. *Eur Respir J.* 2006;27(1):143–50.

192. Suzuki H, Sekine Y, Yoshida S, Suzuki M, Shibuya K, Yonemori Y et al. Risk of acute exacerbation of interstitial pneumonia after pulmonary resection for lung cancer in patients with idiopathic pulmonary fibrosis based on preoperative high-resolution computed tomography. *Surg Today.* 2011;41(7):914–21.

193. Simon-Blancal V, Freynet O, Nunes H, Bouvry D, Naggara N, Brillet PY et al. Acute exacerbation of idiopathic pulmonary fibrosis: Outcome and prognostic factors. *Respiration.* 2012;83(1):28–35.

194. Wootton SC, Kim DS, Kondoh Y, Chen E, Lee JS, Song JW et al. Viral infection in acute exacerbation of idiopathic pulmonary fibrosis. *Am J Respir Crit Care Med.* 2011;183(12):1698–702.

195. Lee JS, Song JW, Wolters PJ, Elicker BM, King TE, Jr., Kim DS et al. Bronchoalveolar lavage pepsin in acute exacerbation of idiopathic pulmonary fibrosis. *Eur Respir J.* 2012;39(2):352–8.

196. Johannson KA, Vittinghoff E, Lee K, Balmes JR, Ji W, Kaplan GG et al. Acute exacerbation of idiopathic pulmonary fibrosis associated with air pollution exposure. *Eur Respir J.* 2014;43(4):1124–31.

197. Sugiura H, Takeda A, Hoshi T, Kawabata Y, Sayama K, Jinzaki M et al. Acute exacerbation of usual interstitial pneumonia after resection of lung cancer. *Ann Thorac Surg.* 2012;93(3):937–43.

198. Sato T, Teramukai S, Kondo H, Watanabe A, Ebina M, Kishi K et al. Impact and predictors of acute exacerbation of interstitial lung diseases after pulmonary resection for lung cancer. *J Thorac Cardiovasc Surg.* 2014;147(5):1604–11e3.

199. Kondoh Y, Taniguchi H, Kitaichi M, Yokoi T, Johkoh T, Oishi T et al. Acute exacerbation of interstitial pneumonia following surgical lung biopsy. *Respir Med.* 2006;100(10):1753–9.

200. Sakamoto K, Taniguchi H, Kondoh Y, Wakai K, Kimura T, Kataoka K et al. Acute exacerbation of IPF following diagnostic bronchoalveolar lavage procedures. *Respir Med.* 2012;106(3):436–42.

201. Ghatol A, Ruhl AP, Danoff SK. Exacerbations in idiopathic pulmonary fibrosis triggered by pulmonary and nonpulmonary surgery: A case series and comprehensive review of the literature. *Lung.* 2012;190(4):373–80.

202. Sekine Y, Ko E. [The influence of intra-operative oxygen inhalation on patients with idiopathic pulmonary fibrosis]. *Masui.* 2011;60(3):307–13.

203. Juarez MM, Chan AL, Norris AG, Morrissey BM, Albertson TE. Acute exacerbation of idiopathic pulmonary fibrosis – A review of current and novel pharmacotherapies. *J Thorac Dis.* 2015;7(3):499–519.

204. Parambil JG, Myers JL, Ryu JH. Histopathologic features and outcome of patients with acute exacerbation of idiopathic pulmonary fibrosis undergoing surgical lung biopsy. *Chest.* 2005;128(5):3310–5.

205. Akira M, Kozuka T, Yamamoto S, Sakatani M. Computed tomography findings in acute exacerbation of idiopathic pulmonary fibrosis. *Am J Respir Crit Care Med.* 2008;178(4):372–8.

206. Ohshimo S, Ishikawa N, Horimasu Y, Hattori N, Hirohashi N, Tanigawa K et al. Baseline KL-6 predicts increased risk for acute exacerbation of idiopathic pulmonary fibrosis. *Respir Med.* 2014;108(7):1031–9.

207. Collard HR, Calfee CS, Wolters PJ, Song JW, Hong SB, Brady S et al. Plasma biomarker profiles in acute exacerbation of idiopathic pulmonary fibrosis. *Am J Physiol Lung Cell Mol Physiol.* 2010;299(1):L3–7.

208. Cao M, Swigris JJ, Wang X, Cao M, Qiu Y, Huang M et al. Plasma leptin is elevated in acute exacerbation of idiopathic pulmonary fibrosis. *Mediators Inflamm.* 2016;2016:6940480.

209. Okuda R, Matsushima H, Aoshiba K, Oba T, Kawabe R, Honda K et al. Soluble intercellular adhesion molecule-1 for stable and acute phases of idiopathic pulmonary fibrosis. *Springerplus.* 2015;4:657.

210. Matsuzawa Y, Kawashima T, Kuwabara R, Hayakawa S, Irie T, Yoshida T et al. Change in serum marker of oxidative stress in the progression of idiopathic pulmonary fibrosis. *Pulm Pharmacol Ther.* 2015;32:1–6.

211. Kakugawa T, Yokota S, Ishimatsu Y, Hayashi T, Nakashima S, Hara S et al. Serum heat shock protein 47 levels are elevated in

acute exacerbation of idiopathic pulmonary fibrosis. *Cell Stress Chaperones.* 2013;18(5):581–90.

212. Tachibana K, Inoue Y, Nishiyama A, Sugimoto C, Matsumuro A, Hirose M et al. Polymyxin-B hemoperfusion for acute exacerbation of idiopathic pulmonary fibrosis: Serum IL-7 as a prognostic marker. *Sarcoidosis Vasc Diffuse Lung Dis.* 2011;28(2):113–22.

213. Lee YH, Kim YS, Lee SN, Lee HC, Oh SJ, Kim SJ et al. Interstitial lung change in pre-radiation therapy computed tomography is a risk factor for severe radiation pneumonitis. *Cancer Res Treat.* 2015;47(4):676–86.

214. Mallick S. Outcome of patients with idiopathic pulmonary fibrosis (IPF) ventilated in intensive care unit. *Respir Med.* 2008;102(10):1355–9.

215. Mura M, Porretta MA, Bargagli E, Sergiacomi G, Zompatori M, Sverzellati N et al. Predicting survival in newly diagnosed idiopathic pulmonary fibrosis: A 3-year prospective study. *Eur Respir J.* 2012;40(1):101–9.

216. Natsuizaka M, Chiba H, Kuronuma K, Otsuka M, Kudo K, Mori M et al. Epidemiologic survey of Japanese patients with idiopathic pulmonary fibrosis and investigation of ethnic differences. *Am J Respir Crit Care Med.* 2014;190(7):773–9.

217. Roberts CM, Barnes S, Lowe D, Pearson MG, Clinical Effectiveness Evaluation Unit RCoP, Audit Subcommittee of the British Thoracic S. Evidence for a link between mortality in acute COPD and hospital type and resources. *Thorax.* 2003;58(11):947–9.

218. Moeller A, Gilpin SE, Ask K, Cox G, Cook D, Gauldie J et al. Circulating fibrocytes are an indicator of poor prognosis in idiopathic pulmonary fibrosis. *Am J Respir Crit Care Med.* 2009;179(7):588–94.

219. Saydain G, Islam A, Afessa B, Ryu JH, Scott JP, Peters SG. Outcome of patients with idiopathic pulmonary fibrosis admitted to the intensive care unit. *Am J Respir Crit Care Med.* 2002;166(6):839–42.

220. Fujimoto K, Taniguchi H, Johkoh T, Kondoh Y, Ichikado K, Sumikawa H et al. Acute exacerbation of idiopathic pulmonary fibrosis: High-resolution CT scores predict mortality. *Eur Radiol.* 2012;22(1):83–92.

221. Oda K, Ishimoto H, Yamada S, Kushima H, Ishii H, Imanaga T et al. Autopsy analyses in acute exacerbation of idiopathic pulmonary fibrosis. *Respir Res.* 2014;15:109.

222. Bhatti H, Girdhar A, Usman F, Cury J, Bajwa A. Approach to acute exacerbation of idiopathic pulmonary fibrosis. *Ann Thorac Med.* 2013;8(2):71–7.

223. Papiris SA, Manali ED, Kolilekas L, Kagouridis K, Triantafillidou C, Tsangaris I et al. Clinical review: Idiopathic pulmonary fibrosis acute exacerbations—Unravelling Ariadne's thread. *Crit Care.* 2010;14(6):246.

224. Papiris SA, Manali ED, Kolilekas L, Triantafillidou C, Tsangaris I, Kagouridis K. Steroids in idiopathic pulmonary fibrosis acute exacerbation: Defenders or killers? *Am J Respir Crit Care Med.* 2012;185(5):587–8.

225. Papiris SA, Kagouridis K, Kolilekas L, Papaioannou AI, Roussou A, Triantafillidou C et al. Survival in idiopathic pulmonary fibrosis acute exacerbations: The non-steroid approach. *BMC Pulm Med.* 2015;15:162.

226. Sakamoto S, Homma S, Miyamoto A, Kurosaki A, Fujii T, Yoshimura K. Cyclosporin A in the treatment of acute exacerbation of idiopathic pulmonary fibrosis. *Intern Med.* 2010;49(2):109–15.

227. Inase N, Sawada M, Ohtani Y, Miyake S, Isogai S, Sakashita H et al. Cyclosporin A followed by the treatment of acute exacerbation of idiopathic pulmonary fibrosis with corticosteroid. *Intern Med.* 2003;42(7):565–70.

228. Horita N, Akahane M, Okada Y, Kobayashi Y, Arai T, Amano I et al. Tacrolimus and steroid treatment for acute exacerbation of idiopathic pulmonary fibrosis. *Intern Med.* 2011;50(3):189–95.

229. Enomoto N, Mikamo M, Oyama Y, Kono M, Hashimoto D, Fujisawa T et al. Treatment of acute exacerbation of idiopathic pulmonary fibrosis with direct hemoperfusion using a polymyxin B-immobilized fiber column improves survival. *BMC Pulm Med.* 2015;15:15.

230. Fumeaux T, Rothmeier C, Jolliet P. Outcome of mechanical ventilation for acute respiratory failure in patients with pulmonary fibrosis. *Intensive Care Med.* 2001;27(12):1868–74.

231. Rangappa P, Moran JL. Outcomes of patients admitted to the intensive care unit with idiopathic pulmonary fibrosis. *Crit Care Resusc.* 2009;11(2):102–9.

232. Al-Hameed FM, Sharma S. Outcome of patients admitted to the intensive care unit for acute exacerbation of idiopathic pulmonary fibrosis. *Can Respir J.* 2004;11(2):117–22.

233. Mollica C, Paone G, Conti V, Ceccarelli D, Schmid G, Mattia P et al. Mechanical ventilation in patients with end-stage idiopathic pulmonary fibrosis. *Respiration.* 2010;79(3):209–15.

234. Gaudry S, Vincent F, Rabbat A, Nunes H, Crestani B, Naccache JM et al. Invasive mechanical ventilation in patients with fibrosing interstitial pneumonia. *J Thorac Cardiovasc Surg.* 2014;147(1):47–53.

235. Knaus WA, Draper EA, Wagner DP, Zimmerman JE. APACHE II: A severity of disease classification system. *Crit Care Med.* 1985;13(10):818–29.

236. Vincent JL, Moreno R, Takala J, Willatts S, De Mendonca A, Bruining H et al. The SOFA (Sepsis-related Organ Failure Assessment) score to describe organ dysfunction/failure. On behalf of the Working Group on Sepsis-Related Problems of the European Society of Intensive Care Medicine. *Intensive Care Med.* 1996;22(7):707–10.

237. The Acute Respiratory Distress Syndrome Network. Ventilation with lower tidal volumes as compared with traditional tidal volumes for acute lung injury and the acute respiratory distress syndrome. *N Engl J Med.* 2000;342(18):1301–8.

238. Fernandez-Perez ER, Yilmaz M, Jenad H, Daniels CE, Ryu JH, Hubmayr RD et al. Ventilator settings and outcome of respiratory failure in chronic interstitial lung disease. *Chest.* 2008;133(5):1113–9.

239. Paone G, Mollica C, Conti V, Vestri A, Cammarella I, Lucantoni G et al. Severity of illness and outcome in patients with end-stage idiopathic pulmonary fibrosis requiring mechanical ventilation. *Chest.* 2010;137(1):241–2; author reply 2.

240. Yokoyama T, Kondoh Y, Taniguchi H, Kataoka K, Kato K, Nishiyama O et al. Noninvasive ventilation in acute exacerbation of idiopathic pulmonary fibrosis. *Intern Med.* 2010;49(15):1509–14.

241. Vianello A, Arcaro G, Battistella L, Pipitone E, Vio S, Concas A et al. Noninvasive ventilation in the event of acute respiratory failure in patients with idiopathic pulmonary fibrosis. *J Crit Care.* 2014;29(4):562–7.

242. Tomii K, Tachikawa R, Chin K, Murase K, Handa T, Mishima M et al. Role of non-invasive ventilation in managing life-threatening acute exacerbation of interstitial pneumonia. *Intern Med.* 2010;49(14):1341–7.

243. Horio Y, Takihara T, Niimi K, Komatsu M, Sato M, Tanaka J et al. High-flow nasal cannula oxygen therapy for acute exacerbation of interstitial pneumonia: A case series. *Respir Investig.* 2016;54(2):125–9.

244. Trudzinski FC, Kaestner F, Schafers HJ, Fahndrich S, Seiler F, Bohmer P et al. Outcome of patients with interstitial lung disease treated with extracorporeal membrane oxygenation for acute respiratory failure. *Am J Respir Crit Care Med.* 2016;193(5):527–33.

245. Simonneau G, Gatzoulis MA, Adatia I, Celermajer D, Denton C, Ghofrani A et al. Updated clinical classification of pulmonary hypertension. *J Am Coll Cardiol.* 2013;62(25 Suppl):D34–41.

246. Nathan SD, Shlobin OA, Ahmad S, Koch J, Barnett SD, Ad N et al. Serial development of pulmonary hypertension in patients with idiopathic pulmonary fibrosis. *Respiration.* 2008;76(3):288–94.

247. Kimura M, Taniguchi H, Kondoh Y, Kimura T, Kataoka K, Nishiyama O et al. Pulmonary hypertension as a prognostic indicator at the initial evaluation in idiopathic pulmonary fibrosis. *Respiration.* 2013;85(6):456–63.

248. Armstrong HF, Schulze PC, Bacchetta M, Thirapatarapong W, Bartels MN. Impact of pulmonary hypertension on exercise performance in patients with interstitial lung disease undergoing evaluation for lung transplantation. *Respirology.* 2014;19(5):675–82.

249. Lettieri CJ, Nathan SD, Barnett SD, Ahmad S, Shorr AF. Prevalence and outcomes of pulmonary arterial hypertension in advanced idiopathic pulmonary fibrosis. *Chest.* 2006;129(3):746–52.

250. Nadrous HF, Pellikka PA, Krowka MJ, Swanson KL, Chaowalit N, Decker PA et al. Pulmonary hypertension in patients with idiopathic pulmonary fibrosis. *Chest*. 2005;128(4):2393–9.

251. Corte TJ, Wort SJ, Gatzoulis MA, Macdonald P, Hansell DM, Wells AU. Pulmonary vascular resistance predicts early mortality in patients with diffuse fibrotic lung disease and suspected pulmonary hypertension. *Thorax*. 2009;64(10):883–8.

252. Nathan SD, Shlobin OA, Ahmad S, Urbanek S, Barnett SD. Pulmonary hypertension and pulmonary function testing in idiopathic pulmonary fibrosis. *Chest*. 2007;131(3):657–63.

253. Minai OA, Santacruz JF, Alster JM, Budev MM, McCarthy K. Impact of pulmonary hemodynamics on 6-min walk test in idiopathic pulmonary fibrosis. *Respir Med*. 2012;106(11):1613–21.

254. Lettieri CJ, Nathan SD, Browning RF, Barnett SD, Ahmad S, Shorr AF. The distance-saturation product predicts mortality in idiopathic pulmonary fibrosis. *Respir Med*. 2006;100(10):1734–41.

255. Nathan SD, Shlobin OA, Barnett SD, Saggar R, Belperio JA, Ross DJ et al. Right ventricular systolic pressure by echocardiography as a predictor of pulmonary hypertension in idiopathic pulmonary fibrosis. *Respir Med*. 2008;102(9):1305–10.

256. Swigris JJ, Olson AL, Shlobin OA, Ahmad S, Brown KK, Nathan SD. Heart rate recovery after six-minute walk test predicts pulmonary hypertension in patients with idiopathic pulmonary fibrosis. *Respirology*. 2011;16(3):439–45.

257. Song JW, Song JK, Kim DS. Echocardiography and brain natriuretic peptide as prognostic indicators in idiopathic pulmonary fibrosis. *Respir Med*. 2009;103(2):180–6.

258. Leuchte HH, Neurohr C, Baumgartner R, Holzapfel M, Giehrl W, Vogeser M et al. Brain natriuretic peptide and exercise capacity in lung fibrosis and pulmonary hypertension. *Am J Respir Crit Care Med*. 2004;170(4):360–5.

259. Zisman DA, Karlamangla AS, Ross DJ, Keane MP, Belperio JA, Saggar R et al. High-resolution chest CT findings do not predict the presence of pulmonary hypertension in advanced idiopathic pulmonary fibrosis. *Chest*. 2007;132(3):773–9.

260. Shin S, King CS, Puri N, Shlobin OA, Brown AW, Ahmad S et al. Pulmonary artery size as a predictor of outcomes in idiopathic pulmonary fibrosis. *Eur Respir J*. 2016;47(5):1445–51.

261. Price LC, Devaraj A, Wort SJ. Central pulmonary arteries in idiopathic pulmonary fibrosis: Size really matters. *Eur Respir J*. 2016;47(5):1318–20.

262. Rivera-Lebron BN, Forfia PR, Kreider M, Lee JC, Holmes JH, Kawut SM. Echocardiographic and hemodynamic predictors of mortality in idiopathic pulmonary fibrosis. *Chest*. 2013;144(2):564–70.

263. McLaughlin VV, Archer SL, Badesch DB, Barst RJ, Farber HW, Lindner JR et al. ACCF/AHA 2009 expert consensus document on pulmonary hypertension a report of the American College of Cardiology Foundation Task Force on Expert Consensus Documents and the American Heart Association developed in collaboration with the American College of Chest Physicians; American Thoracic Society, Inc.; and the Pulmonary Hypertension Association. *J Am Coll Cardiol*. 2009;53(17):1573–619.

264. Galie N, Humbert M, Vachiery JL, Gibbs S, Lang I, Torbicki A et al. 2015 ESC/ERS Guidelines for the diagnosis and treatment of pulmonary hypertension: The Joint Task Force for the Diagnosis and Treatment of Pulmonary Hypertension of the European Society of Cardiology (ESC) and the European Respiratory Society (ERS): Endorsed by: Association for European Paediatric and Congenital Cardiology (AEPC), International Society for Heart and Lung Transplantation (ISHLT). *Eur Heart J*. 2016;37(1):67–119.

265. Navaratnam V, Fogarty AW, McKeever T, Thompson N, Jenkins G, Johnson SR et al. Presence of a prothrombotic state in people with idiopathic pulmonary fibrosis: A population-based case-control study. *Thorax*. 2014;69(3):207–15.

266. Noth I, Anstrom KJ, Calvert SB, de Andrade J, Flaherty KR, Glazer C et al. A

placebo-controlled randomized trial of warfarin in idiopathic pulmonary fibrosis. *Am J Respir Crit Care Med.* 2012;186(1):88–95.

267. Crooks MG, Hart SP. Coagulation and anticoagulation in idiopathic pulmonary fibrosis. *Eur Respir Rev.* 2015;24(137):392–9.

268. Olschewski H, Ghofrani HA, Walmrath D, Schermuly R, Temmesfeld-Wollbruck B, Grimminger F et al. Inhaled prostacyclin and iloprost in severe pulmonary hypertension secondary to lung fibrosis. *Am J Respir Crit Care Med.* 1999;160(2):600–7.

269. Han MK, Bach DS, Hagan PG, Yow E, Flaherty KR, Toews GB et al. Sildenafil preserves exercise capacity in patients with idiopathic pulmonary fibrosis and right-sided ventricular dysfunction. *Chest.* 2013;143(6):1699–708.

270. King TE, Jr., Brown KK, Raghu G, du Bois RM, Lynch DA, Martinez F et al. BUILD-3: A randomized, controlled trial of bosentan in idiopathic pulmonary fibrosis. *Am J Respir Crit Care Med.* 2011;184(1):92–9.

271. Corte TJ, Keir GJ, Dimopoulos K, Howard L, Corris PA, Parfitt L et al. Bosentan in pulmonary hypertension associated with fibrotic idiopathic interstitial pneumonia. *Am J Respir Crit Care Med.* 2014;190(2):208–17.

272. Raghu G, Behr J, Brown KK, Egan JJ, Kawut SM, Flaherty KR et al. Treatment of idiopathic pulmonary fibrosis with ambrisentan: A parallel, randomized trial. *Ann Intern Med.* 2013;158(9):641–9.

273. Darby IA, Hewitson TD. Hypoxia in tissue repair and fibrosis. *Cell Tissue Res.* 2016;365(3):553–62.

274. Kolilekas L, Manali E, Vlami KA, Lyberopoulos P, Triantafillidou C, Kagouridis K et al. Sleep oxygen desaturation predicts survival in idiopathic pulmonary fibrosis. *J Clin Sleep Med.* 2013;9(6):593–601.

275. Lancaster LH, Mason WR, Parnell JA, Rice TW, Loyd JE, Milstone AP et al. Obstructive sleep apnea is common in idiopathic pulmonary fibrosis. *Chest.* 2009;136(3):772–8.

276. Mermigkis C, Stagaki E, Amfilochiou A, Polychronopoulos V, Korkonikitas P, Mermigkis D et al. Sleep quality and associated daytime consequences in patients with idiopathic pulmonary fibrosis. *Med Princ Pract.* 2009;18(1):10–5.

277. Arias MA, Garcia-Rio F, Alonso-Fernandez A, Martinez I, Villamor J. Pulmonary hypertension in obstructive sleep apnoea: Effects of continuous positive airway pressure: A randomized, controlled cross-over study. *Eur Heart J.* 2006;27(9):1106–13.

278. Mermigkis C, Stagaki E, Tryfon S, Schiza S, Amfilochiou A, Polychronopoulos V et al. How common is sleep-disordered breathing in patients with idiopathic pulmonary fibrosis? *Sleep Breath.* 2010;14(4):387–90.

279. Mermigkis C, Bouloukaki I, Antoniou KM, Mermigkis D, Psathakis K, Giannarakis I et al. CPAP therapy in patients with idiopathic pulmonary fibrosis and obstructive sleep apnea: Does it offer a better quality of life and sleep? *Sleep Breath.* 2013;17(4):1137–43.

280. Corrado A, Renda T, Bertini S. Long-term oxygen therapy in COPD: Evidences and open questions of current indications. *Monaldi Arch Chest Dis.* 2010;73(1):34–43.

281. Hardinge M, Suntharalingam J, Wilkinson T, British Thoracic S. Guideline update: The British Thoracic Society Guidelines on home oxygen use in adults. *Thorax.* 2015;70(6):589–91.

282. Raeside DA, Brown A, Patel KR, Welsh D, Peacock AJ. Ambulatory pulmonary artery pressure monitoring during sleep and exercise in normal individuals and patients with COPD. *Thorax.* 2002;57(12):1050–3.

283. Kistler KD, Nalysnyk L, Rotella P, Esser D. Lung transplantation in idiopathic pulmonary fibrosis: A systematic review of the literature. *BMC Pulm Med.* 2014;14:139.

284. Yusen RD, Edwards LB, Kucheryavaya AY, Benden C, Dipchand AI, Goldfarb SB et al. The Registry of the International Society for Heart and Lung Transplantation: Thirty-second Official Adult Lung and Heart-Lung Transplantation Report—2015; Focus Theme: Early Graft Failure. *J Heart Lung Transplant.* 2015;34(10):1264–77.

285. Lederer DJ, Arcasoy SM, Wilt JS, D'Ovidio F, Sonett JR, Kawut SM. Six-minute-walk distance predicts waiting list survival in idiopathic pulmonary fibrosis. *Am J Respir Crit Care Med.* 2006;174(6):659–64.

286. Daccord C, Maher TM. Recent advances in understanding idiopathic pulmonary fibrosis. *F1000Res.* 2016;5.

287. Mizuno K, Mataki H, Seki N, Kumamoto T, Kamikawaji K, Inoue H. MicroRNAs in non-small cell lung cancer and idiopathic pulmonary fibrosis. *J Hum Genet.* 2016;62:57–65.

288. Newton CA, Batra K, Torrealba J, Kozlitina J, Glazer CS, Aravena C et al. Telomere-related lung fibrosis is diagnostically heterogeneous but uniformly progressive. *Eur Respir J.* 2016;48(6):1710–20.

289. Mathai SK, Newton CA, Schwartz DA, Garcia CK. Pulmonary fibrosis in the era of stratified medicine. *Thorax.* 2016;71(12):1154–60.

290. Blanco M, Obeso GA, Duran JC, Rivo JE, Garcia-Fontan E, Pena E et al. Surgical lung biopsy for diffuse lung disease. Our experience in the last 15 years. *Rev Port Pneumol.* 2013;19(2):59–64.

291. Hutchinson JP, McKeever TM, Fogarty AW, Navaratnam V, Hubbard RB. Surgical lung biopsy for the diagnosis of interstitial lung disease in England: 1997–2008. *Eur Respir J.* 2016;48(5):1453–61.

292. Hutchinson JP, Fogarty AW, McKeever TM, Hubbard RB. In-hospital mortality after surgical lung biopsy for interstitial lung disease in the United States. 2000 to 2011. *Am J Respir Crit Care Med.* 2016;193(10):1161–7.

293. Tomassetti S, Wells AU, Costabel U, Cavazza A, Colby TV, Rossi G et al. Bronchoscopic lung cryobiopsy increases diagnostic confidence in the multidisciplinary diagnosis of idiopathic pulmonary fibrosis. *Am J Respir Crit Care Med.* 2016;193(7):745–52.

294. Patel NM, Borczuk AC, Lederer DJ. Cryobiopsy in the diagnosis of interstitial lung disease. A step forward or back? *Am J Respir Crit Care Med.* 2016;193(7):707–9.

295. Win T, Screaton NJ, Porter J, Endozo R, Wild D, Kayani I et al. Novel positron emission tomography/computed tomography of diffuse parenchymal lung disease combining a labeled somatostatin receptor analogue and 2-deoxy-2[18F]fluoro-D-glucose. *Mol Imaging.* 2012;11(2):91–8.

296. Withana NP, Ma X, McGuire HM, Verdoes M, van der Linden WA, Ofori LO et al. Non-invasive imaging of idiopathic pulmonary fibrosis using cathepsin protease probes. *Sci Rep.* 2016;6:19755.

297. Fischer A, Antoniou KM, Brown KK, Cadranel J, Corte TJ, du Bois RM et al. An official European Respiratory Society/ American Thoracic Society research statement: Interstitial pneumonia with autoimmune features. *Eur Respir J.* 2015;46(4):976–87.

298. Oldham JM, Adegunsoye A, Valenzi E, Lee C, Witt L, Chen L et al. Characterisation of patients with interstitial pneumonia with autoimmune features. *Eur Respir J.* 2016;47(6):1767–75.

299. Chartrand S, Swigris JJ, Stanchev L, Lee JS, Brown KK, Fischer A. Clinical features and natural history of interstitial pneumonia with autoimmune features: A single center experience. *Respir Med.* 2016;119:150–4.

300. Luppi F, Wells AU. Interstitial pneumonitis with autoimmune features (IPAF): A work in progress. *Eur Respir J.* 2016;47(6):1622–4.

11

Hypersensitivity pneumonitis

CHRISTINE FIDDLER AND HELEN PARFREY

BACKGROUND

Hypersensitivity pneumonitis (HP), also known as extrinsic allergic alveolitis, is a complex syndrome caused by repeated inhalation of and sensitization to finely dispersed antigens. These antigens encompass a wide variety of organic particles including fungi, bacterial, protozoal, animal and insect proteins, and certain small molecular weight volatile and non-volatile chemical compounds. Pathologically the disease is characterized by a diffuse and predominantly mononuclear cell inflammation of the alveoli, terminal bronchioles and interstitium. However, in some instances, this granulomatous, lymphocytic infiltrate can lead to the development of pulmonary fibrosis.

Magnus, who reported 'a disease of sifters and threshers of grain', made one of the earliest descriptions of HP in 1555. But it was not until 1932 that a detailed account of HP was provided by Campbell, who described the acute symptoms in farmers after working with hay (1). In 1962, Pepys and colleagues observed an association between HP and serum precipitins to hay and mould extracts (2). Similarly others identified 'bird breeder's lung disease' (3) and the occurrence of HP among office workers exposed to thermophilic actinomycete contaminating a central air-conditioning system (4). To date, more than 200 recognized causative agents and sources of antigens have been described (5).

HP can occur in many home, workplace and recreational environments. It varies in intensity, clinical presentation and natural history (6). This may, in part, be related to the amount and duration of exposure to the antigen, the nature of the inhaled particle and the host immune response. However, there is considerable variability between allergen exposure and an individual's susceptibility to develop HP, which is likely due to a complex interaction between environmental triggers and the host genetic background.

Conventionally, HP has been classified into acute, subacute and chronic forms, although there are no agreed diagnostic criteria (7). The clinical manifestations of the prototype of acute HP, farmer's lung, significantly overlap with those of pigeon breeder's lung or bird fancier's lung, which are more representative of subacute and chronic HP, respectively (8,9). Although used in practice, there are limitations to the current classification system. Alternative classification systems have been proposed based upon disease behaviour (10) or a cluster analysis of clinical, radiological and pathological parameters (11). These studies suggest that subacute HP is the most difficult to define; however, they have not been validated.

SCIENTIFIC MECHANISMS IN HP

It remains unclear why only a few exposed individuals develop HP. One current paradigm supports a 'two-hit hypothesis' wherein genetic predisposition or environmental factors (the first hit) increase susceptibility to developing HP when an individual is exposed to an inciting antigen (the second hit).

GENETIC FACTORS

Studies evaluating gene polymorphisms have been undertaken in small cohorts but to date no genetic factors have consistently been associated with HP. One case of familial HP was reported from Japan where summer-type HP occurred in families living in the same house and the affected individuals had HLA-DR9 phenotype (12). Other MHC class II polymorphisms, HLA-DR and DQw3, have been described in HP from populations with diverse genetic backgrounds (13,14). MHC class I has also been implicated in the disease pathogenesis. Polymorphisms in HLA-A2, the immuno-proteasome catalytic subunit β type 8 (PSMB8) that degrades ubiquitinated proteins to generate

antigenic peptides for presentation to cytotoxic T cells (15), and the transporters associated with antigen-processing (TAP) genes responsible for loading peptides onto MHC class I (16) have been identified. These findings highlight the importance of antigen presentation in the pathogenesis of HP.

ENVIRONMENTAL FACTORS

In animal models, concurrent infection with parainfluenza augments the inflammatory response to HP antigens (17). Furthermore, respiratory viruses have been detected in the lower airways in individuals with acute HP (18); however, their role in disease pathogenesis remains to be elucidated. Lipopolysaccharides or exposure to pesticides have also been identified as disease-promoting extrinsic co-factors (19,20).

ASSOCIATION WITH CIGARETTE SMOKING

HP is more prevalent in non-smokers compared to smokers with similar antigenic exposure (21,22). Several studies have demonstrated that pigeon breeders and farmers who smoke have lower levels of specific IgG antibodies than non-smokers and ex-smokers (23–26). Similarly, Arima and colleagues reported that summer-type HP as well as the prevalence of anti–*Trichosporon cutaneum* antibodies were substantially lower in smokers (27). In contrast, non-smokers with HP related to exposure to humidifier antigens have a significantly higher IgG response and more severe lung disease (28). These observations suggest that cigarette smoking suppresses the immunopathologic mechanisms involved in the development of HP. In support of this, nicotine may impair alveolar macrophage function including phagocytosis (29), as well as decrease secretion of the pro-inflammatory cytokines interleukin (IL)-1 and tumour necrosis factor (TNF)α (30,31). It has also been shown to reduce mitogen-induced lymphocyte proliferation, alter the balance between helper (CD4$^+$) and cytotoxic (CD8$^+$) T cells in bronchoalveolar lavage (BAL) fluid (32) and promote Th2 response (33). While experimental models have shown that cigarette smoking reduced the initial inflammatory responses, it delayed the repair processes particularly in the presence of persistent antigen exposure (34). Hence smoking may modify the clinical course to a more insidious, chronic form of HP. This has been observed in farmers who smoke; although farmer's lung occurs less frequently, the combination of antigen exposure and tobacco smoke inhalation may lead to emphysematous change and is associated with a worse prognosis (35,36).

IMMUNOPATHOGENESIS

Although the immunopathogenesis of HP is poorly understood, *in vitro* and *in vivo* studies have demonstrated a role for both humoral and cell-mediated immunity. Inhalation of inciting antigens initiates an inflammatory response mediated by pathogen recognition receptors (PRRs) expressed on alveolar epithelial cells and macrophages. A role for PRR in disease pathogenesis has been suggested from animal studies as mice deficient in dectin-1 (37) or toll-like receptor (TLR) 6 (38) are protected from fungal- and bacterial-induced HP, respectively. Activation of the PRR results in the secretion of several pro-inflammatory cytokines, including IL-8, IL-17 and TNFα as well as complement activation. This leads to an increase in vascular permeability and promotes migration of neutrophils to the lung that can be detected in BAL within 48 hours of an acute antigen exposure (39). If exuberant, this inflammatory response may result in hypoxaemia.

Alveolar macrophages and mature dendritic cells show an enhanced capacity to present the inhaled antigen to naïve $CD4^+$ T cells, which promotes their proliferation and differentiation into a variety of effector cells (40). A Th1 immune response predominates due to regulation by the transcription factor T-bet (41), and the cytokines IL-12 and interferon gamma (IFNγ) (42,43). This contributes to granuloma formation. In addition to the Th1 response, activated B lymphocytes secrete IgG antibodies specific to the causative antigen. It is still unclear whether these antibodies are simply a marker of exposure or if they contribute to disease pathogenesis (44). However, immune complexes (type III hypersensitivity) have been implicated in complement activation and the ensuing lung inflammation in acute HP.

Individuals exposed to an inciting antigen may develop a lymphocytic alveolitis but remain asymptomatic (45), suggesting the development of immune tolerance (10). This is, in part, mediated by regulatory T cells (Tregs), a specific set of $CD4^+$ T cells that down-regulate activation of the immune system and prevent tissue damage and autoimmunity (46). However in HP, isolated Tregs were unable to suppress activated T-cell proliferation, which may contribute to the persistent lymphocyte infiltration observed in subacute and chronic forms (47). Other features associated with chronic HP include an increase in $CD4^+$ T cells and in the $CD4^+/CD8^+$ ratio, a skewing toward Th2 T-cell differentiation and cytokine profile, and an exhaustion of $CD8^+$ T cells (42). More recently, experimental models of HP have demonstrated a role for Th17 cells and IL-17 (48,49), and fibrocytes (50) in collagen deposition and the development of pulmonary fibrosis.

EPIDEMIOLOGY

The prevalence of HP varies considerably around the world due to differences in disease definition, diagnostic methods, type and intensity of exposure, geographical conditions, agricultural and industrial practices and host risk factors. European-based registries reported that HP accounted for 1.5%–12% of incident cases of interstitial lung diseases (ILDs) (51). However, the disease is often unrecognized or misdiagnosed, so it can be difficult to determine how many persons exposed to causative agents develop HP. This is hampered by a lack of a standardized epidemiological approach for assessing the various forms of HP. In a large, UK general-population-based study, the incidence of HP was approximately 1 per 100,000 (52). Similarly, a study of occupational HP in the United Kingdom between 1996 and 2015 reported an annual incidence of 1.4 per million workers (53). However, higher rates may occur among exposed individuals during sporadic outbreaks (54). The disease is relatively uncommon in children with a reported incidence of two per year and a prevalence of 4 per 1,000,000 children (55,56).

CAUSATIVE ANTIGENS

Key to the development of HP is the inhalation of small particulate matter, with an aerodynamic diameter of less than 5 μm, which can penetrate the distal respiratory tract. The time between exposure and disease onset ranges from months to decades (57), which makes it challenging for the clinician to identify the type and source of the antigen, particularly in cases of occult or low-level exposure. Antigens capable of provoking HP are detailed in Table 11.1.

The thermophilic actinomycetes are ubiquitous organisms usually found in contaminated ventilation systems and in decaying compost, hay and sugar cane. Exposure to large quantities of contaminated hay is the most common source of inhalational allergens for farmers and between 1% and 19% will subsequently develop farmer's lung (21). Thus farmer's lung usually occurs in cold, damp climates in late winter and early spring when farmers use stored hay to feed their livestock. However, as farming and industrial practices are changing, new antigens may be introduced. This has been observed in the United Kingdom where occupational HP in machine operators due to contaminated metalworking fluid has increased from 5% to 50%, while the number of cases associated with agricultural work has declined (53).

A variety of low and high molecular weight proteins derived from avian serum, faeces and feathers produce bird fancier's lung, also called pigeon breeder's lung. Studies suggest that up to 20% of individuals exposed to bird droppings will develop bird fancier's lung (60). More recently, a Danish study of 6,920 pigeon breeders confirmed an increased risk of HP with an adjusted hazard ratio of 14.36 (95% CI 8.10–25.44) (61). Pigeons, parakeets, budgerigars and other small cage birds are usually involved, but the disease has been reported in individuals using feather-down duvets and pillows as well as from indirect avian contact in consorts such as through the handling of contaminated clothing.

There is a growing body of evidence to support a role for mycobacterial species in HP. *Mycobacterium avium* complex has been associated with hot tub lung (62) and *Mycobacterium immunogenum* contaminating metalworking fluid aerosols with machine operator's lung in automobile manufacturing and the aerospace industry (63,64). Unlike other bacteria, nontuberculous mycobacteria are capable of surviving such environments due to their thermotolerance and disinfectant resistance. Certain low molecular weight chemicals may cause HP. For example, isocyanates, used for the production of polyurethane polymers in the manufacture of polyurethane foams, paints and plastics, are not antigenic by themselves, but may combine with host proteins, such as albumin, to form haptens (65).

HISTORY AND EXAMINATION

The diagnosis of HP requires a high index of suspicion, and a detailed occupational and environmental exposure history is imperative. Acute HP typically presents following an intense exposure to a sensitizing antigen (58). Constitutional symptoms (i.e. fever, myalgias, lassitude, headache) develop 2–9 hours post-exposure, last from hours to days and usually recur with re-exposure (11,58). Respiratory symptoms including non-productive cough, dyspnoea and chest tightness are common but may also be absent (11). Subacute HP results from repeated or prolonged low-level antigen exposure and presents insidiously over weeks to a few months with cough, fatigue and dyspnoea (5). While chronic HP is characterized by progressive dyspnoea, cough, malaise and weight loss developing over a period of months to years often without recognizable acute episodes (5,58). Identifying an inciting antigen can be particularly difficult in this group and despite an exhaustive search between 30% and 50% of subjects have no identifiable exposure (66).

Physical examination reveals fever, tachypnoea, bibasal fine end-inspiratory crackles and occasionally wheeze in acute HP (5,67). The differential diagnosis includes acute respiratory infection and asthma, particularly in the occupational setting (5). Following a very intense exposure, patients may present with severe hypoxaemia and respiratory failure (68). Crackles in subacute HP can be more diffuse and the characteristic short, high-pitched, end-inspiratory squawks can be audible in both acute and subacute HP (58,67). Patients with chronic HP often develop progressive fibrosis with diffuse crackles, digital clubbing and, in advanced cases, signs of cor pulmonale (5,58).

Subacute and chronic HP may mimic other interstitial lung diseases, particularly idiopathic pulmonary fibrosis (IPF) and fibrotic nonspecific interstitial pneumonia (NSIP), which are important differential diagnoses to consider. Individuals with chronic HP may experience an acute exacerbation, typified by an accelerated decline in

Table 11.1 Hypersensitivity pneumonitis – exposures and antigens

Category	Causative antigen	Source of exposure	Disease association
Bacteria	Thermophilic actinomycetes (*Saccharopolyspora rectivirgula*, *Thermoactinomyces vulgaris*, *T. sacchari*)	Mouldy hay, grain	Farmer's lung
		Mouldy compost	Mushroom worker's lung
		Mouldy hay around potatoes	Potato riddler's lung
		Mouldy compost	Compost worker's lung
		Contaminated forced air systems, water reservoirs	Ventilation pneumonitis, air-conditioner lung
	Lichtheimia corymbifera	Mouldy hay, grain	Farmer's lung
	Streptomyces albus	Mouldy compost	Compost workers
	Klebsiella oxytoca	Contaminated water	Humidifier lung
	Saccharomonospora viridis	Dead grasses and leaves	Thatched roof lung
	Mycobacterium avium-intracellulare and other non-tuberculous mycobacteria	Contaminated water (mist/aerosol)	Spa workers, hot tub lung
	Mycobacterium immunogenum	Contaminated metalworking fluid	Metal worker's lung, Machine operator's lung
	Acinetobacter, Ochrobactrum	Contaminated metalworking fluid	Metal worker's lung
	Bacillus subtilis enzymes	Detergents (during processing or use)	Detergent worker's lung
	Bacillus species	Contaminated water from home humidifier, ultrasonic misting fountains	Humidifier lung
Fungi, yeasts	*Aspergillus* species	Mouldy hay, grain	Farmer's lung
	Aspergillus species	Mouldy mushrooms	Mushroom worker's lung, compost worker's lung
	Aspergillus species	Mouldy compost	
	Aspergillus species	Tobacco plants	Tobacco worker's lung
	Aspergillus fumigatus, Aspergillus clavatus	Mouldy barley	Malt worker's lung
	Trichosporon cutaneum	Contaminated wooden houses	Summer-type HP
	Penicillium species	Mouldy cork	Suberosis
	Penicillium casei	Mouldy cheese or cheese casings	Cheese washer's lung
	Penicillium verrucosum	Contaminated grain and cereals	Food processor's lung
	Alternaria species	Oak, cedar and mahogany dust, pine and spruce pulp or dust	Woodworker's lung
	Cryptostroma corticale	Mouldy maple bark	Maple bark stripper's lung
	Botrytis cinerea	Mould on grapes	Wine maker's lung

(Continued)

Table 11.1 (*Continued*) Hypersensitivity pneumonitis – exposures and antigens

Category	Causative antigen	Source of exposure	Disease association
Animal proteins	Avian droppings, feathers, serum	Parakeets, parrots, budgerigars, pigeons, chickens, turkeys	Pigeon breeder's or bird fancier's lung
	Avian proteins	Feather beds, pillows, duvet	Feather duvet lung
	Fish meal	Fish meal dust	Fish meal worker's lung
	Bat serum protein	Bat droppings	Bat lung
	Rats, gerbils	Urine, serum, pelts	Animal handler's lung, laboratory worker's lung
	Animal fur dust	Animal pelts	Furrier's lung
	Silkworm proteins	Dust from silkworm larvae and cocoons	Silk production HP
Insect proteins	*Sitophilus granarius* (i.e. wheat weevil)	Dust-contaminated grain	Miller's lung
	Carmine (cochineal)	Food dyes	Food industry worker's lung
Plant proteins	Tiger nut	Tiger nut dust	Tiger nut worker's lung
Chemicals	Diisocyanates, trimellitic anhydride	Polyurethane foams, spray paints, dyes, glues	Chemical worker's lung
	Acrylate compounds	Polymer plastics	Dental technicians
Metals	Cobalt	Hard metals	Metal worker's lung
	Zirconium	Zirconium silicate	Ceramic worker's lung
	Zinc	Zinc fumes	Smelters

Source: Adapted from Selman M. In: Schwarz MI, King TE, eds. *Interstitial Lung Disease.* 5th ed. Ashland, OH: People's Medical Publishing House; 2011:597–635; Spagnolo P et al. *J Investig Allergol Clin Immunol.* 2015;25(4):237–50; Quirce S et al. *Allergy.* 2016;71(6):765–79.

respiratory symptoms and new bilateral ground-glass opacities (GGOs) on high-resolution computed tomography (HRCT) scan (69). Although precipitating factors are unknown, exacerbations are more common in those with fewer lymphocytes in BAL, worse pulmonary function and pulmonary fibrosis at the time of diagnosis (70). Histology demonstrates diffuse alveolar damage or organizing pneumonia (OP) superimposed on pre-existing fibrotic lung disease (70). This form is associated with a poorer prognosis.

INVESTIGATIONS

No diagnostic test is pathognomonic for HP. Although various diagnostic criteria have been proposed, none have been prospectively validated (68). The diagnosis of HP therefore depends on the integration of a number of features including history of antigen exposure, clinical, laboratory, radiological and, in some cases, pathological findings.

PULMONARY FUNCTION TESTS

Abnormalities in pulmonary function do not differentiate HP from other ILDs. Hence, their primary role is to determine disease severity at diagnosis and to monitor for progression and response to treatment. A restrictive ventilatory defect and/or reduced carbon monoxide diffusing capacity (DLCO) typify acute HP (67). Hypoxaemia at rest may occur during an acute episode. In subacute and chronic HP a restrictive or mixed obstructive and restrictive ventilatory impairment is accompanied by reduced DLCO (67). Resting and exercise-induced hypoxaemia may develop in severe disease (67). Bronchial hyper-reactivity has been reported in some cases. Generally, however, there is poor correlation between the pulmonary function changes and the magnitude of the radiological changes observed on chest radiograph or HRCT scans.

BASIC LABORATORY INVESTIGATIONS

A peripheral neutrophilia, lymphopenia and rise in non-specific markers of inflammation such as C-reactive protein (CRP) and erythrocyte sedimentation rate (ESR) can occur in acute HP (71). Polyclonal elevation of γ-globulins has frequently been observed in chronic HP and up to 50% of patients have an elevated rheumatoid factor (67,71).

SERUM PRECIPITINS

The detection of specific circulating IgG antibodies (precipitins) to potential antigens was previously regarded as the 'gold standard' for HP diagnosis but it is now understood to signify exposure rather than disease. This is evidenced from studies of asymptomatic farmers where up to 50% have positive precipitins against *Saccharopolyspora rectivirgula,* the bacteria most frequently responsible for farmer's lung (45). Moreover, longitudinal follow-up has demonstrated no increased risk of respiratory sequelae compared to seronegative individuals (45). In the correct clinical context, however, positive precipitins support the diagnosis of HP and are often included in prediction models (8). Rising titres increase the likelihood of HP, while falling titres confirm antigen avoidance (72). Equally the absence of serum precipitins does not exclude HP and false-negative results can occur in acute and chronic HP (5). Furthermore, commercial assays test a limited number of potential antigens and may not take account of geographical and climatic variations in antigen expression (73).

LYMPHOCYTE PROLIFERATION STUDIES

To overcome some of the limitations of precipitin testing, lymphocyte proliferation assays have been studied. Compared to control subjects, individuals with HP respond more frequently and strongly to the inciting antigen distinguishing disease from exposure (6,74). Experience is limited to a few specialized centres and the assay is not routinely used.

INHALATION CHALLENGE

Inhalation challenge studies, similar to those used in occupational asthma, have been examined in HP to determine causality. Following a period of antigen avoidance, a positive test is characterized by cough, dyspnoea, fever, reduced forced vital capacity (FVC) and hypoxaemia developing 8–12 hours after antigen re-exposure (75,76). In the appropriate clinical setting a positive inhalation challenge is diagnostic but false-negative results can occur (75). Due to the risk of severe reaction and the lack of standardization of antigen preparation, inhalation protocols and criteria used to analyse the test result, challenge studies are not widely undertaken and are restricted to specialized or research centres (6).

RADIOLOGY

CHEST RADIOGRAPHY

Chest radiography (CXR) in acute and subacute HP demonstrates nodular opacities and diffuse infiltrates although up to 20% may be normal (8,71). Chronic HP is characterized by volume loss and reticular opacities with a mid- and upper-lobe predilection (71).

HIGH-RESOLUTION COMPUTED TOMOGRAPHY

High resolution computed tomography (HRCT) is more sensitive than CXR and is recommended in the evaluation of suspected HP. Although it can help distinguish between the different clinical forms, it may be normal in 8%–18% of proven cases of HP (8). It is rarely performed in acute HP due to rapid symptom resolution (77). In cases where it has been performed, diffuse GGO is observed, but this is a non-specific finding and has a wide differential including pulmonary oedema, opportunistic infection and cellular NSIP (8,71,78).

In contrast, HRCT changes in subacute HP are more specific and consist of GGO, small poorly defined centrilobular nodules, mosaic perfusion and air trapping (79) (Figure 11.1a–d). Areas of GGO, corresponding pathologically to diffuse interstitial infiltration, can be patchy or diffuse and involve peripheral or central portions of the lung (77,79). Centrilobular nodules (typically <5 mm in diameter) have a mid- and upper-zone predominance and represent interstitial pneumonitis with a peribronchiolar distribution (77,79). Larger, irregular nodules can be present and may be focal areas of OP (79). Mosaic perfusion, seen on inspiratory images as areas of decreased attenuation adjacent

to areas of high attenuation, occurs due to shunting of blood away from poorly ventilated regions of lung as a consequence of bronchiolar obstruction (77). Expiratory images demonstrate lobular areas of air trapping indicative of small airways disease, which are found within and without with areas of mosaic perfusion (77). Thin-walled cysts, that are few in number and range in size from 3 to 25 mm in diameter, have been reported in up to 13% of cases of subacute HP (80).

Chronic HP is characterized by HRCT features of 'fibrosis' (i.e. reticulation, traction bronchiectasis and honeycombing) in a sub-pleural or peri-bronchovascular distribution with basal sparing (77,78) (Figure 11.2a–d). Evidence of active disease, for example, centrilobular nodules and GGO may be superimposed (81). Radiologically the differential diagnosis includes IPF and fibrotic NSIP. Silva and colleagues identified the presence of mosaic attenuation, centrilobular nodules and absence of lower zone predominance as the best CT features to distinguish HP (82). In addition, thin-walled cysts were more frequently observed in chronic HP (39%) compared to IPF (0%) or NSIP (12%) (82). Interestingly, patients with chronic farmer's lung, even lifelong non-smokers, are more likely to develop emphysema than interstitial fibrosis (79,83). The pathogenesis of emphysema in these patients is unknown but may reflect intermittent high-level antigen exposure in contrast to chronic low-level exposure (36).

PATHOLOGY

BRONCHOALVEOLAR LAVAGE

BAL is a sensitive method for detecting lung inflammation and is usually undertaken in those suspected of having subacute or chronic HP. A significant increase in total cell count with a lymphocyte differential count ≥25% (and often ≥50%) is strongly supportive of HP in the correct clinical context (84) (Figure 11.1e). The presence of mast cells, plasma cells and foamy macrophages lend support to the diagnosis (85). A preponderance of CD8$^+$ T cells results in a reduced CD4$^+$/CD8$^+$ ratio, but the utility of evaluating this routinely in clinical practice has been questioned as it

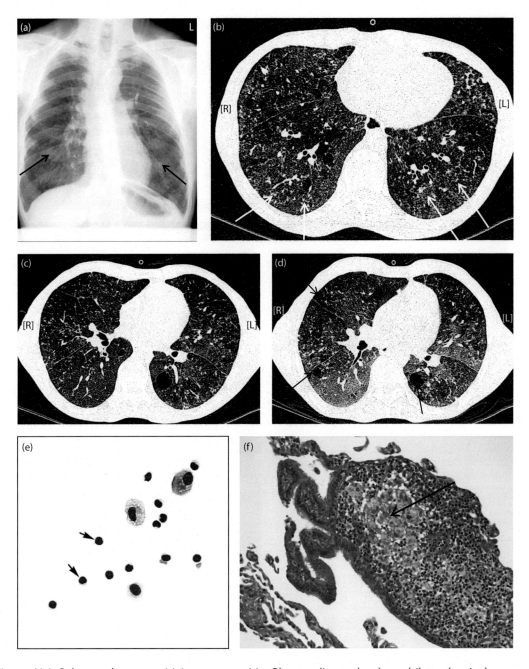

Figure 11.1 Subacute hypersensitivity pneumonitis. Chest radiography shows bilateral reticular change (**a**, *black arrow*). High-resolution computed tomography (HRCT) shows ground-glass opacification and poorly defined centrilobular nodules (**b**, *white arrow*). Inspiratory image demonstrating areas of decreased attenuation adjacent to areas of high attenuation, i.e. mosaic perfusion (**c**). Differences in attenuation are more prominent on expiration and areas of air trapping are identified (**d**, *black arrow*). Photomicrographs of haematoxylin and eosin stained bronchoalveolar lavage fluid (**e**) and transbronchial biopsy (**f**) showing lymphocytes (*arrowhead*) and a poorly formed, non-necrotizing granuloma within a cellular infiltrate (*black arrow*), respectively.

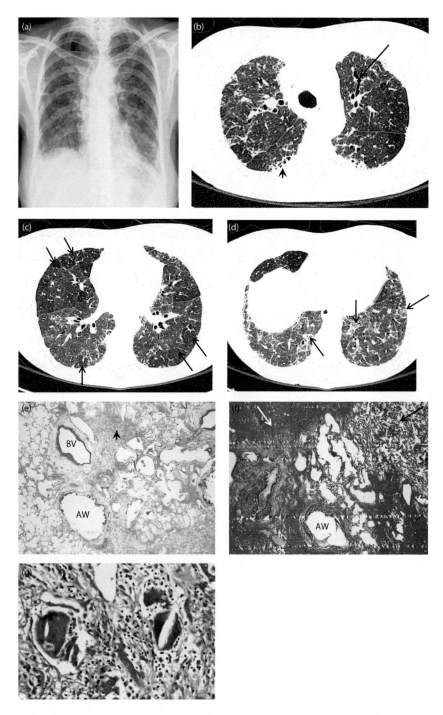

Figure 11.2 Chronic hypersensitivity pneumonitis. Chest radiography shows extensive bilateral reticulation (**a**). High-resolution computed tomography (HRCT) shows honeycombing (**b**, *arrowhead*) and traction bronchiectasis (**b**, *black arrow*). Lobular areas of air trapping indicate small airways disease (**c**, *black arrow*) and diffuse areas of ground-glass opacification are present (**d**, *black arrow*). Photomicrographs of haematoxylin and eosin-stained surgical lung biopsy demonstrating centrilobular fibrosis and a lymphocytic cell infiltration (*arrowhead*) (**e**; BV = blood vessel, AW = airway). Low power magnification shows patchy fibrosis with areas of fibrotic (*white arrow*) and non-fibrotic (*black arrow*) lung (**f**). Interstitial giant cells with cholesterol clefts are present (**g**).

is not specific to HP and is affected by a number of factors including smoking status, corticosteroids and stage of disease (5,42,85). Similar to serum precipitins, a lymphocyte-rich alveolitis can be demonstrated in asymptomatic exposed individuals without long-term sequelae (45). Patients with chronic, fibrotic HP tend to have lower lymphocyte and higher neutrophil counts but a lymphocyte cut-off of 30% was shown to confidently discriminate chronic HP from IPF (86,87).

HISTOPATHOLOGY

Lung biopsy is reserved for cases of diagnostic uncertainty, where the above-mentioned investigations have failed to yield a definitive diagnosis of HP. Although transbronchial biopsies may demonstrate some of the typical histological findings of HP, they can be non-diagnostic and surgical lung biopsy with samples from two different lobes is required (5,88) (Figure 11.1f). Cryobiopsy has recently been shown to yield larger biopsy samples with less crush artefact than transbronchial biopsy but there is insufficient evidence at this time to recommend it as an alternative to surgical biopsy (89,90).

As with HRCT, lung biopsy is rarely performed in acute HP due to rapid symptom resolution. A small case series reported fibrin deposition and a prominent interstitial neutrophilic infiltrate overlaid with some features of subacute HP (91). The differential diagnosis includes acute lung injury, and infection needs to be excluded.

Regardless of the inciting antigen, subacute HP is recognized histologically by the classical triad of bronchiolocentric interstitial pneumonitis, chronic bronchiolitis and poorly formed, non-necrotizing granulomas (92,93). Approximately 75% of cases demonstrate all of these features and any one can predominate (94). The inflammatory infiltrate is composed predominantly of lymphocytes but plasma cells and histiocytes can also be present (92,93). Chronic bronchiolitis can result in associated lymphoid hyperplasia, peribronchiolar metaplasia, bronchiolar wall fibrosis and foci of OP (92,93). A microscopic obstructive pneumonia, indicative of bronchiolitis, is characteristic of HP and consists of clusters of foamy macrophages in the peribronchiolar airspaces (92,93). Granulomas, which occur in up to 80% of surgical lung biopsies, are formed of histiocytes or multinucleated giant cells often containing non-specific cytoplasmic inclusions such as cholesterol clefts and Schaumann bodies (92,93) (Figure 11.2g). Although usually located in the interstitium, granulomas may also be intra-alveolar (95). However numerous compact granulomas should raise the possibility of another diagnosis.

Histologically, chronic HP can overlap with fibrosing NSIP (96), airway-centred interstitial fibrosis (97) and usual interstitial pneumonia (UIP) (87,88,98,99). Features that help to distinguish HP from other ILDs include bronchiolocentric attenuation of inflammation/fibrosis (occasionally with bridging fibrosis between bronchioles), peribronchiolar metaplasia, the presence of granulomas, and a lymphoid infiltrate away from areas of fibrosis (88,100,101) (Figure 11.2e, f). A careful search for these auxiliary findings, particularly in biopsies taken from two different lobes, ensures that in only a minority of cases is the histology indistinguishable from NSIP or UIP.

MANAGEMENT

GENERAL MANAGEMENT

All patients with HP should be advised about the importance of smoking cessation and attending for pneumococcal and flu vaccines. Referral for pulmonary rehabilitation should be discussed and assessment for ambulatory and/or continuous oxygen therapy regularly reviewed.

SPECIFIC ASPECTS OF MANAGEMENT

The cornerstone of HP management is early accurate diagnosis and antigen avoidance. Removal of the suspected or inciting antigen is the most important factor in preventing disease progression, although a small proportion of affected individuals continue to progress even with antigen avoidance measures. In order to reduce occupational exposures appropriate ventilation, dust masks with filters or re-location of the worker may be required (5,102). In bird fancier's lung, despite bird removal and extensive environmental cleaning, high levels of avian antigens can still be detected out to 18 months and may account for disease persistence and/or progression in some instances (103).

Although most cases of acute HP are self-limiting, corticosteroids are often used. In the only placebo-controlled trial to date, corticosteroid therapy resulted in a more rapid improvement in lung function but did not influence the longer-term outcome (104). The optimal pharmacological management of subacute and chronic HP is unknown. Currently, corticosteroids are recommended but their efficacy has not been proven in prospective clinical trials (105). An empirical regime may consist of 0.5 mg/kg/day for 6–8 weeks, followed by a gradual reduction or until a maintenance dose of approximately 10 mg/day is reached (5,10). Symptoms, lung function and radiological changes are key determinants in assessing treatment response.

There are no randomized controlled trials of steroid-sparing agents. However, a retrospective study demonstrated that treatment with mycophenolate mofetil or azathioprine was associated with improvements in DLCO but not FVC in chronic HP (106). Case reports have highlighted a role for biological therapies, such as rituximab, in severe, refractory disease (107). Chronic advanced HP with fibrosis typically fails to respond to immunosuppressive therapy and referral for lung transplantation should be considered. In a recent case series, patients with HP undergoing lung transplantation had excellent outcomes with 1- and 5-year survival of 96% and 89%, respectively (108).

PROGNOSIS

Population-based studies examining HP mortality are limited. Nonetheless, over a 40-year period (1968–2008) in England and Wales mortality rates remained stable at 0.05 per 100,000 for men and 0.03 per 100,000 for women (109). Mortality increased with increasing age, peaking at 0.19 per 100,000 in the 80–84 age group (109). Individuals with acute HP typically have an excellent prognosis if they are correctly diagnosed and re-exposure to the sensitizing antigen avoided. By comparison, patients with subacute/chronic HP, especially those with bird fancier's lung, can progress to irreversible fibrosis and determining the inciting antigen can have a significant impact on prognosis. Fernández Pérez and colleagues, after adjusting for other variables, observed a median survival in patients with chronic HP and an identifiable

antigen of 8.75 years, in contrast to patients with no identifiable antigen where survival was 4.88 years (66). Other factors predictive of a poor prognosis include digital clubbing (110), longer duration of antigen exposure (111), the presence and extent of fibrosis on HRCT (112,113), fibrosis on surgical lung biopsy (70,87,114) and Doppler echocardiography evidence of pulmonary hypertension (sPAP >50 mm Hg) (115).

CURRENT AND FUTURE AREAS OF RESEARCH

The changing environment and the dynamic nature of HP remain challenges for the clinician in establishing not only the diagnosis but also the best treatment strategy. Key to this are a number of important observations that remain unsolved including why certain exposed individuals are more susceptible to HP, why there is considerable variability in the time between antigen exposure and disease development and why the disease progresses even in the absence of antigen exposure. In order to address these issues, there needs to be a consensus statement to define the syndrome of HP including validated clinical, serological, radiological and pathological diagnostic criteria. Rigorous epidemiological studies will be essential to identify and monitor for novel causative antigens, and to define factors that affect both the occurrence and natural history of the disease. There also needs to be a large repository of standardized antigens that can be used in the clinical and research environments. Advances in genomics, epigenetics and proteomics will undoubtedly improve our understanding of the disease pathogenesis leading to candidate diagnostic, prognostic and therapeutic biomarkers. This will be best achieved through multicentre collaborative networks and registries.

Clinical cases

CASE 1

A 46-year-old dairy farmer presented with a 2-month history of exertional dyspnoea. He also described a dry cough, fevers, malaise and weight loss. He was a lifelong non-smoker and had no significant past medical history of note. On chest examination he had bibasal fine inspiratory crackles. There was no digital clubbing or systemic features of autoimmune disease.

Investigations: Lung function showed a mixed restrictive and obstructive defect with an FEV1 40% predicted, FVC 64% predicted and DLCO 50% predicted. CRP and ESR were raised and farmer's lung precipitins were positive. CXR demonstrated bilateral reticular changes and HRCT showed features in keeping with subacute HP (Figure 11.1a–d). Bronchoscopy revealed a lymphocytosis (63%) with CD4/CD8 ratio <1. Transbronchial biopsies showed poorly formed, non-necrotizing granulomas (Figure 11.1e, f).

Management: He was commenced on prednisolone 30 mg daily and advised to use a respirator with filter when performing work on the farm and to avoid contact with hay. His breathlessness and cough significantly improved and this was reflected with an increase in lung function to FEV1 66% predicted, FVC 81% predicted and DLCO 61% predicted. Over the course of 2 years, the prednisolone was gradually weaned and then discontinued with no recurrence of symptoms and lung function remained stable. He continues to use a respirator on the farm.

This is a case of famer's lung with subacute HP that responded to corticosteroids and allergen avoidance measures.

CASE 2

A 57-year-old lady presented with a 3-year history of dry cough and an 18-month history of progressive exertional dyspnoea that limited activities of daily living. She had never smoked and had no features of autoimmune disease. She had kept birds until 10 years ago. Autoimmune serology and avian precipitins were negative. She developed a right-sided pneumothorax which was managed with intercoastal drain insertion. HRCT demonstrated patchy GGO and subpleural reticulation. She proceeded to video-assisted thoracoscopic surgery (VATS) biopsy, which showed features consistent with chronic HP (Figure 11.2e–g). She was commenced on prednisolone 30 mg daily and had received 6 months of treatment before review in the ILD service.

Investigations: Lung function showed a severe restrictive defect with FEV1 43% predicted and FVC 47% predicted. Gas transfer was impaired with DLCO 24% predicted and she desaturated on 6-minute walk test. CXR showed extensive pulmonary fibrosis and HRCT demonstrated changes in keeping with chronic HP (Figure 11.2a–d).

Management: She was commenced on azathioprine, ambulatory oxygen and was referred for pulmonary rehabilitation and a lung transplant opinion. Her lung function stabilized enabling a slow wean of prednisolone to 10 mg daily. One year later she underwent single lung transplant and remains well with an unlimited exercise tolerance.

This is a case of bird fancier's lung and demonstrates progressive chronic HP in the absence of antigen exposure.

ACKNOWLEDGEMENT

We would like to thank Dr Doris Rassl for assistance with the histology images.

REFERENCES

1. Campbell J. Acute symptoms following work with hay. *Br Med J.* 1932;2:1143–4.
2. Pepys J, Riddell R, Citron K, Clayton Y. Precipitins against extracts of hay and moulds in the serum of patients with farmer's lung, aspergillosis, asthma, and sarcoidosis. *Thorax.* 1962;17:366–74.
3. Pearsall HR, Morgan EH, Tesluk H, Beggs D. Parakeet dander pneumonitis. Acute psittacokerato-pneumoconiosis, report of a case. *Bull Mason Clin.* 1960;14:127–37.
4. Banaszak EF, Thiede WH, Fink JN. Hypersensitivity pneumonitis due to contamination of an air conditioner. *N Engl J Med.* 1970;283(6):271–6.
5. Selman M, Pardo A, King TE. Hypersensitivity pneumonitis: Insights in diagnosis and pathobiology. *Am J Respir Crit Care Med.* 2012;186(4):314–24.
6. Fink JN, Ortega HG, Reynolds HY, Cormier YF, Fan LL, Franks TJ et al. Needs and opportunities for research in hypersensitivity pneumonitis. *Am J Respir Crit Care Med.* 2005;171(7):792–8.

7. Richerson HB, Bernstein IL, Fink JN, Hunninghake GW, Novey HS, Reed CE et al. Guidelines for the clinical evaluation of hypersensitivity pneumonitis. Report of the Subcommittee on Hypersensitivity Pneumonitis. *J Allergy Clin Immunol.* 1989 84(5 Pt 2):839–44.

8. Lacasse Y, Selman M, Costabel U, Dalphin J-C, Ando M, Morell F et al. Clinical diagnosis of hypersensitivity pneumonitis. *Am J Respir Crit Care Med.* 2003;168(8):952–8.

9. Girard M, Lacasse Y, Cormier Y. Hypersensitivity pneumonitis. *Allergy.* 2009;64(3):322–34.

10. Selman M. Hypersensitivity pneumonitis. In: Schwarz MI, King TE, eds. *Interstitial Lung Disease.* 5th ed. Ashland, OH: People's Medical Publishing House; 2011:597–635.

11. Lacasse Y, Selman M, Costabel U, Dalphin J-C, Morell F, Erkinjuntti-Pekkanen R et al. Classification of hypersensitivity pneumonitis: A hypothesis. *Int Arch Allergy Immunol.* 2009;149(2):161–6.

12. Asai N, Kaneko N, Ohkuni Y, Aoshima M, Kawamura Y. Familial summer-type hypersensitivity pneumonitis: A review of 25 families and 50 cases in Japan. *Intern Med Tokyo Jpn.* 2016;55(3):279–83.

13. Ando M, Hirayama K, Soda K, Okubo R, Araki S, Sasazuki T. HLA-DQw3 in Japanese summer-type hypersensitivity pneumonitis induced by *Trichosporon cutaneum. Am Rev Respir Dis.* 1989;140(4):948–50.

14. Camarena A, Juárez A, Mejía M, Estrada A, Carrillo G, Falfán R et al. Major histocompatibility complex and tumor necrosis factor-alpha polymorphisms in pigeon breeder's disease. *Am J Respir Crit Care Med.* 2001;163(7):1528–33.

15. Camarena A, Aquino-Galvez A, Falfán-Valencia R, Sánchez G, Montaño M, Ramos C et al. PSMB8 (LMP7) but not PSMB9 (LMP2) gene polymorphisms are associated to pigeon breeder's hypersensitivity pneumonitis. *Respir Med.* 2010;104(6):889–94.

16. Aquino-Galvez A, Camarena A, Montaño M, Juarez A, Zamora AC, González-Avila G et al. Transporter associated with antigen processing (TAP) 1 gene polymorphisms in patients with hypersensitivity pneumonitis. *Exp Mol Pathol.* 2008 Apr;84(2):173–7.

17. Cormier Y, Tremblay GM, Fournier M, Israël-Assayag E. Long-term viral enhancement of lung response to *Saccharopolyspora rectivirgula. Am J Respir Crit Care Med.* 1994;149(2 Pt 1):490–4.

18. Dakhama A, Hegele RG, Laflamme G, Israël-Assayag E, Cormier Y. Common respiratory viruses in lower airways of patients with acute hypersensitivity pneumonitis. *Am J Respir Crit Care Med.* 1999;159(4 Pt 1):1316–22.

19. Fogelmark B, Sjöstrand M, Rylander R. Pulmonary inflammation induced by repeated inhalations of ß(1,3)-D-glucan and endotoxin. *Int J Exp Pathol.* 1994;75(2):85–90.

20. Hoppin JA, Umbach DM, Kullman GJ, Henneberger PK, London SJ, Alavanja MCR et al. Pesticides and other agricultural factors associated with self-reported farmer's lung among farm residents in the Agricultural Health Study. *Occup Environ Med.* 2007;64(5):334–41.

21. Depierre A, Dalphin JC, Pernet D, Dubiez A, Faucompré C, Breton JL. Epidemiological study of farmer's lung in five districts of the French Doubs province. *Thorax.* 1988;43(6):429–35.

22. Warren CP. Extrinsic allergic alveolitis: A disease commoner in non-smokers. *Thorax.* 1977;32(5):567–9.

23. Carrillo T, Rodriguez de Castro F, Cuevas M, Diaz F, Cabrera P. Effect of cigarette smoking on the humoral immune response in pigeon fanciers. *Allergy.* 1991;46(4):241–4.

24. Cormier Y, Bélanger J. Long-term physiologic outcome after acute farmer's lung. *Chest.* 1985;87(6):796–800.

25. Baldwin CI, Todd A, Bourke S, Allen A, Calvert JE. Pigeon fanciers' lung: Effects of smoking on serum and salivary antibody responses to pigeon antigens. *Clin Exp Immunol.* 1998;113(2):166–72.

26. Dalphin JC, Debieuvre D, Pernet D, Maheu MF, Polio JC, Toson B et al. Prevalence and risk factors for chronic bronchitis and farmer's lung in French dairy farmers. *Br J Ind Med.* 1993;50(10):941–4.

27. Arima K, Ando M, Ito K, Sakata T, Yamaguchi T, Araki S et al. Effect of cigarette smoking on prevalence of summer-type hypersensitivity pneumonitis caused by *Trichosporon cutaneum*. *Arch Environ Health*. 1992;47(4):274–8.

28. Baur X, Richter G, Pethran A, Czuppon AB, Schwaiblmair M. Increased prevalence of IgG-induced sensitization and hypersensitivity pneumonitis (humidifier lung) in nonsmokers exposed to aerosols of a contaminated air conditioner. *Respir Int Rev Thorac Dis*. 1992;59(4):211–4.

29. Hocking WG, Golde DW. The pulmonary-alveolar macrophage (first of two parts). *N Engl J Med*. 197913;301(11):580–7.

30. Brown GP, Iwamoto GK, Monick MM, Hunninghake GW. Cigarette smoking decreases interleukin 1 release by human alveolar macrophages. *Am J Physiol*. 1989;256(2 Pt 1):C260–4.

31. Yamaguchi E, Itoh A, Furuya K, Miyamoto H, Abe S, Kawakami Y. Release of tumor necrosis factor-alpha from human alveolar macrophages is decreased in smokers. *Chest*. 1993;103(2):479–83.

32. Costabel U, Bross KJ, Reuter C, Rühle KH, Matthys H. Alterations in immunoregulatory T-cell subsets in cigarette smokers. A phenotypic analysis of bronchoalveolar and blood lymphocytes. *Chest*. 1986;90(1):39–44.

33. Nizri E, Irony-Tur-Sinai M, Lory O, Orr-Urtreger A, Lavi E, Brenner T. Activation of the cholinergic anti-inflammatory system by nicotine attenuates neuroinflammation via suppression of Th1 and Th17 responses. *J Immunol Baltim Md 1950*. 200915;183(10):6681–8.

34. Cormier Y, Gagnon L, Bérubé-Genest F, Fournier M. Sequential bronchoalveolar lavage in experimental extrinsic allergic alveolitis. The influence of cigarette smoking. *Am Rev Respir Dis*. 1988;137(5):1104–9.

35. Emanuel DA, Wenzel FJ, Bowerman CI, Lawton BR. Farmer's lung: Clinical, pathologic and immunologic study of twenty-four patients. *Am J Med*. 1964;37:392–401.

36. Ohtsuka Y, Munakata M, Tanimura K, Ukita H, Kusaka H, Masaki Y et al. Smoking promotes insidious and chronic farmer's lung disease, and deteriorates the clinical outcome. *Intern Med Tokyo Jpn*. 1995;34(10):966–71.

37. Higashino-Kameda M, Yabe-Wada T, Matsuba S, Takeda K, Anzawa K, Mochizuki T et al. A critical role of Dectin-1 in hypersensitivity pneumonitis. *Inflamm Res Off J Eur Histamine Res Soc Al*. 2016;65(3):235–44.

38. Fong DJ, Hogaboam CM, Matsuno Y, Akira S, Uematsu S, Joshi AD. Toll-like receptor 6 drives interleukin-17A expression during experimental hypersensitivity pneumonitis. *Immunology*. 2010;130(1):125–36.

39. Vogelmeier C, Krombach F, Münzing S, König G, Mazur G, Beinert T et al. Activation of blood neutrophils in acute episodes of farmer's lung. *Am Rev Respir Dis*. 1993;148(2):396–400.

40. Girard M, Israël-Assayag E, Cormier Y. Mature CD11c(+) cells are enhanced in hypersensitivity pneumonitis. *Eur Respir J*. 2009;34(3):749–56.

41. Glimcher LH. Trawling for treasure: Tales of T-bet. *Nat Immunol*. 2007;8(5):448–50.

42. Barrera L, Mendoza F, Zuñiga J, Estrada A, Zamora AC, Melendro EI et al. Functional diversity of T-cell subpopulations in subacute and chronic hypersensitivity pneumonitis. *Am J Respir Crit Care Med*. 2008;177(1):44–55.

43. Yamasaki H, Ando M, Brazer W, Center DM, Cruikshank WW. Polarized type 1 cytokine profile in bronchoalveolar lavage T cells of patients with hypersensitivity pneumonitis. *J Immunol Baltim Md 1950*. 1999;163(6):3516–23.

44. Burrell R, Rylander R. A critical review of the role of precipitins in hypersensitivity pneumonitis. *Eur J Respir Dis*. 1981;62(5):332–43.

45. Cormier Y, Létourneau L, Racine G. Significance of precipitins and asymptomatic lymphocytic alveolitis: A 20-yr follow-up. *Eur Respir J*. 2004;23(4):523–5.

46. Bettelli E, Carrier Y, Gao W, Korn T, Strom TB, Oukka M et al. Reciprocal developmental pathways for the generation of pathogenic effector TH17 and regulatory T cells. *Nature*. 2006;441(7090):235–8.

47. Girard M, Israël-Assayag E, Cormier Y. Impaired function of regulatory T-cells in hypersensitivity pneumonitis. *Eur Respir J*. 2011;37(3):632–9.

48. Simonian PL, Roark CL, Wehrmann F, Lanham AK, Diaz del Valle F, Born WK et al. Th17-polarized immune response in a murine model of hypersensitivity pneumonitis and lung fibrosis. *J Immunol Baltim Md 1950*. 2009;182(1):657–65.

49. Joshi AD, Fong DJ, Oak SR, Trujillo G, Flaherty KR, Martinez FJ et al. Interleukin-17-mediated immunopathogenesis in experimental hypersensitivity pneumonitis. *Am J Respir Crit Care Med*. 2009;179(8):705–16.

50. García de Alba C, Buendia-Roldán I, Salgado A, Becerril C, Ramírez R, González Y et al. Fibrocytes contribute to inflammation and fibrosis in chronic hypersensitivity pneumonitis through paracrine effects. *Am J Respir Crit Care Med*. 2015;191(4):427–36.

51. Thomeer MJ, Costabe U, Rizzato G, Poletti V, Demedts M. Comparison of registries of interstitial lung diseases in three European countries. *Eur Respir J Suppl*. 2001;32:114s–118s.

52. Solaymani-Dodaran M, West J, Smith C, Hubbard R. Extrinsic allergic alveolitis: Incidence and mortality in the general population. *QJM Mon J Assoc Physicians*. 2007;100(4):233–7.

53. Barber CM, Wiggans RE, Carder M, Agius R. Epidemiology of occupational hypersensitivity pneumonitis; reports from the SWORD scheme in the UK from 1996 to 2015. *Occup Environ Med*. 2017;74(7):528–30.

54. Bernstein DI, Lummus ZL, Santilli G, Siskosky J, Bernstein IL. Machine operator's lung. A hypersensitivity pneumonitis disorder associated with exposure to metalworking fluid aerosols. *Chest*. 1995;108(3):636–41.

55. Grech V, Vella C, Lenicker H. Pigeon breeder's lung in childhood: Varied clinical picture at presentation. *Pediatr Pulmonol*. 2000;30(2):145–8.

56. Buchvald F, Petersen BL, Damgaard K, Deterding R, Langston C, Fan LL et al. Frequency, treatment, and functional outcome in children with hypersensitivity pneumonitis. *Pediatr Pulmonol*. 2011;46(11):1098–107.

57. Morell F, Roger A, Reyes L, Cruz MJ, Murio C, Muñoz X. Bird fancier's lung: A series of 86 patients. *Medicine (Baltimore)*. 2008;87(2):110–30.

58. Spagnolo P, Rossi G, Cavazza A, Bonifazi M, Paladini I, Bonella F et al. Hypersensitivity pneumonitis: A comprehensive review. *J Investig Allergol Clin Immunol*. 2015;25(4):237–50.

59. Quirce S, Vandenplas O, Campo P, Cruz MJ, de Blay F, Koschel D et al. Occupational hypersensitivity pneumonitis: An EAACI position paper. *Allergy*. 2016;71(6):765–79.

60. Rodríguez de Castro F, Carrillo T, Castillo R, Blanco C, Díaz F, Cuevas M. Relationships between characteristics of exposure to pigeon antigens. Clinical manifestations and humoral immune response. *Chest*. 1993;103(4):1059–63.

61. Cramer C, Schlünssen V, Bendstrup E, Stokholm ZA, Vestergaard JM, Frydenberg M et al. Risk of hypersensitivity pneumonitis and interstitial lung diseases among pigeon breeders. *Eur Respir J*. 2016;48(3):818–25.

62. Sood A, Sreedhar R, Kulkarni P, Nawoor AR. Hypersensitivity pneumonitis-like granulomatous lung disease with nontuberculous mycobacteria from exposure to hot water aerosols. *Environ Health Perspect*. 2007;115(2):262–6.

63. Burton CM, Crook B, Scaife H, Evans GS, Barber CM. Systematic review of respiratory outbreaks associated with exposure to water-based metalworking fluids. *Ann Occup Hyg*. 2012;56(4):374–88.

64. Tillie-Leblond I, Grenouillet F, Reboux G, Roussel S, Chouraki B, Lorthois C et al. Hypersensitivity pneumonitis and metalworking fluids contaminated by mycobacteria. *Eur Respir J*. 2011;37(3):640–7.

65. Baur X. Hypersensitivity pneumonitis (extrinsic allergic alveolitis) induced by isocyanates. *J Allergy Clin Immunol*. 1995;95(5 Pt 1):1004–10.

66. Fernández Pérez ER, Swigris JJ, Forssén AV, Tourin O, Solomon JJ, Huie TJ et al. Identifying an inciting antigen is associated with improved survival in patients with chronic hypersensitivity pneumonitis. *Chest*. 2013;144(5):1644–51.

67. Vogelmeier C. Extrinsic allergic alveolitis. In: Gibson GJ, Geddes DM, Costabel U, Sterk PJ, Corrin B, eds. *Respiratory Medicine*.

3rd ed. Philadelphia, PA: Saunders; 2003:1591–602.

68. Schuyler M, Cormier Y. The diagnosis of hypersensitivity pneumonitis. *Chest.* 1997;111(3):534–6.

69. Olson AL, Huie TJ, Groshong SD, Cosgrove GP, Janssen WJ, Schwarz MI et al. Acute exacerbations of fibrotic hypersensitivity pneumonitis: A case series. *Chest.* 2008;134(4):844–50.

70. Miyazaki Y, Tateishi T, Akashi T, Ohtani Y, Inase N, Yoshizawa Y. Clinical predictors and histologic appearance of acute exacerbations in chronic hypersensitivity pneumonitis. *Chest.* 2008;134(6):1265–70.

71. Kurup VP, Zacharisen MC, Fink JN. Hypersensitivity pneumonitis. *Indian J Chest Dis Allied Sci.* 2006;48(2):115–28.

72. McSharry C, Dye GM, Ismail T, Anderson K, Spiers EM, Boyd G. Quantifying serum antibody in bird fanciers' hypersensitivity pneumonitis. *BMC Pulm Med.* 2006;6:16.

73. Fenoglio CM, Reboux G, Sudre B, Mercier M, Roussel S, Cordier J-F et al. Diagnostic value of serum precipitins to mould antigens in active hypersensitivity pneumonitis. *Eur Respir J.* 2007;29(4):706–12.

74. Hisauchi-Kojima K, Sumi Y, Miyashita Y, Miyake S, Toyoda H, Kurup VP et al. Purification of the antigenic components of pigeon dropping extract, the responsible agent for cellular immunity in pigeon breeder's disease. *J Allergy Clin Immunol.* 1999;103(6):1158–65.

75. Ramírez-Venegas A, Sansores RH, Pérez-Padilla R, Carrillo G, Selman M. Utility of a provocation test for diagnosis of chronic pigeon breeder's disease. *Am J Respir Crit Care Med.* 1998;158(3):862–9.

76. Ohtani Y, Kojima K, Sumi Y, Sawada M, Inase N, Miyake S et al. Inhalation provocation tests in chronic bird fancier's lung. *Chest.* 2000;118(5):1382–9.

77. Patel RA, Sellami D, Gotway MB, Golden JA, Webb WR. Hypersensitivity pneumonitis: Patterns on high-resolution CT. *J Comput Assist Tomogr.* 2000;24(6):965–70.

78. Tateishi T, Ohtani Y, Takemura T, Akashi T, Miyazaki Y, Inase N et al. Serial high-resolution computed tomography findings of acute and chronic hypersensitivity pneumonitis induced by avian antigen. *J Comput Assist Tomogr.* 2011;35(2):272–9.

79. Silva CIS, Churg A, Müller NL. Hypersensitivity pneumonitis: Spectrum of high-resolution CT and pathologic findings. *AJR Am J Roentgenol.* 2007;188(2):334–44.

80. Franquet T, Hansell DM, Senbanjo T, Remy-Jardin M, Müller NL. Lung cysts in subacute hypersensitivity pneumonitis. *J Comput Assist Tomogr.* 2003;27(4):475–8.

81. Silva CIS, Müller NL, Fujimoto K, Kato S, Ichikado K, Taniguchi H et al. Acute exacerbation of chronic interstitial pneumonia: High-resolution computed tomography and pathologic findings. *J Thorac Imaging.* 2007;22(3):221–9.

82. Silva CIS, Müller NL, Lynch DA, Curran-Everett D, Brown KK, Lee KS et al. Chronic hypersensitivity pneumonitis: Differentiation from idiopathic pulmonary fibrosis and non-specific interstitial pneumonia by using thin-section CT. *Radiology.* 2008;246(1):288–97.

83. Malinen AP, Erkinjuntti-Pekkanen RA, Partanen PLK, Rytkönen HT, Vanninen RL. Long-term sequelae of Farmer's lung disease in HRCT: A 14-year follow-up study of 88 patients and 83 matched control farmers. *Eur Radiol.* 2003;13(9):2212–21.

84. Cordeiro CR, Jones JC, Alfaro T, Ferreira AJ. Bronchoalveolar lavage in occupational lung diseases. *Semin Respir Crit Care Med.* 2007;28(5):504–13.

85. Meyer KC, Raghu G, Baughman RP, Brown KK, Costabel U, du Bois RM et al. An official American Thoracic Society clinical practice guideline: The clinical utility of bronchoalveolar lavage cellular analysis in interstitial lung disease. *Am J Respir Crit Care Med.* 2012;185(9):1004–14.

86. Ohshimo S, Bonella F, Cui A, Beume M, Kohno N, Guzman J et al. Significance of bronchoalveolar lavage for the diagnosis of idiopathic pulmonary fibrosis. *Am J Respir Crit Care Med.* 2009;179(11):1043–7.

87. Ohtani Y, Saiki S, Kitaichi M, Usui Y, Inase N, Costabel U et al. Chronic bird fancier's lung: Histopathological and clinical correlation. An application of the 2002 ATS/ERS consensus classification of the idiopathic interstitial pneumonias. *Thorax.* 2005;60(8):665–71.

88. Trahan S, Hanak V, Ryu JH, Myers JL. Role of surgical lung biopsy in separating chronic hypersensitivity pneumonia from usual interstitial pneumonia/idiopathic pulmonary fibrosis: Analysis of 31 biopsies from 15 patients. *Chest*. 2008;134(1):126–32.

89. Pajares V, Puzo C, Castillo D, Lerma E, Montero MA, Ramos-Barbón D et al. Diagnostic yield of transbronchial cryobiopsy in interstitial lung disease: A randomized trial. *Respirology*. 2014;19(6):900–6.

90. Patel NM, Borczuk AC, Lederer DJ. Cryobiopsy in the diagnosis of interstitial lung disease. A step forward or back? *Am J Respir Crit Care Med*. 2016;193(7):707–9.

91. Hariri LP, Mino-Kenudson M, Shea B, Digumarthy S, Onozato M, Yagi Y et al. Distinct histopathology of acute onset or abrupt exacerbation of hypersensitivity pneumonitis. *Hum Pathol*. 2012;43(5):660–8.

92. Myers JL. Hypersensitivity pneumonia: The role of lung biopsy in diagnosis and management. *Mod Pathol Off J U S Can Acad Pathol Inc*. 2012 ;25(Suppl 1):S58–67.

93. Grunes D, Beasley MB. Hypersensitivity pneumonitis: A review and update of histologic findings. *J Clin Pathol*. 2013;66(10):888–95.

94. Costabel U, Bonella F, Guzman J. Chronic hypersensitivity pneumonitis. *Clin Chest Med*. 2012;33(1):151–63.

95. Castonguay MC, Ryu JH, Yi ES, Tazelaar HD. Granulomas and giant cells in hypersensitivity pneumonitis. *Hum Pathol*. 2015;46(4):607–13.

96. Vourlekis JS, Schwarz MI, Cool CD, Tuder RM, King TE, Brown KK. Nonspecific interstitial pneumonitis as the sole histologic expression of hypersensitivity pneumonitis. *Am J Med*. 2002;112(6):490–3.

97. Churg A, Myers J, Suarez T, Gaxiola M, Estrada A, Mejia M et al. Airway-centered interstitial fibrosis: A distinct form of aggressive diffuse lung disease. *Am J Surg Pathol*. 2004;28(1):62–8.

98. Takemura T, Akashi T, Kamiya H, Ikushima S, Ando T, Oritsu M et al. Pathological differentiation of chronic hypersensitivity pneumonitis from idiopathic pulmonary fibrosis/usual interstitial pneumonia. *Histopathology*. 2012;61(6):1026–35.

99. Morell F, Villar A, Montero M-Á, Muñoz X, Colby TV, Pipvath S et al. Chronic hypersensitivity pneumonitis in patients diagnosed with idiopathic pulmonary fibrosis: A prospective case-cohort study. *Lancet Respir Med*. 2013;1(9):685–94.

100. Akashi T, Takemura T, Ando N, Eishi Y, Kitagawa M, Takizawa T et al. Histopathologic analysis of sixteen autopsy cases of chronic hypersensitivity pneumonitis and comparison with idiopathic pulmonary fibrosis/usual interstitial pneumonia. *Am J Clin Pathol*. 2009;131(3):405–15.

101. Churg A, Sin DD, Everett D, Brown K, Cool C. Pathologic patterns and survival in chronic hypersensitivity pneumonitis. *Am J Surg Pathol*. 2009;33(12):1765–70.

102. Müller-Wening D, Repp H. Investigation on the protective value of breathing masks in farmer's lung using an inhalation provocation test. *Chest*. 1989;95(1):100–5.

103. Craig TJ, Hershey J, Engler RJ, Davis W, Carpenter GB, Salata K. Bird antigen persistence in the home environment after removal of the bird. *Ann Allergy*. 1992;69(6):510–2.

104. Kokkarinen JI, Tukiainen HO, Terho EO. Effect of corticosteroid treatment on the recovery of pulmonary function in farmer's lung. *Am Rev Respir Dis*. 1992;145(1):3–5.

105. Bradley B, Branley HM, Egan JJ, Greaves MS, Hansell DM, Harrison NK et al. Interstitial lung disease guideline: The British Thoracic Society in collaboration with the Thoracic Society of Australia and New Zealand and the Irish Thoracic Society. *Thorax*. 2008;63 (Suppl 5):v1–58.

106. Morisset J, Johannson KA, Vittinghoff E, Aravena C, Elicker BM, Jones KD et al. Use of mycophenolate mofetil or azathioprine for the management of chronic hypersensitivity pneumonitis. *Chest*. 2017;151(3):619–25.

107. Lota HK, Keir GJ, Hansell DM, Nicholson AG, Maher TM, Wells AU et al. Novel use of rituximab in hypersensitivity pneumonitis refractory to conventional treatment. *Thorax*. 2013;68(8):780–1.

108. Kern RM, Singer JP, Koth L, Mooney J, Golden J, Hays S et al. Lung transplantation for hypersensitivity pneumonitis. *Chest*. 2015;147(6):1558–65.

109. Hanley A, Hubbard RB, Navaratnam V. Mortality trends in asbestosis, extrinsic allergic alveolitis and sarcoidosis in England and Wales. *Respir Med.* 2011;105(9):1373–9.

110. Sansores R, Salas J, Chapela R, Barquin N, Selman M. Clubbing in hypersensitivity pneumonitis. Its prevalence and possible prognostic role. *Arch Intern Med.* 1990;150(9):1849–51.

111. de Gracia J, Morell F, Bofill JM, Curull V, Orriols R. Time of exposure as a prognostic factor in avian hypersensitivity pneumonitis. *Respir Med.* 1989;83(2):139–43.

112. Hanak V, Golbin JM, Hartman TE, Ryu JH. High-resolution CT findings of parenchymal fibrosis correlate with prognosis in hypersensitivity pneumonitis. *Chest.* 2008;134(1):133–8.

113. Mooney JJ, Elicker BM, Urbania TH, Agarwal MR, Ryerson CJ, Nguyen MLT et al. Radiographic fibrosis score predicts survival in hypersensitivity pneumonitis. *Chest.* 2013;144(2):586–92.

114. Vourlekis JS, Schwarz MI, Cherniack RM, Curran-Everett D, Cool CD, Tuder RM et al. The effect of pulmonary fibrosis on survival in patients with hypersensitivity pneumonitis. *Am J Med.* 2004;116(10):662–8.

115. Koschel DS, Cardoso C, Wiedemann B, Höffken G, Halank M. Pulmonary hypertension in chronic hypersensitivity pneumonitis. *Lung.* 2012;190(3):295–302.

12

Idiopathic interstitial pneumonias other than idiopathic pulmonary fibrosis

TOBY M MAHER

INTRODUCTION

The idiopathic interstitial pneumonias (IIPs) represent a group of diffuse parenchymal lung diseases comprising a number of distinct clinic–pathological entities. The most common of the IIPs, idiopathic pulmonary fibrosis (IPF) is dealt with elsewhere in this book. The remaining entities were first formally classified in an American Thoracic Society and European Respiratory Society joint guideline published in 2002 with a further update published in 2013 (1,2). The genesis for the 2002 guidelines was the observation that distinct histopathologic forms of idiopathic interstitial lung disease manifest distinct clinical syndromes with differences in radiologic appearances and, importantly, prognosis. The 2013 update reflected improved understanding of the IIPs gained following publication of the 2002 document. The key changes were the separation of IIPs into groups of major and rare disorders with further sub-division of the major group into chronic fibrosing, smoking-related and acute/subacute IIPs. With this in mind, this chapter provides an overview of the currently accepted IIP diagnostic entities with a focus on clinical presentation, diagnosis, clinical course and treatment (with the caveat that there are no approved or evidence-based treatments for this disparate group of disorders).

CHRONIC FIBROSING IIPs

Usual interstitial pneumonia (UIP)/idiopathic pulmonary fibrosis (IPF) and non-specific interstitial pneumonia (NSIP) have overlapping features and carry a worse prognosis than other chronic IIPs. IPF has been dealt with extensively in other chapters and has its own separate international consensus guidelines (3). As with other IIPs both UIP and NSIP occur in the context of a range of systemic diseases, especially connective tissue disease. As such diagnosis of the idiopathic form of the condition requires careful exclusion of other disorders.

NON-SPECIFIC INTERSTITIAL PNEUMONIA

NSIP as a distinct entity was introduced in the 2002 classification as a provisional terminology having first been described histologically in 1994 by Katzenstein and Fiorelli (Figure 12.1a) (4). It was noted at this time that NSIP had a histologic appearance distinct from desquamative interstitial pneumonitis (DIP), cryptogenic organizing pneumonia (COP) and acute interstitial pneumonia (AIP) and a better prognosis than UIP/IPF. In their original description, Katzenstein and Fiorelli divided NSIP into three groups: group 1, latterly known as cellular NSIP, characterized by interstitial inflammation only while group 3, referred to as fibrotic NSIP, is characterized by fibrosis with minimal inflammation. Group 2 is intermediate between groups 1 and 3 and describes individuals with mixed cellular and fibrotic NSIP. It remains unclear whether there is a continuum between cellular and fibrotic NSIP (i.e. does persistent cellular NSIP inevitably progress to fibrosis) or whether these are distinct lesions with overlapping patterns of distribution.

The decision to include NSIP as a separate IIP was, and remains, controversial given that there is no distinct clinical phenotype to identify individuals with this histologic lesion. In the years since 2002 it has been shown that NSIP and UIP can separately be found in the lungs of the same individual

(a) (b)

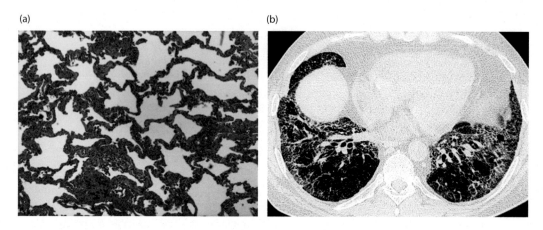

Figure 12.1 Typical histologic (a) and radiologic (b) appearances of NSIP. (a) Haematoxylin and eosin (H&E) section of surgical biopsy from 48-year-old lady with NSIP. Section shows homogeneous thickening of the intra-alveolar septae due to fibrosis but with preservation of overall lung architecture. (b) Demonstrates sections through lung bases of 54-year-old woman with NSIP. The image demonstrates basal and peripheral reticulation with ground-glass change and traction bronchiectasis but an absence of honeycombing.

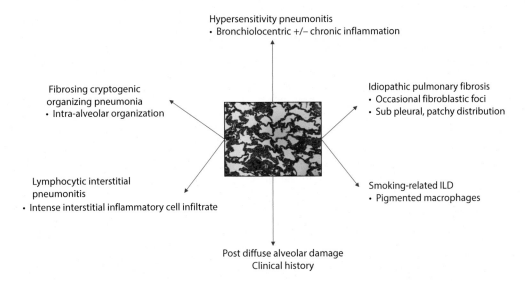

Figure 12.2 Important differential diagnoses to be considered in individuals presenting with NSIP. Each box highlights histopathologic features pointing to a diagnosis other than idiopathic NSIP.

undergoing biopsy (5). In some cases NSIP appears to progress radiologically and histologically to resemble UIP while in other cases the predominant lesion remains that of NSIP even in end-stage disease (6). A 2008 ATS workshop aiming to better define idiopathic NSIP illustrated a number of the challenges inherent in identifying and diagnosing the condition (7). Of 305 cases submitted by expert centres around the world only 6% fulfilled a multi-disciplinary team (MDT) consensus-classification of idiopathic NSIP. Of the 67 cases felt to have definite or probable NSIP a significant proportion had symptoms, signs or autoantibodies suggestive of an underlying connective tissue disease. Subsequent studies have demonstrated that both expert radiologists and expert pathologists struggle to reach agreement when trying to classify NSIP radiologically or histologically. This is then reflected in large variations between international centres in classifying the same cases NSIP at MDT discussion.

These issues of classification notwithstanding, NSIP can also be seen as a component of other IIPs, chronic hypersensitivity pneumonitis and drug-induced ILD. It is also the histologic lesion seen in 95% of cases of scleroderma-associated ILD and the majority of cases of mixed connective tissue disease-associated ILD. For these reasons, when NSIP is identified care should be taken to exclude other potential diagnoses. Figure 12.2 describes the important disease associations and highlights features which point to a diagnosis other than idiopathic NSIP.

Clinical features

The clinical characteristics of idiopathic NSIP overlap with those of IPF. Patients typically present with inexorably progressive breathlessness and cough. Clinical findings include clubbing in a minority and bilateral and basal Velcro-type crepitations. The average age of onset is younger than IPF with affected individuals typically being in their fifth decade. Unlike IPF there is no clear gender predilection. A proportion of patients present with symptoms and signs suggestive of autoimmune disease without fulfilling diagnostic criteria for a defined connective tissue disease. It has been proposed that such individuals be classified as having idiopathic pneumonia with auto-immune features (IPAF) (8). In some cases NSIP may be the presenting feature of a defined disorder such as scleroderma. Longitudinal disease behaviour is often important in defining such diagnoses and as such idiopathic NSIP should be periodically reviewed. The bronchoalveolar lavage profile of NSIP is indistinguishable from UIP. A finding of lymphocytosis suggests a diagnosis other than idiopathic NSIP.

Radiologic features

NSIP has a similar pattern of distribution radiographically to UIP/IPF being predominantly subpleural and basal with the key differences being an absence of honeycomb change and the presence of ground-glass attenuation (Figure 12.1b). In fibrotic NSIP there is evidence of fibrotic change within the ground-glass regions with reticulation and traction bronchiectasis. Consolidation is sometimes seen in cases of connective tissue disease-associated NSIP but is unusual in idiopathic cases.

Histologic features

In contrast to UIP, NSIP tends to demonstrate temporal and spatial uniformity with relative preservation of the alveolar architecture (Figure 12.1a). Fibrotic NSIP demonstrates marked septal thickening and fibrosis with mild or moderate associated inflammation. Fibroblastic foci, if present are sparse in number compared with UIP. Cellular NSIP demonstrates mild-to-moderate interstitial inflammation but an absence of fibrosis but with overlying type II pneumocyte hyperplasia. Pertinent negative findings are presented in Figure 12.2.

Clinical course and prognosis

NSIP carries a better prognosis than UIP/IPF. Nonetheless, fibrotic NSIP tends to be progressive and ultimately results in death from respiratory failure. Median survival is approximately 5–7 years from diagnosis. Cellular NSIP has a better prognosis and frequently resolves without long-term sequelae. Optimal therapy for NSIP remains to be defined. Cellular NSIP frequently responds to corticosteroid and/or immunosuppressant therapy. Treatment of fibrotic NSIP is typically less satisfactory with no consensus on best therapy. Many expert centres tend to tailor treatment according to which condition the individual with NSIP most resembles. In cases where there are autoimmune features then treatment mirroring that used for scleroderma ILD (i.e. low-dose corticosteroids, mycophenolate mofetil, cyclophosphamide or rituximab) is generally considered. In individuals more closely resembling IPF (e.g. older males or those with more rapidly progressive fibrosis) then treatment with anti-fibrotic drugs may be beneficial. It is hoped that the issue of best treatment will be addressed in forthcoming clinical trials.

SMOKING-RELATED IIPs

Respiratory-bronchiolitis-associated interstitial lung disease (RBILD) and DIP are diseases of macrophage accumulation with overlapping histologic appearances. Almost all cases of RBILD and the majority of cases of DIP occur in current smokers and for this reason these disorders are frequently viewed as being smoking related. Despite the similarities between RBILD and DIP there are sufficient differences between these disorders for them to be considered separate entities.

RESPIRATORY-BRONCHIOLITIS-ASSOCIATED INTERSTITIAL LUNG DISEASE

Clinical features

Respiratory bronchiolitis, characterized by the presence of pigmented intra-luminal macrophages within first- and second-generation bronchioles is a near universal finding in active cigarette smokers. In general it is associated with few, if any, symptoms but may contribute to small airway dysfunction. In a tiny minority of cigarette smokers RB progresses to cause ILD.

RBILD most commonly occurs in active cigarette smokers in their fourth or fifth decades. The majority of sufferers have a substantial cigarette exposure history (on average >30 pack-years). In most cases, the condition is associated with relatively minor symptoms. Those affected by the condition most frequently complain of mild but gradually progressive breathlessness and an exaggerated 'smoker's cough' productive of non-purulent sputum. In keeping with historic smoking patterns, men are more commonly affected than women. Clinical findings are often unremarkable with an absence of auscultatory abnormalities. In contrast with DIP finger clubbing is unusual.

Because of co-existent emphysema affected individuals may have a mixed obstructive and restrictive defect on spirometry with an associated moderate reduction in gas transfer. Bronchoalveolar lavage demonstrates pigmented macrophages indistinguishable from those seen in healthy cigarette smokers. An absence of pigmented macrophages should lead to consideration of an alternate diagnosis.

Radiographic features

The cardinal computed tomography (CT) findings in RBILD include thickening of the walls of central and peripheral bronchi, patchy ground-glass attenuation, centrilobular nodules and, less frequently, evidence of gas trapping. Because of the association with cigarette smoking mild-to-moderate centrilobular emphysema is a frequent co-existent finding (9). The nodules seen on CT correspond pathologically with macrophage accumulation and chronic inflammation of the respiratory bronchioles. Radiologically, important differential diagnoses to consider are hypersensitivity pneumonitis (which would be unusual in a current smoker), DIP and NSIP.

Histologic features

RB is characterized by clusters of dusty brown or golden macrophages within respiratory bronchioles, alveolar ducts and peribronchiolar alveolar spaces. These macrophages are accompanied by patchy sub-mucosal and peribronchiolar infiltrates of histiocytes and lymphocytes. The ILD component is characterized by peribronchiolar and alveolar septal fibrosis which becomes lined by hyperplastic type II pneumocytes and cuboidal bronchiolar-type epithelium. Coexistent centrilobular emphysema is also frequently seen.

Treatment and prognosis

RBILD is typically self-limiting and improves spontaneously with smoking cessation. Anecdotally, corticosteroids have been reported to be effective in individuals with symptomatic or progressive disease. Rare cases of progression to end-stage fibrosis are seen but this is unusual and for the majority prognosis is excellent if smoking cessation can be achieved (10).

DESQUAMATIVE INTERSTITIAL PNEUMONITIS

Clinical features

DIP is named based on a misnomer. The condition is characterized by alveoli filled with abundant foamy macrophages. Early descriptions of the disease mis-identified these macrophages as sloughed-off epithelium, hence use of the term 'desquamative'. While the condition most frequently occurs in active cigarette smokers, 20%–40% of those affected are non-smokers. In these individuals the condition may be associated with autoimmune disease or environmental exposure including passive cigarette smoke exposure.

Individuals afflicted by the disease tend to be in their fourth or fifth decade with men more frequently affected than women. Most present with progressive breathlessness and cough. Unlike RBILD, DIP can progress to end-stage fibrosis. Approximately a third of those affected develop progressive fibrosis resembling UIP/IPF which then often results in respiratory failure and premature death. Approximately 50% of individuals with DIP have finger clubbing. Lung function testing typically demonstrates restrictive spirometry with impaired gas transfer. Bronchoalveolar lavage demonstrates markedly increased numbers of pigmented macrophages with occasional corresponding increases in the numbers of neutrophils, eosinophils and lymphocytes.

Radiographic features

The cardinal CT feature of DIP is patchy ground-glass attenuation. This is more often basal and peripheral but with marked areas of geographic sparing (Figure 12.3a). In a minority of cases interlobular septal thickening may also be seen. In more advanced cases the basal ground-glass change evolves into honeycombing indicative of progressive fibrosis. In a small proportion of smokers there are overlapping radiologic features of DIP and RBILD.

Histologic features

DIP is characterized by abundant filling of the alveolar spaces with pigmented macrophages (Figure 12.3b). Additionally, there is often alveolar septal thickening with a sparse inflammatory cell infiltrate of plasma cells and eosinophils. The alveolar spaces are typically lined by plump, hyperplastic epithelial cells. In distinction from RBILD, DIP tends to be more uniform and lacks a bronchocentric pattern of distribution.

Treatment and prognosis

The majority of individuals with smoking-related DIP show improvement following smoking cessation (10). Best treatment of those with progressive or auto-immune-related DIP remains to be

(a)   (b)

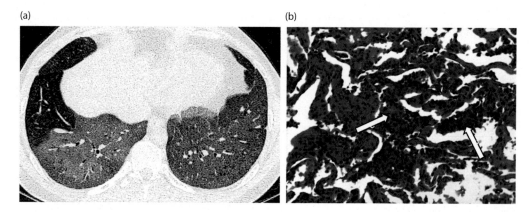

Figure 12.3 Typical CT (a) and histologic (b) appearances of desquamative interstitial pneumonia. CT (a) through the lung bases of a 41-year-old male smoker demonstrates diffuse patchy ground-glass attenuation with areas of spared normal lung and an absence of any features of fibrosis. Biopsy demonstrates preservation of lung architecture with alveolar spaces filled with abundant pigmented macrophages (*white arrows*).

defined. However, in most cases corticosteroids and, where necessary, other immunosuppressants appear to have a positive effect on the condition. Approximately a third of patients with DIP will develop end-stage fibrosis with associated respiratory impairment or failure. Survival at 10 years is approximately 70%; however, given the potential of the condition to progress it is important that patients are monitored appropriately to identify those most at need of treatment with the goal of preventing complications from disease progression.

ACUTE/SUBACUTE IIPs

AIP and COP are, for the most part, distinguishable from other IIPS by their relatively rapid onset of symptoms which develop over a period of days to a few weeks. Although the conditions have differing aetiologies both are grouped in the current classification based on their rapidity of onset. It should also be noted that other IIPs, most frequently UIP but also, albeit to a lesser extent, NSIP, can be complicated by acute exacerbations which resemble AIP (11). When assessing an acute-onset IIP it should therefore be borne in mind that the diagnosis may be one of a hitherto undiagnosed chronic IIP presenting with an acute exacerbation.

ACUTE INTERSTITIAL PNEUMONITIS

Clinical features

AIP is a rapidly progressive IIP characterized by widespread diffuse alveolar damage, which tends to result in hypoxaemic respiratory failure. The condition is similar to acute respiratory distress syndrome (ARDS) albeit without a cause. AIP is often preceded by a viral-type prodrome. Affected individuals, who tend to be in their fifth decade with no gender predilection, initially develop dyspnoea sometimes associated with a dry cough. This progresses over a few days to a few weeks to fulminant respiratory failure. The majority require mechanical ventilation.

Radiographic features

The CT features of AIP mirror those of ARDS with an early exudative phase, characterized by diffuse ground-glass attenuation, progressing to consolidation in a dependent distribution (Figure 12.4a). This then leads to an organizing stage with traction bronchiectasis and distortion of bronchovascular bundles with areas of consolidation being replaced by ground-glass attenuation. Occasional cysts are seen, often in anterior regions of initially spared lung tissue. Those who survive typically demonstrate full or near-complete resolution of the radiographic changes

(a)

(b)

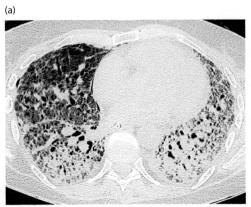
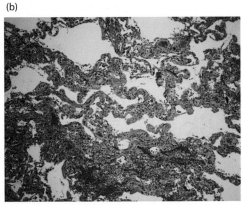

Figure 12.4 CT (a) and biopsy specimen (b) from a 63-year-old lady presenting with acute interstitial pneumonia. CT scan (a) obtained 2 weeks into the illness demonstrates dense consolidation with a gravitational gradient. The condition is beginning to organize as demonstrated by traction bronchiectasis. The biopsy (b) demonstrates the typical features of diffuse alveolar damage with inflammatory cell infiltrate, oedema and blood in the alveolar spaces together with hyaline membranes.

over time. If present residual abnormalities tend to comprise sub-pleural reticulation anteriorly in the mid- and upper zones. In the acute phase the finding of established fibrosis points to a pre-existing IIP with an acute exacerbation being the first presentation of disease.

Histologic features

The cardinal histologic abnormality in AIP is diffuse alveolar damage (Figure 12.4b). This is characterized by diffuse, temporally homogeneous alveolar epithelial injury, airway oedema and hyaline membranes with diffuse inflammatory cell infiltrate. Later in the organizing phase of the disease alveolar septal thickening and airspace organization can be seen. Important negative findings are an absence of granulomas, viral inclusions, micro-organisms or neutrophilic abscesses, all of which suggest alternate diagnoses.

Treatment and prognosis

Three-month mortality from AIP exceeds 50%. At present best treatment mirrors that administered to individuals with ARDS, with lung protective ventilation and careful attention to nutrition, glycaemic control and appropriate antimicrobial therapy. The role of corticosteroids and immunosuppression is controversial. A proportion of individuals with AIP have disease which later evolves into anti-synthetase syndrome or related autoimmune disorders. Where an underlying autoimmune disorder is strongly suspected there may be some merit in considering appropriate immunosuppressive strategies.

CRYPTOGENIC ORGANIZING PNEUMONIA

The 2002 IIP guidelines unified the nomenclature used to describe cryptogenic organizing pneumonia. Prior to the introduction of the guidelines COP was, in some countries, referred to as bronchiolitis obliterans organizing pneumonia (BOOP). COP was chosen as the preferred term as it more closely reflects the central histopathological lesion characterizing the condition. Since the publication of the 2002 guidelines there has been a growing understanding of the wide range of conditions which give rise to organizing pneumonia (Table 12.1). As such the number of truly cryptogenic cases of organizing pneumonia are diminishing as causation can be better ascribed. For instance, many of the previously observed treatment-resistant cases of COP have been shown to represent forms of anti-synthetase syndrome (12). This observation has been driven by the discovery of hitherto unrecognized anti-synthetase antibodies such as anti-PL7 and anti-mdm5. It is also now appreciated that the histologic lesion of organizing pneumonia can also be seen as a component of other disorders including

Table 12.1 Conditions associated with organizing pneumonia pattern on histology

Connective tissue disease (especially idiopathic inflammatory myositis and anti-synthetase syndrome)

Post radiotherapy (especially for breast cancer)

Distal to proximal obstruction

Inflammatory bowel disease

Post-infective/sequelae of aspiration pneumonitis

As part of other processes, e.g. vasculitis, abscesses, neoplasia

Acute hypersensitivity pneumonitis

Drugs (including chemotherapeutics, cocaine and gold salts)

Following bone marrow, lung, kidney and stem cell transplants

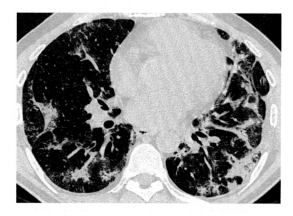

Figure 12.5 CT scan of a 38-year-old man with biopsy proving cryptogenic organizing pneumonia. Section from the lung base demonstrates patchy, multi-focal consolidation. The differential diagnosis for this appearance includes infection.

acute hypersensitivity pneumonitis and acute exacerbations of IPF. Organizing pneumonia can also be seen as an epi-phenomenon in infection and surrounding tumours or areas of vasculitic inflammation. This evolving understanding of the causes of OP makes interpretation of the COP literature especially challenging as historic observations undoubtedly include a number of now separate disorders.

Clinical features

COP occurs most frequently in non-smokers with a median age of onset in the sixth decade and with an equal gender predilection. Affected individuals frequently report a history of a few weeks to a few months of pneumonic-type symptoms with productive cough, worsening breathlessness, fatigue, malaise and weight loss. It is not unusual that individuals with COP will have had one or more unsuccessful treatment courses with antibiotics. On examination chest auscultation typically discloses coarse crepitations. Clubbing is not a feature of COP. Attention should be paid to ancillary features suggestive of an underlying condition associated with the organizing pneumonia, e.g. mechanics hands which would suggest dermatomyositis or an anti-synthetase syndrome. Resting hypoxaemia is common in COP and is often disproportionate to the extent of disease. This phenomenon may reflect shunting of blood through non-functioning consolidated regions of the lung.

Radiographic features

The principal finding in COP is airspace consolidation (Figure 12.5). This may be peripheral or peribronchial in distribution. It is more often multifocal and basal in distribution. In up to two-thirds of cases ground-glass attenuation may be seen in regions surrounding the consolidation. Pleural effusions are rare. Features of fibrosis including reticulation or traction bronchiectasis suggest an alternate diagnosis as does cavitation. Important radiologic differential diagnoses include community-acquired pneumonia, atypical mycobacterial disease, alveolar cell carcinoma, vasculitis, lymphoma or sarcoidosis. For this reason, and unlike many of the other IIPs, a diagnosis of COP can rarely be made on imaging alone. In the absence of an identified systemic disease such as anti-synthetase syndrome a tissue biopsy is generally required to confirm the presence of OP.

Histologic features

The key feature of organizing pneumonia is intraluminal organization comprising fibroblasts and connective tissue within alveoli, alveolar ducts and bronchioles with preservation of the underlying lung architecture. There is often a mild inflammatory cell infiltrate but an absence of granulomas, microorganisms, neutrophils or eosinophils. As noted, OP can occur in the context of other IIPs and so the presence of a UIP or NSIP pattern should be excluded.

Treatment and prognosis

COP tends to be responsive to corticosteroids (13). The vast majority of individuals affected recover fully following a tapering course of prednisolone or equivalent. A small proportion of individuals relapse following corticosteroid discontinuation and in such cases prolonged (12–24 months) therapy with low-dose corticosteroids combined with azathioprine or mycophenolate mofetil tends to be effective. Repeated relapse or progression of COP to fibrosis should prompt clinical re-evaluation with a particular emphasis on excluding an underlying systemic autoimmune disorder.

RARE IIPs

The concept of major and rare IIPs was introduced with the 2013 update of the IIP guidelines. This was done to reflect increased knowledge gained regarding the IIPs following the 2002 classification and to incorporate the newly recognized entity of pleuro-parenchymal fibroelastosis (PPFE) (14).

LYMPHOCYTIC INTERSTITIAL PNEUMONITIS

Lymphocytic interstitial pneumonitis was first described by Leibow and Carrington in 1969 and was included in the 2002 IIP guidelines as an idiopathic condition. It has, however, been increasingly recognized that LIP occurs either in the context of autoimmune disease (especially Sjögren syndrome [15]) or in certain immunodeficiency diseases including infection with human immunodeficiency virus (HIV) and severe combined immunodeficiency (SCID). Furthermore, in certain circumstances LIP appears to be a premalignant condition capable of developing into non-Hodgkin low grade B-cell mucosa-associated lymphoid tissue (MALT) lymphoma. With this in mind extreme caution should be exercised in concluding that any case of LIP is truly idiopathic.

Clinical features

LIP is more common in women than men and classically arises in the fourth or fifth decade. The most prominent early symptom is frequently an intractable dry cough. This is often followed by very insidiously worsening breathlessness. In keeping with the fact that most cases are auto-immune related, systemic features including fever, weight loss, sicca syndrome and arthralgia are common. Clinical findings are often sparse but occasionally fine crepitations are heard on auscultation of the chest. Bronchoalveolar lavage demonstrates a marked non-clonal lymphocytic infiltrate with lymphocytes usually accounting for more than 50% of the cell differential.

Radiologic features

The appearances of LIP are frequently quite varied. The most common finding is diffuse ground-glass change often with associated lung nodules and small thin-walled cysts (Figure 12.6). Upwards of 50% of affected individuals may have sub-pleural reticular changes and in a minority of cases honeycomb change is seen. Nodules increasing in size over time should raise the possibility of lymphoma and these should be investigated accordingly.

Histologic findings

The cardinal finding in LIP is extensive lymphoplasmocytic infiltration of the alveolar septae. Lymphoid follicles, often with germinal centres,

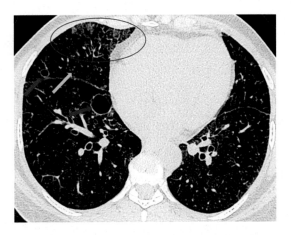

Figure 12.6 CT scan from a 56-year-old woman with Sjögren's related lymphocytic interstitial pneumonia. A section from the lung bases shows typical features of thin-walled cysts (*red arrows*), nodules (*green arrow*) and ground-glass attenuation with distraction of the underlying airways (*red circle*).

are frequently seen and these tend to follow the distribution of pulmonary lymphatics. Fibrosis of the alveolar septum together with occasional non-necrotizing granulomas may also be seen as may intra-alveolar organization and macrophage accumulation. The histologic differential diagnosis primarily includes MALT lymphoma or cellular NSIP.

Treatment and prognosis

Treatment in general should be targeted at the underlying cause of the LIP. In idiopathic cases corticosteroids and other immunosuppressants including hydroxychloroquine, mycophenolate mofetil and rituximab can be considered. A minority of cases progress to end-stage disease and the role of treatment in preventing such progression remains unclear. As noted LIP can progress to lymphoma and appropriate surveillance should be undertaken to exclude the development of this disease-related complication.

PLEURO-PARENCHYMAL FIBROELASTOSIS

Clinical features

PPFE is a new entity recognized for the first time in the 2013 guideline update. As the name suggests the condition is characterized by fibrosis of both the pleura and sub-pleural lung. It typically occurs in the upper lobes but may be associated with other histologic sub-types of IIP most usually UIP. In reported series it arises in individuals in the fifth and sixth decades of life with no gender predilection (16). Many individuals with the disease report a history of recurrent lower respiratory tract infection. A number of familial cases have been described and these tend to occur at an earlier age (17). PPFE has also been reported as a late complication of bone marrow transplant and as a form of chronic rejection following lung transplantation. Clinical findings are often unremarkable. Signs, when present, tend to be in the upper zone and may comprise crepitations or, in advanced cases, bronchial breathing. Spirometry tends to demonstrate a marked restrictive defect with relative preservation of diffusion capacity.

Radiologic appearance

PPFE results in sub-pleural fibrosis usually in an upper lobe distribution. As the disease advances the upper lobes lose considerable volume with elevation of the hilae and tenting of the diaphragms (Figure 12.7a, b). The fibrosis in places becomes confluent giving the appearance of patchy consolidation with traction bronchiectasis

(a)   (b)

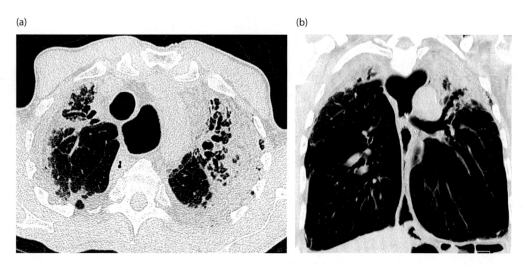

Figure 12.7 Axial (a) and coronal (b) CT reconstructions from a 68-year-old man with pleuroparenchymal fibroelastosis. Axial CT scan demonstrates dense pleural and sub-pleural fibrosis characterized by elements of consolidation admixed with reticulation and traction bronchiectasis. The coronal section (b) illustrates the upper lobe nature of the condition with marked loss of volume of the upper lobes with a shift in the position of the hilae and tenting of the diaphragm.

and distortion of the lung architecture. In up to a third of cases there may be co-existent changes suggestive of UIP/IPF or chronic hypersensitivity pneumonitis.

Histologic appearances

The characteristic appearance of PPFE is elastotic fibrosis of pleura and sub-pleural lung. In addition to alveolar septal involvement there tends to be evidence of intra-alveolar organization. These changes can best be appreciated using specific elastin stains.

Treatment and prognosis

The clinical course of PPFE remains to be fully defined. As many as 40%–60% of patients have progressive disease culminating in respiratory failure and premature death. Given the apparent roles played by infection and immune dysregulation in the pathogenesis of PPFE many centres advocate therapy with prophylactic antimicrobials (antibiotics and/or antifungals) and low-dose immunomodulation (in the form of either low-dose corticosteroids or hydroxychloroquine).

UNCLASSIFIABLE ILD

The ATS/ERS guidelines acknowledge that even in circumstances where all available clinical investigations are performed some cases of IIP defy multidisciplinary team classification according to the current guideline criteria. In some further cases it is not possible to undertake more invasive investigations, particularly surgical biopsy. Difficulty in classifying IIPs can be driven by (1) discordant clinical, radiologic and pathological data; (2) overlapping histologic entities either at the point of diagnosis or on serial images; or (3) modification of the underlying disease process by partial therapy. Interstitial pneumonia with auto-immune features has been proposed as a diagnostic classification for the subset of individuals who are unclassifiable due to the presence of auto-immune features in the absence of a defined connective tissue disease. The relevance of this classifier has yet to be confirmed in prospective studies.

In retrospective studies from dedicated ILD centres it has been estimated that 10%–15% of individuals presenting with idiopathic ILD have an unclassifiable condition (18). Outcomes in this group tend to be intermediate between IPF and non-IPF IIPs. At present guidelines advocate treating individuals with unclassifiable ILD based on a working diagnosis which approximates the condition to the IIP which it most closely resembles. Clinical trials are ongoing assessing the utility of anti-fibrotic drugs in this sub-group of patients (NCT02999178).

DECLARATIONS OF INTEREST

Toby M Maher has no declarations directly related to this manuscript. He has, however, received industry-academic research funding from GlaxoSmithKline R&D, UCB and Novartis and has received consultancy or speakers fees from Astra Zeneca, Bayer, Biogen Idec, Boehringer Ingelheim, Cipla, Dosa, Galapagos, GlaxoSmithKline R&D, ProMetic, Roche (and previously InterMune), Sanofi-Aventis, Takeda and UCB.

ACKNOWLEDGEMENTS

Toby Maher is supported by an NIHR Clinician Scientist Fellowship (NIHR Ref: CS-2013-13-017).

REFERENCES

1. ATS/ERS. American Thoracic Society/ European Respiratory Society International Multidisciplinary Consensus Classification of the Idiopathic Interstitial Pneumonias. This joint statement of the American Thoracic Society (ATS), and the European Respiratory Society (ERS) was adopted by the ATS board of directors, June 2001 and by the ERS Executive Committee, June 2001. *Am J Respir Crit Care Med.* 2002;165(2):277–304.
2. Travis WD, Costabel U, Hansell DM, King TE, Jr., Lynch DA, Nicholson AG et al. An official American Thoracic Society/ European Respiratory Society statement: Update of the international multidisciplinary classification of the idiopathic interstitial pneumonias. *Am J Respir Crit Care Med.* 2013;188(6):733–48.
3. Raghu G, Collard HR, Egan JJ, Martinez FJ, Behr J, Brown KK et al. An official ATS/ERS/ JRS/ALAT statement: idiopathic pulmonary

fibrosis: Evidence-based guidelines for diagnosis and management. *Am J Respir Crit Care Med.* 2011;183(6):788–824.

4. Katzenstein AL, Fiorelli RF. Nonspecific interstitial pneumonia/fibrosis. Histologic features and clinical significance. *Am J Surg Pathol.* 1994;18(2):136–47.

5. Flaherty KR, Travis WD, Colby TV, Toews GB, Kazerooni EA, Gross BH et al. Histopathologic variability in usual and non-specific interstitial pneumonias. *Am J Respir Crit Care Med.* 2001;164(9):1722–7.

6. Katzenstein AL, Zisman DA, Litzky LA, Nguyen BT, Kotloff RM Usual interstitial pneumonia: histologic study of biopsy and explant specimens. *Am J Surg Pathol.* 2002;26(12):1567–77.

7. Travis WD, Hunninghake G, King TE, Jr., Lynch DA, Colby TV, Galvin JR et al. Idiopathic nonspecific interstitial pneumonia: Report of an American Thoracic Society project. *Am J Respir Crit Care Med.* 2008;177(12):1338–47.

8. Luppi F, Wells AU. Interstitial pneumonitis with autoimmune features (IPAF): A work in progress. *Eur Respir J.* 2016;47(6):1622–4.

9. Attili AK, Kazerooni EA, Gross BH, Flaherty KR, Myers JL, Martinez FJ. Smoking-related interstitial lung disease: Radiologic-clinical-pathologic correlation. *Radiographics.* 2008;28(5):1383–96; discussion 1396–8.

10. Craig PJ, Wells AU, Doffman S, Rassl D, Colby TV, Hansell DM et al. Desquamative interstitial pneumonia, respiratory bronchiolitis and their relationship to smoking. *Histopathology.* 2004;45(3):275–82.

11. Collard HR, Ryerson CJ, Corte TJ, Jenkins G, Kondoh Y, Lederer DJ et al. Acute exacerbation of Idiopathic pulmonary fibrosis.

An International Working Group report. *Am J Respir Crit Care Med.* 2016;194(3):265–75.

12. Fischer A, Swigris JJ, du Bois RM, Lynch DA, Downey GP, Cosgrove GP et al. Antisynthetase syndrome in ANA and anti-Jo-1 negative patients presenting with idiopathic interstitial pneumonia. *Respir Med.* 2009;103(11):1719–24.

13. Lazor R, Vandevenne A, Pelletier A, Leclerc P, Court-Fortune I, Cordier JF Cryptogenic organizing pneumonia. Characteristics of relapses in a series of 48 patients. The Groupe d'Etudes et de Recherche sur les Maladles 'Orphelines' Pulmonaires (GERM'O'P). *Am J Respir Crit Care Med.* 2000;162(2 Pt 1):571–7.

14. Kokosi MA, Nicholson AG, Hansell DM, Wells AU. Rare idiopathic interstitial pneumonias: LIP and PPFE and rare histologic patterns of interstitial pneumonias: AFOP and BPIP. *Respirology.* 2016;21(4):600–14.

15. Parambil JG, Myers JL, Lindell RM, Matteson EL, Ryu JH. Interstitial lung disease in primary Sjogren syndrome. *Chest.* 2006;130(5):1489–95.

16. Reddy TL, Tominaga M, Hansell DM, von der Thusen J, Rassl D, Parfrey H et al. Pleuroparenchymal fibroelastosis: a spectrum of histopathological and imaging phenotypes. *Eur Respir J.* 2012;40(2):377–85.

17. Newton CA, Batra K, Torrealba J, Kozlitina J, Glazer CS, Aravena C et al. Telomere-related lung fibrosis is diagnostically heterogeneous but uniformly progressive. *Eur Respir J.* 2016;48(6):1710–20.

18. Ryerson CJ, Urbania TH, Richeldi L, Mooney JJ, Lee JS, Jones KD et al. Prevalence and prognosis of unclassifiable interstitial lung disease. *Eur Respir J.* 2013;42(3):750–7.

13

Eosinophilic interstitial lung disorders

VINCENT COTTIN AND CLAUDIA VALENZUELA

BACKGROUND

Eosinophilic lung diseases are a group of diffuse parenchymal lung diseases characterized by the prominent infiltration by polymorphonuclear eosinophils into the lung interstitium and the alveolar spaces. Eosinophilic lung diseases usually respond dramatically to systemic corticosteroids. As the lung architecture is preserved, healing occurs without any sequelae in almost all cases.

Regardless of possible causes, the main clinical radiologic presentations include acute pneumonia (symptoms for less than 1 month), chronic pneumonia, eosinophilic lung disease in the context of systemic conditions or the transient Löffler syndrome, generally of parasitic origin.

Blood *eosinophilia* is defined by an eosinophil blood cell count greater than 0.5×10^9/L, and *hypereosinophilia* by an eosinophil blood cell count greater than 1.5×10^9 on two examinations with at least a 1-month interval (1–3). Alveolar eosinophilia is defined by differential cell count greater than 25% eosinophils at bronchoalveolar lavage (BAL) (and preferably greater than 40%) (2). BAL eosinophilia is especially diagnostic when eosinophils represent the predominant cell in BAL, macrophages excepted.

Following differentiation of precursors in the bone marrow under the action of interleukin (IL)-5, IL-3, and granulocyte macrophage colony-stimulating factor, eosinophils are recruited in the blood and tissue in response to circulating IL-5, eotaxins, and the C-C chemokine receptor-3. Because recruitment of eosinophils to tissues is organ specific, tissue and blood eosinophilia are not necessarily associated. Eosinophils are major players in immunity against parasites and pathogenesis of allergic diseases, however may also cause normal tissue injury. The prominence of IL-5 in eosinophil differentiation and recruitment has led to the development of anti-IL-5 monoclonal antibodies to selectively target the eosinophil lineage in humans.

Eosinophils interact with the majority of lung cells through cell membrane signalling molecules and receptors including toll-like receptors and receptors for cytokines, immunoglobulins and complement. They participate to innate immunity and produce numerous pro-inflammatory mediators. Eosinophilic cationic proteins released by degranulation of activated eosinophils exert direct cytotoxicity, up-regulate chemoattraction and expression of adhesion molecules, regulate vascular permeability and induce the contraction of smooth muscle cells, thereby causing inflammation and tissue damage. Importantly, eosinophils are also involved in adaptive immunity against bacteria, viruses and tumours through interaction with T-lymphocytes, present antigens to T helper-2 cells, and amplify the T helper-2 response in the lung through a positive feedback loop mediated by IL-4, IL-5 and IL-13.

IDIOPATHIC CHRONIC EOSINOPHILIC PNEUMONIA

SCIENTIFIC MECHANISMS

Idiopathic chronic eosinophilic pneumonia (ICEP) directly reflects the reversible infiltration of the lungs by activated eosinophils, which release numerous pro-inflammatory molecules and express activation markers. Recent studies have suggested a possible role for clonal blood and lung tissue T cells, similar to the lymphocytic variant of the idiopathic HES, however without clinical implication to date.

EPIDEMIOLOGY

Idiopathic chronic eosinophilic pneumonia (ICEP) is a rare disease, and represents less than 3% of cases of all interstitial lung diseases (ILDs). However, it is the most common of the eosinophilic pneumonias in non-tropical areas. It predominates in women (2:1 female/male ratio) (4,5). The median age at diagnosis is 45 years. No genetic predisposition has been identified. Two-thirds of the patients have a prior history of asthma, and half have a history of atopy (4,5). Most patients are non-smokers (4–6).

HISTORY AND EXAMINATION

ICEP is characterized by the onset over a few weeks of cough, dyspnoea, malaise and weight loss, with diffuse pulmonary infiltrates (7). The onset of ICEP is progressive or subacute, with several weeks or months between the onset of symptoms and the diagnosis (4,5). Shortness of breath is the prominent clinical manifestation, present in 60%–90% of patients. Cough (90%), rhinitis or sinusitis (20%) and rarely chest pain or haemoptysis (10% or less) may be present (4,5). Respiratory failure requiring mechanical ventilation is exceptional, in contrast with idiopathic acute eosinophilic pneumonia (IAEP). Wheezes or crackles are found in one third of patients at auscultation.

About 75% of the patients with ICEP experience asthma at some time throughout the course of disease. Asthma can precede the onset of ICEP, occur concomitantly (8) or present as long-term persistent airflow obstruction despite oral and inhaled corticosteroid therapy (8).

Systemic symptoms are frequently seen with fatigue, malaise, fever, anorexia, night sweats and weight loss (occasionally severe) (4,5). Extrathoracic manifestations should be absent, although non-abundant pericardial effusion or arthralgia (4,7) have been reported.

INVESTIGATIONS

BAL eosinophilia greater than 25% confirms the diagnosis of eosinophilic lung disease in the appropriate setting. It is present in all patients with ICEP who have not yet received systemic corticosteroids. The BAL eosinophil count is commonly greater than 40%, with a mean of 58% in large series. High-level peripheral blood eosinophilia is common, with mean values of 5000–6000/mm³ (5), but may be lacking in patients who have received systemic corticosteroids. Blood C-reactive protein and total immunoglobulin (Ig) E levels are elevated but have no specificity.

Approximately half the patients with ICEP have airflow obstruction, and the other half have a restrictive ventilatory defect associated with multiple consolidations at imaging. Carbon monoxide transfer factor and coefficient are frequently reduced. Mild hypoxemia may be present (4,5).

Working diagnostic criteria for ICEP are found in Table 13.1 (2). In the setting of a characteristic clinical and radiologic presentation, the presence of eosinophilia at BAL (>25% [2]) confirms the diagnosis and obviates the need for lung biopsy. Particular attention must be paid to thoroughly investigate for potential causes of eosinophilia before the condition can be considered idiopathic, especially drug intake, exposure to toxins, illicit drug use and infections with parasites and fungi. Markedly elevated peripheral blood eosinophilia together with typical clinical radiologic features also strongly suggest the diagnosis of ICEP, and BAL may not be mandatory in such cases.

RADIOLOGY

As imaging abnormalities rapidly resolve upon corticosteroid therapy (12), it is important that they be obtained before initiation of treatment. The imaging features of ICEP typically consist of bilateral alveolar infiltrates with ill-defined margins. The characteristic peripheral predominance (negative of pulmonary oedema), and the spontaneous migration of the opacities (also observed in cryptogenic organizing pneumonia) are each observed in about 25% of cases (4).

On high-resolution computed tomography (HRCT) (4,13), typical features consist of confluent consolidations and ground-glass opacities (Figure 13.1), almost always bilateral and predominating in the upper lobes and peripheral sub-pleural areas. This pattern is sufficiently typical to suggest the diagnosis of ICEP in about 75% of cases in the appropriate setting (14). Septal line thickening, band-like opacities parallel to the chest, mediastinal lymph node enlargement or mild pleural effusion, may be found, but cavitary lesions are exceedingly rare.

PATHOLOGY

The diagnosis of ICEP does not require a lung biopsy, which therefore is performed only in rare cases when the diagnosis was not suspected and BAL was not done prior to treatment. Pathology is characterized by prominent infiltration of the lung interstitium and the alveolar spaces by eosinophils (5,7) accompanied by a fibrinous exudate, with preservation of the lung architecture. Occasional lesions of eosinophilic microabscesses, non-necrotizing vasculitis, or multinucleated giant cells can also be found, but granulomas are absent.

GENERAL MANAGEMENT

Spontaneous resolution can occur, but drug therapy is usually preferred to simple observation because of marked symptoms and dramatic response to corticosteroids (clinical improvement within 2 days, clearing of chest opacities within 1 week [4,5]).

To induce remission of disease, oral prednisone may be initiated at a dose of 0.5 mg/kg/day for 2 weeks, followed by 0.25 mg/kg/day for 2 weeks, then progressively reduced over a total duration of about 3 to 6 months and stopped (2,4,15). A recent study found no difference in the relapse rate between a 3-month and a 6-month treatment regimen (16).

Table 13.1 Working diagnostic criteria.

Idiopathic chronic eosinophilic pneumonia	1. Diffuse pulmonary alveolar consolidation with air bronchograms and/or ground-glass opacities at chest imaging, especially with peripheral predominance
	2. Eosinophilia at BAL differential cell count ≥40% (or peripheral blood eosinophilias ≥1000/mm³)
	3. Respiratory symptoms present for at least 2–4 weeks
	4. Absence of other known causes of eosinophilic lung disease (especially exposure to drug susceptible to induce pulmonary eosinophilia)
Idiopathic acute eosinophilic pneumonia	1. Acute onset with febrile respiratory manifestations (≤1 month, and especially ≤7 days duration before medical examination)
	2. Bilateral diffuse infiltrates on imaging
	3. Pao_2 on room air ≤60 mm Hg (8 kPa), or Pao_2/Fio_2 ≤300 mm Hg (40 kPa), or oxygen saturation on room air <90%
	4. Lung eosinophilia, with ≥25% eosinophils at BAL differential cell count (or eosinophilic pneumonia at lung biopsy when done)
	5. Absence of determined cause of acute eosinophilic pneumonia (including infection or exposure to drugs known to induce pulmonary eosinophilia); recent onset of tobacco smoking or exposure to inhaled dusts may be present
Eosinophilic granulomatosis with polyangiitis[a]	1. Asthma
	2. Peripheral blood eosinophilia >1500/mm³ and/or alveolar eosinophilia >25%
	3. Extrapulmonary clinical manifestations of disease (other than rhinosinusitis), with at least one of the following:
	a. Systemic manifestation typical of the disease: mononeuritis multiplex or cardiomyopathy confidently attributed to the eosinophilic disorder or palpable purpura
	b. Any extrapulmonary manifestation with histopathological evidence of vasculitis as demonstrated especially by skin, muscle or nerve biopsy
	c. Any extrapulmonary manifestation with evidence of antineutrophil cytoplasmic antibodies with antimyeloperoxidase or antiproteinase 3 specificity
Allergic bronchopulmonary aspergillosis (in patients with asthma and central bronchiectasis)	1. Asthma
	2. Central bronchiectasis (inner 2/3 of chest CT field)
	3. Immediate cutaneous reactivity to Aspergillus
	4. Total serum IgE concentration >417 kU/L (1000 mg/mL)
	5. Elevated serum IgE-Aspergillus fumigatus and/or IgG-A. fumigatus (Infiltrates on chest radiograph and serum precipitating antibodies to A. fumigatus may be present but are not minimal essential diagnostic criteria.)

(Continued)

Table 13.1 (*Continued*) Working diagnostic criteria.

Allergic bronchopulmonary aspergillosis (in patients with asthma (ABPA–seropositive)	Patients with the above criteria 1, 3, 4, 5 (Infiltrates on chest radiograph may be present but are not a minimal essential diagnostic criteria.)
Allergic bronchopulmonary aspergillosis (in patients with cystic fibrosis)	1. Clinical deterioration (increased cough, wheezing, exercise intolerance, increase sputum, decrease in pulmonary function) 2. Immediate cutaneous reactivity to *Aspergillus* or presence of IgE-A. *fumigatus* 3. Total serum IgE concentration ≥1000 kU/L 4. Precipitating antibodies to A. *fumigatus* or serum IgG-A. *fumigatus* 5. Abnormal chest radiograph (infiltrates, mucus plugging, or a change from earlier films)
Hypereosinophilic obliterative bronchiolitis	1. Demonstration of bronchiolitis, by lung biopsy and/or HRCT showing direct signs of bronchiolitis (centrilobular nodules and branching opacities) 2. Peripheral blood and/or alveolar eosinophilia, 3. Persistent airflow obstruction despite high-dose inhaled bronchodilators and corticosteroids

Source: Adapted from Cottin V, Cordier JF. *Orphan Lung Diseases: A Clinical Guide to Rare Lung Disease.* London, UK: Springer-Verlag; 2015:227–51; Cottin V et al. *Autoimmun Rev.* 2017;16:1–9; Agarwal R et al. *Clin Exp Allergy.* 2013;43:850–73; Cordier JF et al. *Eur Respir J.* 2013;41:1126–34.

[a] When a single extrapulmonary manifestation attributable to the systemic disease is present, disease may be called forme *fruste* of eosinophilic granulomatosis with polyangiitis.

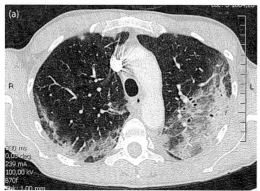

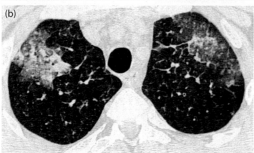

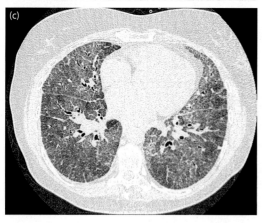

Figure 13.1 **(a)** Chest CT of a patient with idiopathic chronic eosinophilic pneumonia, demonstrating peripheral airspace consolidation predominating in the upper lobes. **(b)** Chest CT of a patient with eosinophilic granulomatosis with polyangiitis, demonstrating peripheral airspace consolidation predominating in the upper lobes. **(c)** Chest CT of a patient with eosinophilic iatrogenic interstitial lung disease related to flecainide, showing diffuse ground-glass attenuation and some reticulation.

Relapses occur in more than half the patients while decreasing or after stopping corticosteroids, and patients should be informed of this possibility. Relapses respond very well to prednisone, which can be resumed at a dose of 20 mg/day, then progressively tapered and then stopped. Such approach of accepting some risk of relapse reduces the patient's overall exposure to long-term corticosteroids and minimizes their side effects.

SPECIFIC ASPECTS OF MANAGEMENT

Patients with ICEP and asthma should receive inhaled corticosteroids. Whether inhaled corticosteroids may be useful in non-asthmatic patients with ICEP is unknown.

PROGNOSIS AND LONG-TERM OUTLOOK

There are no long-term sequelae or death of ICEP. Long-term follow-up is however necessary (4) (a) to minimize treatment with oral corticosteroids, (b) to manage adverse events related to corticosteroids, and (c) to monitor possible persistent airflow obstruction that may develop despite bronchodilators and inhaled corticosteroids and often oral low-dose corticosteroids (17).

IDIOPATHIC ACUTE EOSINOPHILIC PNEUMONIA

SCIENTIFIC MECHANISMS

The mechanisms that lead to the acute onset of eosinophilic infiltration of the lung with a presentation distinct from that of ICEP are unknown.

EPIDEMIOLOGY

IAEP occurs acutely in previously healthy young adults, with a mean age of about 30 years, male predominance (18–23), and usually no history of asthma. Two-thirds of patients are smokers.

The disease can be triggered by various respiratory exposures related to

- Tobacco smoking: a recent initiation of tobacco smoking, a change in smoking habits, smoking large quantities, restarting to smoke or even short-term passive smoking. (22–24)
- Non-specific environmental inhaled contaminants, especially when inhaled acutely. (15)

Table 13.2 Distinctive features between idiopathic chronic eosinophilic pneumonia (ICEP) and idiopathic acute eosinophilic pneumonia (IAEP)

	ICEP	IAEP
Onset	>2–4 weeks	<1 month
History of asthma	Yes	No
Smoking history	10% of smokers	Two-thirds of smokers, often recent initiation
Respiratory failure	No	Usual
Initial blood eosinophilia	Yes, on admission	No (delayed)
BAL eosinophilia	>25%	>25%
Chest imaging	Homogeneous, peripheral airspace consolidation	Bilateral patchy areas of ground-glass attenuation, airspace consolidation, interlobular septal thickening, bilateral pleural effusion
Relapse	Yes	No

The term 'idiopathic' is debatable in such cases with identifiable triggers (2). In addition, parasites, fungi, viruses, red spiders, drugs, over-the-counter medications, illicit drugs, allogenic hematopoietic stem cell transplantation and acquired immunodeficiency virus infection are possible aetiologies of AEP (2,15).

HISTORY AND EXAMINATION

IAEP is both dramatic and frequently misdiagnosed, because it mimics infectious pneumonia or acute respiratory distress syndrome in previously healthy individuals (18,19). It differs from ICEP by its acute onset (symptoms since less than 1 month and usually less than 7 days [20,21]), the severity of hypoxemia, the usual lack of blood eosinophilia at the onset of disease and the absence of relapse (Table 13.2).

IAEP is characterized by acute onset of dyspnoea (100%), fever usually moderate (100%), cough (80%–100%) and thoracic pain (50%–70%) mostly pleuritic, sometimes with myalgias (30%–50%) or abdominal complaints (25%) (2). Acute respiratory failure is frequent (23), often meeting criteria for acute lung injury or for acute respiratory distress syndrome, and admission to the intensive care unit and mechanical ventilation are often required (20,22). Crackles are present in most patients at lung auscultation.

INVESTIGATIONS

Importantly, blood eosinophil count is *normal* at presentation in most cases of IAEP even untreated (21, 22), a feature that further contributes to potential misdiagnosis of IAEP as infectious pneumonia.

Within days after presentation, the eosinophil count rises to high values (20–22), a finding very evocative of IAEP. Given the usual lack of initial blood eosinophilia, BAL eosinophilia >25% is key to the diagnosis (20–22). BAL further shows negative cultures. BAL eosinophilia usually resolves with corticosteroid therapy, but may persist for several weeks. Causes listed under the epidemiology section must be ruled out.

Pulmonary function tests performed in the less severe cases show a restrictive ventilatory defect, with reduced carbon monoxide transfer capacity, and increased alveolar–arterial oxygen gradient of PO_2. Arterial blood gas demonstrates hypoxemia which is often severe.

Diagnostic criteria are listed in Table 13.1.

RADIOLOGY

The chest radiograph shows bilateral infiltrates, with mixed alveolar and interstitial opacities, especially Kerley lines (21,25,26). Chest HRCT demonstrates the typical combination of poorly defined nodules of ground-glass opacity (100%), interlobular septal thickening (90%), bilateral pleural effusion (76%) and airspace consolidation (55%) (27), which suggests the diagnosis in the appropriate setting. Thickening of bronchovascular bundles, lymph node enlargement and centrilobular nodules may also be found.

PATHOLOGY

A lung biopsy is only performed in rare cases when the diagnosis of eosinophilic pneumonia has not been suspected. It shows acute and organizing diffuse alveolar damage together with interstitial alveolar and bronchiolar infiltration by eosinophils, intra-alveolar eosinophils and interstitial oedema.

GENERAL MANAGEMENT

Treatment with systemic corticosteroids is recommended with a starting dose of oral prednisone of 30 mg/day, or 1–2 mg/kg/day of intravenous methylprednisolone in patients with respiratory failure. A total duration of 2 weeks may be sufficient (23). Clinical recovery occurs within 3 days on corticosteroid treatment (23,28). Imaging (20,21,23,26) and pulmonary function abnormalities (20,21) resolve within less than a month.

PROGNOSIS AND LONG-TERM OUTLOOK

IAEP has been lethal on very exceptional cases through extra-pulmonary organ failure or shock. Extracorporeal membrane oxygenation has been used occasionally.

In contrast with ICEP, IAEP does not relapse, unless tobacco smoking is resumed, in which case IAEP may or may not recur. Patients must be strongly encouraged to definitively quit smoking.

EOSINOPHILIC GRANULOMATOSIS WITH POLYANGIITIS

BACKGROUND

Eosinophilic granulomatosis with polyangiitis (EGPA, formerly, Churg–Strauss syndrome) was historically described mainly from autopsied cases (29), and is classified in the group of small-vessel vasculitides (30). It is defined as an eosinophil-rich and granulomatous inflammation often involving the respiratory tract, and necrotizing vasculitis predominantly affecting small-to-medium-sized vessels which is associated with asthma and eosinophilia. EGPA is associated in about 40% of cases to antineutrophil cytoplasmic antibodies (ANCA) and therefore belongs to the pulmonary ANCA-associated vasculitides.

SCIENTIFIC MECHANISMS

Although the cause for EGPA has not been identified, several triggering or adjuvant factors have been identified or suspected (15,31,32): infectious agents (*Aspergillus*, *Candida*, *Ascaris*, *Actinomyces*), bird exposure, cocaine, drugs (sulphonamides used together with antiserum, diflunisal, macrolides, diphenylhydantoin and omalizumab), allergic hyposensitizations and vaccinations. Clonal T cells may also play a role.

EPIDEMIOLOGY

The incidence of EGPA has been estimated as 0.5–6.8 cases/million inhabitants/year, and the prevalence as 10.7–13 cases/million (32). EGPA predominates between 30 and 50 years of age, with no gender predominance (33–36). A genetic predisposition has been linked to the major histopathology complex DRB4 allele, and polymorphisms have been correlated with presence of ANCA. Familial cases are exceedingly rare.

A definite history of allergy or atopy is found in less than 30% of patients (37,38). When present, allergy mainly consists of perennial allergies especially to *Dermatophagoides*. Seasonal allergies are less frequent than in control asthmatics (37,38).

The association between leukotriene-receptor antagonists (montelukast, zafirlukast, pranlukast) and EGPA has been well established, however whether there is causal relationship with a direct effect of these drugs on the vasculitis pathogenesis is uncertain (2,39). EGPA may be precipitated by reducing the dose of oral or inhaled corticosteroids in subjects with smouldering pre-existing disease (32,40). It is generally advisable to avoid leukotriene-receptor antagonists in asthmatics with eosinophilia.

HISTORY AND EXAMINATION

The natural course of EGPA has been described to follow three phases (34) with rhinosinusitis and asthma, blood and tissue eosinophilia and eventually systemic vasculitis, but these often overlap in time. Asthma is always present in EGPA, occurring at a mean age of about 35 years, generally severe and becoming rapidly corticodependent (34,36,38), and preceding the onset of the vasculitis by 3 to 9 years (33–36,38,41,42). Asthma may attenuate once the vasculitis is treated using systemic corticosteroids (34,38,42–44).

In addition to asthma, patients frequently present with eosinophilic pneumonia, similar to ICEP in presentation or more acute in onset. The eosinophilic pneumonia rapidly resolves upon corticosteroid treatment, and may be missed.

Chronic rhinosinusitis (75% of cases) lacks specificity and may consist of chronic paraseptal sinusitis, crusty rhinitis, nasal obstruction or nasal polyposis. When performed, biopsies demonstrate eosinophilic infiltration of the sinusal mucosa. Septal nasal perforation does not occur.

General symptoms are present in two-thirds of patients (asthenia, weight loss, fever, arthralgias, myalgias). Any organ system can be affected by the systemic disease through eosinophilic infiltration and/or granulomatous vasculitis. Heart and kidney involvement are frequently insidious and must be systematically investigated due to potential morbidity and mortality (9).

Cardiac involvement is due to eosinophilic myocarditis and less commonly to coronary arteritis. The spectrum of manifestations ranges from asymptomatic cardiac involvement to sudden death as well as acute or chronic cardiac failure. Any patient with suspected EGPA should undergo a systematic cardiac evaluation with electrocardiogram, echocardiography, N-terminal pro-brain natriuretic peptide and serum level of troponin I. Magnetic resonance imaging of the heart may be useful when cardiac involvement is suspected, although the clinical significance of subclinical abnormalities is unknown.

INVESTIGATIONS

Peripheral blood eosinophilia is particularly marked, with values of 5 to 20,000/mm^3 at diagnosis (34,36,38,42). BAL eosinophilia may be present even in the absence of consolidation on the chest CT. Increase in serum IgE and C-reactive protein levels is nonspecific.

Although EGPA is one of the ANCA-associated pulmonary vasculitides, ANCA are found in only 40% of patients, and their absence certainly does not exclude the diagnosis. When present, ANCAs are mainly perinuclear-ANCA with myeloperoxidase specificity (35,36,45–47), which support the diagnosis of EGPA. Different clinical phenotypes of

disease have been reported in ANCA-positive and ANCA-negative patients (45–49), and in patients with or without definite features of systemic vasculitis (*polyangiitis*) (9).

Airflow obstruction is present in 70% of patients at diagnosis despite inhaled bronchodilator and high-dose inhaled corticosteroid therapy for asthma (38,43).

The diagnosis may be difficult in patients with asthma, blood eosinophilia and mild or single-organ extrathoracic manifestations, i.e. with the '*formes frustes*' of EGPA, or in subjects already receiving corticosteroids. It is crucial that the diagnosis be established before severe organ involvement (especially cardiac) is present. Working diagnostic criteria have recently been proposed (Table 13.1).

RADIOLOGY

Chest imaging abnormalities in patients with EGPA are twofold:

- Pulmonary infiltrates (50%–70%) corresponding to eosinophilic pneumonia and consisting of ill-defined opacities, sometimes migratory, with peripheral predominance or random distribution, and density varying from ground-glass opacities to airspace consolidation (14,50) (Figure 13.1). These abnormalities rapidly disappear upon corticosteroid therapy.
- Airways abnormalities including centrilobular nodules, bronchial wall thickening and bronchiectasis (14,51).

Interlobular septal thickening, hilar or mediastinal lymphadenopathy, pleural effusion or pericardial effusion may also be seen. Pleural effusion may correspond to eosinophilic pleural effusion or to a transudate caused by cardiomyopathy.

PATHOLOGY

Because the diagnosis of EGPA is frequently made on the clinical presentation and marked eosinophilia, a lung biopsy is seldom necessary. When performed, a biopsy located in skin, nerve or muscle (9) may demonstrate some or all three of the characteristic features:

- Vasculitis, necrotizing or not, involving mainly the medium-sized pulmonary arteries
- Granulomata
- Eosinophilic tissular infiltration with palisading histiocytes and giant cells

GENERAL MANAGEMENT

Corticosteroids are the mainstay of treatment of EGPA and are always necessary once the diagnosis is secure. Oral prednisone may be initiated at a dose of 1 mg/kg/day for 3–4 weeks, then tapered progressively to reach 5–10 mg/day at 12 months of therapy (32).

In severe cases, an initial methylprednisolone infusion (15 mg/kg/day for 1–3 days) is useful. Cyclophosphamide therapy (0.6–0.7 g/m^2 intravenously at day 1, 15, 30, then every 3 weeks) should be added to corticosteroids to induce remission in patients with manifestations that could result in mortality or severe morbidity especially heart failure, with one or more of the following criteria (revised five factor score): age >65 years; cardiac symptoms; gastrointestinal involvement; renal insufficiency with serum creatinine >150 μg/L; and absence of ear, nose and throat manifestation.

Experience with rituximab is limited in EGPA (32,52), with a possible risk of bronchospasm (52,53). Other therapies are reserved for cases refractory to corticosteroids and may consist in subcutaneous interferon alpha, high-dose intravenous immunoglobulins, plasma exchange and cyclosporine.

Maintenance therapy to prevent relapses must be maintained for 18–24 months after remission. Patients without poor prognosis criteria are generally treated by corticosteroids alone, whereas those with poor prognosis criteria generally receive azathioprine (32).

SPECIFIC MANAGEMENT

The titre of ANCAs should not be used to monitor disease activity or to take treatment decisions.

PROGNOSIS AND LONG-TERM OUTLOOK

Nearly half of patients experience at least one relapse, consisting in asthma exacerbation with peripheral eosinophilia (two-thirds of cases), or to new onset systemic manifestations (one-third of cases) (38). The 5-year overall survival in EGPA is currently greater than 95%, with most deaths occurring during the first year of treatment due to cardiac involvement.

Long-term morbidity is related to (1) side effects of corticosteroids and severe immunosuppression, because low dose long-term oral corticosteroids are required for asthma in most patients in addition to inhaled therapy; and (2) difficult asthma with persistent airflow obstruction present in nearly half the patients (38,43,54).

CURRENT AND FUTURE AREAS OF RESEARCH

In a retrospective multicentric study, omalizumab (used alone or in association with other immunosuppressive agents), provided some efficacy in severe steroid-dependent asthma and corticosteroid sparing effect, but severe flares occurred in a quarter of patients (55).

Promising preliminary results have been obtained using the anti-IL5 antibody mepolizumab (56–58) (and clinicaltrials.gov, NCT02281318). Drugs that target the eosinophil cell lineage may become part of the treatment strategy in the near future.

EOSINOPHILIC PNEUMONIAS INDUCED BY DRUGS AND TOXICS

The search for a cause of eosinophilic ILD is of paramount importance especially when investigating causative drugs (15). A thorough investigation must be conducted for drugs taken in the weeks or days prior to an eosinophilic lung disease.

Although many drugs have been incriminated (www.pneumotox.com), causality has been established in about 20. Those are mostly antibiotics (ethambutol, fenbufen, minocycline, nitrofurantoin, penicillins, pyrimethamine, sulfamides, sulfonamides, trimethoprim-sulfamethoxazole) and non-steroid anti-inflammatory drugs and related drugs. Other drugs can be involved in eosinophilic ILD of varying presentation such as captopril, carbamazepine and many others, as well as illicit drugs especially cocaine or heroin but also cannabis.

An acute onset similar to the presentation to IAEP is suggestive of drug-induced ILD, especially due to minocycline or nitrofurantoin. However, a more chronic onset similar to that of ICEP is possible. Pleural effusion or extrapulmonary manifestations when present, further suggest the possibility of drug-induced ILD, especially cutaneous rash. Acute eosinophilic pneumonia may occur in the context of drug rash with eosinophilia and systemic symptoms (DRESS).

OTHER EOSINOPHILIC LUNG DISEASES

ALLERGIC BRONCHOPULMONARY ASPERGILLOSIS

Allergic bronchopulmonary aspergillosis (ABPA) belongs to the spectrum of eosinophilic lung diseases (59), however it only rarely presents as ILD. It occurs almost exclusively in subjects with a prior history of asthma or cystic fibrosis, with isolated cases reported in patients with chronic obstructive pulmonary disease. Patients with ABPA experience chronic cough, dyspnoea, expectoration of brown or tan sputum plugs, low-grade fever or chronic rhinitis.

Imaging abnormalities often suggest the diagnosis (14) and include central cylindrical bronchiectasis (including in the upper lobes), bronchial wall thickening, mucous plugging (mucoid impaction) with 'finger in glove' pattern, ground-glass attenuation and airspace consolidation suggesting eosinophilic pneumonia, and features of bronchiolitis with centrilobular nodules and tree-in-bud pattern. Pulmonary infiltrates may only be present during the acute phase or recurrent exacerbations of the disease, and at a late 'fibrotic' stage consisting of bronchiectasis with adjacent lung remodelling, with frequently segmental or lobar atelectasis caused by mucus plugging and chronic consolidation. ABPA rarely progresses to chronic respiratory failure requiring oxygen supplementation.

The diagnosis is based on a combination of criteria (10). Treatment mainly relies on corticosteroids during ABPA exacerbations, preferably with oral prednisolone 0.5 mg/kg/day for 2 weeks followed

by 0.5 mg/kg on alternate days for 8 weeks, then taper by 5 mg every 2 weeks and discontinue after 3–5 months. Oral itraconazole prescribed for 16–32 weeks in adjunction to prednisolone, allows to reduce its dose, and decreases the frequency of exacerbations. Persistent airflow obstruction may develop over the years despite inhaled and oral corticosteroids, which frequently need to be maintained on the long term to prevent frequent symptomatic attacks or progressive lung damage.

IDIOPATHIC HYPEREOSINOPHILIC SYNDROMES

The idiopathic hypereosinophilic syndromes include

- The 'lymphocytic variant' (about 30% of cases), resulting from clonal Th2 lymphocytes bearing an aberrant antigenic surface phenotype
- Chronic eosinophilic leukaemia or the 'myeloproliferative variant' (about 20% of cases) due to an interstitial chromosomal deletion in 4q12 encoding a constitutively activated tyrosine kinase fusion protein (*Fip1L1-PDGFRα*)
- A large proportion of cases which remain idiopathic and unclassified

Clinical manifestations mainly comprise fatigue, weight loss and non-respiratory involvement especially targeting the skin, mucosa, heart and nervous system. Respiratory manifestations are generally of mild severity. Eosinophilic pneumonia is rare. Chronic dry cough can be remarkable and may be a presenting feature (60). Patchy ground-glass attenuation, consolidation and small nodules may be found at chest imaging.

IDIOPATHIC HYPEREOSINOPHILIC OBLITERATIVE BRONCHIOLITIS

Hypereosinophilic obliterative bronchiolitis is a recently individualized entity (Table 13.1) (11). Whitish tracheal and bronchial granulations or bronchial ulcerative lesions can be present with prominent eosinophilia at bronchial biopsy (11). It can be idiopathic, or occur in the setting of

EGPA, ABPA, drug-induced eosinophilic lung disease (such as minocycline) and possibly in severe asthma.

EOSINOPHILIC PNEUMONIAS ASSOCIATED WITH PARASITIC INFECTION

Parasitic infection is the main cause of eosinophilic pneumonia in the world but is less frequent in Europe and North America. A detailed description can be found elsewhere (15). Frequent causes include infection with

* *Ascaris lumbricoides* mainly causing Löffler syndrome (mild eosinophilic pneumonia with transient cough, wheezing, fever, high blood eosinophilia and pulmonary infiltrates)
* *Toxocara canis* causing visceral larva migrans syndrome with fever, seizures, fatigue, blood eosinophilia and Löffler syndrome
* *Strongyloides stercoralis* responsible for hyperinfection syndrome in immunocompromised patients
* Filarial parasites *Wuchereria bancrofti* and *Brugia malayi* responsible for tropical pulmonary eosinophilia

RADIATION THERAPY

A condition similar to ICEP has been reported after radiation therapy for breast cancer in women (similar to the syndrome of radiation-induced organizing pneumonia), with a median delay of 3.5 months after completion of radiotherapy and possible relapses (61).

MISCELLANEOUS

ICEP may overlap with, or mimic cryptogenic organizing pneumonia. Eosinophilia may be found in other ILDs, including bronchocentric granulomatosis, isolated cases of idiopathic pulmonary fibrosis, desquamative interstitial pneumonia, pulmonary Langerhans cell histiocytosis and sarcoidosis.

CONCLUSION: A PRACTICAL APPROACH IN EOSINOPHILIC ILD

The diagnosis of eosinophilic ILD is based on characteristic clinical-imaging features and the demonstration of alveolar eosinophilia by BAL. Lung biopsy is generally not necessary. Peripheral blood eosinophilia when present suggests the diagnosis but may be absent at presentation, especially in IAEP and in patients who have already received corticosteroid treatment. Possible causes must be searched for, especially drugs, toxins and parasitic infection including fungi, taking into account the epidemiology of parasites. Biological investigations for ABPA should be prompted by the presence of proximal bronchiectasis in patients with asthma or cystic fibrosis. Extrathoracic manifestations are key to the diagnosis of EGPA. Treatment of eosinophilic ILD involves oral corticosteroids in most cases, withdrawal of the offending agent when appropriate and cyclophosphamide in severe cases of EGPA. In the future, anti-IL-5 monoclonal antibodies may complement available therapeutic approaches, with however still very limited experience in eosinophilic ILD.

REFERENCES

1. Valent P, Klion AD, Horny HP, Roufosse F, Gotlib J, Weller PF et al. Contemporary consensus proposal on criteria and classification of eosinophilic disorders and related syndromes. *J Allergy Clin Immunol.* 2012;130:607–12.
2. Cottin V, Cordier JF. Eosinophilic pneumonia. In: Cottin V, Cordier JF, Richeldi L, eds. *Orphan Lung Diseases: A Clinical Guide to Rare Lung Disease.* London, UK: Springer-Verlag; 2015:227–51.
3. Cottin V, Cordier JF. Eosinophilic pneumonia. In: Mason RJ, Ernst JD, King Jr TE, Lazarus SC, Murray BW, Nadel JA, Slutsky AS, Gotway MB, eds. *Murray and Nadel's Textbook of Respiratory Medicine.* 6th ed. Philadelphia, PA: Elsevier Saunders; 2016:1221–42.

4. Marchand E, Reynaud-Gaubert M, Lauque D, Durieu J, Tonnel AB, Cordier JF. Idiopathic chronic eosinophilic pneumonia. A clinical and follow-up study of 62 cases. The Groupe d'Etudes et de Recherche sur les Maladies 'Orphelines' Pulmonaires (GERM'O'P). *Medicine (Baltimore)*. 1998;77:299–312.

5. Jederlinic PJ, Sicilian L, Gaensler EA. Chronic eosinophilic pneumonia. A report of 19 cases and a review of the literature. *Medicine (Baltimore)*. 1988;67:154–62.

6. Naughton M, Fahy J, FitzGerald MX. Chronic eosinophilic pneumonia. A long-term follow-up of 12 patients. *Chest*. 1993;103:162–5.

7. Carrington CB, Addington WW, Goff AM, Madoff IM, Marks A, Schwaber JR, Gaensler EA. Chronic eosinophilic pneumonia. *N Engl J Med*. 1969;280:787–98.

8. Marchand E, Etienne-Mastroianni B, Chanez P, Lauque D, Leclerq P, Cordier JF. Idiopathic chronic eosinophilic pneumonia and asthma: How do they influence each otherThe Groupe d'Etudes et de Recherche sur les Maladies 'Orphelines' Pulmonaires (GERM'O'P). *Eur Respir J*. 2003;22:8–13.

9. Cottin V, Bel E, Bottero P, Dalhoff K, Humbert M, Lazor R et al. Revisiting the systemic vasculitis in eosinophilic granulomatosis with polyangiitis (Churg-Strauss): A study of 157 patients by the Groupe d'Etudes et de Recherche sur les Maladies Orphelines Pulmonaires and the European Respiratory Society Taskforce on eosinophilic granulomatosis with polyangiitis (Churg-Strauss). *Autoimmun Rev*. 2017;16:1–9.

10. Agarwal R, Chakrabarti A, Shah A, Gupta D, Meis JF, Guleria R et al. Allergic bronchopulmonary aspergillosis: Review of literature and proposal of new diagnostic and classification criteria. *Clin Exp Allergy*. 2013;43:850–73.

11. Cordier JF, Cottin V, Khouatra C, Revel D, Proust C, Freymond N et al. Hypereosinophilic obliterative bronchiolitis: A distinct, unrecognised syndrome. *Eur Respir J*. 2013;41:1126–34.

12. Ebara H, Ikezoe J, Johkoh T, Kohno N, Takeuchi N, Kozuka T, Ishida O. Chronic eosinophilic pneumonia: Evolution of chest radiograms and CT features. *J Comput Assist Tomogr*. 1994;18:737–44.

13. Arakawa H, Kurihara Y, Niimi H, Nakajima Y, Johkoh T, Nakamura H. Bronchiolitis obliterans with organizing pneumonia versus chronic eosinophilic pneumonia: High-resolution CT findings in 81 patients. *AJR Am J Roentgenol*. 2001;176:1053–8.

14. Johkoh T, Muller NL, Akira M, Ichikado K, Suga M, Ando M et al. Eosinophilic lung diseases: Diagnostic accuracy of thin-section CT in 111 patients. *Radiology*. 2000;216:773–80.

15. Cordier JF, Cottin V. Eosinophilic pneumonias. In: Schwarz MI, King TE, Jr, eds. *Interstitial lung Disease*. 5th ed. Shelton, CT: People's Medical Publishing House-USA; 2011:833–93.

16. Oyama Y, Fujisawa T, Hashimoto D, Enomoto N, Nakamura Y, Inui N et al. Efficacy of short-term prednisolone treatment in patients with chronic eosinophilic pneumonia. *Eur Respir J*. 2015;45:1624–31.

17. Durieu J, Wallaert B, Tonnel AB. Long term follow-up of pulmonary function in chronic eosinophilic pneumonia. *Eur Respir J*. 1997;10:286–91.

18. Allen JN, Pacht ER, Gadek JE, Davis WB. Acute eosinophilic pneumonia as a reversible cause of noninfectious respiratory failure. *N Engl J Med*. 1989;321:569–74.

19. Badesch DB, King TE, Schwartz MI. Acute eosinophilic pneumonia: A hypersensitivity phenomenon? *Am Rev Respir Dis*. 1989;139:249–52.

20. Philit F, Etienne-Mastroianni B, Parrot A, Guerin C, Robert D, Cordier JF. Idiopathic acute eosinophilic pneumonia: A study of 22 patients. The Groupe d'Etudes et de Recherche sur les Maladies 'Orphelines' Pulmonaires (GERM'O'P). *Am J Respir Crit Care Med*. 2002;166:1235–9.

21. Pope-Harman AL, Davis WB, Allen ED, Christoforidis AJ, Allen JN. Acute eosinophilic pneumonia. A summary of 15 cases and review of the literature. *Medicine (Baltimore)*. 1996;75:334–42.

22. Shorr AF, Scoville SL, Cersovsky SB, Shanks GD, Ockenhouse CF, Smoak BL et al. Acute eosinophilic pneumonia among US military personnel deployed in or near Iraq. *JAMA*. 2004;292:2997–3005.

23. Rhee CK, Min KH, Yim NY, Lee JE, Lee NR, Chung MP, Jeon K. Clinical characteristics and corticosteroid treatment of acute eosinophilic pneumonia. *Eur Respir J.* 2013;41:402–9.
24. Uchiyama H, Suda T, Nakamura Y, Shirai M, Gemma H, Shirai T et al. Alterations in smoking habits are associated with acute eosinophilic pneumonia. *Chest.* 2008;133:1174–80.
25. Cheon JE, Lee KS, Jung GS, Chung MH, Cho YD. Acute eosinophilic pneumonia: Radiographic and CT findings in six patients. *AJR.* 1996;167:1195–9.
26. King MA, Pope-Harman AL, Allen JN, Christoforidis GA, Christoforidis AJ. Acute eosinophilic pneumonia: Radiologic and clinical features. *Radiology.* 1997;203: 715–9.
27. Daimon T, Johkoh T, Sumikawa H, Honda O, Fujimoto K, Koga T et al. Acute eosinophilic pneumonia: Thin-section CT findings in 29 patients. *Eur J Radiol.* 2008;65:462–7.
28. Jhun BW, Kim SJ, Kim K, Lee JE. Outcomes of rapid corticosteroid tapering in acute eosinophilic pneumonia patients with initial eosinophilia. *Respirology.* 2015;20:1241–7.
29. Churg J, Strauss L. Allergic granulomatosis, allergic angiitis, and periarteritis nodosa. *Am J Pathol.* 1951;27:277–301.
30. Jennette JC, Falk RJ, Bacon PA, Basu N, Cid MC, Ferrario F et al. 2012 revised International Chapel Hill Consensus Conference Nomenclature of Vasculitides. *Arthritis Rheum.* 2013;65:1–11.
31. Cottin V, Bonniaud P. Drug-induced infiltrative lung disease. *Eur Respir Mon.* 2009;46:287–318.
32. Dunogué B, Pagnoux C, Guillevin L. Churg-Strauss syndrome: Clinical symptoms, complementary investigations, prognosis and outcome, and treatment. *Semin Respir Crit Care Med.* 2011;32:298–309.
33. Mouthon L, le Toumelin P, Andre MH, Gayraud M, Casassus P, Guillevin L. Polyarteritis nodosa and Churg-Strauss angiitis: Characteristics and outcome in 38 patients over 65 years. *Medicine (Baltimore).* 2002;81:27–40.
34. Lanham JG, Elkon KB, Pusey CD, Hughes GR. Systemic vasculitis with asthma and eosinophilia: A clinical approach to the Churg-Strauss syndrome. *Medicine (Baltimore).* 1984;63:65–81.
35. Keogh KA, Specks U. Churg-Strauss syndrome: Clinical presentation, antineutrophil cytoplasmic antibodies, and leukotriene receptor antagonists. *Am J Med.* 2003;115:284–90.
36. Guillevin L, Cohen P, Gayraud M, Lhote F, Jarrousse B, Casassus P. Churg-Strauss syndrome. Clinical study and long-term follow-up of 96 patients. *Medicine (Baltimore).* 1999;78:26–37.
37. Bottero P, Bonini M, Vecchio F, Grittini A, Patruno GM, Colombo B, Sinico RA. The common allergens in the Churg-Strauss syndrome. *Allergy.* 2007;62:1288–94.
38. Cottin V, Bel E, Bottero P, Dalhoff K, Humbert M, Lazor R et al. Respiratory manifestations of eosinophilic granulomatosis with polyangiitis (Churg-Strauss). *Eur Respir J.* 2016;48:1429–41.
39. Bibby S, Healy B, Steele R, Kumareswaran K, Nelson H, Beasley R. Association between leukotriene receptor antagonist therapy and Churg-Strauss syndrome: An analysis of the FDA AERS database. *Thorax.* 2010;65:132–8.
40. Hauser T, Mahr A, Metzler C, Coste J, Sommerstein R, Gross WL et al. The leukotriene-receptor antagonist montelukast and the risk of Churg-Strauss syndrome: A case-crossover study. *Thorax.* 2008;63(8):677–82.
41. Reid AJ, Harrison BD, Watts RA, Watkin SW, McCann BG, Scott DG. Churg-Strauss syndrome in a district hospital. *Qjm.* 1998;91:219–29.
42. Chumbley LC, Harrison EG, Jr., DeRemee RA. Allergic granulomatosis and angiitis (Churg-Strauss syndrome). Report and analysis of 30 cases. *Mayo Clin Proc.* 1977;52:477–84.
43. Cottin V, Khouatra C, Dubost R, Glerant JC, Cordier JF. Persistent airflow obstruction in asthma of patients with Churg-Strauss syndrome and long-term follow-up. *Allergy.* 2009;64:589–95.

44. Szczeklik W, Sokolowska BM, Zuk J, Mastalerz L, Szczeklik A, Musial J. The course of asthma in Churg-Strauss syndrome. *J Asthma*. 2011;48:183–7.

45. Sablé-Fourtassou R, Cohen P, Mahr A, Pagnoux C, Mouthon L, Jayne D et al. Antineutrophil cytoplasmic antibodies and the Churg-Strauss syndrome. *Ann Intern Med*. 2005;143:632–8.

46. Sinico RA, Di Toma L, Maggiore U, Bottero P, Radice A, Tosoni C et al. Prevalence and clinical significance of antineutrophil cytoplasmic antibodies in Churg-Strauss syndrome. *Arthritis Rheum*. 2005;52:2926–35.

47. Healy B, Bibby S, Steele R, Weatherall M, Nelson H, Beasley R. Antineutrophil cytoplasmic autoantibodies and myeloperoxidase autoantibodies in clinical expression of Churg-Strauss syndrome. *J Allergy Clin Immunol*. 2013;131:571–6 e1–6.

48. Comarmond C, Pagnoux C, Khellaf M, Cordier JF, Hamidou M, Viallard JF et al. Eosinophilic granulomatosis with polyangiitis (Churg-Strauss): Clinical characteristics and long-term followup of the 383 patients enrolled in the French Vasculitis Study Group cohort. *Arthritis Rheum*. 2013;65:270–81.

49. Sokolowska BM, Szczeklik WK, Wludarczyk AA, Kuczia PP, Jakiela BA, Gasior JA et al. ANCA-positive and ANCA-negative phenotypes of eosinophilic granulomatosis with polyangiitis (EGPA): Outcome and long-term follow-up of 50 patients from a single Polish center. *Clin Exp Rheumatol*. 2014;32:S41–7.

50. Choi YH, Im JG, Han BK, Kim JH, Lee KY, Myoung NH. Thoracic manifestation of Churg-Strauss syndrome: Radiologic and clinical findings. *Chest*. 2000;117:117–24.

51. Furuiye M, Yoshimura N, Kobayashi A, Tamaoka M, Miyazaki Y, Ohtani Y et al. Churg-Strauss syndrome versus chronic eosinophilic pneumonia on high-resolution computed tomographic findings. *J Comput Assist Tomogr*. 2010;34:19–22.

52. Mohammad AJ, Hot A, Arndt F, Moosig F, Guerry MJ, Amudala N et al. Rituximab for the treatment of eosinophilic granulomatosis with polyangiitis (Churg-Strauss). *Ann Rheum Dis*. 2016;75:396–401.

53. Bouldouyre MA, Cohen P, Guillevin L. Severe bronchospasm associated with rituximab for refractory Churg-Strauss syndrome. *Ann Rheum Dis*. 2009;68:606.

54. Ribi C, Cohen P, Pagnoux C, Mahr A, Arene JP, Lauque D et al. Treatment of Churg-Strauss syndrome without poor-prognosis factors: A multicenter, prospective, randomized, open-label study of seventy-two patients. *Arthritis Rheum*. 2008;58:586–94.

55. Jachiet M, Samson M, Cottin V, Kahn JE, Le Guenno G, Bonniaud P et al. for the French Vasculitis Study Group (FVSG). Anti-IgE monoclonal antibody in refractory and relapsing eosinophilic granulomatosis with polyangiitis (Churg-Strauss): Data from 17 patients. *Arthritis Rheumatol*. 2016;68(9):2274–82.

56. Kahn JE, Grandpeix-Guyodo C, Marroun I, Catherinot E, Mellot F, Roufosse F, Bletry O. Sustained response to mepolizumab in refractory Churg-Strauss syndrome. *J Allergy Clin Immunol*. 2010;125:267–70.

57. Kim S, Marigowda G, Oren E, Israel E, Wechsler ME. Mepolizumab as a steroid-sparing treatment option in patients with Churg-Strauss syndrome. *J Allergy Clin Immunol*. 2010;125:1336–43.

58. Moosig F, Gross WL, Herrmann K, Bremer JP, Hellmich B. Targeting interleukin-5 in refractory and relapsing Churg-Strauss syndrome. *Ann Intern Med*. 2011;155:341–3.

59. Cottin V. Eosinophilic lung diseases. *Clin Chest Med*. 2016;37:535–56.

60. Roufosse F, Heimann P, Lambert F, Sidon P, Bron D, Cottin V, Cordier JF. Severe prolonged cough as presenting manifestation of FIP1L1-PDGFRA+ chronic eosinophilic leukaemia: A widely ignored association. *Respiration*. 2016;91:374–9.

61. Cottin V, Frognier R, Monnot H, Levy A, DeVuyst P, Cordier JF. Chronic eosinophilic pneumonia after radiation therapy for breast cancer. *Eur Respir J*. 2004;23:9–13.

14

Interstitial lung disease associated with connective tissue disorders

DEBORAH ASSAYAG AND ARYEH FISCHER

BACKGROUND

Interstitial lung disease (ILD) often arises within the context of an underlying connective tissue disease (CTD) and is often associated with significant morbidity and mortality (1). The CTDs are a group of systemic autoimmune disorders with significant clinical heterogeneity characterized by immune-mediated organ dysfunction (Table 14.1), and the lung is a frequent target. All CTD patients are at risk for developing ILD, and those with systemic sclerosis (SSc), poly-/dermatomyositis (PM/DM) and rheumatoid arthritis (RA) are at particularly high risk. ILD may develop at any point in the natural history of CTD, is most frequently identified within the context of an established CTD and may also be the first clinically apparent manifestation of occult CTD (2–4). Furthermore, some individuals may have 'interstitial pneumonia with autoimmune features' (IPAF), defined by the presence of ILD and features suggestive of (but not diagnostic for) underlying CTD (5). Determining whether a patient has a diagnosis of CTD-associated ILD (CTD-ILD) is important, as this knowledge may impact treatment decisions, can guide surveillance for other concomitant clinical features and can help with prognostication (1).

Table 14.1 List of connective tissue diseases

Rheumatoid arthritis (RA)
Systemic sclerosis (SSc)
Systemic lupus erythematosus (SLE)
Idiopathic inflammatory myopathies (IIM)
Primary Sjögren syndrome (SjS)
Mixed connective tissue disease (MCTD)
Undifferentiated connective tissue disease (UCTD)

SCIENTIFIC MECHANISMS

CTDs likely develop due to a complex and incompletely understood interplay of genetic factors, environmental exposures and immune dysregulation. Recent data suggest that immune cells (T cells, neutrophils, macrophages and fibrocytes) and soluble mediators (cytokines and chemokines) are central to development of ILD, and innate or adaptive immune mechanisms contribute to fibrogenesis at several cellular and noncellular levels (6). Further, excessive deposition of extracellular matrix proteins results in fibrotic remodelling, alveolar destruction and resultant loss of lung function (6).

Numerous gaps exist in our understanding of why certain CTD populations are more likely to develop ILD, but certain phenotypic risk factors have been identified. In RA, these include older age, cigarette smoking, male gender, RF positivity, CCP positivity and more severe articular disease (7,8). In SSc, autoantibodies serve as the most reliable predictor of ILD, with anti-Scl-70 being one of the strongest predictors (9–11). Other autoantibodies associated with higher risk of ILD development include Th/To, U3-RNP and U11/12 RNP (9,12,13). It is noteworthy that skin thickening in SSc is not a reliable predictor of ILD development – as severe ILD frequently occurs with limited or no skin involvement. In PM/DM, autoantibody profiles also are useful predictors of ILD. Of particular relevance are the anti-synthetase antibodies (e.g. JO-1, PL-7, PL-12, others), anti-PM-Scl antibody and anti-MDA-5 antibody. Anti-synthetase antibody positive or PM-Scl-positive patients typically manifest with non-specific interstitial pneumonia (NSIP) with overlapping organizing pneumonia (OP) and an array of often-subtle cutaneous and musculoskeletal manifestations as part of the 'anti-synthetase syndrome' (14–17). Original reports have shown that anti-MDA-5 antibody is associated with rapidly progressive, often fatal, diffuse alveolar damage with clinical amyopathic dermatomyositis (18) but more recent data suggest this antibody may also be associated with less severe ILD (19). Reliable risk factors for ILD development in the other CTDs are lacking.

EPIDEMIOLOGY

Prevalence rates of CTD-ILD are influenced by the methods of detection. Studies that define the presence of ILD based on plain chest roentgenogram will find lower prevalence rates compared with studies that define its presence by thoracic high-resolution computed tomography (HRCT) or autopsy. Recent studies demonstrate that increasing prevalence rates of CTD-ILD may in part be due to the technological advances and wider availability of HRCT.

The prevalence of interstitial lung disease (ILD) in SSc is at least 55% with autopsy estimates of prevalence closer to 74% (20,21). For PM/DM, clinically significant ILD appears to occur in approximately 30%, whereas HRCT evidence may be present in over 70% of patients (22–24). The reported prevalence of RA-ILD varies greatly and depends on the diagnostic method used to identify ILD and the patient population studied (25–27). Clinically significant ILD likely occurs in approximately 10% of RA patients (28), but approximately 50% will have radiographic evidence of interstitial lung abnormalities on HRCT (29–32). The clinical impact of these radiographic abnormalities remains to be determined and is the focus of ongoing research (30). Reliable estimates of prevalence rates for the other CTDs are lacking, but it is worth noting that chronic ILD is surprisingly rare in systemic lupus erythematosus (SLE) compared to other CTDs (33).

HISTORY AND EXAMINATION

Patients with ILD most commonly present with insidious and progressive dyspnoea on exertion

Table 14.2 Suggested categories of ILD patients who require further rheumatologic evaluation

1. Women, particularly those younger than 50
2. Any patient with extra-thoracic manifestations highly suggestive of CTD
   a. Raynaud phenomenon, oesophageal hypomotility, inflammatory arthritis of the metacarpal–phalangeal joints or wrists, digital oedema, or symptomatic keratoconjunctivitis sicca
3. All cases of NSIP, LIP, or any ILD pattern with secondary histopathology features that might suggest CTD
   a. Extensive pleuritis, dense perivascular collagen, lymphoid aggregates with germinal centre formation, or prominent plasmacytic infiltration
4. Patients with a positive ANA or RF in high titre (generally considered to be ANA > 1:320 or RF > 60 IU/mL), a nucleolar-staining ANA at any titre, or any positive autoantibody specific to a particular CTD
   a. Anti-CCP, Anti-Scl-70, Anti-Ro, Anti-La, Anti-dsDNA, Anti-Smith, Anti-RNP, Anti-tRNA synthetase

Source: Fischer A, du Bois RM. In: Baughman RP, du Bois RM, eds. 2nd ed. New York, NY: Springer; 2012:217–37.

as their predominant symptoms. Dyspnoea is a significant predictor of psychological well-being (34) as well as physical and global functioning in CTD-ILD (35). New onset of dyspnoea or change in exercise capacity, especially with physical examination findings of crackles on chest auscultation, should prompt a thorough evaluation for ILD. Identification of ILD in patients with pre-existing CTD mandates a comprehensive evaluation to explore all potential aetiologies (e.g. infection, medication toxicity, environmental exposures, etc.). Determining whether the ILD is associated with the pre-existing CTD must be done via a thorough process of elimination. In particular, respiratory infection and drug-induced lung disease are almost always in the differential and require detailed assessment.

Identifying occult CTD among patients diagnosed with a presumed 'idiopathic' interstitial pneumonia (IIP) is common: a recent study from a multidisciplinary ILD program evaluated 114 consecutive ILD patients, of which 17 (15%) were confirmed to have a new CTD diagnosis (36). There is no standardized approach to this evaluation, and current guidelines recommend performing a thorough history and physical examination and testing for a panel of autoantibodies (37–39). Many centres have also found that a multidisciplinary evaluation that includes rheumatologic consultation is useful (14,34,40,41). However, because it is both unrealistic and impractical to have rheumatologic evaluation for all cases of IIP, it is left up to the individual provider to decide when to engage rheumatology,

and certain guidelines have been suggested (41) (Table 14.2).

Demographic features should not be overlooked, as they may heighten suspicion for underlying CTD. In comparison to IPF, patients with CTD-ILD are more likely to be younger and female (42). Certain specific clinical features lend more support for the presence of an underlying CTD than others. Raynaud phenomenon is often of significance and should raise suspicions for underlying CTD in general, especially for SSc (with or without overt skin thickening) or the PM/DM spectrum. Performing nailfold capillary microscopy may be useful in this context, as the presence of dilated or tortuous capillary loops or significant capillary dropout may be helpful and lend additional support for CTD. The presence of synovitis should also lend consideration for underlying CTD. The cutaneous manifestations of SSc and the anti-synthetase syndrome are worthy of special mention, because these disorders are commonly associated with ILD and have specific (yet often subtle) extra-thoracic features. The 'mechanic hands' of anti-synthetase syndrome (or with PM-Scl antibody or MDA-5 positive patients) may manifest with only mild distal digital fissuring, palmar telangiectasia may be few and difficult to appreciate on quick inspection (Figure 14.1) and generalized digital oedema may go unnoticed. Nonetheless, these examination features should be looked for in those with presumed IIP, and such findings, if present, are highly suggestive of underlying CTD (3,13–15).

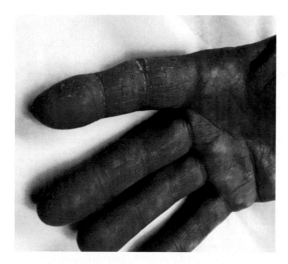

Figure 14.1 Distal digital fissuring – most prominently seen on the medial aspect of the second
digit – consistent with 'mechanic hands' of the
anti-synthetase syndrome.

Table 14.3 Useful autoantibodies to consider as
part of CTD evaluation in those with ILD

Autoantibody	Most common CTD association
High-titre ANA (>1:320)	Many types
RF (>60 IU/mL)	Many types/RA
Anti-centromere	SSc
Nucleolar-ANA	SSc
Anti-CCP	RA
Anti-Scl-70	SSc
Anti-Ro (SS-A)	Many types
Anti-tRNA synthetase (Jo-1, PL-7, PL-12, others)	PM/DM
Anti-PM-Scl	SSc/PM overlap
Anti-La (SS-B)	Sjögren's, SLE
Anti-dsDNA	SLE
Anti-RNP	MCTD, SLE/SSc
Anti-Smith	SLE
Anti-MDA-5	CADM

Source: Fischer A, Richeldi L Semin Respir Crit Care
Med. 2014;35(2):159–65.

INVESTIGATIONS

AUTOANTIBODIES

Autoantibody assessment is an important part of
the ILD evaluation, but serologic positivity often
requires clinical interpretation (often rheumatologic consultation), and, to be candid, autoantibody detection sometimes generates more
questions than answers. For patients with ILD in
whom there is clinical suspicion of an underlying
CTD, a broad panel of autoantibodies is recommended to ensure that the full spectrum of CTD
is encompassed (Table 14.3) (39,40). The preferred
method for the anti-nuclear antibody (ANA) assay
is by indirect immunofluorescence, which allows
for reporting of ANA titre and staining pattern
(43). The enzyme-linked immunosorbent assay
(ELISA) assay for ANA testing is less reliable, has
been shown to be falsely negative in subsets of
patients with SSc, does not allow for staining pattern reporting and does not provide a titre (44). The
pattern of immunofluorescence when the ANA is
positive can be helpful, as the nucleolar-staining
ANA pattern in patients with ILD may suggest the
SSc spectrum of disease (13,45). Myositis antibody
panel assessment for anti-synthetase antibodies

and specifically assessing for anti-SSA (and Ro-52)
is of particular importance in those with NSIP and/
or OP, and one should recall that many of these
patients are ANA negative (14,15). It may also be
worth testing for the anti-MDA5 antibody in cases
of rapidly progressive ILD, especially if 'idiopathic'
diffuse alveolar damage is identified.

DYSPNOEA AND QUALITY-OF-LIFE MEASURES

Reproducible, subjective indicators of a patient's
level of breathlessness, exercise capacity and
quality of life may be useful as part of the ILD
assessment and with determining general functionality. In a clinical setting, the Modified
Medical Research Council scale can be used easily and quickly to assess dyspnoea and associated functional limitations (46). This scale was
initially developed and validated in patients with
chronic obstructive pulmonary disease but has
been shown to be associated with activity limitation, anxiety and depression in ILD (47,48). In one
study, the self-reported measures of the Multi-
Dimensional Health Assessment Questionnaire,

University of California San Diego Dyspnea Questionnaire and Dypsnea-12 Questionnaire were found to be useful in the assessment of patients with a wide spectrum of CTD-ILD (35). A number of other dyspnoea indices have been validated in a variety of respiratory diseases, and the choice of which index to use for CTD-ILD is likely to be less important than their consistent implementation.

PULMONARY PHYSIOLOGY

Full pulmonary function tests (PFTs) should be done routinely in all patients to screen for presence of ILD and to monitor disease progression. However, PFT values can be normal in the presence of mild ILD, especially if previous tests showed supra-normal values, highlighting the importance of serial testing over time (49). Early on in the disease course, a low diffusion capacity for carbon monoxide (DLCO) may be the only abnormality and precede the appearance of a restrictive pattern. In rare cases with airway-centric disease, a mixed restrictive and obstructive pattern can be seen (50,51). Assessment of forced vital capacity (FVC) and DLCO allows for objective quantification of the degree of respiratory impairment due to ILD and may provide clues about the presence of co-existent pulmonary vasculopathy as well (e.g. when the DLCO is disproportionately low relative to the FVC). The 6-minute walk test (6MWT) can also provide important information about ILD severity, functional limitations, disease progression and potential need for supplemental oxygen therapy.

BRONCHOALVEOLAR LAVAGE

Select cases of CTD-ILD may require bronchoalveolar lavage (BAL), and this is determined on a case-by-case basis. Routine BAL assessment is no longer recommended, as recent data demonstrate that BAL neutrophilia is not a reliable predictor of progression and rarely influences treatment decisions (52–54). However, because CTD patients are frequently immunocompromised, BAL may be indicated to reliably exclude infection. BAL analysis is also useful when diffuse alveolar haemorrhage is a concern.

RADIOLOGY AND PATHOLOGY

HIGH-RESOLUTION COMPUTED TOMOGRAPHY

Plain chest radiographs are not specific or sensitive for the evaluation of ILD in CTD (55). They can be part of the initial evaluation for pulmonary disease in CTD to identify alternate causes for respiratory symptoms or signs as well as to identify non-ILD pulmonary disease associated with CTD (e.g. pleural effusion, pneumonia, etc.). The radiologic gold standard for making a diagnosis of CTD-ILD is thoracic high-resolution computed tomography (HRCT) of the chest. HRCT can reliably diagnose or exclude ILD and is essential in the evaluation of patients with suspected ILD. HRCT imaging plays an integral role in the characterization of ILD by providing detailed information on the pattern, distribution and extent of the ILD, assessing disease severity and detecting the presence of extra-parenchymal abnormalities (56–58). The HRCT can also help when evaluating patients with presumed IIP for possible occult CTD. Individuals with CTD are more likely to have a HRCT pattern suggestive of NSIP when compared to those without CTD. Compared with IIP, patients with CTD-ILD are more likely to have ground-glass abnormalities, pleural effusions, pericardial effusions, pericardial thickening and oesophageal dilatation (56). Overlapping patterns suggestive of UIP/NSIP or NSIP/OP are not unusual and can be considered almost routine in disorders such as PM/DM (Figure 14.2). Lymphocytic interstitial pneumonia (LIP) with cystic lung disease may be the presenting manifestation of Sjögren's syndrome (59) (Figure 14.3).

ROLE OF SURGICAL LUNG BIOPSY

The role of surgical lung biopsy (SLB) in CTD-ILD is controversial for several reasons: (a) In contrast to IIP, it remains to be determined whether lung histopathology impacts prognosis for CTD-ILD (60). (b) It has been shown in SSc-ILD that lung physiology and HRCT disease extent carry more prognostic significance than histopathology, and this may apply to other forms of CTD-ILD (61).

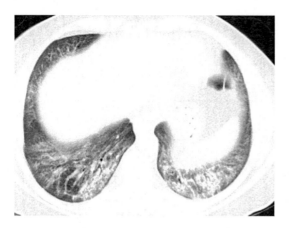

Figure 14.2 Thoracic high-resolution computed tomography image demonstrating a pattern suggestive of NSIP with component of OP in a patient with PL-7 positive anti-synthetase syndrome.

(c) Patients with CTD-ILD tend to be treated with systemic immunosuppression (targeting both ILD and extra-thoracic inflammatory features) irrespective of the specific lung injury pattern on SLB specimens.

Performing a SLB may be appropriate in patients with pre-existing CTD when there are significant concerns for an alternative ILD diagnosis (e.g. hypersensitivity pneumonitis), when the HRCT is 'atypical' or suggests the presence of malignancy or infection (e.g. progressive nodules, cavitation, or consolidation). Ultimately, the decision of whether to perform a SLB is individualized for each patient and should only be performed following due consideration for its associated risks and whether its findings will impact management and prognosis (62).

LUNG HISTOPATHOLOGY

Lung tissue obtained via SLB may provide specific clues about whether the ILD is CTD-associated. Histopathologic features considered to be highly associated with (though not specific for) CTD include the patterns of NSIP, OP and LIP and the secondary features of interstitial lymphoid aggregates with germinal centres and diffuse lymphoplasmacytic infiltration with or without lymphoid follicles (63). A histopathologic pattern of UIP may be seen in CTD as well, but is not specific for CTD. When compared to IPF, lung tissue biopsies from patients with CTD-UIP have fewer fibroblast foci and less honeycombing, but more germinal centre formation and more evidence of inflammation is present (64,65).

THORACIC MULTICOMPARTMENT INVOLVEMENT

Thoracic multicompartment involvement, as manifested by unexplained intrinsic airways disease (e.g. bronchiolitis or bronchiectasis), pleural or pericardial effusion or thickening or pulmonary vasculopathy may be encountered with CTD, and these findings should alert clinicians to the possibility that an occult CTD is present (5).

In summary, confirming a diagnosis of CTD requires the integration of clinical features, serologies and thoracic morphologic features identified by imaging and/or histopathology. Ideally, the evaluation of patients with suspected CTD-ILD is comprehensive and multidisciplinary in nature.

INTERSTITIAL PNEUMONIA WITH AUTOIMMUNE FEATURES

Despite undergoing a thorough evaluation, it is not uncommon to encounter patients with IIP that have certain (but often subtle) features suggesting an underlying autoimmune process and

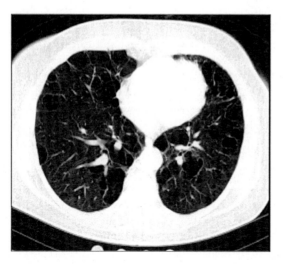

Figure 14.3 Thoracic high-resolution computed tomography image demonstrating extensive peribronchovascular cysts in a pattern suggestive of LIP in a patient with primary Sjögren syndrome.

yet do not meet established diagnostic criteria for any of the characterizable CTDs (5,42,66–69). Although the patient may have an 'autoimmune flavour,' in the absence of specific characterizable features of a defined CTD, the patient is considered to have IIP by default. The European Respiratory Society and American Thoracic Society Task Force on Undifferentiated Forms of CTD-ILD proposed that the name, 'interstitial pneumonia with autoimmune features' (IPAF),

can be used to identify such patients (5). The classification of IPAF requires the *a priori* exclusion of alternative aetiologies for ILD along with the presence of at least one feature from at least two of three primary domains: clinical, serologic and intra-thoracic morphology (Table 14.4) (5). Future research studies of IPAF are needed to refine the diagnostic criteria, determine its natural history and identify the clinical implications of such a classification.

Table 14.4 Classification criteria for interstitial pneumonia with autoimmune features (IPAF)

1. Presence of an interstitial pneumonia (by HRCT or surgical lung biopsy) *and*
2. Exclusion of alternative aetiologies *and*
3. Does not meet criteria of a defined CTD *and*
4. At least one feature from at least two of these domains:

A. Clinical domain	B. Serologic domain	C. Morphologic domain

1. Distal digital fissuring (i.e. 'mechanic hands')
 2. Distal digital tip ulceration
 3. Inflammatory arthritis or polyarticular morning joint stiffness >60 minutes
 4. Palmar telangiectasia
 5. Raynaud phenomenon
 6. Unexplained digital oedema
 7. Unexplained fixed rash on the digital extensor surfaces (i.e. 'Gottron sign')
	1. ANA, either diffuse, speckled, or homogeneous patterns at >1:320 titre *or* ANA nucleolar pattern at any titre *or* ANA centromere pattern at any titre
	 2. RF > 2 X ULN
	 3. Anti-CCP
	 4. Anti-dsDNA
	 5. Anti-Ro (SS-A)
	 6. Anti-La (SS-B)
	 7. Anti-ribonucleoprotein
	 8. Anti-Smith
	 9. Anti-topoisomerase (Scl-70)
	 10. Anti-tRNA synthetase (e.g. Jo-1, PL-7, PL-12, EJ, OJ, KS, Zo, tRS)
	 11. Anti-PM-Scl
	 12. Anti-MDA5 (CADM-40)
		1. Suggestive radiology patterns by HRCT:
		   a. NSIP
		   b. OP
		   c. NSIP with OP overlap
		   d. LIP
		 2. Histopathology patterns or features by surgical lung biopsy:
		   a. NSIP
		   b. OP
		   c. NSIP with OP overlap
		   d. LIP
		   e. Interstitial lymphoid aggregates with germinal centres
		   f. Diffuse lympho-plasmacytic infiltration (with or without lymphoid follicles)
		 3. Unexplained multicompartment involvement[a]:
		   a. Pleural effusion or thickening
		   b. Pericardial effusion or thickening
		   c. Intrinsic airways disease
		   d. Pulmonary vasculopathy

Source: Fischer A et al. *Eur Respir J.* 2015;46(4):976–87.

[a] Either by: thoracic imaging, lung histopathology, right heart catheterization, pulmonary physiology.

GENERAL MANAGEMENT

The decision to treat is usually based on whether the patient is clinically impaired by the ILD, whether there is evidence of progression of the ILD, and what extra-thoracic features require therapy. Not all patients with CTD-ILD require immunosuppressive therapy, and, in many cases, immunosuppression may only be needed for the extra-thoracic inflammatory disease features. Determining the degree of impairment or disease activity is typically based on integration of subjective factors plus objective parameters of functional capacity assessment, pulmonary physiology and HRCT findings. Identifying potential contraindications to therapy, comorbid conditions and potential drug–drug interactions all need to be taken into consideration.

A long-term approach to therapy is often indicated in CTD-ILD, and for disorders other than SSc-ILD, management is often 'experience based' rather than 'evidence based'. Initial therapy often includes high doses of corticosteroids (CS) along with early initiation of a steroid-sparing agent. This approach may be particularly indicated in those with more rapid progression of disease. Considering the pace of the disease, the underlying CTD and the specific histopathologic pattern may impact intensity and duration of CS therapy. Treatment decisions are made on an individualized basis by weighing pros and cons of specific therapeutic regimes. The more chronic phase of treatment usually consists of CS tapering and long-term use of a steroid-sparing agent. *Pneumocystis jiroveci* pneumonia (PjP) prophylaxis is usually recommended when two immunosuppressive therapies (including CS $\geq$ 20 mg/day of prednisone equivalent) are used (70), and some clinicians employ this approach when using CS at $\geq$20 mg/day of prednisone equivalent alone for any sustained period of time. Ultimately, the decision when to initiate PjP prophylaxis is individualized. Ideally, the treatment plan should be comprehensive in nature and balance a combination of pharmacologic therapies and non-pharmacologic strategies (71,72).

Supplemental oxygen needs should be assessed at rest, with exercise and during sleep, and oxygen therapy should be implemented in patients who demonstrate hypoxemia. Pulmonary rehabilitation can be an important adjunctive modality, as it provides a structured exercise and education programme that can have positive effects on exercise tolerance, quality of life and depression for patients with ILD or other chronic lung diseases (73). It is important to encourage and emphasize smoking cessation in all patients with CTD, and especially those with ILD. Appropriate vaccinations should be administered unless otherwise contraindicated. The seasonal inactivated *Influenza A* vaccine should be administered annually, and appropriate *Pneumococcal* vaccines (Prevnar© and Pneumovax©) should also be administered (74–76). *Herpes zoster* vaccine should be considered in CTD-ILD patients independently of age (74); however, because this is a live attenuated vaccine, administering the *herpes zoster* vaccine to those on chronic immunosuppressive therapy may be relatively contraindicated, and seeking expert input (such as with an infectious disease specialist) may be helpful to guide immunization decisions (71,75).

SPECIFIC ASPECTS OF MANAGEMENT

CORTICOSTEROIDS

Corticosteroids have broad anti-inflammatory and immunosuppressive effects and have served as an initial and mainstay of therapy for CTD-ILD (62). There are some small case series supporting the use of CS for CTD-ILD (77–79), but no controlled studies exist. The toxicity and adverse side effects associated with long-term use of CS are numerous and frequently limit their use. Corticosteroids are commonly introduced early in the treatment course at a moderate-to-high dose in order to obtain early improvement in symptoms. As steroid-sparing agents are added and dose-escalated, CS are slowly tapered towards a lower maintenance dose to minimize the cumulative toxicity of the CS. In many cases, CS may be tapered to complete discontinuation. Because of concerns that SSc patients treated with moderate-to-high dose CS may be at increased risk of scleroderma renal crisis, one caveat to this strategy is that the daily prednisone dose is often maintained at less than 15 mg/day for patients with SSc-ILD, although this is determined on a case-by-case basis. CS may be particularly effective in those with acute interstitial pneumonia (AIP) or more cellular forms of NSIP or OP. In such scenarios an intense up-front course of intravenous CS (such as with a several day course of pulse dosing) followed by a more prolonged taper may be indicated (71,72).

AZATHIOPRINE

Azathioprine (AZA) is a commonly used steroid-sparing agent for ILD but the data for AZA in CTD-ILD are largely limited to small and retrospective series (80–85). A recent randomized trial compared response to treatment with AZA versus cyclophosphamide (CYC) in SSc-ILD (86). In this 18-month study, 30 patients were treated with oral CYC (2 mg/kg/day for 12 months and then maintained on 1 mg/kg/day) and 30 patients were treated with oral AZA (2.5 mg/kg daily for 12 months and then maintained on 2 mg/kg daily). Both arms were also treated with low-dose prednisolone during the first 6 months of the trial. The FVC and DLCO were unchanged following treatment in the CYC arm, but both significantly declined in the AZA treatment arm (86). Nonetheless, AZA is a 'familiar' drug to many pulmonary practitioners, is well tolerated and, even in the absence of strong evidence, remains a popular choice as a steroid-sparing agent for a diverse array of CTD-ILD (71,72).

Prior to initiating AZA, it may be useful to test for thiopurine methyltransferase (TPMT) enzymes. Patients with absent or low levels of TPMT activity are at high risk for myelosuppression, whereas patients with normal or high levels of enzyme activity have a lower frequency of toxicity (87). In patients with normal TPMT levels in whom AZA is considered the agent of choice, therapy may be initiated at a low initial oral dose of 50 mg daily, and dose escalation performed based upon individual safety and tolerability with close drug-specific monitoring towards a target, goal maintenance dose of ~2 mg/kg/day. Dosing regimens should be tailored to the individual patient's tolerance of the agent, disease severity and disease responsiveness, and based on safety demonstrated by periodic serologic monitoring for myelosuppression and hepatotoxicity (88). Of note, because allopurinol substantially potentiates the effects of AZA, the combination of these two drugs is relatively contraindicated.

CYCLOPHOSPHAMIDE

Cyclophosphamide (CYC) is one of the most potent CS-sparing immunosuppressive medications and is often used to treat a variety of organ-threatening CTD manifestations. A number of small prospective (89–91) and retrospective (92–94) studies have suggested that CYC may lead to stabilization or improvement in lung function in CTD-ILD, and CYC is often considered first-line therapy for CTD patients with severe ILD (71,72).

The Scleroderma Lung Study (SLS) I (95) was a prospective clinical trial in which 158 subjects with SSc-ILD were randomized to oral CYC or placebo for 12 months. The FVC difference (ΔFVC) at 12 months was +2.53% of predicted ($p < 0.03$) in favour of the CYC group, which remained significant at 18 months from time of CYC initiation. However, by 24 months, the treated group had regressed to a similar FVC as the placebo arm (96). Those with FVC <70% predicted (96), higher fibrosis scores on thoracic high-resolution computed tomography (HRCT) scan or more skin thickening, had a more robust response to CYC (97).

The Fibrosing Alveolitis in Scleroderma Trial (FAST) (81) randomized patients with SSc-ILD to treatment ($n = 22$) with monthly IV CYC for 6 months followed by oral AZA for 6 months along with background low-dose oral prednisolone or to placebo ($n = 23$). The ΔFVC in the treatment group compared to the placebo group was not significantly different (ΔFVC +4.19% between groups; $p = 0.08$) (81). However, the ΔFVC was actually more pronounced in FAST than in SLS (+4.2% versus +2.5%, respectively), but the smaller number of subjects in FAST ($n = 45$) compared with SLS ($n = 158$) likely limited the ability of the results to achieve statistical significance in FAST.

Given the substantial toxicity associated with CYC (e.g. bone marrow suppression, infection risk, malignancy risk, bladder toxicity), it is usually considered a short-term option, and its use is often limited to those with more severe forms of CTD-ILD (62). CYC is equally effective in either oral or intravenous form. The intravenous form has less bladder toxicity and is generally considered as a safer option than the oral form. With intravenous therapy, a typical first infusion dose is 500 mg/m². and subsequent infusions are dose escalated based on tolerability and the white blood cell count nadir. Peak dosing is often ~750–1000 mg/m². Commonly, MESNA (administered at approximately 40% of the cumulative CYC dose before and after each CYC infusion) and robust hydration are utilized to minimize bladder toxicity. Judicious use of anti-emetic therapy is often required. Given the potential for adverse side effects and nuances associated with dose escalation, and institution of anti-emetics, infusions are often coordinated via rheumatology and infused in experienced centres. When CYC is given orally, the initial dose begins at 25–50 mg/day and dose-escalated as tolerated towards a recommended goal maintenance dose of ~2 mg/kg/day. The dosing regimen should be carefully titrated to individual tolerance, disease responsiveness and disease severity. Frequent assessment of the complete blood count and urinalysis is important to assess for myelosuppression and bladder toxicity, respectively (88).

MYCOPHENOLATE MOFETIL

Mycophenolate mofetil (MMF) has become an increasingly popular treatment in CTD-ILD. A number of small retrospective series suggested a beneficial role of MMF for CTD-ILD (98–100). The largest retrospective study of MMF use for CTD-ILD (101) consisted of a heterogeneous cohort of 125 CTD-ILD patients (44 SSc-ILD, 32 myositis-ILD, 18 RA-ILD), treated with MMF over a 3-year period. MMF treatment was found to be well tolerated, associated with effective CS dose tapering (from a median of 20 mg/day to 5 mg/day of prednisone at 12 months from MMF initiation [$p < 0.0001$]) and with longitudinal improvements in FVC and DLCO (101).

SLS II is a recently completed, randomized controlled trial that enrolled subjects with SSc-ILD to one of two arms: oral CYC ($n = 73$) for 1 year or MMF ($n = 69$) for 2 years (102). The adjusted percentage predicted FVC improved from baseline to 24 months by 2.19 with MMF and 2.88 with CYC and did not differ significantly between the two groups. Leukopenia (30 versus 4 patients) occurred more often with CYC, fewer patients in the MMF arm prematurely withdrew from the study (20 versus 32), and time to treatment cessation was shorter in the CYC group ($p = 0.019$) (102). Taken together, these data support the use of either CYC or MMF for SSc-ILD and a general preference for MMF because of its better tolerability and toxicity profile.

MMF is usually initiated at a low starting dosage (250–500 mg twice daily) and dose-escalated with close drug-specific monitoring towards a target dose of 1–1.5 g twice daily as tolerated. Periodic

serologic monitoring for myelosuppression, hepatotoxicity and other potential adverse effects of the drug should be instituted (88). In patients with gastrointestinal intolerance to MMF, a dose reduction of the MMF or a switch to mycophenolic acid (Myfortic©) may be considered.

OTHER AGENTS

The calcineurin inhibitors, cyclosporine and tacrolimus, are commonly used to treat a variety of CTD-ILD, and both drugs are well-tolerated and suitable steroid-sparing therapies. A number of retrospective studies suggest beneficial roles of cyclosporine and tacrolimus in CTD-ILD in general, and they may be particularly helpful in treating myositis-associated ILD (e.g. the anti-synthetase syndrome) in particular (103–109). Retrospective data suggest a possible role for rituximab in select forms of CTD-ILD (66,67) including anti-synthetase syndrome (110–113) or as 'rescue therapy' for severe forms of ILD. Rituximab is currently under investigation in a randomized, double-blind controlled trial compared to intravenous CYC therapy in patients with diverse forms of CTD-ILD (ClinicalTrials.gov Identifier: NCT01862926).

Longitudinal assessment

Assessments of medication tolerance, development of comorbidities and determination of disease progression are important for the longitudinal monitoring of patients with CTD-ILD and help guide therapeutic decision making and potential modification or cessation of therapy. Implementation of reproducible, subjective indicators of a patient's level of breathlessness, exercise capacity and quality of life can provide clinically important information and helps in the assessment of respiratory disease progression and general functionality. Serial assessment of FVC and DLCO are useful in assessing the degree of respiratory impairment due to ILD and may provide clues about the development of co-existent pulmonary vasculopathy. These pulmonary physiology parameters are particularly helpful when trying to assess for disease progression and response to therapy. Longitudinal decline in FVC is associated with survival in IPF, and FVC is commonly used as a surrogate marker for response to therapy in ILD in general (114). The 6MWT is generally a useful test to perform longitudinally for clinical purposes, is relatively inexpensive and easy to perform and provides an additional objective measure of exercise capacity that can be used to help plot the longitudinal clinical course of a patient's lung disease. Periodic HRCT scanning is also a valuable objective test for longitudinal monitoring of CTD-ILD by providing detailed information on the pattern, distribution and extent of the ILD, an assessment of disease severity, and the development of extra-parenchymal abnormalities.

LUNG TRANSPLANTATION

Lung transplantation is reserved for select patients who progress despite conventional therapy and is considered a last-resort option for CTD-ILD. The presence of co-morbid conditions (e.g. gastro-oesophageal reflux disease [GERD], pulmonary hypertension, cardiovascular disease, disability, etc.) and extra-pulmonary manifestations of their underlying CTD may adversely affect allograft function and survival following transplantation (115,116). Among carefully selected patients, survival after lung transplantation for patients with SSc-ILD may be similar to that for recipients with IPF complicated by pulmonary arterial hypertension (117,118), and similar survival findings have been found for patients with RA-ILD who have undergone lung transplantation as well as improvements in respiratory-related quality of life (119).

CURRENT AND FUTURE AREAS OF RESEARCH

With the recent approval of two novel anti-fibrotic agents (pirfenidone and nintedanib) for the treatment of idiopathic pulmonary fibrosis (IPF), there is a pressing need to evaluate their efficacy in fibrotic forms of CTD-ILD. Studies of these agents in SSc-ILD are already underway. The safety and tolerability of pirfenidone was tested in the LOTUSS (Safety and Tolerability of Pirfenidone in Patients with Systemic Sclerosis-Associated Interstitial Lung Disease) study (120). This open-label, phase II, 16-week study enrolled 63 patients, and 64% of the study participants were on background MMF.

Pirfenidone was found to be safe and generally well tolerated. However, LOTUSS was not designed to determine whether the drug is effective in treating SSc-ILD. A double-blind, randomized, placebo-controlled trial evaluating efficacy and safety of oral nintedanib treatment for at least 52 weeks in patients with SSc-ILD is actively enrolling (ClinicalTrials.gov Identifier: NCT02597933) and should help determine whether nintedanib has a role in the management of SSc-ILD. Beyond SSc-ILD, other forms of fibrotic CTD-ILD need to be studied.

Without the implementation of well-designed, thoughtful clinical trials, we are unable to address a number of fundamental questions. Can we extrapolate the findings from the studies of SSc-ILD to other forms of CTD-ILD? Should the presence of specific autoimmune features (i.e. a classification of IPAF) impact management decisions? Should we base management decisions in CTD-ILD independent of the specific patterns of ILD (e.g. NSIP versus UIP)? What is the role of rituximab in managing CTD-ILD? Are there other biologic disease-modifying anti-rheumatic drugs (DMARDs) worthy of consideration for treating CTD-ILD? Should specific therapies vary based on specific CTD, specific ILD histopathologic type or both? Obtaining answers to these and other questions requires a sustained and co-coordinated multicentre network approach to perform prospective, adequately powered clinical trials.

Other areas of research in CTD-ILD relate to identifying predictors of development and/or progression of ILD in specific CTD populations and enhancing HRCT technology with quantifiable HRCT interpretation to help guide treatment responsiveness. Most importantly, more effective therapeutic options are desperately needed. Finally, prospective studies are needed to validate and/or refine the IPAF classification criteria and to determine the natural history and clinical implications of such a classification.

PROGNOSIS AND LONG-TERM OUTLOOK

ILD has a significant impact on mortality in CTD populations. In patients with SSc, ILD has emerged as the leading cause of mortality (121), and ILD is one of the leading causes of death for patients with PM/DM (122). The presence of ILD conveys a threefold higher risk of death for patients with RA and accounts for 7% of all RA-associated deaths (123). In comparison to IIP and IPF in particular, a number of studies have shown that patients with CTD-ILD generally have a better survival experience; in part, this difference is based on an improved survival with CTD-UIP compared with idiopathic UIP (i.e. IPF) (60). The only exception may be RA, as several studies have demonstrated that the natural history of RA-UIP resembles that of IPF (7,124,125). However, the small sample sizes in the existing studies of RA-ILD, which contain inherent referral and cohort selection biases, and the presence of conflicting data limit our ability to draw firm conclusions concerning prognosis in comparison to that of patients with IPF.

For patients with SSc-ILD, older age, lower FVC and lower DLCO predicted mortality in more than one study (126). Male sex, extent of disease on thoracic HRCT scan, presence of honeycombing, elevated KL-6 values and increased alveolar epithelial permeability were identified as predictors of both mortality and ILD progression on unadjusted analyses. The extent of disease on HRCT scan was the only variable that independently predicted both mortality and ILD progression (61,126). Exertional hypoxia on 6MWT has been shown to be associated with mortality, probably reflecting its utility as a surrogate for disease severity and/or the presence of co-existing pulmonary hypertension (127).

For RA-ILD, Significant predictors of increased mortality risk on multivariate analysis were older age, male gender, lower DLCO, greater extent of fibrosis on HRCT and the presence of a UIP pattern (7). In one study of 114 patients with PM/DM-ILD, an acute/subacute form of ILD, lower FVC % predicted, higher age, higher percentage of neutrophils in BAL fluid, and a diagnosis of clinical amyopathic DM (CADM) were significantly associated with worse outcome in univariate Cox proportional hazards models. Multivariate Cox proportional hazards analysis validated acute/subacute ILD, %FVC, age and diagnosis of CADM (versus PM) as significant predictors of overall mortality. Patients with acute/subacute ILD had a much lower survival rate than those with chronic forms, and patients with CADM-ILD had a lower survival rate than those with PM-ILD (128). Because there are shared patient-specific and ILD-specific clinical,

physiologic, radiographic and pathologic indicators of prognosis across the various CTDs, composite score models, such as the ILD-GAP model, may be useful to predict mortality in CTD-ILD using easily obtained clinical variables (129). Given the substantial morbidity and mortality of CTD-ILD we need to expand our knowledge base to move forward for the benefit of our patients.

Clinical cases

CASE 1

A 38-year-old woman presented with progressive cough, exertional dyspnoea and fever that has been unresponsive to three courses of oral antibiotics. Her plain chest roentgenogram demonstrates bibasilar infiltrates, and a follow-up thoracic HRCT scan reveals features suggestive of NSIP and OP. The patient lacks arthralgias, arthritis, myalgias or myopathy, and she has not recently travelled or had sick contacts. She reports mild GERD as well as recent-onset Raynaud phenomenon. On physical exam, she has coarseness of the skin on the lateral aspect of the digits compatible with 'mechanic hands' and a fixed rash over the metacarpal and proximal inter-phalangeal joints. A complete blood count, comprehensive metabolic panel, erythrocyte sedimentation rate and creatine phosphokinase are all normal. Her ANA, RF, CCP and Scl-70 are negative but the SS-A and JO-1 antibody are positive.

This patient has an anti-synthetase syndrome, which is characterized by constitutional symptoms, myositis, Raynaud phenomenon, mechanic hands, non-erosive arthritis and interstitial lung disease (ILD). Other features such as a heliotrope rash, Gottron's papules and GERD may also be present. It is not uncommon to see this syndrome present in an incomplete manner, as some patients will lack the myositis or the ILD (or some of the other features described above).

CASE 2

A 63-year-old man with RA reports several months of exertional dyspnoea and cough. He is an active, long-time cigarette smoker. He has been treated with methotrexate and combinations of biologic DMARDs for the past 10 years, and he has also been maintained on prednisone 10 mg daily for the past 3 months due to an increase in his synovitis. A HRCT scan shows a few scattered areas of nodularity as well as ground-glass opacities that are predominantly in the upper lung zones. He is referred for further evaluation.

Patients with CTD are at risk for pulmonary diseases and various forms of ILD in particular, but they also have multiple other risk factors for lung disease. In this patient with RA, medication-related pneumonitis, smoking-related ILD, and infection must be included in differential diagnostic considerations. The HRCT is described as atypical for RA-ILD, and a thorough evaluation is needed to arrive at an accurate diagnosis that explains the HRCT abnormalities.

CASE 3

A 47-year-old woman with a 3-year history of limited cutaneous SSc presents with progressive dyspnoea over the past few months. She has Raynaud phenomenon, limited skin thickening and well-controlled GERD. The FVC % predicted values have decreased over the past 12 months from 88% to 75%, and the DLCO has decreased from 73% to 65% of predicted. The thoracic HRCT scan shows mild progression of a lower lobe, non-specific interstitial pneumonia-type pattern, with an estimated disease extent of approximately 15%. You are asked to recommend specific therapeutic agents for management of progressive SSc-ILD.

This patient presents with evidence of progression of SSc-ILD and should be treated with immunosuppressive therapy. Based on the existing data from controlled trials, the best therapy for SSc-ILD is either mycophenolate mofetil or cyclophosphamide. Due to the better tolerability associated with MMF, and because MMF appears to be equally effective as CYC, she is initiated on MMF 500 mg twice daily with a plan to titrate to a target dose of 1500 mg twice daily.

REFERENCES

1. Fischer A, du Bois R. Interstitial lung disease in connective tissue disorders. *Lancet.* 2012;380(9842):689–98.
2. Cottin V. Interstitial lung disease: Are we missing formes frustes of connective tissue disease? *Eur Respir J.* 2006;28(5):893–6.
3. Tzelepis GE, Toya SP, Moutsopoulos HM. Occult connective tissue diseases mimicking idiopathic interstitial pneumonias. *Eur Respir J.* 2008;31(1):11–20.
4. Fischer A, Brown KK. Interstitial lung disease in undifferentiated forms of connective tissue disease. *Arthritis Care Res (Hoboken).* 2015;67(1):4–11.
5. Fischer A, Antoniou KM, Brown KK, Cadranel J, Corte TJ, du Bois RM et al. An official European Respiratory Society/American Thoracic Society research statement: Interstitial pneumonia with autoimmune features. *Eur Respir J.* 2015;46(4):976–87.
6. Kolahian S, Fernandez IE, Eickelberg O, Hartl D. Immune mechanisms in pulmonary fibrosis. *Am J Respir Cell Mol Biol.* 2016;55(3):309–22.
7. Assayag D, Lubin M, Lee JS, King TE, Collard HR, Ryerson CJ. Predictors of mortality in rheumatoid arthritis-related interstitial lung disease. *Respirology.* 2014;19(4):493–500.
8. Yunt ZX, Solomon JJ. Lung disease in rheumatoid arthritis. *Rheum Dis Clin North Am.* 2015;41(2):225–36.
9. Steen VD. Autoantibodies in systemic sclerosis. *Semin Arthritis Rheum.* 2005;35(1):35–42.
10. Steen VD. The lung in systemic sclerosis. *J Clin Rheumatol.* 2005;11(1):40–6.
11. Wells AU, Margaritopoulos GA, Antoniou KM, Denton C. Interstitial lung disease in systemic sclerosis. *Semin Respir Crit Care Med.* 2014;35(2):213–21.
12. Fertig N, Domsic RT, Rodriguez-Reyna T, Kuwana M, Lucas M, Medsger TA, Jr. et al. Anti-U11/U12 RNP antibodies in systemic sclerosis: A new serologic marker associated with pulmonary fibrosis. *Arthritis Rheum.* 2009;61(7):958–65.
13. Fischer A, Meehan RT, Feghali-Bostwick CA, West SG, Brown KK. Unique characteristics of systemic sclerosis sine scleroderma-associated interstitial lung disease. *Chest.* 2006;130(4):976–81.
14. Chartrand S, Swigris JJ, Peykova L, Chung J, Fischer A. A multidisciplinary evaluation helps identify the antisynthetase

syndrome in patients presenting as idiopathic interstitial pneumonia. *J Rheumatol.* 2016;43(5):887–92.

15. Fischer A, Swigris JJ, du Bois RM, Lynch DA, Downey GP, Cosgrove GP et al. Antisynthetase syndrome in ANA and anti-Jo-1 negative patients presenting with idiopathic interstitial pneumonia. *Respir Med.* 2009;103(11):1719–24.

16. Lega JC, Cottin V, Fabien N, Thivolet-Bejui F, Cordier JF. Interstitial lung disease associated with anti-PM/Scl or anti-aminoacyl-tRNA synthetase autoantibodies: A similar condition? *J Rheumatol.* 2010;37(5):1000–9.

17. Lega JC, Fabien N, Reynaud Q, Durieu I, Durupt S, Dutertre M et al. The clinical phenotype associated with myositis-specific and associated autoantibodies: A meta-analysis revisiting the so-called antisynthetase syndrome. *Autoimmun Rev.* 2014;13(9): 883–91.

18. Sato S, Kuwana M, Fujita T, Suzuki Y. Amyopathic dermatomyositis developing rapidly progressive interstitial lung disease with elevation of anti-CADM-140/MDA5 autoantibodies. *Mod Rheumatol.* 2012;22(4):625–9.

19. Suzuki A, Kondoh Y, Taniguchi H, Tabata K, Kimura T, Kataoka K et al. Lung histopathological pattern in a survivor with rapidly progressive interstitial lung disease and anti-melanoma differentiation-associated gene 5 antibody-positive clinically amyopathic dermatomyositis. *Respir Med Case Rep.* 2016;19:5–8.

20. Winklehner A, Berger N, Maurer B, Distler O, Alkadhi H, Frauenfelder T. Screening for interstitial lung disease in systemic sclerosis: The diagnostic accuracy of HRCT image series with high increment and reduced number of slices. *Ann Rheum Dis.* 2012;71(4):549–52.

21. D'Angelo WA, Fries JF, Masi AT, Shulman LE. Pathologic observations in systemic sclerosis (scleroderma). A study of fifty-eight autopsy cases and fifty-eight matched controls. *Am J Med.* 1969;46(3):428–40.

22. Schnabel A, Hellmich B, Gross WL. Interstitial lung disease in polymyositis and dermatomyositis. *Curr Rheumatol Rep.* 2005;7(2):99–105.

23. Schnabel A, Reuter M, Biederer J, Richter C, Gross WL. Interstitial lung disease in polymyositis and dermatomyositis: Clinical course and response to treatment. *Semin Arthritis Rheum.* 2003;32(5):273–84.

24. Schwarz MI. The lung in polymyositis. *Clin Chest Med.* 1998;19(4):701–12, viii.

25. Bongartz T, Nannini C, Medina-Velasquez YF, Achenbach SJ, Crowson CS, Ryu JH et al. Incidence and mortality of interstitial lung disease in rheumatoid arthritis: A population-based study. *Arthritis Rheum.* 2010;62(6):1583–91.

26. Dawson JK, Fewins HE, Desmond J, Lynch MP, Graham DR. Fibrosing alveolitis in patients with rheumatoid arthritis as assessed by high resolution computed tomography, chest radiography, and pulmonary function tests. *Thorax.* 2001;56(8):622–7.

27. Nannini C, Ryu JH, Matteson EL. Lung disease in rheumatoid arthritis. *Curr Opin Rheumatol.* 2008;20(3):340–6.

28. Olson AL, Swigris JJ, Sprunger DB, Fischer A, Fernandez-Perez ER, Solomon J et al. Rheumatoid arthritis-interstitial lung disease-associated mortality. *Am J Respir Crit Care Med.* 2011;183(3):372–8.

29. Chen J, Doyle TJ, Liu Y, Aggarwal R, Wang X, Shi Y et al. Biomarkers of rheumatoid arthritis-associated interstitial lung disease. *Arthritis Rheumatol.* 2015;67(1):28–38.

30. Doyle TJ, Dellaripa PF, Batra K, Frits ML, Iannaccone CK, Hatabu H et al. Functional impact of a spectrum of interstitial lung abnormalities in rheumatoid arthritis. *Chest.* 2014;146(1):41–50.

31. Doyle TJ, Hunninghake GM, Rosas IO. Subclinical interstitial lung disease: Why you should care. *Am J Respir Crit Care Med.* 2012;185(11):1147–53.

32. Doyle TJ, Patel AS, Hatabu H, Nishino M, Wu G, Osorio JC et al. Detection of rheumatoid arthritis-interstitial lung disease is enhanced by serum biomarkers. *Am J Respir Crit Care Med.* 2015;191(12):1403–12.

33. Castelino FV, Varga J. Interstitial lung disease in connective tissue diseases: Evolving concepts of pathogenesis and management. *Arthritis Res Ther.* 2010;12(4):213.

34. Castelino FV, Goldberg H, Dellaripa PF. The impact of rheumatological evaluation in the management of patients with interstitial lung disease. *Rheumatology (Oxford)*. 2011;50(3):489–93.

35. Swigris JJ, Yorke J, Sprunger DB, Swearingen C, Pincus T, du Bois RM et al. Assessing dyspnea and its impact on patients with connective tissue disease-related interstitial lung disease. *Respir Med*. 2010;104(9):1350–5.

36. Mittoo S, Gelber AC, Christopher-Stine L, Horton MR, Lechtzin N, Danoff SK. Ascertainment of collagen vascular disease in patients presenting with interstitial lung disease. *Respir Med*. 2009;103(8):1152–8.

37. ATS/ERS. American Thoracic Society/European Respiratory Society International Multidisciplinary Consensus Classification of the Idiopathic Interstitial Pneumonias. This joint statement of the American Thoracic Society (ATS), and the European Respiratory Society (ERS) was adopted by the ATS board of directors, June 2001 and by the ERS Executive Committee, June 2001. *Am J Respir Crit Care Med*. 2002;165(2):277–304.

38. Raghu G, Collard HR, Egan JJ, Martinez FJ, Behr J, Brown KK et al. An official ATS/ERS/JRS/ALAT statement: Idiopathic pulmonary fibrosis: Evidence-based guidelines for diagnosis and management. *Am J Respir Crit Care Med*. 2011;183(6):788–824.

39. Bahmer T, Romagnoli M, Girelli F, Claussen M, Rabe KF. The use of auto-antibody testing in the evaluation of interstitial lung disease (ILD): A practical approach for the pulmonologist. *Respir Med*. 2016;113:80–92.

40. Fischer A, Richeldi L. Cross-disciplinary collaboration in connective tissue disease-related lung disease. *Semin Respir Crit Care Med*. 2014;35(2):159–65.

41. Fischer A, du Bois RM. A practical approach to connective tissue disease-associated lung disease. In: Baughman RP, du Bois RM, eds. *Diffuse Lung Disease*. 2nd ed. New York, NY: Springer, 2012. p. 217–37.

42. Corte TJ, Copley SJ, Desai SR, Zappala CJ, Hansell DM, Nicholson AG et al. Significance of connective tissue disease features in idiopathic interstitial pneumonia. *Eur Respir J*. 2012;39(3):661–8.

43. Solomon DH, Kavanaugh AJ, Schur PH, American College of Rheumatology Ad Hoc Committee on Immunologic Testing G. Evidence-based guidelines for the use of immunologic tests: Antinuclear antibody testing. *Arthritis Rheum*. 2002;47(4):434–44.

44. Shanmugam VK, Swistowski DR, Saddic N, Wang H, Steen VD. Comparison of indirect immunofluorescence and multiplex antinuclear antibody screening in systemic sclerosis. *Clin Rheumatol*. 2011;30(10):1363–8.

45. Fischer A, Pfalzgraf FJ, Feghali-Bostwick CA, Wright TM, Curran-Everett D, West SG et al. Anti-Th/To-positivity in a cohort of patients with idiopathic pulmonary fibrosis. *J Rheumatol*. 2006;33(8):1600–5.

46. Papiris SA, Daniil ZD, Malagari K, Kapotsis GE, Sotiropoulou C, Milic-Emili J et al. The Medical Research Council dyspnea scale in the estimation of disease severity in idiopathic pulmonary fibrosis. *Respir Med*. 2005;99(6):755–61.

47. Holland AE, Fiore JF, Jr., Bell EC, Goh N, Westall G, Symons K et al. Dyspnoea and comorbidity contribute to anxiety and depression in interstitial lung disease. *Respirology*. 2014;19(8):1215–21.

48. Kozu R, Jenkins S, Senjyu H. Evaluation of activity limitation in patients with idiopathic pulmonary fibrosis grouped according to Medical Research Council dyspnea grade. *Arch Phys Med Rehabil*. 2014;95(5):950–5.

49. Suliman YA, Dobrota R, Huscher D, Nguyen-Kim TD, Maurer B, Jordan S et al. Brief report: Pulmonary function tests: High rate of false-negative results in the early detection and screening of scleroderma-related interstitial lung disease. *Arthritis Rheumatol*. 2015;67(12):3256–61.

50. Nogueira CR, Napolis LM, Bagatin E, Terra-Filho M, Muller NL, Silva CI et al. Lung diffusing capacity relates better to short-term progression on HRCT abnormalities than spirometry in mild asbestosis. *Am J Ind Med*. 2011;54(3):185–93.

51. Pellegrino R, Viegi G, Brusasco V, Crapo RO, Burgos F, Casaburi R et al. Interpretative strategies for lung function tests. *Eur Respir J.* 2005;26(5):948–68.

52. Goh NS, Veeraraghavan S, Desai SR, Cramer D, Hansell DM, Denton CP et al. Bronchoalveolar lavage cellular profiles in patients with systemic sclerosis-associated interstitial lung disease are not predictive of disease progression. *Arthritis Rheum.* 2007;56(6):2005–12.

53. Kowal-Bielecka O, Kowal K, Highland KB, Silver RM. Bronchoalveolar lavage fluid in scleroderma interstitial lung disease: Technical aspects and clinical correlations: Review of the literature. *Semin Arthritis Rheum.* 2012;40(1):73–88.

54. Strange C, Bolster MB, Roth MD, Silver RM, Theodore A, Goldin J et al. Bronchoalveolar lavage and response to cyclophosphamide in scleroderma interstitial lung disease. *Am J Respir Crit Care Med.* 2008;177(1):91–8.

55. Mathieson JR, Mayo JR, Staples CA, Muller NL. Chronic diffuse infiltrative lung disease: Comparison of diagnostic accuracy of CT and chest radiography. *Radiology.* 1989; 171(1):111–6.

56. Hwang JH, Misumi S, Sahin H, Brown KK, Newell JD, Lynch DA. Computed tomographic features of idiopathic fibrosing interstitial pneumonia: Comparison with pulmonary fibrosis related to collagen vascular disease. *J Comput Assist Tomogr.* 2009;33(3):410–5.

57. Lynch DA. Quantitative CT of fibrotic interstitial lung disease. *Chest.* 2007;131(3):643–4.

58. Lynch DA, Travis WD, Muller NL, Galvin JR, Hansell DM, Grenier PA et al. Idiopathic interstitial pneumonias: CT features. *Radiology.* 2005;236(1):10–21.

59. Gupta N, Wikenheiser-Brokamp KA, Fischer A, McCormack FX. Diffuse cystic lung disease as the presenting manifestation of Sjogren syndrome. *Ann Am Thorac Soc.* 2016;13(3):371–5.

60. Park JH, Kim DS, Park IN, Jang SJ, Kitaichi M, Nicholson AG et al. Prognosis of fibrotic interstitial pneumonia: Idiopathic versus collagen vascular disease-related subtypes. *Am J Respir Crit Care Med.* 2007;175(7):705–11.

61. Goh NS, Desai SR, Veeraraghavan S, Hansell DM, Copley SJ, Maher TM et al. Interstitial lung disease in systemic sclerosis: A simple staging system. *Am J Respir Crit Care Med.* 2008;177(11):1248–54.

62. Fischer A, Chartrand S. Assessment and management of connective tissue disease-associated interstitial lung disease. *Sarcoidosis Vasc Diffuse Lung Dis.* 2015;32(1):2–21.

63. Leslie KO, Trahan S, Gruden J. Pulmonary pathology of the rheumatic diseases. *Semin Respir Crit Care Med.* 2007;28(4):369–78.

64. Flaherty KR, Colby TV, Travis WD, Toews GB, Mumford J, Murray S et al. Fibroblastic foci in usual interstitial pneumonia: Idiopathic versus collagen vascular disease. *Am J Respir Crit Care Med.* 2003;167(10):1410–5.

65. Song JW, Do KH, Kim MY, Jang SJ, Colby TV, Kim DS. Pathologic and radiologic differences between idiopathic and collagen vascular disease-related usual interstitial pneumonia. *Chest.* 2009;136(1): 23–30.

66. Fischer A, West SG, Swigris JJ, Brown KK, du Bois RM. Connective tissue disease-associated interstitial lung disease: A call for clarification. *Chest.* 2010;138(2):251–6.

67. Fujita J, Ohtsuki Y, Yoshinouchi T, Yamadori I, Bandoh S, Tokuda M et al. Idiopathic non-specific interstitial pneumonia: As an 'autoimmune interstitial pneumonia'. *Respir Med.* 2005;99(2):234–40.

68. Kinder BW, Collard HR, Koth L, Daikh DI, Wolters PJ, Elicker B et al. Idiopathic nonspecific interstitial pneumonia: Lung manifestation of undifferentiated connective tissue disease? *Am J Respir Crit Care Med.* 2007;176(7):691–7.

69. Vij R, Noth I, Strek ME. Autoimmune-featured interstitial lung disease: A distinct entity. *Chest.* 2011;140(5):1292–9.

70. Vananuvat P, Suwannalai P, Sungkanuparph S, Limsuwan T, Ngamjanyaporn P, Janwityanujit S. Primary prophylaxis for

Pneumocystis jirovecii pneumonia in patients with connective tissue diseases. *Semin Arthritis Rheum.* 2011;41(3):497–502.

71. Chartrand S, Fischer A. Management of connective tissue disease-associated interstitial lung disease. *Rheum Dis Clin North Am.* 2015;41(2):279–94.

72. Lee JS, Fischer A. Current and emerging treatment options for interstitial lung disease in patients with rheumatic disease. *Expert Rev Clin Immunol.* 2016;12(5):509–20.

73. Ryerson CJ, Cayou C, Topp F, Hilling L, Camp PG, Wilcox PG et al. Pulmonary rehabilitation improves long-term outcomes in interstitial lung disease: A prospective cohort study. *Respir Med.* 2014;108(1):203–10.

74. Bridges CB, Coyne-Beasley T. Advisory committee on immunization practices recommended immunization schedule for adults aged 19 years or older: United States, 2014. *Ann Intern Med.* 2014;160(3):190.

75. van Assen S, Agmon-Levin N, Elkayam O, Cervera R, Doran MF, Dougados M et al. EULAR recommendations for vaccination in adult patients with autoimmune inflammatory rheumatic diseases. *Ann Rheum Dis.* 2011;70(3):414–22.

76. Bombardier C, Hazlewood GS, Akhavan P, Schieir O, Dooley A, Haraoui B et al. Canadian Rheumatology Association recommendations for the pharmacological management of rheumatoid arthritis with traditional and biologic disease-modifying antirheumatic drugs: Part II safety. *J Rheumatol.* 2012;39(8):1583–602.

77. Holgate ST, Glass DN, Haslam P, Maini RN, Turner-Warwick M. Respiratory involvement in systemic lupus erythematosus. A clinical and immunological study. *Clin Exp Immunol.* 1976;24(3):385–95.

78. Patterson CD, Harville WE, Pierce JA. Rheumatoid lung disease. *Ann Intern Med.* 1965;62:685–97.

79. Sullivan WD, Hurst DJ, Harmon CE, Esther JH, Agia GA, Maltby JD et al. A prospective evaluation emphasizing pulmonary involvement in patients with mixed connective tissue disease. *Medicine (Baltimore).* 1984;63(2):92–107.

80. Mira-Avendano IC, Parambil JG, Yadav R, Arrossi V, Xu M, Chapman JT et al. A retrospective review of clinical features and treatment outcomes in steroid-resistant interstitial lung disease from polymyositis/dermatomyositis. *Respir Med.* 2013;107(6):890–6.

81. Hoyles RK, Ellis RW, Wellsbury J, Lees B, Newlands P, Goh NS et al. A multicenter, prospective, randomized, double-blind, placebo-controlled trial of corticosteroids and intravenous cyclophosphamide followed by oral azathioprine for the treatment of pulmonary fibrosis in scleroderma. *Arthritis Rheum.* 2006;54(12):3962–70.

82. Berezne A, Ranque B, Valeyre D, Brauner M, Allanore Y, Launay D et al. Therapeutic strategy combining intravenous cyclophosphamide followed by oral azathioprine to treat worsening interstitial lung disease associated with systemic sclerosis: A retrospective multicenter open-label study. *J Rheumatol.* 2008;35(6):1064–72.

83. Dheda K, Lalloo UG, Cassim B, Mody GM. Experience with azathioprine in systemic sclerosis associated with interstitial lung disease. *Clin Rheumatol.* 2004;23(4):306–9.

84. Poormoghim H, Rezaei N, Sheidaie Z, Almasi AR, Moradi-Lakeh M, Almasi S et al. Systemic sclerosis: Comparison of efficacy of oral cyclophosphamide and azathioprine on skin score and pulmonary involvement- a retrospective study. *Rheumatol Int.* 2014;34(12):1691–9.

85. Deheinzelin D, Capelozzi VL, Kairalla RA, Barbas Filho JV, Saldiva PH, de Carvalho CR. Interstitial lung disease in primary Sjogren's syndrome. Clinical-pathological evaluation and response to treatment. *Am J Respir Crit Care Med.* 1996;154 (3 Pt 1):794–9.

86. Nadashkevich O, Davis P, Fritzler M, Kovalenko W. A randomized unblinded trial of cyclophosphamide versus azathioprine in the treatment of systemic sclerosis. *Clin Rheumatol.* 2006;25(2):205–12.

87. Stolk JN, Boerbooms AM, de Abreu RA, de Koning DG, van Beusekom HJ, Muller WH et al. Reduced thiopurine methyltransferase activity and development of side

effects of azathioprine treatment in patients with rheumatoid arthritis. *Arthritis Rheum.* 1998;41(10):1858–66.

88. Furst DE, Clements PJ. Immunosuppressives. In: Hochberg MC, Silman AJ, Smolen JS, Weinblatt ME, Weisman MH, eds. *Rheumatology.* 3rd ed. St. Louis, MO: Mosby; 2003:439–48.

89. Silver RM, Warrick JH, Kinsella MB, Staudt LS, Baumann MH, Strange C. Cyclophosphamide and low-dose prednisone therapy in patients with systemic sclerosis (scleroderma) with interstitial lung disease. *J Rheumatol.* 1993;20(5):838–44.

90. Schnabel A, Reuter M, Gross WL. Intravenous pulse cyclophosphamide in the treatment of interstitial lung disease due to collagen vascular diseases. *Arthritis Rheum.* 1998;41(7):1215–20.

91. Akesson A, Scheja A, Lundin A, Wollheim FA. Improved pulmonary function in systemic sclerosis after treatment with cyclophosphamide. *Arthritis Rheum.* 1994;37(5):729–35.

92. White B, Moore WC, Wigley FM, Xiao HQ, Wise RA. Cyclophosphamide is associated with pulmonary function and survival benefit in patients with scleroderma and alveolitis. *Ann Intern Med.* 2000;132(12):947–54.

93. Steen VD, Lanz JK, Jr., Conte C, Owens GR, Medsger TA, Jr. Therapy for severe interstitial lung disease in systemic sclerosis. A retrospective study. *Arthritis Rheum.* 1994;37(9):1290–6.

94. Yamasaki Y, Yamada H, Yamasaki M, Ohkubo M, Azuma K, Matsuoka S et al. Intravenous cyclophosphamide therapy for progressive interstitial pneumonia in patients with polymyositis/dermatomyositis. *Rheumatology (Oxford).* 2007;46(1):124–30.

95. Tashkin DP, Elashoff R, Clements PJ, Goldin J, Roth MD, Furst DE et al. Cyclophosphamide versus placebo in scleroderma lung disease. *N Engl J Med.* 2006;354(25):2655–66.

96. Tashkin DP, Elashoff R, Clements PJ, Roth MD, Furst DE, Silver RM et al. Effects of 1-year treatment with cyclophosphamide on outcomes at 2 years in scleroderma lung disease. *Am J Respir Crit Care Med.* 2007;176(10):1026–34.

97. Roth MD, Tseng CH, Clements PJ, Furst DE, Tashkin DP, Goldin JG et al. Predicting treatment outcomes and responder subsets in scleroderma-related interstitial lung disease. *Arthritis Rheum.* 2011;63(9):2797–808.

98. Gerbino AJ, Goss CH, Molitor JA. Effect of mycophenolate mofetil on pulmonary function in scleroderma-associated interstitial lung disease. *Chest.* 2008;133(2):455–60.

99. Swigris JJ, Olson AL, Fischer A, Lynch DA, Cosgrove GP, Frankel SK et al. Mycophenolate mofetil is safe, well tolerated, and preserves lung function in patients with connective tissue disease-related interstitial lung disease. *Chest.* 2006;130(1):30–6.

100. Liossis SN, Bounas A, Andonopoulos AP. Mycophenolate mofetil as first-line treatment improves clinically evident early scleroderma lung disease. *Rheumatology (Oxford).* 2006;45(8):1005–8.

101. Fischer A, Brown KK, Du Bois RM, Frankel SK, Cosgrove GP, Fernandez-Perez ER et al. Mycophenolate mofetil improves lung function in connective tissue disease-associated interstitial lung disease. *J Rheumatol.* 2013;40(5):640–6.

102. Tashkin DP, Roth MD, Clements PJ, Furst DE, Khanna D, Kleerup EC et al. Mycophenolate mofetil versus oral cyclophosphamide in scleroderma-related interstitial lung disease (SLS II): A randomised controlled, double-blind, parallel group trial. *Lancet Respir Med.* 2016;4(9):708–19.

103. Cavagna L, Caporali R, Abdi-Ali L, Dore R, Meloni F, Montecucco C. Cyclosporine in anti-Jo1-positive patients with corticosteroid-refractory interstitial lung disease. *J Rheumatol.* 2013;40(4):484–92.

104. Harigai M, Hara M, Kamatani N, Kashiwazaki S. [Nation-wide survey for the treatment with cyclosporin A of interstitial pneumonia associated with collagen diseases]. *Ryumachi [Rheumatism].* 1999;39(6):819–28.

105. Kurita T, Yasuda S, Oba K, Odani T, Kono M, Otomo K et al. The efficacy of tacrolimus in patients with interstitial lung diseases complicated with polymyositis or dermatomyositis. *Rheumatology.* 2015;54(1):39–44.

106. Ochi S, Nanki T, Takada K, Suzuki F, Komano Y, Kubota T et al. Favorable outcomes with tacrolimus in two patients with refractory interstitial lung disease associated with polymyositis/dermatomyositis. *Clin Exp Rheumatol.* 2005;23(5):707–10.

107. Oddis CV, Sciurba FC, Elmagd KA, Starzl TE. Tacrolimus in refractory polymyositis with interstitial lung disease. *Lancet.* 1999;353(9166):1762–3.

108. Takada K, Nagasaka K, Miyasaka N. Polymyositis/dermatomyositis and interstitial lung disease: A new therapeutic approach with T-cell-specific immunosuppressants. *Autoimmunity.* 2005;38(5):383–92.

109. Wilkes MR, Sereika SM, Fertig N, Lucas MR, Oddis CV. Treatment of antisynthetase-associated interstitial lung disease with tacrolimus. *Arthritis Rheum.* 2005;52(8):2439–46.

110. Andersson H, Sem M, Lund MB, Aalokken TM, Gunther A, Walle-Hansen R et al. Long-term experience with rituximab in anti-synthetase syndrome-related interstitial lung disease. *Rheumatology (Oxford).* 2015;54(8):1420–8.

111. Unger L, Kampf S, Luthke K, Aringer M. Rituximab therapy in patients with refractory dermatomyositis or polymyositis: Differential effects in a real-life population. *Rheumatology (Oxford).* 2014;53(9):1630–8.

112. Sem M, Molberg O, Lund MB, Gran JT. Rituximab treatment of the anti-synthetase syndrome: A retrospective case series. *Rheumatology (Oxford).* 2009;48(8):968–71.

113. Marie I, Dominique S, Janvresse A, Levesque H, Menard JF. Rituximab therapy for refractory interstitial lung disease related to antisynthetase syndrome. *Respir Med.* 2012;106(4):581–7.

114. du Bois RM, Weycker D, Albera C, Bradford WZ, Costabel U, Kartashov A et al. Forced vital capacity in patients with idiopathic pulmonary fibrosis: Test properties and minimal clinically important difference. *Am J Respir Crit Care Med.* 2011;184(12):1382–9.

115. Fisichella PM, Jalilvand A. The role of impaired esophageal and gastric motility in end-stage lung diseases and after lung transplantation. *J Surg Res.* 2014;186(1):201–6.

116. Diamond JM, Lee JC, Kawut SM, Shah RJ, Localio AR, Bellamy SL et al. Clinical risk factors for primary graft dysfunction after lung transplantation. *Am J Respir Crit Care Med.* 2013;187(5):527–34.

117. Sottile PD, Iturbe D, Katsumoto TR, Connolly MK, Collard HR, Leard LA et al. Outcomes in systemic sclerosis-related lung disease after lung transplantation. *Transplantation.* 2013;95(7):975–80.

118. Bernstein EJ, Peterson ER, Sell JL, D'Ovidio F, Arcasoy SM, Bathon JM et al. Survival of adults with systemic sclerosis following lung transplantation: A nationwide cohort study. *Arthritis Rheumatol.* 2015;67(5):1314–22.

119. Yazdani A, Singer LG, Strand V, Gelber AC, Williams L, Mittoo S. Survival and quality of life in rheumatoid arthritis-associated interstitial lung disease after lung transplantation. *J Heart Lung Transplant.* 2014;33(5):514–20.

120. Khanna D, Albera C, Fischer A, Khalidi N, Raghu G, Chung L et al. Safety and tolerability of pirfenidone in patients with systemic sclerosis-associated interstitial lung disease—The LOTUSS study. *Am J Respir Crit Care Med.* 2012(191):A1175.

121. Tyndall AJ, Bannert B, Vonk M, Airo P, Cozzi F, Carreira PE et al. Causes and risk factors for death in systemic sclerosis: A study from the EULAR Scleroderma Trials and Research (EUSTAR) database. *Ann Rheum Dis.* 2010;69(10):1809–15.

122. Amaral Silva M, Cogollo E, Isenberg DA. Why do patients with myositis die? A retrospective analysis of a single-centre cohort. *Clin Exp Rheumatol.* 2016;34(5):820–6.

123. Brown KK. Rheumatoid lung disease. *Proc Am Thorac Soc.* 2007;4(5):443–8.

124. Kim EJ, Collard HR, King TE, Jr. Rheumatoid arthritis-associated interstitial lung disease: The relevance of histopathologic and radiographic pattern. *Chest.* 2009;136(5):1397–405.

125. Kim EJ, Elicker BM, Maldonado F, Webb WR, Ryu JH, Van Uden JH et al. Usual interstitial pneumonia in rheumatoid arthritis-associated interstitial lung disease. *Eur Respir J.* 2010;35(6):1322–8.

126. Ryerson CJ, O'Connor D, Dunne JV, Schooley F, Hague CJ, Murphy D et al. Predicting mortality in systemic sclerosis-associated interstitial lung disease using risk prediction models derived from idiopathic pulmonary fibrosis. *Chest.* 2015;148(5):1268–75.

127. Rizzi M, Sarzi-Puttini P, Airoldi A, Antivalle M, Battellino M, Atzeni F. Performance capacity evaluated using the 6-minute walk test: 5-year results in patients with diffuse systemic sclerosis and initial interstitial lung disease. *Clin Exp Rheumatol.* 2015;33(4 Suppl 91):S142–7.

128. Fujisawa T, Hozumi H, Kono M, Enomoto N, Hashimoto D, Nakamura Y et al. Prognostic factors for myositis-associated interstitial lung disease. *PLoS One.* 2014;9(6):e98824.

129. Ryerson CJ, Vittinghoff E, Ley B, Lee JS, Mooney JJ, Jones KD et al. Predicting survival across chronic interstitial lung disease: The ILD-GAP model. *Chest.* 2014;145(4):723–8.

15

Pulmonary sarcoidosis

DAVID R MOLLER AND LING-PEI HO

BACKGROUND

Sarcoidosis is a multisystem disease that affects the lungs in over 90% of individuals. With an incidence of ~10–64/100,000 people in the United States and Europe, pulmonary sarcoidosis is one of the most common causes of interstitial lung disease (1). Systemic sarcoidosis is characterized by tremendous heterogeneity in disease manifestations, with variable extra-pulmonary involvement and a clinical course and healthcare burden that vary widely. The diagnosis can be challenging and with uncommon exceptions, requires a confirmatory biopsy and exclusion of competing diagnoses. Pulmonary sarcoidosis may manifest with intra-thoracic lymphadenopathy, pulmonary nodules, infiltrates and/or masses that vary in distribution. Pulmonary hypertension and advanced fibrocystic disease can result

in respiratory insufficiency and death. Systemic manifestations such as cardiac, neurologic, abdominal, skin or ocular involvement may dominate the clinical picture and drive treatment approaches (discussed in Chapter 16). We review the scientific basis of sarcoidosis and consensus approaches to manage pulmonary sarcoidosis.

SCIENTIFIC MECHANISMS

IMMUNOBIOLOGY

The defining pathology in pulmonary sarcoidosis is the active immune granuloma which comprise coalescing macrophages forming epithelioid cells, and which are usually non-caseating. Generation of these well-defined cellular entities require a minimum combination of (a) monocytes possibly with higher sensitivity of homing receptors (CCR2) and pathogen recognition receptors causing heightened activity and homing capabilities to tissue where they differentiate into macrophages (b) an appropriate class of antigen (poorly degradable) to provide a nidus for formation of granuloma and (c) activated CD4+ Th1 lymphocytes to drive activation of local macrophages. The role of CD8+ T cells, B cells and granulocytes which are less commonly seen within sarcoidosis granulomas, is uncertain.

There are immunologic hallmarks that underlie the granulomatous inflammation in sarcoidosis (2). Bronchoalveolar lavage studies demonstrate an increased number and proportion of CD4+ T cells in pulmonary sarcoidosis that express specific T-cell receptor genes, consistent with an antigen-driven disorder. The immunologic profile at sites of disease such as the lung is characterized by a highly polarized Th1 immune responses characterized by the upregulated expression of INFγ, TNF, IL12 and IL18. Recent studies suggest that classic Th17 effector cells that produce IL17 and Th17.1 effector cells that produce INFγ also localize to sarcoidosis tissues (3–5). Deficiencies in iNKT cell and regulatory T-cell function associated with reduced regulatory capabilities have been described that likely contribute to the heightened polarized Th1/Th17.1/Th17 responses in affected tissues (6,7). Aberrant responses of innate immune receptors such as Toll-like receptors likely play a critical role in immunopathogenesis but remain poorly understood (8). The mechanism of pulmonary fibrosis in sarcoidosis remains poorly understood, but may involve transition of lung macrophages to a fibrosis-promoting alternatively activated phenotype (9,10).

CLINICAL ASSOCIATIONS

There are known clinical associations with sarcoidosis that support the premise that sarcoidosis is a Th1 disorder. Examples include the association of new-onset or recurrent sarcoidosis in patients treated with Th1-promoting therapies such as INFα, INFγ, immune checkpoint inhibitors (anti-CTLA4, anti-PD1) and immune reconstitution scenarios such as following anti-retroviral therapy in HIV disease or chemotherapy for cancer. Because of these associations, clinicians should carefully review the patient's medicines for biologic agents or drugs that promote

Th1 responses since removal of these therapies may be associated with disease remission.

GENETICS

Sarcoidosis is not considered a monogenetic disease, but there is a genetic susceptibility to sarcoidosis. The U.S. multicenter ACCESS study found an approximate fivefold increased risk in all first- and second-degree relatives, with significantly higher familial relative risk in Caucasian compared to African American cases (11). Since sarcoidosis is considered a 'rare' disease, there is consensus that such an increased risk does not justify routine testing of family members. The genetic linkage in sarcoidosis is dominantly through associations with genes of the MHC locus and specifically, the HLA genes (12,13). Limited single loci association studies and more recently Genome Wide Association Studies have implicated multiple other genetic loci linked to sarcoidosis, but these genetic links often differ by ancestry or link only to specific clinical manifestations such as Löfgren syndrome (14,15).There are no genetic tests that have been validated for use in the clinic.

AETIOLOGY

Patients invariably ask what causes sarcoidosis. There is substantial evidence for microbial triggers in sarcoidosis, with mycobacterial or propionibacterial organisms most commonly implicated by research studies. Evidence for microbial triggers include the presence of microbial DNA and protein antigens in sarcoidosis tissues and antigen-specific Th1/Th17 immune responses to these antigens in the lung and blood of sarcoidosis patients (16–20). Despite this link, experienced clinicians find there is no clinical, microbiologic or pathologic evidence that sarcoidosis is associated with an active replicating infection at any time in the clinical course despite the use of corticosteroid, immunosuppressive and anti-TNF therapy.

The ACCESS study found a ~1.5-fold increased risk in a few environmental factors such as mold/mildew or insecticide exposure at work but no consistent large size effect (odds ratio >2) from any specific environmental exposure found in >5% of subjects (21). Whether unusual environmental exposures such as experienced by first responders in the World Trade Center tragedy may trigger sarcoidosis remains uncertain though this cohort has been found to have an increased frequency of granulomatous lung disease (22,23). Beryllium exposure may cause a granulomatous pneumonitis that mimics pulmonary sarcoidosis in a subset of people who develop hypersensitivity to the metal. However, the differences between the diseases (e.g. absence of extra-pulmonary disease in chronic beryllium disease) leads many investigators to conclude that beryllium and other metals that cause granulomatous pneumonitis should not be classified as a cause of systemic sarcoidosis.

PROTEIN AGGREGATION HYPOTHESIS

Given the lack of clinical or pathologic evidence that chronic sarcoidosis is caused by an active replicating microbial infection, what is the mechanism that links a microbial trigger to sarcoidosis pathobiology? One of the authors (DM) and his colleagues report the protein aggregation of serum amyloid A (SAA) within sarcoidosis granulomas unlike in other granulomatous diseases (24). Because SAA is an amyloid precursor protein, an immune adjuvant and is highly induced following microbial infections, they hypothesize the pathobiology of sarcoidosis involves the progressive aggregation of SAA within granulomas with subsequent release of SAA fragments that promotes the feed-forward amplification of local CD4+ T cell responses to pathogenic tissue antigens (25). This scenario is compatible and synergistic with new research studies that document a role for specific tissue autoantigens such as vimentin in sarcoidosis immunopathology (26,27). Reconceptualizing sarcoidosis as a protein aggregation disorder is consistent with the known clinical biology of sarcoidosis and has implications for novel therapeutic approaches to this disease.

EPIDEMIOLOGY

There is wide variation in the reported frequency of sarcoidosis, with most studies finding incident rates ranging from 10–64/100,000 people (28). Higher frequencies are seen in Black populations in the United States and in women. Although these figures suggest sarcoidosis is a rare disease, lifetime estimates suggest the risk for Black populations may be >2% and ≥1% for White populations in Europe and the United States (29). Most cases are diagnosed between the ages of 20 and 50 years, with a later peak >65 years old; sarcoidosis is rarely diagnosed in children. The frequency of specific manifestations of sarcoidosis varies with ancestry. For example, lupus pernio which causes disfiguring facial lesions is more frequent in patients of African descent, while Löfgren syndrome (defined by the presence of constitutional symptoms, bilateral hilar lymphadenopathy, acute arthritis most commonly involving the ankles, feet, Achilles tendon, +/− erythema nodosum, and often uveitis) is more frequent in Scandinavian and Irish patients. Mortality rates approximate 1%–6% with advanced pulmonary, cardiac and neurologic manifestations responsible for most deaths.

HISTORY AND EXAMINATION

There is tremendous heterogeneity of clinical manifestations in systemic sarcoidosis. The snowflake is a symbol of sarcoidosis reflecting that every sarcoidosis patient is different. Extra-pulmonary manifestations (discussed in Chapter 16) often result in management challenges, but initially may provide a clue to the diagnosis. For example, uveitis, cranial neuropathy, or skin nodules may lead to testing for sarcoidosis.

Pulmonary manifestations are seen in >90% of patients. Respiratory symptoms are non-specific and include cough, shortness of breath, chest tightness, occasionally wheezing or haemoptysis. Many sarcoidosis patients are initially diagnosed as having asthma, bronchitis or chronic obstructive pulmonary disease (COPD). Sarcoidosis patients often see multiple physicians until new manifestations or a chest radiograph is obtained that instigate further diagnostic evaluation. Physical exam of the lungs is usually unremarkable with crackles heard in <10% of patients; this may be due to the fact that nodules and infiltrates in sarcoidosis tend to be central in location along bronchovascular bundles rather than peripheral as in IPF, where crackles are typically heard.

INVESTIGATIONS

BLOOD TESTS

There are no diagnostic blood tests for sarcoidosis. Consensus recommendations for an initial evaluation include a complete blood count and comprehensive metabolic panel with liver, kidney function and calcium levels (1). A urinalysis, electrocardiogram and ophthalmologic exam are also recommended. The serum angiotensin-converting enzyme lacks the specificity and sensitivity to serve as a diagnostic test or clinical biomarker and is not used in all centres. Serologic testing for rheumatologic conditions, vasculitis, infectious and other chronic inflammatory disorders may be helpful in distinguishing competing diagnoses. Specific organ testing (e.g. cardiac, neurologic) is indicated on a case-by-case basis when symptoms or manifestations suggest these organs may be involved (discussed in Chapter 16).

PULMONARY FUNCTION TESTS

Pulmonary function testing may show restriction, obstruction and/or a reduction in diffusing capacity or a mixture of physiologic impairments. Pulmonary function testing should include spirometry with or without bronchodilators, and a diffusion capacity. This latter test is necessary to identify a subset of patients with pulmonary sarcoidosis who have dominant reduction in gas transfer that may be associated with normal or near normal spirometry. Lung volumes are helpful if restriction is suggested by spirometry but usually

do not impact management during clinical follow-up examinations.

RADIOLOGY

Computer tomography (CT) imaging is central to the diagnosis and management of patients with pulmonary sarcoidosis. In the last 10 years, high-resolution CT scan has gradually superseded chest x-ray in its ability to diagnose, stage, measure disease activity and subtype pulmonary sarcoidosis (30).

Chest x-rays

Chest x-rays are useful in suggesting the diagnosis of pulmonary sarcoidosis. The four most common findings are bilateral hilar lymphadenopathy (BHL), nodular shadowing which can be described as micronodular or reticulonodular; and fibrosis (represented as architectural distortion, volume loss – typically upper lobes, linear bands and masses). These changes are encompassed in the Scadding CXR description, which provides the stages of disease and some information on prognosis (Table 15.1) (31). However, chest radiographs are limited by their low sensitivity to subdefine nodular changes, identify stigmata of progression to fibrosis and differentiate between active and inactive ('burnt out') fibrosis. They also have low specificity for diagnosis.

High-resolution CT

High-resolution CT (HRCT) scanning is more sensitive than chest x-rays in identifying and characterizing intra-thoracic lymph nodes, lung parenchymal and airway-related abnormalities. There are

Table 15.1 Scadding CXR stages and prognosis at initial presentation

Stage	CXR appearance	% at presentation	Prognosis (approximate % remission)
0	Normal	5–10	Uncertain (usually extra-pulmonary)
I	Lymphadenopathy only	50	70%
II	Lymphadenopathy and parenchymal lung disease	25–30	50%
III	Parenchymal disease only	10–15	20%
IV	Pulmonary fibrosis	5	<5%

highly typical constellations of abnormalities which can be used by experienced thoracic radiologists to make the diagnosis of pulmonary sarcoidosis. First, the presence of bilateral symmetrical, well-defined and uniformly enhancing hilar and mediastinal lymphadenopathy with areas of amorphous calcification is highly suggestive of sarcoidosis. In contrast asymmetry, presence of supraclavicular, anterior and cervical or internal mammary lymph node enlargement raises suspicions of alternative diagnoses like tuberculosis or lymphoma. Lymphadenopathy in sarcoidosis is almost never unilateral. Second, lung parenchymal findings of nodularity, typically in the perilymphatic distribution (fissural, peribronchovascular and interlobular nodularity) and along perihilar or mid- and upper lung zone distribution are almost pathognomonic of pulmonary sarcoidosis (Figure 15.1).

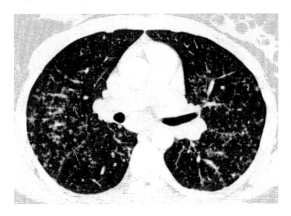

Figure 15.1 Typical CT scan for pulmonary sarcoidosis demonstrating florid micronodules with fissural nodularity (*arrows*), hilar lymphadenopathy. This could be termed 'simple pulmonary sarcoidosis' and many patients resolve with or without corticosteroids.

HRCT scans also have the added value of sub-defining the changes into those with good prognosis (high likelihood of resolution with or without treatment, low risk of developing progressive fibrosis) and those with poor prognosis (high risk of developing progressive fibrosis) (Table 15.2) (Figure 15.2). Importantly, CT scans allow the identification of complications of pulmonary sarcoidosis – bronchiectasis, severe fibrocystic disease, mycetomas, bullous lung disease and secondary pulmonary hypertension. Finally, CT scans can differentiate inactive, resolved fibrotic disease (linear reticulation with or without volume loss only) with active fibrosis (additional presence of nodularity, interlobular septal thickening, ground-glass appearance and consolidation) (Figure 15.2) (32). At least 20% of patients with pulmonary sarcoidosis progress to fibrotic disease. The most common pattern is fibrocystic changes which can be caused by cysts, bullae or paracicatricial emphysema. Honeycombing and usual interstitial pneumonia (UIP) CT pattern are uncommon but portend to a poor prognosis, particularly if there is also evidence of ground-glass opacities with or without traction bronchiectasis (33).

DIAGNOSIS

Confirming a diagnosis of sarcoidosis requires biopsy support in most cases. The exceptions may include (1) patients in non-histoplasmosis endemic areas manifesting with acute sarcoidosis or classic Löfgren syndrome; (2) Heerfordt syndrome or uveoparotid fever with bilateral hilar lymphadenopathy, parotitis, often with associated salivary

Table 15.2 Subtyping of pulmonary disease by HRCT

Subtype of pulmonary disease	CT parenchymal findings
Good prognosis or simple pulmonary sarcoidosis	• Micronodules (2–4 mm in diameter; well defined, bilateral) • Macronodules (≥5 mm in diameter, coalescing) • Perilymphatic distribution: peribronchovascular, subpleural, interlobular septal • Upper- and mid-zone predominance
Poor prognosis or risk of developing progressive fibrosis	• Masses, perihilar consolidation or conglomeration, ground-glass changes
Established fibrotic disease	• Typically, fibrocystic, honeycombing and/or ground-glass opacification and traction bronchiectasis

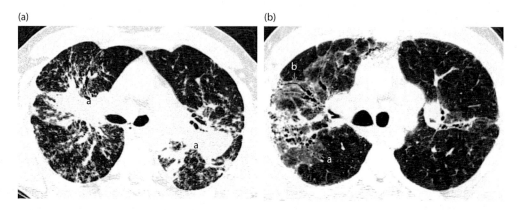

Figure 15.2 Two CT scans showing disease with poorer prognosis. **(a)** Disease with propensity for fibrosis. Note perihilar consolidation (also known as conglomeration) (marked a), florid nodularity, areas of early traction bronchiectasis (*arrow*). **(b)** CT scan showing active fibrosis. Note ground-glass opacity **(a)**, traction bronchodilation **(b)** and perihilar distribution.

gland involvement with sicca symptoms, uveitis with or without cranial neuropathy (most commonly V or VIIn); (3) long-standing presumed pulmonary sarcoidosis with a typical HRCT scan and a compatible clinical course that includes a lack of evidence of malignancy or chronic infection over a time period sufficient to reasonably exclude these alternative possibilities.

Except in these uncommon situations, a confirmatory biopsy and exclusion of alternative diagnoses are necessary to establish a confident diagnosis of sarcoidosis. A biopsy of the most easily accessible tissue that appears to be involved (e.g. skin or conjunctival nodule, peripheral lymph node) is usually recommended as a first step. If the nature of the lung disease is uncertain, or there is an absence of superficially accessible tissue to biopsy, a bronchoscopic approach is recommended when there is chest radiographic evidence of intrathoracic involvement. In experienced hands, an endobronchial ultrasound (EBUS)–directed transbronchial biopsy of mediastinal or hilar lymph nodes may avoid the need for a transbronchial lung biopsy with its greater risk of pneumothorax or serious bleeding, but should be included if the preliminary lymph node biopsies are non-diagnostic. A bronchial biopsy should always be considered given its relative safety and in some studies, 50% or greater sensitivity even without visual evidence of abnormality. Occasionally, a fluorodeoxyglucose-positron emission tomography (FDG-PET) scan can be useful to look for areas of inflammation that may be amenable to biopsy to help confirm a diagnosis

of sarcoidosis, particularly in cardiac or neurosarcoidosis cases or when investigating possible rare manifestations of sarcoidosis.

PATHOLOGY

Sarcoidosis-type granulomas are compact, non-caseating epithelioid granulomas that are most commonly found in the draining lymph nodes and perilymphatic and perivascular distribution in the lung parenchyma (34). In the lungs, the bronchial mucosa and vascular interstitium can also contain granulomas. Pathology in pulmonary sarcoidosis is directly related to the granuloma burden and its location. For example, a high burden of granulomas and accompanying lymphocytes cause disturbance of alveolar gas exchange; granulomas localized to the endothelium can lead to pulmonary hypertension.

Sarcoidosis-type granulomas are non-specific lesions and in the absence of an identifiable aetiologic agent, are not diagnostic of sarcoidosis or any other specific disease. Among the diseases to be excluded are mycobacterial, fungal, and parasitic infections, chronic beryllium disease and other pneumoconioses, hypersensitivity pneumonitis, and Wegener granulomatosis. The presence of granulomas, with an increased number and proportion of CD4+ T cells in bronchoalveolar lavage and the absence of infectious agents provide a strong basis for diagnosing sarcoidosis. However, these findings also require a typical CT scan for a secure diagnosis of pulmonary sarcoidosis. Non-caseating granulomas can also be seen in areas of cancer, including lymphoma at sites of infection such as fungal or mycobacterial disease, aspiration pneumonia or hypersensitivity pneumonitis. Rare poorly formed granulomas are occasionally seen in COP, NSIP or acute lung injury. Physicians should be aware that fibrinoid necrosis is seen in a subset of sarcoidosis pathology. However, necrotizing 'caseation' necrosis or extensive fibrinoid necrosis should always lead to consideration of infection (e.g. mycobacterial, fungal) over sarcoidosis.

In fibrotic pulmonary sarcoidosis, granulomas become less prevalent. The fibrotic changes occur surrounding the granuloma and then extend within the granuloma. Very few, if any, fibroblastic foci are found, and the overall histology pattern is distinct from UIP, often comprising acellular collagen with interstitial inflammation.

GENERAL MANAGEMENT

A systematic approach to patients with suspected sarcoidosis is recommended. First, the physician should establish a confident diagnosis. A firm diagnosis requires compatible clinical and radiology manifestations and in most cases, a compatible biopsy as well as the exclusion of other known causes of granulomatous inflammation. If such evidence is not available, then the clinician is advised to diagnose probable or possible sarcoidosis, reflecting the uncertainty so that alternative diagnoses are considered depending on the clinical course.

Second, physicians should define clinically important organ involvement. A consensus initial evaluation includes chest radiology, pulmonary function tests, blood tests (described above), ophthalmology exam, electrocardiogram (EKG) and in most patients, purified protein derivative (PPD) or blood test for latent tuberculosis (TB). Other organ-specific testing is indicated for clinically apparent manifestations that may reflect involvement of these organs (see Chapter 16).

Third, physicians need to determine indications for immediate treatment or whether a period of observation is indicated. Fourth, if treatment is indicated, physicians must consider treatment options. Fifth, the physician should plan a follow-up strategy depending on the expected clinical course.

A framework for an approach to treatment of pulmonary sarcoidosis can be based on the known clinical biology of the underlying granulomatous inflammation. First, in >95% of cases, untreated granulomatous inflammation progresses in a slow monophasic progression with a rate that varies among patients. Treatment such as corticosteroid (CS) therapy can suppress the inflammation temporarily, but tapering below an effective dose results in recurrent inflammation with a similar monophasic progression in those patients who have not undergone remission. The development of new or worsening granulomas takes weeks to develop, so there is typically a gap of weeks to months before evidence of progression is clinically apparent.

Second, organ involvement typically defines itself in the early stages of disease. For example, the ACCESS study found less than 20% of newly diagnosed patients had evidence of new organ involvement at a 2-year follow-up evaluation. Third, with few exceptions, patients follow one of two mutually exclusive courses: the disease undergoes remission, generally within the first 2–3 years, or the clinical course is chronic, unremitting with only rare 'late' remissions.

The initial clinical manifestations associate with different prognoses. For example, acute sarcoidosis or Löfgren syndrome is associated with remission in 70%–80% of patients, though in the authors' experience, African Americans with this syndrome do not enjoy such a good prognosis. Other presentations associated with a good prognosis for remission include those with a stage 1 chest radiograph on initial diagnosis. Multiorgan disease (e.g. five or more organs), pulmonary fibrosis, and lupus pernio carry a poor prognosis with typically chronic, lifelong disease. True remitting/relapsing sarcoidosis is usually seen only in subsets of neurologic, ocular or non-lupus skin disease.

SPECIFIC ASPECTS OF MANAGEMENT

CORTICOSTEROID THERAPY

A consensus view is that CS are first-line therapies for progressive pulmonary sarcoidosis (Box 15.1)

BOX 15.1: Consensus approach to treatment of sarcoidosis*

Stage 1 CXR, normal PFTs: no treatment, observation

Asymptomatic patient with pulmonary infiltrates and mildly abnormal lung function with stable disease: no treatment, observation

Symptomatic patient, stage 2 or 3 CXR, impaired PFTs: Oral corticosteroids effective

Oral corticosteroids are first-line therapy in progressive disease (pulmonary or extrapulmonary disease)

Inhaled corticosteroids are ineffective

Steroid-sparing drugs have undefined role

Methotrexate [or azathioprine] usually first line

Lung and heart transplantation for end-stage disease

*Adapted from Bradley et al. *Thorax.* 2008;63 (Suppl. 5):v1–58.

(1,35). There is a lack of clinical studies that help define the optimal dose and duration of therapy for pulmonary sarcoidosis so recommendations are based on expert consensus. It is likely that the wide spectrum of disease severity and rate of progression complicate evidence-based recommendations. Often, a period of observation is indicated to confirm disease progression. For initial treatment, most experts suggest prednisone 20–40 mg/day followed after several weeks by a slow taper regimen over several months. Most patients are treated for 6–12 months and then tapered to assess whether the patient has undergone remission. Several studies indicate recurrent pulmonary disease occurs in 50% or more of patients as therapy is tapered. In this case, resuming therapy is indicated with subsequent taper to a minimum dose needed for stable lung function and symptoms. Periodic attempts at tapering are recommended in the first several years of disease to assess for remission, though many of these patients will have chronic sarcoidosis requiring long-term treatment.

For chronic pulmonary sarcoidosis there is typically a precisely defined dose that is effective for long-term control, where even prednisone 1–2 mg/day difference in dose may result in stable

suppression versus progression. For pulmonary sarcoidosis, this minimum effective dose typically ranges between prednisone 5 and 15 mg/day, usually 10–15 mg/day; higher doses are rarely needed. Alternate day CS therapy is frequently *ineffective* in patients who will respond to daily dosing. There is consensus that inhaled CS therapy (ICS) is ineffective as monotherapy for long-term control of pulmonary sarcoidosis but can be useful in some patients with cough or symptoms of bronchial hyperreactivity. Corticosteroid (and other CS-sparing therapies) are not curative, but result in only temporary suppression, with recurrent progression when the CS dose is tapered below an effective dose or tapered off.

For patients on chronic maintenance CS, minimizing adverse effects is critical. Monitoring of blood sugar, blood pressure, bone density, and nutritional status is indicated. Education regarding adverse effects and steps to minimize their effects such as dietary restraint should be provided at every visit.

STEROID-SPARING THERAPIES

Because CS degrade quality of life in those who require chronic maintenance therapy, steroid-sparing therapies are typically employed. Hydroxychloroquine is relatively safe compared to more potent cytotoxic therapies (though with risk of ocular toxicity), and can be tried but the common experience is that this drug typically does not have significant benefit for pulmonary sarcoidosis. In the authors' experience, one exception may be a subgroup of patients with mild symptoms, typically mid-upper lung zone infiltrates and dominant obstruction characterized by slow progression over several years, whose pulmonary sarcoidosis may be stabilized by the combination of hydroxychloroquine plus high-dose ICS (unproven regimen). Several other relatively safe drugs (pentoxifylline, tetracyclines, melatonin) have been reported useful in case reports or small clinical trials, but more widespread experience indicates these drugs do not appear to have a significant benefit in pulmonary sarcoidosis.

Potent steroid-sparing therapies are frequently recommended in those patients with significant adverse effects from CS therapy (2,36). The most commonly used therapies include methotrexate, azathioprine, mycophenolate and possibly, leflunomide in some centres. Cyclophosphamide is used only in severe cases of neurologic or ocular sarcoidosis given its higher risk profile.

Given the lack of comparison clinical trials, expert consensus but not evidence-based recommendations can be made regarding these therapies. Methotrexate is most commonly used as a first-line potent steroid-sparing therapy, though some centres use azathioprine initially. One retrospective study showed similar effectiveness of these drugs with a slightly higher frequency of infections with azathioprine (37). Potential adverse effects of methotrexate include hepatic, pulmonary and bone marrow toxicity. Azathioprine is more immunosuppressive with risk of infection and increased risk of cancer (as for all immunosuppressive therapies). There is less experience with mycophenolate and leflunomide, but small case series indicate they may be beneficial in a subset of pulmonary sarcoidosis, though in the authors' experience, these drugs appear to be less frequently effective than methotrexate or azathioprine (perhaps because they are used after failure on these latter therapies).

ANTI-TNF THERAPIES

One large randomized clinical trial of infliximab showed improvement in FVC over 6 months compared to placebo (38). The effect was modest (2.5% improvement) and of uncertain clinical significance. More recent clinical trials involving the anti-TNF golimumab and the anti-IL12/IL23 ustekinumab were negative (39). Both clinical trials mandated that all patients were continued on their maintenance dose CS for the primary study which likely hampered interpretation of the study results (40). There have been no formal clinical trials with adalimumab, though some small case series suggest benefit in pulmonary sarcoidosis. In the authors' experience, however, adalimumab is rarely effective for pulmonary sarcoidosis, but may be steroid sparing in subgroups with extra-pulmonary sarcoidosis. Several small clinical trials show etanercept is *not* effective for pulmonary or ocular sarcoidosis and is not recommended. Interestingly, this class of therapy has been associated with new-onset or recurrent sarcoidosis. Other serious potential adverse effects include infection risk and increased risk of cancer. For these reasons, as well as their higher cost, anti-TNF therapy is generally used after CS-sparing drugs have been tried and found ineffective for pulmonary sarcoidosis or was poorly tolerated.

Accumulated experience in the clinic suggests that all steroid-sparing therapies, including the biologics, share similar characteristics. First, these therapies are steroid sparing in only a subset of patients, perhaps 60%–65% of patients (i.e. they do not always work). Second, these therapies have potentially serious adverse effects different than CS so the recommendation to transition to these therapies must be based both on a risk/benefit analysis versus CS therapy while accounting for an individualized assessment of their risk in an individual patient. Third, these drugs typically take months to become maximally effective (e.g. methotrexate 3–6 months, azathioprine or mycophenolate 2–3 months), so premature CS taper may be associated with recurrent inflammation. Fourth, these CS-sparing therapies often need a small dose of prednisone to be effective (i.e. their effectiveness as monotherapy is lower) (37); we counsel our patients regarding this possibility as part of an individualized risk assessment. If a steroid-sparing therapy is not found to be clinically effective or is not tolerated, we recommend stopping the drug and trying an alternative therapy rather than adding another drug.

There are several myths related to pulmonary sarcoidosis that unfortunately are oft repeated:

1. *Myth*: CS-resistant pulmonary sarcoidosis exists. Clinical and radiologic evidence indicate moderate high-dose steroid therapy is almost always/always effective for pulmonary sarcoidosis. This myth probably derived from an imprecise use of CS resistance to refer to patients who do not tolerate a dose of CS that is sufficient to effectively treat the inflammation. It is not that the pulmonary inflammation is CS resistant (i.e. cannot be biologically suppressed). Steroid-sparing therapy is recommended for CS-intolerant patients by consensus opinion though their role remains undefined (41).

2. *Myth*: Fibrotic pulmonary sarcoidosis 'burns out'. This myth probably originated from the lack of response of some patients to a steroid trial. Typically the steroid trial was too short (lasting weeks instead of 2–3 months) or used an insufficient dose (<15–20 mg/day) or the lack of response was due to pre-existing

pulmonary fibrosis which of course is unresponsive to anti-inflammatory therapies. For example, there is radiographic and FDG-PET scan evidence that >80%–85% of patients with advanced fibrocystic sarcoidosis have active disease (42,43). The goal of treatment in this group is to prevent further progression of their advanced pulmonary impairment, not to expect dramatic improvement.

3. *Myth*: Pulmonary sarcoidosis can undergo 'flares' or 'exacerbations'. This is biologically unsound – underlying granulomatous inflammation cannot 'flare' as granulomas take weeks to develop. Respiratory exacerbations occur in pulmonary sarcoidosis but are typically due to superimposed infection, congestive heart failure, pulmonary embolism or other secondary cause. Inadequately treated pulmonary sarcoidosis may result in bronchial hyperreactivity with bronchospasm but is uncommon in those on effective maintenance therapy. For those patients with respiratory exacerbations, we recommend treatment based on the underlying cause. Empiric antibiotics and a temporary small increase in prednisone dose for 1–2 weeks (to reduce bronchial hyperreactivity) may hasten resolution when respiratory infection is the likely cause.

PULMONARY HYPERTENSION

There are multiple causes of pulmonary hypertension in sarcoidosis – advanced fibrocystic pulmonary disease, LV failure (e.g. from cardiac sarcoidosis), pulmonary arterial compression (e.g. by mediastinal lymph nodes) or rarely veno-occlusive disease from mediastinal lymphadenopathy or fibrosis. Other causes include sleep apnoea (often worsened by steroid-associated weight gain) and thromboembolic disease. An important, often overlooked cause of pulmonary hypertension is a subgroup of patients with radiographic subtle pulmonary vascular disease with minimal interstitial lung disease and well-preserved spirometry; this phenotype is seen in up to 20% of patients with pulmonary sarcoidosis and is detected by a dominant reduction in diffusing capacity compared to spirometry. These patients typically present with progressive dyspnoea on exertion not explained by the relatively normal spirogram or cardiac causes.

Pulmonary hypertension is the best predictor of survival in patients with advanced lung disease awaiting lung transplant (44). In the authors' experience, those with dominant pulmonary vascular involvement will respond to anti-inflammatory treatment if detected before severe impairment is present (likely implying irreversible fibrosis) but may require higher doses of prednisone (e.g. 20 mg/day) and/or CS-sparing therapy. Several studies have examined the effect of pulmonary arterial vasodilator therapy, noting improvements in dyspnoea and measures of pulmonary hypertension; a survival benefit has not been established (45,46).

MYCETOMA IN FIBROCYSTIC SARCOIDOSIS

Patients with fibrocystic sarcoidosis may develop mycetomas, most commonly from aspergillus, that colonize pre-existing cavities. Severe or chronic haemoptysis may develop, usually from the associated bronchiectasis and not from semi-invasive or invasive aspergillosis, based on the clinical experience prior to the advent of oral anti-fungal agents that antibiotics, bed rest, and cough suppression were usually effective in controlling the exacerbation. Bronchial artery embolization is recommended for management of severe or recurrent haemoptysis. A course of oral azole antifungal therapy is usually recommended in current practice but there is a lack of consensus and a lack of data regarding the optimal duration of therapy since the cavities are not sterilized and mycetomas can recur after antifungal treatment is stopped. For this reason, we often recommend a 6–8 week course initially for haemoptysis (rather than a 6 month or longer course with attempt at sterilization) with longer-term prophylaxis for those with recurrent episodes of haemoptysis (unproven approach). Many patients exist with their mycetomas without problems as long as their CS therapy or CS-sparing therapies are not overly immunosuppressive.

PROGNOSIS AND LONG-TERM OUTLOOK

The prognosis of sarcoidosis varies in different groups. Recent studies show worse outcomes in women of African descent in the United States compared to other groups. Overall, 50%–65% of patients with pulmonary sarcoidosis may undergo remission, typically within the first 2–3 years. Management during this period should include attempts at tapering CS or other therapies to determine whether the patient has undergone remission. For patients with chronic pulmonary sarcoidosis, maintenance daily CS results in better preservation of lung function than intermittent use of CS based on respiratory symptoms (47). CS-sparing therapy is recommend in patients with chronic disease whose quality of life is sufficiently impaired to warrant the potential risks of these therapies. The timing of initiating CS-sparing therapy however, should remain individualized given the wide range of patient ages, fitness and co-morbid conditions.

There is consensus that patients with advanced pulmonary sarcoidosis should be considered for lung transplantation if appropriate as candidates. Studies suggest overall survival rates are similar to lung transplantation for non-sarcoidosis lung disease (48). Recurrent granulomas are found in up to 50% of patients but typically respond to an increase in CS dosing. Note that the calcineurin inhibitors have not been found to be effective in sarcoidosis, and that mycophenolate and azathioprine work in only 60%–65% of patients as discussed above. Thus, a typical lung transplant anti-rejection regimen with a calcineurin inhibitor, immunosuppressive and prednisone 5 mg/day may not be effective treatment for recurrent pulmonary sarcoidosis but can respond to higher doses of CS. (This calculation is also relevant to other organ transplantations in sarcoidosis.)

CURRENT AND FUTURE AREAS OF RESEARCH

The sarcoidosis community has multiple needs. There is a lack of a simple diagnostic test to avoid the risk and expense of biopsy procedures, and a lack of biomarkers to assist the clinician in monitoring and predicting the clinical course and assess treatment responses. There is also a lack of safe, effective therapies and no cure in sight.

A multicentre US study called GRADS (Genomic Research in Alpha-1 Antitrypsin Deficiency and Sarcoidosis) is a state-of-the-art microbiome and genomic study of these diseases that is currently in the analysis phase (49). The genomic and microbiome profiles of lung (BAL) and blood are being examined in different clinical phenotypes with different expected clinical outcomes to explore the molecular basis of clinical heterogeneity in sarcoidosis and to search for clinically useful biomarkers.

Research is ongoing regarding the immunopathogenesis of sarcoidosis, and biologics targeting relevant inflammatory pathways are being explored. Unfortunately, current therapies under investigation do not have a significantly improved safety profile compared to current therapies. Novel strategies include targeting the SAA pathway, innate immune receptors, autoantigen-specific T cells and using antibiotics for their anti-inflammatory properties. The promise of better therapies for chronic sarcoidosis remains on the horizon.

ACKNOWLEDGEMENT

We thank Dr Rachel Benamore, Thoracic Radiologist, Oxford University Hospitals NHS Foundation Trust, Oxford, United Kingdom, for discussion on radiology of sarcoidosis and providing CT scan figures.

REFERENCES

1. Statement on sarcoidosis. Joint Statement of the American Thoracic Society (ATS), the European Respiratory Society (ERS) and the World Association of Sarcoidosis and Other Granulomatous Disorders (WASOG) adopted by the ATS Board of Directors and by the ERS Executive Committee, February 1999. *Am J Respir Crit Care Med.* 1999;160(2):736–55.
2. Valeyre D, Prasse A, Nunes H, Uzunhan Y, Brillet PY, Muller-Quernheim J. Sarcoidosis. *Lancet.* 2014;383(9923):1155–67.
3. Ramstein J, Broos CE, Simpson LJ, Ansel KM, Sun SA, Ho ME et al. Interferon-gamma-producing Th17.1 cells are increased in sarcoidosis and more prevalent than Th1 cells. *Am J Respir Crit Care Med.* 2015;193(11):1281–91.

4. Facco M, Cabrelle A, Teramo A, Olivieri V, Gnoato M, Teolato S et al. Sarcoidosis is a Th1/Th17 multisystem disorder. *Thorax.* 2011;66(2):144–50.

5. Kaiser Y, Lepzien R, Kullberg S, Eklund A, Smed-Sorensen A, Grunewald J. Expanded lung T-bet+RORγT+ CD4+ T-cells in sarcoidosis patients with a favourable disease phenotype. *Eur Respir J.* 2016;48(2):484–94.

6. Taflin C, Miyara M, Nochy D, Valeyre D, Naccache JM, Altare F et al. FoxP3+ regulatory T cells suppress early stages of granuloma formation but have little impact on sarcoidosis lesions. *Am J Pathol.* 2009;174(2):497–508.

7. Crawshaw A, Kendrick YR, McMichael AJ, Ho LP. Abnormalities in iNKT cells are associated with impaired ability of monocytes to produce IL-10 and suppress T-cell proliferation in sarcoidosis. *Eur J Immunol.* 2014;44(7):2165–74.

8. Gabrilovich MI, Walrath J, van Lunteren J, Nethery D, Seifu M, Kern JA et al. Disordered Toll-like receptor 2 responses in the pathogenesis of pulmonary sarcoidosis. *Clin Exp Immunol.* 2013;173(3):512–22.

9. Boot RG, Hollak CE, Verhoek M, Alberts C, Jonkers RE, Aerts JM. Plasma chitotriosidase and CCL18 as surrogate markers for granulomatous macrophages in sarcoidosis. *Clin Chim Acta.* 2010;411(1–2):31–6.

10. Prasse A, Pechkovsky DV, Toews GB, Jungraithmayr W, Kollert F, Goldmann T et al. A vicious circle of alveolar macrophages and fibroblasts perpetuates pulmonary fibrosis via CCL18. *Am J Respir Crit Care Med.* 2006;173(7):781–92.

11. Rybicki BA, Iannuzzi MC, Frederick MM, Thompson BW, Rossman MD, Bresnitz EA et al. Familial aggregation of sarcoidosis. A case-control etiologic study of sarcoidosis (ACCESS). *Am J Respir Crit Care Med.* 2001;164(11):2085–91.

12. Fischer A, Grunewald J, Spagnolo P, Nebel A, Schreiber S, Muller-Quernheim J. Genetics of sarcoidosis. *Semin Respir Crit Care Med.* 2014;35(3):296–306.

13. Fischer A, Ellinghaus D, Nutsua M, Hofmann S, Montgomery CG, Iannuzzi MC et al. Identification of immune-relevant factors conferring sarcoidosis genetic risk. *Am J Respir Crit Care Med.* 2015;192(6):727.

14. Rybicki BA, Walewski JL, Maliarik MJ, Kian H, Iannuzzi MC, Group AR. The BTNL2 gene and sarcoidosis susceptibility in African Americans and Whites. *Am J Hum Genet.* 2005;77(3):491–9.

15. Valentonyte R, Hampe J, Huse K, Rosenstiel P, Albrecht M, Stenzel A et al. Sarcoidosis is associated with a truncating splice site mutation in BTNL2. *Nat Genet.* 2005;37(4):357–64.

16. Gupta D, Agarwal R, Aggarwal AN, Jindal SK. Molecular evidence for the role of mycobacteria in sarcoidosis: A meta-analysis. *Eur Respir J.* 2007;30(3):508–16.

17. Song Z, Marzilli L, Greenlee BM, Chen ES, Silver RF, Askin FB et al. Mycobacterial catalase-peroxidase is a tissue antigen and target of the adaptive immune response in systemic sarcoidosis. *J Exp Med.* 2005;201(5):755–67.

18. Chen ES, Wahlstrom J, Song Z, Willett MH, Wiken M, Yung RC et al. T cell responses to mycobacterial catalase-peroxidase profile a pathogenic antigen in systemic sarcoidosis. *J Immunol.* 2008;181(12):8784–96.

19. Drake WP, Dhason MS, Nadaf M, Shepherd BE, Vadivelu S, Hajizadeh R et al. Cellular recognition of Mycobacterium tuberculosis ESAT-6 and KatG peptides in systemic sarcoidosis. *Infect Immun.* 2007;75(1):527–30.

20. Eishi Y, Suga M, Ishige I, Kobayashi D, Yamada T, Takemura T et al. Quantitative analysis of mycobacterial and propionibacterial DNA in lymph nodes of Japanese and European patients with sarcoidosis. *J Clin Microbiol.* 2002;40(1):198–204.

21. Newman LS, Rose CS, Bresnitz EA, Rossman MD, Barnard J, Frederick M et al. A case control etiologic study of sarcoidosis: Environmental and occupational risk factors. *Am J Respir Crit Care Med.* 2004;170(12):1324–30.

22. Izbicki G, Chavko R, Banauch GI, Weiden MD, Berger KI, Aldrich TK et al. World Trade Center 'sarcoid-like' granulomatous pulmonary disease in New York City Fire Department rescue workers. *Chest.* 2007;131(5):1414–23.

23. Crowley LE, Herbert R, Moline JM, Wallenstein S, Shukla G, Schechter C et al. 'Sarcoid like' granulomatous pulmonary disease in World Trade Center disaster responders. *Am J Ind Med.* 2011;54(3):175–84.

24. Chen ES, Song Z, Willett MH, Heine S, Yung RC, Liu MC et al. Serum amyloid A regulates granulomatous inflammation in sarcoidosis through Toll-like receptor-2. *Am J Respir Crit Care Med.* 2010;181(4):360–73.

25. Chen ES, Moller DR. Sarcoidosis—Scientific progress and clinical challenges. *Nat Rev Rheumatol.* 2011;7(8):457–67.

26. Wahlstrom J, Dengjel J, Winqvist O, Targoff I, Persson B, Duyar H et al. Autoimmune T cell responses to antigenic peptides presented by bronchoalveolar lavage cell HLA-DR molecules in sarcoidosis. *Clin Immunol.* 2009;133(3):353–63.

27. Eberhardt C, Thillai M, Parker R, Siddiqui N, Potiphar L, Goldin R et al. Proteomic analysis of kveim reagent identifies targets of cellular immunity in sarcoidosis. *PLoS One.* 2017;12(1):e0170285.

28. Rybicki BA, Iannuzzi MC. Epidemiology of sarcoidosis: Recent advances and future prospects. *Semin Respir Crit Care Med.* 2007;28(1):22–35.

29. Rybicki BA, Major M, Popovich J Jr., Maliarik MJ, Iannuzzi MC. Racial differences in sarcoidosis incidence: A 5-year study in a health maintenance organization. *Am J Epidemiol.* 1997;145(3):234–41.

30. Hawtin KE, Roddie ME, Mauri FA, Copley SJ. Pulmonary sarcoidosis: The 'Great Pretender'. *Clin Radiol.* 2010;65(8):642–50.

31. Scadding JG. Prognosis of intrathoracic sarcoidosis in England. A review of 136 cases after five years' observation. *Br Med J.* 1961;2(5261):1165–72.

32. Benamore R, Kendrick YR, Repapi E, Helm E, Cole SL, Taylor S et al. CTAS: A CT score to quantify disease activity in pulmonary sarcoidosis. *Thorax.* 2016;71:1161–3.

33. Abehsera M, Valeyre D, Grenier P, Jaillet H, Battesti JP, Brauner MW. Sarcoidosis with pulmonary fibrosis: CT patterns and correlation with pulmonary function. *AJR Am J Roentgenol.* 2000;174(6):1751–7.

34. Rossi G, Cavazza A, Colby TV. Pathology of sarcoidosis. *Clin Rev Allergy Immunol.* 2015;49(1):36–44.

35. Bradley B, Branley HM, Egan JJ, Greaves MS, Hansell DM, Harrison NK et al. Interstitial lung disease guideline: The British Thoracic Society in collaboration with the Thoracic Society of Australia and New Zealand and the Irish Thoracic Society. *Thorax.* 2008;63:v1–58.

36. Baughman RP, Lower EE. Treatment of sarcoidosis. *Clin Rev Allergy Immunol.* 2015;49(1):79–92.

37. Vorselaars AD, Wuyts WA, Vorselaars VM, Zanen P, Deneer VH, Veltkamp M et al. Methotrexate vs azathioprine in second-line therapy of sarcoidosis. *Chest.* 2013;144(3):805–12.

38. Baughman RP, Drent M, Kavuru M, Judson MA, Costabel U, du Bois R et al. Infliximab therapy in patients with chronic sarcoidosis and pulmonary involvement. *Am J Respir Crit Care Med.* 2006;174(7):795–802.

39. Judson MA, Baughman RP, Costabel U, Drent M, Gibson KF, Raghu G et al. Safety and efficacy of ustekinumab or golimumab in patients with chronic sarcoidosis. *Eur Respir J.* 2014;44(5):1296–307.

40. Moller DR. Negative clinical trials in sarcoidosis: Failed therapies or flawed study design? *Eur Respir J.* 2014;44(5): 1123–6.

41. Bradley B, Branley HM, Egan JJ, Greaves MS, Hansell DM, Harrison NK et al. Interstitial lung disease guideline: the British Thoracic Society in collaboration with the Thoracic Society of Australia and New Zealand and the Irish Thoracic Society. *Thorax.* 2008;63(Suppl. 5):v1–58.

42. Hours S, Nunes H, Kambouchner M, Uzunhan Y, Brauner MW, Valeyre D et al. Pulmonary cavitary sarcoidosis: Clinico-radiologic characteristics and natural history of a rare form of sarcoidosis. *Medicine (Baltimore).* 2008;87(3):142–51.

43. Mostard RL, Verschakelen JA, van Kroonenburgh MJ, Nelemans PJ, Wijnen PA, Voo S et al. Severity of pulmonary involvement and (18)F-FDG PET activity in sarcoidosis. *Respir Med.* 2013;107(3): 439–47.

44. Arcasoy SM, Christie JD, Pochettino A, Rosengard BR, Blumenthal NP, Bavaria JE et al. Characteristics and outcomes of patients with sarcoidosis listed for lung transplantation. *Chest*. 2001;120(3):873–80.

45. Bonham CA, Oldham JM, Gomberg-Maitland M, Vij R. Prostacyclin and oral vasodilator therapy in sarcoidosis-associated pulmonary hypertension: A retrospective case series. *Chest*. 2015;148(4):1055–62.

46. Barnett CF, Bonura EJ, Nathan SD, Ahmad S, Shlobin OA, Osei K et al. Treatment of sarcoidosis-associated pulmonary hypertension. A two-center experience. *Chest*. 2009;135(6):1455–61.

47. Gibson GJ, Prescott RJ, Muers MF, Middleton WG, Mitchell DN, Connolly CK et al. British Thoracic Society sarcoidosis study: Effects of long term corticosteroid treatment. *Thorax*. 1996;51(3):238–47.

48. Taimeh Z, Hertz MI, Shumway S, Pritzker M. Lung transplantation for pulmonary sarcoidosis. Twenty-five years of experience in the USA. *Thorax*. 2016;71(4):378–9.

49. Moller DR, Koth LL, Maier LA, Morris A, Drake W, Rossman M et al. Rationale and design of the genomic research in alpha-1 antitrypsin deficiency and sarcoidosis (GRADS) study. Sarcoidosis protocol. *Ann Am Thorac Soc*. 2015;12(10):1561–71.

16

Sarcoidosis extra-pulmonary manifestations

DOMINIQUE VALEYRE, HILARIO NUNES, FLORENCE JENY,
MATTHIEU MAHÉVAS AND MARC A JUDSON

BACKGROUND AND EPIDEMIOLOGY

Extra-pulmonary organ involvement depends upon epidemiological factors, the means used for diagnosis and biases in recruitment. The World Association of Sarcoidosis and Other Granulomatous Disorders (WASOG) Organ Assessment Instrument may be useful to identify clinical scenarios consistent with sarcoidosis organ involvement (1). Using very sensitive tests that are not required in most patients like 18F-fluorodeoxyglucose-positron emission tomography (^{18F}FDG-PET) may unveil unexpected latent localizations (2). While pulmonary involvement is observed in 80%–95% of cases, the presence of any

extra-pulmonary organ involvement is observed in around 50%, meaning that extra-pulmonary involvement is rarely isolated (8%–20%) and most often associated with pulmonary sarcoidosis (3). Parasarcoidosis syndromes observed in up to 70% of patients may be responsible for persistent disabling symptoms. Skin and eye involvement and peripheral lymphadenopathy are most frequent, 20% each in a worldwide series (4) and slightly lower in a multicentre US study (Table 16.1) (3). Lymph node, eye, bone marrow and skin involvement are more frequent in Blacks than in Caucasians. Eye and neurologic involvement are more frequent in women than men. Hypercalcaemia is more frequent in Caucasian males older than 40 (3). In Japan, uveitis and cardiac involvement are far more

Table 16.1 Sarcoidosis extra-pulmonary involved organs: influence of epidemiological factors, prevalence and severity

Organs	Variations with epidemiology	Prevalence	Severity
Eye	++	Frequent	Occasionally
Skin (specific)	+++	Frequent	Rare
Erythema nodosum	++++	Frequent or not, depending on patient demographics	Not
Liver		Frequent	Rare
Nervous system	+++	Low-moderate	Often
Heart	++	Low-moderate	Often
Kidney		Rare	Often
Nose, larynx		Rare	Often
Salivary glands		Low frequency	Not
Skeleton		Rare	Rare
Endocrine glands		Rare	Occasionally
Digestive tract		Rare	Rare
Spleen		Moderate	Rare

prevalent than elsewhere and muscle involvement is more common in females (5). Erythema nodosum is most often observed in females while bilateral ankle arthritis without skin lesions is more frequent in males (6). Erythema nodosum is very frequent in the United Kingdom and northern Europe populations while it is moderately frequent in Blacks and in Japanese (5,7). In children, liver, spleen and eye involvement and fever and weight loss are frequent (8,9). In elder patients, eye and specific skin lesions are unexpectedly frequent (10).

Number of involved organs: In the ACCESS study, half of the patients had single-organ involvement that was mainly thoracic; however, 30% had two organs involved, 13% three organs involved, 5% had four organs involved and 2% had five or more involved organs (3).

HISTORY AND EXAMINATION AND INVESTIGATIONS

EXTRA-PULMONARY ORGAN INVOLVEMENT

Sarcoidosis often presents with erythema nodosum, specific skin lesions, arthralgia, uveitis, peripheral lymphadenopathy and general symptoms while other manifestations are scarcely observed (e.g. parotid swelling). Other manifestations appear at any time during the course from onset to several years later (e.g. heart, lupus pernio). Skin lesions can lead to a rapid diagnosis (11). Erythema nodosum and parotid involvement tend to abate rapidly while lupus pernio, heart, central nervous system, nasosinusal and renal involvement are usually persistent for a long duration.

Biopsies are justified to confirm a sarcoidosis diagnosis or to confirm an extra-pulmonary manifestation of sarcoidosis. Skin lesions (except for erythema nodosum), peripheral lymphadenopathy (12) or conjunctival nodules are targets for biopsy. Evidence of abnormal [18F]FDG uptake may guide the biopsy. Accessory salivary gland biopsy may be helpful. Other biopsy sites may be recommended for confirming specific involvement of the liver, bone marrow, nose, larynx, kidney, muscle, skeleton or nervous system.

SCREENING STUDIES FOR ORGAN INVOLVEMENT

Sarcoidosis is present in more organs than is clinically apparent (13). However, often, sarcoidosis organ involvement has no clinical impact, no long-term consequences and does not require therapy (14). Therefore, patient care is not optimized by identifying every possible organ involved with sarcoidosis (13). It is imperative to detect sarcoidosis organ involvement that results in significant symptoms or impairment of function or quality of life. This requires all patients diagnosed with sarcoidosis to undergo a complete medical history and physical examination. As sarcoidosis may affect any organ in the body, any symptom may represent a manifestation of sarcoidosis. Obviously, knowledge of typical and atypical presentations of sarcoidosis is useful to determine the likelihood that a specific sign or symptom warrants further evaluation for sarcoidosis. Descriptions of such presentations are available in the literature (15,16).

Sarcoidosis involvement of certain organs does need to be detected even if the patient has no obvious symptoms because serious potential complications may be avoided. This includes involvement of the eyes, heart and vitamin D dysregulation.

The eye is one of the most frequent organs involved with sarcoidosis (14). If active eye inflammation is effectively treated, permanent vision impairment can be averted (17,18). Although anterior uveitis, a common manifestation of eye sarcoidosis (19), may cause red eye, eye pain and photophobia, one-third of patients with an acute anterior uveitis have no eye symptoms (20). For this reason, all individuals diagnosed with sarcoidosis should undergo an ophthalmologic evaluation even in the absence of eye symptoms (15). This examination should include a slit-lamp examination to detect an anterior uveitis and a funduscopic examination to detect an intermediate and posterior uveitis as well as evaluate the optic nerve. The lacrimal glands should also be evaluated, as they are commonly involved with sarcoidosis (21) and may cause dry eyes that may adversely affect vision.

Symptomatic cardiac sarcoidosis occurs in approximately 5% of sarcoidosis patients (22). Cardiac sarcoidosis is responsible for a significant percentage of deaths attributable to sarcoidosis (23). Contrary to deaths caused from pulmonary sarcoidosis that usually occur many years after the diagnosis from fibrotic accumulation resulting in respiratory failure (24), acute granulomatous inflammation strategically positioned in the heart can be suddenly life threatening, leading to heart failure, heart block, arrhythmias and sudden death (24,25). For these reasons, it is imperative that all patients with sarcoidosis be screened for cardiac involvement. Screening for cardiac sarcoidosis is not standardized. All of the following tests have been advocated in various combinations for screening: eliciting cardiac symptoms (palpitations, pre-syncope, syncope, symptoms of heart failure), electrocardiogram, Holter monitor and echocardiogram (13). The sensitivity of each of these individual screening tests has been shown to be poor at 50% or less (26). However, if any one of the aforementioned screening tests is abnormal, the sensitivity for cardiac sarcoidosis approaches 100% (26). Experts recommend that all patients with sarcoidosis undergo a history of significant cardiac symptoms, and a 12-lead electrocardiogram to screen for cardiac sarcoidosis (22,27). It is controversial whether an echocardiogram should be an additional cardiac sarcoidosis screening test (27). If any of these screening tests is abnormal, the patient should undergo a 'diagnostic test' for sarcoidosis, usually cardiac magnetic resonance imaging (MRI) (28,29) or [18F]FDG-PET. These 'surrogate tests' are usually preferred over endomyocardial biopsy because they are minimally invasive and endomyocardial biopsy has a poor diagnostic yield (30).

Vitamin D dysregulation in sarcoidosis is related to increased 1-α hydroxylase activity in sarcoidosis macrophages that converts 25-hydroxy vitamin D, to 1,25-dihydroxy vitamin D, the active form of the vitamin (31,32). This may lead to hypercalciuria, hypercalcemia, nephrolithiasis, nephrocalcinosis, acute kidney injury and chronic kidney disease (33). Sarcoidosis-induced hypercalciuria is three times as common as hypercalcemia (33,34). The serum 25-hydroxy vitamin D levels are usually low in this condition, and the serum 1,25-dihydroxy vitamin D levels tend to be in the high-normal to elevated range. Serum PTH levels are usually low as they are suppressed by the elevated 1,25-dihydroxyvitamin D levels (35).

Currently, there are no accepted guidelines for the assessment of vitamin D metabolism in sarcoidosis patients (36). Both 25-hydroxy vitamin D and 1,25-dihydroxy vitamin D serum levels should be measured (36). If both the 25-hydroxy vitamin D is low and the 1,25-dihydroxy vitamin D is high-normal or high, we recommend obtaining a serum PTH level as it should be low in sarcoidosis-induced vitamin D dysregulation and high in primary hyperparathyroidism. A 24-hour urine for calcium is not recommended as a screening test for hypercalciuria because isolated hypercalciuria is not an indication for corticosteroid therapy (37).

Blood tests of renal function, hepatic function and complete blood count are recommended as routine screening tests for specific sarcoidosis organ involvement (13).

SCREENING STUDIES FOR PARASARCOIDOSIS SYNDROMES

Sarcoidosis may cause symptoms or dysfunction that is not directly related to the deposition of granulomas in tissues. These entities are collectively known as parasarcoidosis syndromes (16). Most parasarcoidosis syndromes are thought to be the result of a systemic release of inflammatory mediators from the sarcoidosis granuloma (38). Common parasarcoidosis syndromes are listed in Table 16.2.

Small fibre neuropathy (SFN) occurs in up to 40% of sarcoidosis patients (39) and is often disabling. This neuropathy involves the unmyelinated C and thinly myelinated Aδ fibres (40) and typically causes pain, numbness, burning, vibrating

Table 16.2 Parasarcoidosis syndromes

- Small fibre neuropathy
  - Painful neuropathy
    - Character: pain, numbness, burning, vibrating and electric shock sensations
    - Distribution: distal, or patchy, non-contiguous
  - Autonomic neuropathy
    - Palpitations, orthostatic hypotension, hyper- and hypohidrosis, nausea, constipation, diarrhoea, flushing, sexual dysfunction and bowel/bladder disturbances
- Fatigue
- Cognitive decline
- Pain syndromes
- Depression
- Erythema nodosum[a]
- Vitamin D dysregulation[b]

[a] Often considered a form of skin sarcoidosis but technically, this is a parasarcoidosis syndrome that is thought to be related to inflammatory mediators involved in the granulomatous inflammation from sarcoidosis.

[b] Could be considered a parasarcoidosis syndrome in that this results from activation of 1-α hydroxylase in activated macrophages involved in granuloma formation.

and electric shock sensations (16). Although this neuropathy can start in the distal extremities, it may be patchy and have a noncontiguous distribution in other parts of the body (16). Sarcoidosis small fibre neuropathy may also cause an autonomic neuropathy resulting in palpitations, orthostatic hypotension, sweating patterns (hyper- and hypohidrosis), gastrointestinal problems (nausea, constipation, diarrhoea), flushing, sexual dysfunction and bowel/bladder disturbances (38,39,41). The diagnosis of SFN is problematic and not standardized (40). Suggested diagnostic approaches have included neurophysiological tests (contact heat-evoked potentials [42], laser-evoked potentials [43], and quantitative sudomotor axon reflex testing [QSART] [44]), psychophysical tests (temperature sensation thresholds) (45), results from skin or nerve biopsies (intraepidermal nerve fibre quantification [46,47]) and nerve fibre estimates from *in vivo* confocal microscopy (48). Treatment of SFN is also not standardized. Anti-sarcoidosis therapy may be beneficial, but not always (38). Infliximab (49) and intravenous immunoglobulin (41) have been useful in small cases series. Alternative therapies include medications prescribed for neuropathic pain, such as antidepressants and anti-epileptics, as well as lifestyle modifications including exercise, nutrition and mind–body therapies (e.g. meditation and tai chi) (38,50,51).

Fever may occur in sarcoidosis that is associated with erythema nodosum (Löfgren syndrome) or Heerfordt syndrome or in some paediatric cases (9). It also has been described with liver, renal or meningeal involvement (37). Short of that, fever is rare in sarcoidosis and alternative causes of fever should be considered including infections.

Weight loss may be observed, particularly with acute initial presentations.

Fatigue is common in sarcoidosis with an estimated prevalence of 50%–70% (52). Fatigue may be conjectured to be a consequence of inflammatory mediators released by granulomatous inflammation (53). However, fatigue in sarcoidosis may also be related to an adverse effect of corticosteroid or other anti-sarcoidosis therapy, corticosteroid withdrawal or sleep-disordered breathing that is commonly associated with sarcoidosis (54). If these potential alternative causes of fatigue have been reasonably excluded, the patient may be considered to have the parasarcoidosis syndrome of sarcoidosis-associated fatigue (54). Corticosteroids and other anti-sarcoid medications appear to be <50% effective for this problem (55,56). Potentially effective therapies for sarcoidosis-associated fatigue include stimulants such as dexmethylphenidate (53), methylphenidate (57) and armodafinil (58), as well as physical training (59).

Cognitive decline, pain syndromes and depression are often related to the presence of a chronic disease/chronic impairment and are not specific for sarcoidosis (60). However, the fact that some sarcoidosis patients with cognitive decline have responded to anti-tumour necrosis alpha therapy (61) suggests that some of them may have a parasarcoidosis syndrome (62,63).

Depression has been reported in 23%–66% of sarcoidosis cohorts (63–66). Depression is more common in sarcoidosis patients who are female, have dyspnoea, and have poor access to medical care, and who have a greater number of organs involved (65–67). Depression is also less common in sarcoidosis patients diagnosed within the previous 6 months compared to those diagnosed earlier (64,65). Depressed patients perceive more serious consequences of sarcoidosis than those who are not depressed (66). Depression, fatigue and anxiety appear to all be inter-related in sarcoidosis such that each disorder may be caused or influenced by the others (65,68,69). Sleep apnoea is common in sarcoidosis (54) and may also cause anxiety, fatigue and depression (67). Therefore, the treatment of depression and other psychiatric disorders in sarcoidosis is complex, as fatigue and its potential causes such as anxiety, and obstructive sleep apnoea require different treatments.

Pain is reported by over 70% of sarcoidosis patients, with arthralgia as the most common pain complaint (70). Chest pain, headache and muscle pain are reported by more than one-quarter of all sarcoidosis patients (70). Sarcoidosis-associated pain may be related to emotional and psychological issues, fatigue (71), depression or immobility (72). At least a portion of these sarcoidosis-associated pain syndromes represent parasarcoidosis syndromes, such as the peri-arthritis associated with Löfgren syndrome (73).

Because parasarcoidosis syndromes may adversely affect health-related quality of life, they require specialized tools for screening, detection and the assessment of therapy. *Health-related quality of life* (HLQOL) patient-reported outcome

(PRO) measures involve HRQOL reports coming directly from the patient without interpretation of physicians or others (74,75). General and sarcoidosis-specific HRQOL PROs have been successfully used in sarcoidosis (76).

SPECIFIC ASPECTS OF MANAGEMENT

ERYTHEMA NODOSUM

Erythema nodosum (EN) occurs in 5%–30% of patients with sarcoidosis. Typical skin lesions are associated with arthritis, ankle oedema, fever and weight loss. EN is often associated with intrathoracic bilateral hilar lymphadenopathy in sarcoidosis and is described as Löfgren syndrome. Prognosis is favourable with rapid spontaneous recovery but some rare cases of persistent or severe disease have been described, particularly in Blacks or in association with some HLA DR subtypes (77).

OCULAR SARCOIDOSIS

The eye is one of the most common organs involved with sarcoidosis (3,14). Uveitis is the most common manifestation of eye sarcoidosis (19). The inflammation of anterior uveitis occurs in the portion of the uveal tract extending forward from the iris and ciliary body and may cause a red eye, painful eye and photophobia. However, one-third of sarcoidosis patients with anterior uveitis will not present with any symptoms (13). Slit-lamp examination in sarcoid anterior uveitis typically reveals keratic precipitates that are globules of coalesced inflammatory cells suspended in the anterior chamber or as sediment at the chamber's base (78). Chronic anterior uveitis may lead to glaucoma or cataracts. An intermediate uveitis involves the accumulation of inflammatory cells along the pars plana, vitreous or peripheral retina (78), leading to the development of a string of pearls or snow banking. An intermediate uveitis may cause the patient to experience floaters or other visual disturbances. A posterior uveitis occurs over the central portions of the retina. A sarcoidosis posterior uveitis manifests as a venulitis that causes exudation of protein from retinal veins, leading to an appearance of candle wax drippings (78,79). This may result in retinal scarring and permanent vision loss. Optic neuritis is a rare but potentially vision-threatening manifestation of eye sarcoidosis (80,81). Patients present with sudden loss of vision or color vision (78). Funduscopic examination shows papilloedema, papillitis and/or neovascularization with resultant optic atrophy (81). Lacrimal gland involvement in sarcoidosis occurs in up to one-quarter of cases and may present as lacrimal gland enlargement and/or dry eyes ('sicca') syndrome (82,83).

Topical corticosteroid eye drops are commonly used to treat anterior sarcoid uveitis (84). Cycloplegics eye drops are often added to relieve pain from ciliary spasm or prevent posterior synechiae (84). For uveitis deeper than the anterior chamber, systemic corticosteroids are often required. Prednisone is usually used at an initial dose of 1–1.5 mg/kg day, and then tapered (84). Intra-ocular injections and implants can also be considered (84). Several immunosuppressive agents have been successfully used for sarcoid uveitis including methotrexate, azathioprine, leflunomide, cyclophosphamide, infliximab and adalimumab (85). Most of these medications are added on to corticosteroids, and then the corticosteroids are attempted to be weaned off (85). High-dose corticosteroids (up to 1 g/day of IV methylprednisolone for 3 days) and infliximab are often used for sudden loss of vision from optic neuritis.

CUTANEOUS SARCOIDOSIS

The skin has been reported as the second-most common organ involved next to the lung in two large sarcoidosis cohorts (3,14). Sarcoidosis skin lesions are classified as 'specific,' in that they demonstrate granulomatous inflammation histologically, or 'non-specific', without granulomatous inflammation (86). Non-specific lesions include erythema nodosum.

Specific sarcoidosis lesions typically cause cosmetic disfigurement and rarely other symptoms such as pruritus or pain (87). Although the most common specific sarcoidosis skin lesion is a papule 2–5 mm in diameter that is often translucent red-brown or yellow-brown in colour (87), these lesions may have quite a varied appearance including psoriaform, annular, plaques, intradermal nodules and ulcerations (88). Lupus pernio is a specific sarcoidosis skin lesion that is a disfiguring red

to violaceous indurated lesion affecting the nose, cheeks, perioral areas and forehead (73). These lesions are relatively refractory to treatment (89). Sarcoidosis skin lesions have a predilection to form over scars, tattoos, skin piercings and other sites of trauma (90).

Although topical corticosteroids are sometimes considered to be beneficial for sarcoidosis skin lesions, evidence of their efficacy is scant (88). Intra-lesional injections of triamcinolone acetonide may be more effective than topical preparations (91). However, topical or intra-lesional corticosteroids are impractical for cases with widespread lesions (92).

Systemic corticosteroids are the drug of choice for sarcoidosis skin lesions not amenable to corticosteroid injection (88,92). These agents work quickly. Other effective drugs include hydroxychloroquine and chloroquine. However, these agents work slowly, occasionally requiring more than 1 year of therapy for maximum effect and carry a risk of ocular toxicity, higher for chloroquine (93). Often, these drugs are used concomitantly with corticosteroids, with the corticosteroids being tapered as the anti-malarial drugs take effect. Methotrexate (94), leflunomide (95), tetracyclines (96), thalidomide (97) and apremilast (98) have also been shown useful for the treatment of skin sarcoidosis in selected cases. Infliximab and adalimumab are also useful for skin sarcoidosis in some patients, including for lupus pernio that is relatively refractory to other forms of anti-sarcoidosis therapy (99–101).

PERIPHERAL LYMPHADENOPATHY

Peripheral lymph node enlargement occurs in sarcoidosis, often as an initial manifestation. The enlarged lymph nodes often regress requiring no treatment. Persistent discomforting or disfiguring peripheral lymphadenopathy is seen in <5% of patients, and is responsive to corticosteroid therapy.

HEPATIC SARCOIDOSIS

Abnormalities in liver function tests are encountered in 20%–40% of patients but clinical expression and relevance of such findings are variable, and not well studied in the literature (3,102,103). Granulomatosis can cause both intra-hepatic and, more rarely, extra-hepatic cholestasis due to mechanical obstruction or periductal fibrosis mimicking sclerosing fibrosis (103–105). Sarcoidosis inflammation can lead to a non-specific hepatitis with cell necrosis. These mechanisms can either coexist or evolve independently, elicit fibrosis, nodular regeneration and ultimately cirrhosis. Because histologic features of hepatic sarcoidosis mimic other primary liver diseases, alternative causes of cholestasis and/or hepatitis (infection, drugs, metabolites, auto-immune disease) should be excluded before establishing a diagnosis of sarcoidosis. In patients with chronic sarcoidosis who develop progressive severe liver involvement, these alternative diagnoses should be carefully excluded, especially in patients on steroids or immunosuppressive therapy (106). Severe serum liver function test abnormalities defined as three or four tests with three or more times the upper limit of normal during a minimum of 3 months, strongly suggest fibrosis (107). A liver biopsy is then recommended to assess the disease severity and guide the treatment approach. In hepatic sarcoidosis, non-invasive explorations with CT scan or MRI usually show diffuse hepatic and splenic parenchymal heterogeneity due to countless microscopic granulomas associated with bands of fibrosis (108). In most cases, hepatic sarcoidosis is benign and spontaneously resolves. The efficacy of corticosteroids on the course of hepatic sarcoidosis is not well established; results of uncontrolled reports are variable with a resulting lack of consensus. The evolution towards cirrhosis appears unpredictable (102–106).

NEUROSARCOIDOSIS

Symptomatic neurosarcoidosis occurs in 5%–13% of sarcoidosis patients (109). Manifestations of neurosarcoidosis typically are seen within the first two years of the initial diagnosis of sarcoidosis (110). Only half of sarcoidosis patients with neurologic problems have neurosarcoidosis (111); therefore, alternative causes for neurologic symptoms need to be carefully excluded.

Sarcoidosis can affect any portion of the nervous system. Cranial neuropathies are the most common, being present in 50%–75% of neurosarcoidosis patients (112); a facial nerve palsy is the most common of these and often predates the diagnosis of sarcoidosis (113). Sarcoidosis may cause an acute sterile meningitis and present with fever, stiff neck and headache (114). Cerebral spinal fluid (CSF) studies in such cases typically reveal a lymphocytic pleocytosis with elevated protein levels. Hypoglycorrhachia occurs in about one-third of meningitis cases (113). The CSF angiotensin-converting enzyme level is thought not sensitive or specific enough to diagnose sarcoidosis-associated meningitis (110). Parenchymal brain lesions occur in up to 50% of neurosarcoidosis patients (115). Clinical presentations of such lesions depend on their anatomic location. Neurosarcoidosis has a predilection for the base of the brain, and approximately 15% of patients with central nervous system (CNS) disease develop neuroendocrine-related symptoms due to involvement of the hypothalamic and pituitary glands (116) such as diabetes insipidus (117). Sarcoidosis may involve the spinal cord, and the presence of spinal cord lesions on neuroimaging extending more than three spine segments strongly suggests neurosarcoidosis rather than multiple sclerosis (118). Additional manifestations of neurosarcoidosis include seizures (111), cognitive and behavioural disorders (that may possibly be related to granulomatous CNS inflammation and respond to anti-sarcoidosis therapy) (119), peripheral neuropathy (120) and hydrocephalus as the result of scarring from meningeal involvement (113).

Although the gold standard for the diagnosis of neurosarcoidosis requires histologic confirmation of neural tissue, this is an invasive procedure. Because patients with neurosarcoidosis have extra-neural sarcoidosis in approximately 90% of cases (111,121), the diagnosis of neurosarcoidosis is usually made by demonstrating surrogate evidence of neural sarcoidosis involvement coupled with histologic or strong clinical evidence of extra-neural sarcoidosis. Several algorithms have been proposed for the diagnosis of neurosarcoidosis that incorporate extra-neural evidence of sarcoidosis plus the presence of certain neurologic symptoms, signs and/or laboratory findings (1,122,123). Magnetic resonance imaging (MRI) without and with intravenous gadolinium is the imaging technique of choice in the evaluation of neurosarcoidosis (113). CNS neuroimaging involvement may be diffuse, focal or multifocal, with a predilection for the basal meninges (113). Sarcoidosis lesions, especially around the meninges, usually require gadolinium enhancement to be visualized (124). Other studies that may be useful for the diagnosis of neurosarcoidosis include CSF findings, and less commonly positron emission tomography scans (125) and neurophysiologic tests (e.g. electroencephalography electromyography and nerve-conduction studies) (119).

Neurosarcoidosis rarely spontaneously remits with the exception of facial nerve palsy (111). Corticosteroids are the drug of choice for neurosarcoidosis (110,113). The dose of corticosteroids for neurosarcoidosis is not standardized, with initial doses of 20–100 mg/day of prednisone or the equivalent recommended for mild-to-moderate disease and 500–1000 mg of intravenous methyl prednisolone daily for several days recommended for severe disease (110). In general, neurosarcoidosis is not as responsive to corticosteroid therapy as extraneural sarcoidosis (126). A significant percentage of neurosarcoidosis patients are refractory to corticosteroids or relapse when corticosteroids are tapered to lower doses (126,127). Additional agents that have been found useful for neurosarcoidosis in case series and case reports include hydroxychloroquine (128), chloroquine (128), mycophenolate (129), methotrexate (126) and cyclophosphamide (126,130). In most instances, these agents are corticosteroid sparing but corticosteroids are often unable to be discontinued. Although the medical evidence is limited, infliximab, a tumour necrosis factor-alpha (TNF-α) antagonist, appears to have excellent activity for neurosarcoidosis (131). Adalimumab, another TNF-α antagonist, has also been found beneficial for neurosarcoidosis in case reports (132). Neurosurgery should be reserved for life-threatening complications such as hydrocephalus and mass lesions causing increased intracranial pressure (133). Although radiotherapy for neurosarcoidosis has been reported to have potential benefit (134), it should also be considered a manoeuver of last resort in patients who have severe disease and cannot tolerate chemotherapy.

Muscle involvement in sarcoidosis usually manifests in three forms. Nodular intramuscular granulomatous lesions may form that are usually painless (110), are not associated with muscle weakness (135) and do not cause an elevation in serum muscle enzymes (135). Sarcoidosis may cause an acute myositis resulting in muscle swelling and pain affecting proximal muscles symmetrically that progresses to muscle contracture, hardening and hypertrophy (135,136). Serum muscle enzymes are typically elevated in this condition (135). Finally, sarcoidosis may cause a chronic myopathy that usually presents with a slowly progressing weakness and atrophy in proximal symmetric muscles (135). Serum muscle enzymes are usually normal in chronic sarcoid myopathy (135). There are limited data concerning the treatment of sarcoidosis muscle involvement, but corticosteroids appear to be the drug of choice (135,136). Other causes of chronic myopathy such as caused by corticosteroid therapy must be considered in the proper clinical context.

CARDIAC SARCOIDOSIS

While autopsy studies reveal heart lesions in 20%–30% of sarcoid patients, less than 5% suffer from clinical disease. Cardiac sarcoidosis (CS) is much more prevalent in Japan, reaching 23%–58%, particularly in women older than 50 (137,138).

The myocardium is much more likely to be damaged, with a predilection for the base of the interventricular septum and the left ventricular (LV) free wall. The pericardium and endocardium may also be affected (137,138). The histologic process is patchy in space and time throughout the heart, combining oedema, granulomatous infiltration and scarring (137,138).

Cardiac manifestations are various and include most frequently (a) aberrations of atrioventricular or intraventricular conduction, either silent or symptomatic; (b) ventricular arrhythmias; (c) subacute congestive heart failure (up to 30% of cases), which may be rapidly progressive within a few weeks or months and is often accompanied by conduction or rhythmic abnormalities; and (d) sudden death (137,138).

When heart involvement is symptomatic, it is usually inaugural of sarcoidosis (88% of cases). About 50% of patients have associated lung involvement and 25% have eye, skin or peripheral nodes involvement. Sarcoidosis can be confined to the heart, making the diagnosis problematic (137,138).

All sarcoidosis patients should be screened for CS at first work-up and during follow-up (137,138). In patients with suspected CS, further investigations are aimed at confirming diagnosis and evaluating risk stratification. CS is a diagnostic challenge, as no gold standard exists (137,138) (Table 16.1). Endomyocardial biopsy is an invasive procedure with poor sensitivity. Patients with suspected CS should undergo transthoracic echocardiography (TTE) and 24-hour Holter monitoring. TTE findings suggestive of CS include wall motion abnormalities, basal septal thinning and ventricular dysfunction (137,138). Ambulatory ECG allows detection of more severe conduction or rhythmic abnormalities than basal ECG and characterization of ventricular tachycardia (sustained or nonsustained) (137,138). Either cardiac MRI or [18]FDG PET scanning is now viewed as the best test for CS diagnosis. The keystone feature is late gadolinium enhancement (LGE) on cardiac MRI. However, there is no specific pattern of LGE that is pathognomonic for CS and LGE does not distinguish granulomatous inflammation and fibrosis (137,138). Positive T2 enhancement on cardiac MRI is suggestive of oedema and active disease. [18]FDG PET may be more sensitive but less specific for cardiac sarcoidosis. Concomitant perfusion scanning, such as with the use of perfusion tracer [82]Rubidium improves the diagnostic yield of PET (22,138). A multimodal approach is useful to classify patients with active (LGE on CMRI and PET positive) or non-active CS (LGE on CMRI and PET negative) to help make therapeutic decisions (139).

CS accounts for 13%–25% of sarcoidosis-related deaths in Western countries and is the leading cause of mortality in Japan (22,138). Contemporary outcomes are better than previously reported (140), with transplantation-free survival of 83% at 10 years (141). The main prognostic indicators are New York Heart Association (NYHA) functional class, heart failure, left ventricular (LV) ejection fraction (EF) <35%, LV enlargement and sustained ventricular tachycardia (140,141). LGE on CMRI and PET abnormal perfusion and/or metabolism have been independently associated with the occurrence of severe cardiac events in prospective studies (142,143). However, the true significance of clinically silent LGE remains controversial (144).

Treatment is based on systemic steroids with an initial dose between 30 mg/day and 1 mg/kg/day, which is usually maintained for at least 24 months (137). Ventricular arrhythmias can persist despite steroids, atrioventricular or intraventricular blocks are inconstantly reversed; however, improvement in LV ejection fraction is often observed in subjects with mild-to-moderate LV dysfunction and even patients with low EFs may show significant improvement in cardiac function (141). The role of other immunosuppressive agents is not determined but is often tried because of steroid adverse effects. Specific cardiac drugs are important to improve cardiac function and ameliorate arrhythmias. Indications for cardiac procedures, including pacemaker or implantable cardiac defibrillator, have been proposed in a recent consensus statement though wide consensus is still lacking (138). Cardiac transplantation is rarely required but consensus is that cardiac sarcoidosis should be considered in appropriate candidates, with survival rates similar to many other causes of advanced cardiac disease.

RENAL SARCOIDOSIS

Sarcoidosis renal manifestations include abnormal calcium/vitamin D metabolism, nephrocalcinosis and nephrolithiasis, but also granulomatous tubulointerstitial nephritis which can be associated with acute renal failure, which may require haemodialysis (145). Renal failure commonly ranges from 0.7% to 4.3% of cases in previous clinical series (146). In most cases, renal involvement is observed at onset of sarcoidosis, but can also be delayed (about 20% of cases), justifying regular assessment of renal parameters in follow-up. The clinical phenotype of renal sarcoidosis does not differ significantly from that of patients without renal involvement according to the prevalence of thoracic and extrathoracic involvement; however, fever is frequent (147) and the prevalence of hypercalcemia is high (30%) (148). Renal function impairment is associated with mild proteinuria, and more rarely, with aseptic leucocyturia and microscopic haematuria. Pseudo-tumoral infiltration of the kidney is described. Granulomatous conditions that can mimic renal sarcoidosis include allergic reactions due to medications, neoplasia and autoimmune disorders (e.g. granulomatosis with polyangiitis or Wegener granulomatosis) and should be excluded. Steroids are very effective in improving renal function (147,148). Nevertheless, an incomplete response and renal insufficiency are observed in two-thirds of patients. Importantly, the renal function outcome is inversely related to the severity of interstitial renal fibrosis; long-term renal response to treatment is related to the response at 1 month (37). Treatment must be initiated early to avoid long-term renal insufficiency.

SINONASAL AND LARYNGEAL SARCOIDOSIS

Sinonasal sarcoidosis (SN) has been estimated at 1.6% of patients. SN involvement can precede sarcoidosis diagnosis in about 60% of cases and be strictly isolated in 20% (149). The most common symptoms are stuffiness (90%), anosmia (70%), rhinorrhea (70%), crusting (55%) and epistaxis (30%) (149). Local examination shows hypertrophy (75%) and a violaceous colouring of the nasal mucosa with granulations (50%) in the septum and/or inferior turbinates (149). On sinus CT, patients typically have mucosal hyperplasia and opacification of the maxillary and/or anterior ethmoidal sinuses, and there is evidence of perforation or lytic lesions, mainly of the septum and/or the turbinates, in about half the cases (149). Laryngeal sarcoidosis is rare and manifests with hoarseness (77%), inspiratory dyspnoea (38%), dysphagia (38%) and sleep disorder/snoring (15%) (150). SN and laryngeal involvement frequently coexist, and both have an increased association with lupus pernio (50% and 25%, respectively) (150). SN and laryngeal sarcoidosis are associated with chronic and severe disease requiring more frequent and longer systemic treatment, and local relapses are common (149,150). High-dose pulse intravenous steroids are useful for life-threatening manifestations; surgery including temporary tracheostomy, is rarely required (150).

SALIVARY GLANDS

Bilateral parotid swelling is seen in less than 5% of patients. This occurs most often at disease onset, and often spontaneously resolves in 8–12 weeks independently of the general course of the disease. Submaxillary and sublingual glands may also be involved. Parotid involvement may be an element of Heerfordt syndrome.

SKELETAL SARCOIDOSIS

The skeleton may be involved in three different ways: abnormal vitamin D and calcium metabolism (see below), osseous sarcoidosis and corticosteroid-induced osteoporosis or fragility fractures (151–153). The prevalence of osseous sarcoidosis is usually low (0.5%–1.5%) but may be higher (15%) in some series where sensitive investigations were performed (3,154). Although skeletal involvement commonly causes no symptoms and is detected coincidentally on imaging performed for other reasons, typical symptoms include tenderness, swelling, stiffness, deformity and redness affecting fingers and toes. Standard radiography and CT findings include moth-eaten, lytic lesions, trabeculations, marginal scalloping and cystic lesions (154). Axial lesions may involve the spine and pelvis; these lesions are often asymptomatic, as they are usually discovered on [18]FDG-PET and MRI necessitating sometimes a differential diagnosis with metastasis (2,154). Fracture fragility and osteoporosis are frequent, due to diverse causes, and in particular with the use of long-term corticosteroid therapy (155).

ENDOCRINE SARCOIDOSIS

The hypothalamus is the most involved of all endocrine glands with hormonal deficiencies including most often hypogonadism and diabetes insipidus with abnormal MRI imaging (156). Thyroid and pancreas are rarely involved. Diabetes mellitus stems from corticosteroid therapy.

DIGESTIVE TRACT SARCOIDOSIS

Digestive tract involvement is rare. The main digestive clinical features are abdominal pain, weight loss, nausea, vomiting and gastrointestinal bleeding (157). Endoscopy shows that the stomach is most commonly involved with an absence of ileum or colonic macroscopic lesions that is typically found in Crohn disease.

GENITOURINARY SYSTEM

Genitourinary sarcoidosis is rare, with the epididymis being the most common localization for men and the uterus for women, with no deleterious effect on pregnancy and fertility. Breast tissue may also be involved with subcutaneous nodules and raise concern of possible breast cancer.

CALCIUM METABOLISM IN SARCOIDOSIS

Calcium metabolism is abnormal in around 40% of cases due to abnormal vitamin D metabolism, discussed above (158,159). Severe clinical consequences of (a) hypercalcemia, (b) renal stones (151) and (c) nephrocalcinosis causing renal insufficiency in subsets of patients are less common (160).

Abnormalities of parathyroid hormone mediators including PTH-rp have been associated with the abnormal vitamin D dysregulation in sarcoidosis (161). Marked hypercalcemia is typically rapidly corrected by oral corticosteroids which block calcium absorption. Sun exposure, vitamin D and calcium supplements are contraindicated in patients with active sarcoidosis when calcium metabolism is abnormal.

HAEMATOLOGICAL SARCOIDOSIS

Sarcoidosis-associated cytopenias (anaemia, neutropenia and thrombocytopenia) may occur by the following main mechanisms: hypersplenism, bone marrow infiltration and associated immune-mediated processes such as immune thrombocytopenia (ITP) and auto-immune haemolytic anaemia. Splenomegaly, which has been reported to occur in 10% of sarcoidosis patients (162), can induce hypersplenism with a splenic sequestration leading to platelet destruction, moderate anaemia and neutropenia. Common variable immunodeficiency (CVID) is associated with cases of systemic sarcoidosis, but can also mimic sarcoidosis by causing bronchiectasis with typically poorly formed granulomas on bronchial biopsy. In this setting, contrary to sarcoidosis, with CVID there is often a history of recurrent infections, hypogammaglobulinemia and different thoracic presentations (163,164). The cause for the association of sarcoidosis with ITP remains unknown, and the clinical course of ITP and sarcoidosis may differ. (165,166). ITP presentation is usually severe, but response to treatment is favorable in most cases (166). The clinical course of sarcoidosis in those with associated ITP is often severe with chronic multiple organ involvement.

REFERENCES

1. Judson MA, Costabel U, Drent M, Wells A, Maier L, Koth L et al. The WASOG Sarcoidosis Organ Assessment Instrument: An update of a previous clinical tool. *Sarcoidosis Vasc Diffuse Lung Dis Off J WASOG World Assoc Sarcoidosis Granulomatous Disord.* 2014;31(1):19–27.
2. Soussan M, Augier A, Brillet P-Y, Weinmann P, Valeyre D. Functional imaging in extrapulmonary sarcoidosis: FDG-PET/CT and MR features. *Clin Nucl Med.* 2014;39(2):e146–59.
3. Baughman RP, Teirstein AS, Judson MA, Rossman MD, Yeager H Jr., Bresnitz EA et al. Clinical characteristics of patients in a case control study of sarcoidosis. *Am J Respir Crit Care Med.* 2001;164(10):1885–9.
4. Siltzbach LE, James DG, Neville E, Turiaf J, Battesti JP, Sharma OP et al. Course and prognosis of sarcoidosis around the world. *Am J Med.* 1974;57(6):847–52.
5. Morimoto T, Azuma A, Abe S, Usuki J, Kudoh S, Sugisaki K et al. Epidemiology of sarcoidosis in Japan. *Eur Respir J.* 2008;31(2):372–9.
6. Grunewald J, Eklund A. Löfgren's syndrome: Human leukocyte antigen strongly influences the disease course. *Am J Respir Crit Care Med.* 2009;179(4):307–12.
7. Hillerdal G, Nöu E, Osterman K, Schmekel B. Sarcoidosis: Epidemiology and prognosis. A 15-year European study. *Am Rev Respir Dis.* 1984;130(1):29–32.
8. Hoffmann AL, Milman N, Byg KE. Childhood sarcoidosis in Denmark 1979–1994: Incidence, clinical features and laboratory results at presentation in 48 children. *Acta Paediatr Oslo Nor 1992.* 2004;93(1):30–6.
9. Nathan N, Marcelo P, Houdouin V, Epaud R, de Blic J, Valeyre D et al. Lung sarcoidosis in children: Update on disease expression and management. *Thorax.* 2015;70(6):537–42.
10. Varron L, Cottin V, Schott A-M, Broussolle C, Sève P. Late-onset sarcoidosis: A comparative study. *Medicine (Baltimore).* 2012;91(3):137–43.
11. Judson MA, Thompson BW, Rabin DL, Steimel J, Knattereud GL, Lackland DT et al. The diagnostic pathway to sarcoidosis. *Chest.* 2003;123(2):406–12.
12. Boussouar S, Medjhoul A, Bernaudin JF, Tayebjee O, Soussan M, Uzunhan Y et al. Diagnostic efficacy of ultrasound-guided core-needle biopsy of peripheral lymph nodes in sarcoidosis. *Sarcoidosis Vasc Diffuse Lung Dis Off J WASOG World Assoc Sarcoidosis Granulomatous Disord.* 2015;32(3):188–93.
13. Judson MA. The three tiers of screening for sarcoidosis organ involvement. *Respir Med.* 2016;113:42–9.

14. Judson MA, Boan AD, Lackland DT. The clinical course of sarcoidosis: Presentation, diagnosis, and treatment in a large white and black cohort in the United States. *Sarcoidosis Vasc Diffuse Lung Dis Off J WASOG World Assoc Sarcoidosis Granulomatous Disord.* 2012;29(2):119–27.

15. Hunninghake GW, Costabel U, Ando M, Baughman R, Cordier JF, du Bois R et al. ATS/ERS/WASOG statement on sarcoidosis. American Thoracic Society/European Respiratory Society/World Association of Sarcoidosis and other Granulomatous Disorders. *Sarcoidosis Vasc Diffuse Lung Dis Off J WASOG.* 1999;16(2):149–73.

16. Judson MA. The clinical features of sarcoidosis: A comprehensive review. *Clin Rev Allergy Immunol.* 2015;49(1):63–78.

17. Dana MR, Merayo-Lloves J, Schaumberg DA, Foster CS. Prognosticators for visual outcome in sarcoid uveitis. *Ophthalmology.* 1996;103(11):1846–53.

18. Baughman RP, Lower EE, Kaufman AH. Ocular sarcoidosis. *Semin Respir Crit Care Med.* 2010;31(4):452–62.

19. Evans M, Sharma O, LaBree L, Smith RE, Rao NA. Differences in clinical findings between Caucasians and African Americans with biopsy-proven sarcoidosis. *Ophthalmology.* 2007;114(2):325–33.

20. Rothova A, Alberts C, Glasius E, Kijlstra A, Buitenhuis HJ, Breebaart AC. Risk factors for ocular sarcoidosis. *Doc Ophthalmol Adv Ophthalmol.* 1989;72(3–4):287–96.

21. Sulavik SB, Palestro CJ, Spencer RP, Swyer AJ, Goldsmith SJ, Tierstein AS. Extrapulmonary sites of radiogallium accumulation in sarcoidosis. *Clin Nucl Med.* 1990;15(12):876–8.

22. Birnie DH, Sauer WH, Bogun F, Cooper JM, Culver DA, Duvernoy CS et al. HRS expert consensus statement on the diagnosis and management of arrhythmias associated with cardiac sarcoidosis. *Heart Rhythm.* 2014;11(7):1305–23.

23. Huang CT, Heurich AE, Sutton AL, Lyons HA. Mortality in sarcoidosis. A changing pattern of the causes of death. *Eur J Respir Dis.* 1981;62(4):231–8.

24. Hamzeh N, Steckman DA, Sauer WH, Judson MA. Pathophysiology and clinical management of cardiac sarcoidosis. *Nat Rev Cardiol.* 2015;12(5):278–88.

25. Kim JS, Judson MA, Donnino R, Gold M, Cooper LT, Prystowsky EN et al. Cardiac sarcoidosis. *Am Heart J.* 2009;157(1):9–21.

26. Mehta D, Lubitz SA, Frankel Z, Wisnivesky JP, Einstein AJ, Goldman M et al. Cardiac involvement in patients with sarcoidosis: Diagnostic and prognostic value of outpatient testing. *Chest.* 2008;133(6):1426–35.

27. Hamzeh NY, Wamboldt FS, Weinberger HD. Management of cardiac sarcoidosis in the United States: A Delphi study. *Chest.* 2012;141(1):154–62.

28. Ichinose A, Otani H, Oikawa M, Takase K, Saito H, Shimokawa H et al. MRI of cardiac sarcoidosis: Basal and subepicardial localization of myocardial lesions and their effect on left ventricular function. *AJR Am J Roentgenol.* 2008;191(3):862–9.

29. Cummings KW, Bhalla S, Javidan-Nejad C, Bierhals AJ, Gutierrez FR, Woodard PK. A pattern-based approach to assessment of delayed enhancement in non-ischemic cardiomyopathy at MR imaging. *Radiogr Rev Publ Radiol Soc N Am Inc.* 2009;29(1):89–103.

30. Ardehali H, Howard DL, Hariri A, Qasim A, Hare JM, Baughman KL et al. A positive endomyocardial biopsy result for sarcoid is associated with poor prognosis in patients with initially unexplained cardiomyopathy. *Am Heart J.* 2005;150(3):459–63.

31. Bell NH, Stern PH, Pantzer E, Sinha TK, DeLuca HF. Evidence that increased circulating 1 alpha, 25-dihydroxyvitamin D is the probable cause for abnormal calcium metabolism in sarcoidosis. *J Clin Invest.* 1979;64(1):218–25.

32. Adams JS, Gacad MA. Characterization of 1 alpha-hydroxylation of vitamin D3 sterols by cultured alveolar macrophages from patients with sarcoidosis. *J Exp Med.* 1985;161(4):755–65.

33. Sharma OP. Vitamin D and sarcoidosis. *Curr Opin Pulm Med.* 2010;16(5):487–8.

34. Rizzato G, Colombo P. Nephrolithiasis as a presenting feature of chronic sarcoidosis: A prospective study. *Sarcoidosis Vasc Diffuse Lung Dis Off J WASOG.* 1996;13(2):167–72.

35. Vucinic V, Skodric-Trifunovic V, Ignjatović S. How to diagnose and manage difficult problems of calcium metabolism in sarcoidosis: An evidence-based review. *Curr Opin Pulm Med.* 2011;17(5):297–302.

36. Burke RR, Rybicki BA, Rao DS. Calcium and vitamin D in sarcoidosis: How to assess and manage. *Semin Respir Crit Care Med.* 2010;31(4):474–84.

37. Mahévas M, Lescure FX, Boffa JJ, Delastour V, Belenfant X, Chapelon C et al. Renal sarcoidosis: Clinical, laboratory, and histologic presentation and outcome in 47 patients. *Medicine (Baltimore).* 2009;88(2):98–106.

38. Tavee J, Culver D. Sarcoidosis and small-fiber neuropathy. *Curr Pain Headache Rep.* 2011;15(3):201–6.

39. Hoitsma E, Marziniak M, Faber CG, Reulen JPH, Sommer C, De Baets M et al. Small fibre neuropathy in sarcoidosis. *Lancet Lond Engl.* 2002;359(9323):2085–6.

40. Devigili G, Tugnoli V, Penza P, Camozzi F, Lombardi R, Melli G et al. The diagnostic criteria for small fibre neuropathy: From symptoms to neuropathology. *Brain J Neurol.* 2008;131(Pt 7):1912–25.

41. Parambil JG, Tavee JO, Zhou L, Pearson KS, Culver DA. Efficacy of intravenous immunoglobulin for small fiber neuropathy associated with sarcoidosis. *Respir Med.* 2011;105(1):101–5.

42. Atherton DD, Facer P, Roberts KM, Misra VP, Chizh BA, Bountra C et al. Use of the novel Contact Heat Evoked Potential Stimulator (CHEPS) for the assessment of small fibre neuropathy: Correlations with skin flare responses and intra-epidermal nerve fibre counts. *BMC Neurol.* 2007;7:21.

43. Truini A, Galeotti F, Romaniello A, Virtuoso M, Iannetti GD, Cruccu G. Laser-evoked potentials: Normative values. *Clin Neurophysiol Off J Int Fed Clin Neurophysiol.* 2005;116(4):821–6.

44. Low PA, Caskey PE, Tuck RR, Fealey RD, Dyck PJ. Quantitative sudomotor axon reflex test in normal and neuropathic subjects. *Ann Neurol.* 1983;14(5):573–80.

45. Reulen JPH, Lansbergen MDI, Verstraete E, Spaans F. Comparison of thermal threshold tests to assess small nerve fiber function: Limits vs. levels. *Clin Neurophysiol Off J Int Fed Clin Neurophysiol.* 2003;114(3):556–63.

46. Ebenezer GJ, Hauer P, Gibbons C, McArthur JC, Polydefkis M. Assessment of epidermal nerve fibers: A new diagnostic and predictive tool for peripheral neuropathies. *J Neuropathol Exp Neurol.* 2007;66(12):1059–73.

47. Lauria G, Cornblath DR, Johansson O, McArthur JC, Mellgren SI, Nolano M et al. EFNS guidelines on the use of skin biopsy in the diagnosis of peripheral neuropathy. *Eur J Neurol.* 2005;12(10):747–58.

48. Bucher F, Schneider C, Blau T, Cursiefen C, Fink GR, Lehmann HC et al. Small-fiber neuropathy is associated with corneal nerve and dendritic cell alterations: An in vivo confocal microscopy study. *Cornea.* 2015;34(9):1114–9.

49. Hoitsma E, Faber CG, van Santen-Hoeufft M, De Vries J, Reulen JPH, Drent M. Improvement of small fiber neuropathy in a sarcoidosis patient after treatment with infliximab. *Sarcoidosis Vasc Diffuse Lung Dis Off J WASOG.* 2006;23(1):73–7.

50. Tavee J, Rensel M, Planchon SM, Butler RS, Stone L. Effects of meditation on pain and quality of life in multiple sclerosis and peripheral neuropathy: A pilot study. *Int J MS Care.* 2011;13(4):163–8.

51. Smith AG, Russell J, Feldman EL, Goldstein J, Peltier A, Smith S et al. Lifestyle intervention for pre-diabetic neuropathy. *Diabetes Care.* 2006;29(6):1294–9.

52. Drent M, Lower EE, De Vries J. Sarcoidosis-associated fatigue. *Eur Respir J.* 2012;40(1):255–63.

53. Lower EE, Harman S, Baughman RP. Double-blind, randomized trial of dexmethylphenidate hydrochloride for the treatment of sarcoidosis-associated fatigue. *Chest.* 2008;133(5):1189–95.

54. Lal C, Medarov BI, Judson MA. Interrelationship between sleep-disordered breathing and sarcoidosis. *Chest.* 2015;148(4):1105–14.

55. De Kleijn WPE, De Vries J, Lower EE, Elfferich MDP, Baughman RP, Drent M. Fatigue in sarcoidosis: A systematic review. *Curr Opin Pulm Med.* 2009;15(5):499–506.

56. Gerke AK. Morbidity and mortality in sarcoidosis. *Curr Opin Pulm Med.* 2014;20(5):472–8.

57. Wagner MT, Marion SD, Judson MA. The effects of fatigue and treatment with methylphenidate on sustained attention in sarcoidosis. *Sarcoidosis Vasc Diffuse Lung Dis Off J WASOG.* 2005;22(3):235.

58. Lower EE, Malhotra A, Surdulescu V, Baughman RP. Armodafinil for sarcoidosis-associated fatigue: A double-blind, placebo-controlled, crossover trial. *J Pain Symptom Manage.* 2013;45(2):159–69.

59. Marcellis R, Van der Veeke M, Mesters I, Drent M, De Bie R, De Vries G et al. Does physical training reduce fatigue in sarcoidosis? *Sarcoidosis Vasc Diffuse Lung Dis Off J WASOG.* 2015;32(1):53–62.

60. Katon W, Lin EHB, Kroenke K. The association of depression and anxiety with medical symptom burden in patients with chronic medical illness. *Gen Hosp Psychiatry.* 2007;29(2):147–55.

61. Elfferich MD, Nelemans PJ, Ponds RW, De Vries J, Wijnen PA, Drent M. Everyday cognitive failure in sarcoidosis: The prevalence and the effect of anti-TNF-alpha treatment. *Respir Int Rev Thorac Dis.* 2010;80(3):212–9.

62. Korenromp IHE, Grutters JC, van den Bosch JMM, Zanen P, Kavelaars A, Heijnen CJ. Reduced Th2 cytokine production by sarcoidosis patients in clinical remission with chronic fatigue. *Brain Behav Immun.* 2011;25(7):1498–502.

63. Cox CE, Donohue JF, Brown CD, Kataria YP, Judson MA. Health-related quality of life of persons with sarcoidosis. *Chest.* 2004;125(3):997–1004.

64. Yeager H, Rossman MD, Baughman RP, Teirstein AS, Judson MA, Rabin DL et al. Pulmonary and psychosocial findings at enrollment in the ACCESS study. *Sarcoidosis Vasc Diffuse Lung Dis Off J WASOG.* 2005;22(2):147–53.

65. Chang B, Steimel J, Moller DR, Baughman RP, Judson MA, Yeager H et al. Depression in sarcoidosis. *Am J Respir Crit Care Med.* 2001;163(2):329–34.

66. Ireland J, Wilsher M. Perceptions and beliefs in sarcoidosis. *Sarcoidosis Vasc Diffuse Lung Dis Off J WASOG.* 2010;27(1):36–42.

67. Hinz A, Fleischer M, Brähler E, Wirtz H, Bosse-Henck A. Fatigue in patients with sarcoidosis, compared with the general population. *Gen Hosp Psychiatry.* 2011;33(5):462–8.

68. De Boer S, Kolbe J, Wilsher ML. The relationships among dyspnoea, health-related quality of life and psychological factors in sarcoidosis. *Respirol Carlton Vic.* 2014;19(7):1019–24.

69. De Kleijn WPE, Drent M, De Vries J. Nature of fatigue moderates depressive symptoms and anxiety in sarcoidosis. *Br J Health Psychol.* 2013;18(2):439–52.

70. Hoitsma E, De Vries J, van Santen-Hoeufft M, Faber CG, Drent M. Impact of pain in a Dutch sarcoidosis patient population. *Sarcoidosis Vasc Diffuse Lung Dis Off J WASOG.* 2003;20(1):33–9.

71. De Vries J, Wirnsberger RM. Fatigue, quality of life and health status in sarcoidosis. *Eur Respir Mon.* 2005;10:92–104.

72. Gvozdenovic BS, Mihailovic-Vucinic V, Ilic-Dudvarski A, Zugic V, Judson MA. Differences in symptom severity and health status impairment between patients with pulmonary and pulmonary plus extrapulmonary sarcoidosis. *Respir Med.* 2008;102(11):1636–42.

73. Eklund A, Rizzato G. Skin manifestations in sarcoidosis. *Eur Respir Mon.* 2005;32:150–63.

74. U.S. Department of Health and Human Services FDA Center for Drug Evaluation and Research, U.S. Department of Health and Human Services FDA Center for Biologics Evaluation and Research, U.S. Department of Health and Human Services FDA Center for Devices and Radiological Health. Guidance for industry: Patient-reported outcome measures: Use in medical product development to support labeling claims: Draft guidance. *Health Qual Life Outcomes.* 2006;4:79.

75. Patrick DL, Burke LB, Powers JH, Scott JA, Rock EP, Dawisha S et al. Patient-reported outcomes to support medical product labeling claims: FDA perspective. *Value Health J Int Soc Pharmacoeconomics Outcomes Res.* 2007;10 (Suppl 2):S125–37.

76. Judson MA. Quality of life assessment in sarcoidosis. *Clin Chest Med.* 2015;36(4):739–50.

77. Berlin M, Fogdell-Hahn A, Olerup O, Eklund A, Grunewald J. HLA-DR predicts the prognosis in Scandinavian patients with pulmonary sarcoidosis. *Am J Respir Crit Care Med.* 1997;156(5):1601–5.

78. Ohara K, Judson MA, Baughman RP. Clinical aspects of ocular sarcoidosis. *Eur Respir Mon.* 2005;32:188–209.

79. Rothova A. Ocular involvement in sarcoidosis. *Br J Ophthalmol.* 2000;84(1):110–6.

80. Bradley D, Baughman RP, Raymond L, Kaufman AH. Ocular manifestations of sarcoidosis. *Semin Respir Crit Care Med.* 2002;23(6):543–8.

81. Mayers M. Ocular sarcoidosis. *Int Ophthalmol Clin.* 1990;30(4):257–63.

82. Jabs DA, Johns CJ. Ocular involvement in chronic sarcoidosis. *Am J Ophthalmol.* 1986;102(3):297–301.

83. Yanardag H, Pamuk ON. Lacrimal gland involvement in sarcoidosis. The clinical features of 9 patients. *Swiss Med Wkly.* 2003;133(27–28):388–91.

84. Pasadhika S, Rosenbaum JT. Ocular sarcoidosis. *Clin Chest Med.* 2015;36(4):669–83.

85. Baughman RP, Lower EE, Ingledue R, Kaufman AH. Management of ocular sarcoidosis. *Sarcoidosis Vasc Diffuse Lung Dis Off J WASOG World Assoc Sarcoidosis Granulomatous Disord.* 2012;29(1):26–33.

86. Mañá J, Salazar A, Manresa F. Clinical factors predicting persistence of activity in sarcoidosis: A multivariate analysis of 193 cases. *Respir Int Rev Thorac Dis.* 1994;61(4):219–25.

87. Marchell RM, Judson MA. Chronic cutaneous lesions of sarcoidosis. *Clin Dermatol.* 2007;25(3):295–302.

88. Haimovic A, Sanchez M, Judson MA, Prystowsky S. Sarcoidosis: A comprehensive review and update for the dermatologist: Part I. Cutaneous disease. *J Am Acad Dermatol.* 2012;66(5):699.e1–18; quiz 717–8.

89. Neville E, Walker AN, James DG. Prognostic factors predicting the outcome of sarcoidosis: An analysis of 818 patients. *Q J Med.* 1983;52(208):525–33.

90. Antonovich DD, Callen JP. Development of sarcoidosis in cosmetic tattoos. *Arch Dermatol.* 2005;141(7):869–72.

91. Callen JP. Intralesional corticosteroids. *J Am Acad Dermatol.* 1981;4(2):149–51.

92. Badgwell C, Rosen T. Cutaneous sarcoidosis therapy updated. *J Am Acad Dermatol.* 2007;56(1):69–83.

93. Siltzbach LE, Teirstein AS. Chloroquine therapy in 43 patients with intrathoracic and cutaneous sarcoidosis. *Acta Med Scand Suppl.* 1964;425:302–8.

94. Baughman RP, Lower EE. Evidence-based therapy for cutaneous sarcoidosis. *Clin Dermatol.* 2007;25(3):334–40.

95. Sahoo DH, Bandyopadhyay D, Xu M, Pearson K, Parambil JG, Lazar CA et al. Effectiveness and safety of leflunomide for pulmonary and extrapulmonary sarcoidosis. *Eur Respir J.* 2011;38(5):1145–50.

96. Bachelez H, Senet P, Cadranel J, Kaoukhov A, Dubertret L. The use of tetracyclines for the treatment of sarcoidosis. *Arch Dermatol.* 2001;137(1):69–73.

97. Baughman RP, Judson MA, Teirstein AS, Moller DR, Lower EE. Thalidomide for chronic sarcoidosis. *Chest.* 2002;122(1):227–32.

98. Baughman RP, Judson MA, Ingledue R, Craft NL, Lower EE. Efficacy and safety of apremilast in chronic cutaneous sarcoidosis. *Arch Dermatol.* 2012;148(2):262–4.

99. Stagaki E, Mountford WK, Lackland DT, Judson MA. The treatment of lupus pernio: Results of 116 treatment courses in 54 patients. *Chest.* 2009;135(2):468–76.

100. Baughman RP, Judson MA, Lower EE, Drent M, Costabel U, Flavin S et al. Infliximab for chronic cutaneous sarcoidosis: A subset analysis from a double-blind randomized clinical trial. *Sarcoidosis Vasc Diffuse Lung Dis Off J WASOG.* 2016;32(4):289–95.

101. Judson MA. Successful treatment of lupus pernio with adalimumab. *Arch Dermatol.* 2011;147(11):1332–3.

102. Karagiannidis A, Karavalaki M, Koulaouzidis A. Hepatic sarcoidosis. *Ann Hepatol.* 2006;5(4):251–6.

103. Ebert EC, Kierson M, Hagspiel KD. Gastrointestinal and hepatic manifestations of sarcoidosis. *Am J Gastroenterol.* 2008;103(12):3184–92; quiz 3193.

104. Rudzki C, Ishak KG, Zimmerman HJ. Chronic intrahepatic cholestasis of sarcoidosis. *Am J Med.* 1975;59(3):373–87.

105. Murphy JR, Sjogren MH, Kikendall JW, Peura DA, Goodman Z. Small bile duct abnormalities in sarcoidosis. *J Clin Gastroenterol.* 1990;12(5):555–61.

106. Kennedy PTF, Zakaria N, Modawi SB, Papadopoulou AM, Murray-Lyon I, du Bois RM et al. Natural history of hepatic sarcoidosis and its response to treatment. *Eur J Gastroenterol Hepatol.* 2006;18(7):721–6.

107. Cremers J, Drent M, Driessen A, Nieman F, Wijnen P, Baughman R et al. Liver-test abnormalities in sarcoidosis. *Eur J Gastroenterol Hepatol.* 2012;24(1):17–24.

108. Fetzer DT, Rees MA, Dasyam AK, Tublin ME. Hepatic sarcoidosis in patients presenting with liver dysfunction: Imaging appearance, pathological correlation and disease evolution. *Eur Radiol.* 2016;26(9):3129–37.

109. Nozaki K, Judson MA. Neurosarcoidosis. *Curr Treat Options Neurol.* 2013;15(4):492–504.

110. Nozaki K, Judson MA. Neurosarcoidosis: Clinical manifestations, diagnosis and treatment. *Presse Medicale Paris Fr 1983.* 2012;41(6 Pt 2):e331–48.

111. Stern BJ, Krumholz A, Johns C, Scott P, Nissim J. Sarcoidosis and its neurological manifestations. *Arch Neurol.* 1985;42(9):909–17.

112. Nowak DA, Widenka DC. Neurosarcoidosis: A review of its intracranial manifestation. *J Neurol.* 2001;248(5):363–72.

113. Terushkin V, Stern BJ, Judson MA, Hagiwara M, Pramanik B, Sanchez M et al. Neurosarcoidosis: Presentations and management. *The Neurologist.* 2010;16(1):2–15.

114. Plotkin GR, Patel BR. Neurosarcoidosis presenting as chronic lymphocytic meningitis. *Pa Med.* 1986;89(7):36–7.

115. Lower EE, Weiss KL. Neurosarcoidosis. *Clin Chest Med.* 2008;29(3):475–92, ix.

116. Murialdo G, Tamagno G. Endocrine aspects of neurosarcoidosis. *J Endocrinol Invest.* 2002;25(7):650–62.

117. Konrad D, Gartenmann M, Martin E, Schoenle EJ. Central diabetes insipidus as the first manifestation of neurosarcoidosis in a 10-year-old girl. *Horm Res.* 2000;54(2):98–100.

118. Sohn M, Culver DA, Judson MA, Scott TF, Tavee J, Nozaki K. Spinal cord neurosarcoidosis. *Am J Med Sci.* 2014;347(3):195–8.

119. Hoitsma E, Faber CG, Drent M, Sharma OP. Neurosarcoidosis: A clinical dilemma. *Lancet Neurol.* 2004;3(7):397–407.

120. Galassi G, Gibertoni M, Mancini A, Nemni R, Volpi G, Merelli E et al. Sarcoidosis of the peripheral nerve: Clinical, electrophysiological and histological study of two cases. *Eur Neurol.* 1984;23(6):459–65.

121. Christoforidis GA, Spickler EM, Recio MV, Mehta BM. MR of CNS sarcoidosis: Correlation of imaging features to clinical symptoms and response to treatment. *AJNR Am J Neuroradiol.* 1999;20(4):655–69.

122. Zajicek JP, Scolding NJ, Foster O, Rovaris M, Evanson J, Moseley IF et al. Central nervous system sarcoidosis—Diagnosis and management. *QJM Mon J Assoc Physicians.* 1999;92(2):103–17.

123. Judson MA, Baughman RP, Teirstein AS, Terrin ML, Yeager H. Defining organ involvement in sarcoidosis: The ACCESS proposed instrument. ACCESS Research Group. A case control etiologic study of sarcoidosis. *Sarcoidosis Vasc Diffuse Lung Dis Off J WASOG.* 1999;16(1):75–86.

124. Sherman JL, Stern BJ. Sarcoidosis of the CNS: Comparison of unenhanced and enhanced MR images. *AJR Am J Roentgenol.* 1990;155(6):1293–301.

125. Aide N, Benayoun M, Kerrou K, Khalil A, Cadranel J, Talbot JN. Impact of [18F]-fluorodeoxyglucose ([18F]-FDG) imaging in sarcoidosis: Unsuspected neurosarcoidosis discovered by [18F]-FDG PET and early metabolic response to corticosteroid therapy. *Br J Radiol.* 2007;80(951):e67–71.

126. Lower EE, Broderick JP, Brott TG, Baughman RP. Diagnosis and management of neurological sarcoidosis. *Arch Intern Med.* 1997;157(16):1864–8.

127. Agbogu BN, Stern BJ, Sewell C, Yang G. Therapeutic considerations in patients with refractory neurosarcoidosis. *Arch Neurol.* 1995;52(9):875–9.

128. Sharma OP. Effectiveness of chloroquine and hydroxychloroquine in treating selected patients with sarcoidosis with

neurological involvement. *Arch Neurol.* 1998;55(9):1248–54.

129. Androdias G, Maillet D, Marignier R, Pinède L, Confavreux C, Broussolle C et al. Mycophenolate mofetil may be effective in CNS sarcoidosis but not in sarcoid myopathy. *Neurology.* 2011;76(13):1168–72.

130. Doty JD, Mazur JE, Judson MA. Treatment of corticosteroid-resistant neurosarcoidosis with a short-course cyclophosphamide regimen. *Chest.* 2003;124(5):2023–6.

131. Sodhi M, Pearson K, White ES, Culver DA. Infliximab therapy rescues cyclophosphamide failure in severe central nervous system sarcoidosis. *Respir Med.* 2009;103(2):268–73.

132. Marnane M, Lynch T, Scott J, Stack J, Kelly PJ. Steroid-unresponsive neurosarcoidosis successfully treated with adalimumab. *J Neurol.* 2009;256(1):139–40.

133. Sharma OP. Neurosarcoidosis: A personal perspective based on the study of 37 patients. *Chest.* 1997;112(1):220–8.

134. Menninger MD, Amdur RJ, Marcus RB. Role of radiotherapy in the treatment of neurosarcoidosis. *Am J Clin Oncol.* 2003;26(4):e115–8.

135. Fayad F, Lioté F, Berenbaum F, Orcel P, Bardin T. Muscle involvement in sarcoidosis: A retrospective and followup studies. *J Rheumatol.* 2006;33(1):98–103.

136. Berger C, Sommer C, Meinck H-M. Isolated sarcoid myopathy. *Muscle Nerve.* 2002;26(4):553–6.

137. Nunes H, Freynet O, Naggara N, Soussan M, Weinman P, Diebold B et al. Cardiac sarcoidosis. *Semin Respir Crit Care Med.* 2010;31(4):428–41.

138. Birnie DH, Nery PB, Ha AC, Beanlands RSB. Cardiac sarcoidosis. *J Am Coll Cardiol.* 2016;68(4):411–21.

139. Soussan M, Brillet P-Y, Nunes H, Pop G, Ouvrier M-J, Naggara N et al. Clinical value of a high-fat and low-carbohydrate diet before FDG-PET/CT for evaluation of patients with suspected cardiac sarcoidosis. *J Nucl Cardiol Off Publ Am Soc Nucl Cardiol.* 2013;20(1):120–7.

140. Yazaki Y, Isobe M, Hiroe M, Morimoto S, Hiramitsu S, Nakano T et al. Prognostic determinants of long-term survival in Japanese patients with cardiac sarcoidosis treated with prednisone. *Am J Cardiol.* 2001;88(9):1006–10.

141. Kandolin R, Lehtonen J, Airaksinen J, Vihinen T, Miettinen H, Ylitalo K et al. Cardiac sarcoidosis: Epidemiology, characteristics, and outcome over 25 years in a nationwide study. *Circulation.* 2015;131(7):624–32.

142. Patel MR, Cawley PJ, Heitner JF, Klem I, Parker MA, Jaroudi WA et al. Detection of myocardial damage in patients with sarcoidosis. *Circulation.* 2009;120(20):1969–77.

143. Greulich S, Deluigi CC, Gloekler S, Wahl A, Zürn C, Kramer U et al. CMR imaging predicts death and other adverse events in suspected cardiac sarcoidosis. *JACC Cardiovasc Imaging.* 2013;6(4):501–11.

144. Nagai T, Kohsaka S, Okuda S, Anzai T, Asano K, Fukuda K. Incidence and prognostic significance of myocardial late gadolinium enhancement in patients with sarcoidosis without cardiac manifestation. *Chest.* 2014;146(4):1064–72.

145. Bergner R, Hoffmann M, Waldherr R, Uppenkamp M. Frequency of kidney disease in chronic sarcoidosis. *Sarcoidosis Vasc Diffuse Lung Dis Off J WASOG.* 2003;20(2):126–32.

146. Milman N, Selroos O. Pulmonary sarcoidosis in the Nordic countries 1950–1982. Epidemiology and clinical picture. *Sarcoidosis.* 1990;7(1):50–7.

147. Rajakariar R, Sharples EJ, Raftery MJ, Sheaff M, Yaqoob MM. Sarcoid tubulo-interstitial nephritis: Long-term outcome and response to corticosteroid therapy. *Kidney Int.* 2006;70(1):165–9.

148. Kettritz R, Goebel U, Fiebeler A, Schneider W, Luft F. The protean face of sarcoidosis revisited. *Nephrol Dial Transplant Off Publ Eur Dial Transpl Assoc—Eur Ren Assoc.* 2006;21(10):2690–4.

149. Aubart FC, Ouayoun M, Brauner M, Attali P, Kambouchner M, Valeyre D et al. Sinonasal involvement in sarcoidosis: A case-control study of 20 patients. *Medicine (Baltimore).* 2006;85(6):365–71.

150. Duchemann B, Lavolé A, Naccache J-M, Nunes H, Benzakin S, Lefevre M et al. Laryngeal sarcoidosis: A case-control

study. *Sarcoidosis Vasc Diffuse Lung Dis Off J WASOG World Assoc Sarcoidosis Granulomatous Disord.* 2014;31(3):227–34.

151. Rizzato G. Clinical impact of bone and calcium metabolism changes in sarcoidosis. *Thorax.* 1998;53(5):425–9.

152. Porter N, Beynon HL, Randeva HS. Endocrine and reproductive manifestations of sarcoidosis. *QJM Mon J Assoc Physicians.* 2003;96(8):553–61.

153. Sweiss NJ, Lower EE, Korsten P, Niewold TB, Favus MJ, Baughman RP. Bone health issues in sarcoidosis. *Curr Rheumatol Rep.* 2011;13(3):265–72.

154. Sparks JA, McSparron JI, Shah N, Aliabadi P, Paulson V, Fanta CH et al. Osseous sarcoidosis: Clinical characteristics, treatment, and outcomes—Experience from a large, academic hospital. *Semin Arthritis Rheum.* 2014;44(3):371–9.

155. Saidenberg-Kermanac'h N, Semerano L, Nunes H, Sadoun D, Guillot X, Boubaya M et al. Bone fragility in sarcoidosis and relationships with calcium metabolism disorders: A cross sectional study on 142 patients. *Arthritis Res Ther.* 2014;16(2):R78.

156. Bihan H, Christozova V, Dumas J-L, Jomaa R, Valeyre D, Tazi A et al. Sarcoidosis: Clinical, hormonal, and magnetic resonance imaging (MRI) manifestations of hypothalamic-pituitary disease in 9 patients and review of the literature. *Medicine (Baltimore).* 2007;86(5):259–68.

157. Ghrenassia E, Mekinian A, Chapelon-Albric C, Levy P, Cosnes J, Sève P et al. Digestive-tract sarcoidosis: French nationwide case-control study of 25 cases. *Medicine (Baltimore).* 2016;95(29):e4279.

158. Conron M, Young C, Beynon HL. Calcium metabolism in sarcoidosis and its clinical implications. *Rheumatol Oxf Engl.* 2000; 39(7):707–13.

159. Meyrier A, Valeyre D, Bouillon R, Paillard F, Battesti JP, Georges R. Resorptive versus absorptive hypercalciuria in sarcoidosis: Correlations with 25-hydroxy vitamin D3 and 1,25-dihydroxy vitamin D3 and parameters of disease activity. *Q J Med.* 1985;54(215):269–81.

160. Muther RS, McCarron DA, Bennett WM. Renal manifestations of sarcoidosis. *Arch Intern Med.* 1981;141(5):643–5.

161. Zeimer HJ, Greenaway TM, Slavin J, Hards DK, Zhou H, Doery JC et al. Parathyroid-hormone-related protein in sarcoidosis. *Am J Pathol.* 1998;152(1):17–21.

162. Fordice J, Katras T, Jackson RE, Cagle PT, Jackson D, Zaleski H et al. Massive splenomegaly in sarcoidosis. *South Med J.* 1992;85(7):775–8.

163. Bouvry D, Mouthon L, Brillet P-Y, Kambouchner M, Ducroix J-P, Cottin V et al. Granulomatosis-associated common variable immunodeficiency disorder: A case-control study versus sarcoidosis. *Eur Respir J.* 2013;41(1):115–22.

164. Michel M, Chanet V, Galicier L, Ruivard M, Levy Y, Hermine O et al. Autoimmune thrombocytopenic purpura and common variable immunodeficiency: Analysis of 21 cases and review of the literature. *Medicine (Baltimore).* 2004;83(4):254–63.

165. Mahévas M, Le Page L, Salle V, Lescure F-X, Smail A, Cevallos R et al. Thrombocytopenia in sarcoidosis. *Sarcoidosis Vasc Diffuse Lung Dis Off J WASOG.* 2006;23(3):229–35.

166. Mahévas M, Chiche L, Uzunhan Y, Khellaf M, Morin AS, Le Guenno G et al. Association of sarcoidosis and immune thrombocytopenia: Presentation and outcome in a series of 20 patients. *Medicine (Baltimore).* 2011;90(4):269–78.

17

Smoking and interstitial lung disease

JOSHUA J SOLOMON AND KEVIN K BROWN

BACKGROUND

The first documented reports of tobacco use date to the Mayans in Pre-Columbian times. Subsequently brought to Spain by Columbus, it gained popularity in Western Europe during the sixteenth and seventeenth centuries as something to be chewed or smoked in a pipe. The cigarette was not introduced until the 1840s, but by the early decades of the 1900s, cigarette smoking had gained wide acceptance in the Western world (1). Cigarette smoking in the United States likely peaked sometime between 1955 and 1965 at over 40% of the adult population, but it has since declined in all socio-demographic subpopulations to approximately 16.8% of US adults (2) and 14% of high school students (3). Unfortunately, worldwide consumption of tobacco has continued to grow with over 1 billion active users at present (4).

Cigarette smoke is a known toxin. It contains over 4,000 compounds, approximately 1,017 oxidant molecules per puff and over 60 tumour initiators, promoters and carcinogens (5,6). Long suspected to cause illness, it was not until the 1950s that research directly linked tobacco use to disease (7), with diseases of the lung the first to be recognized (7,8).

In 1964, the U.S. Surgeon General concluded that smoking was the primary cause of lung cancer (9), and 90% of current lung cancer deaths worldwide are estimated to be linked to tobacco use (10). The link between cigarettes and chronic obstructive pulmonary disease (COPD) was established in the 1970s (11). Tobacco use is now a recognized risk factor in six of the eight leading worldwide causes of death, including respiratory cancers, chronic obstructive pulmonary disease (COPD), heart disease, stroke, pneumonia and tuberculosis (12). It is estimated that tobacco use leads to 443,000 premature deaths and $193 billion yearly in healthcare expenditures and productivity loss (13).

It has recently been recognized that less common lung diseases may be caused or exacerbated by tobacco smoke. This chapter reviews the impact of cigarette use on a variety of these interstitial lung diseases (Table 17.1).

RESPIRATORY BRONCHIOLITIS INTERSTITIAL LUNG DISEASE

HISTORY

In 1974, Niewoehner et al. described pathologic changes in the small airways of young smokers (14). All had abnormalities of the respiratory bronchioles consisting of 'clusters of brown macrophages in the first- and second-order respiratory bronchiole distal to the terminal membranous bronchiole...frequently associated with oedema, fibrosis and epithelial hyperplasia in the adjacent bronchiolar and alveolar walls'. The authors concluded that these changes were a possible precursor to centriacinar emphysema, responsible for physiologic abnormalities seen in asymptomatic smokers, and likely reversible with smoking

Table 17.1 Smoking-related interstitial lung diseases

	RB-ILD	DIP	PLCH	CPFE
Age of onset	40s to 50s	30s to 40s	30s to 40s	50s to 70s
M:F ratio	3:2	1:1	1:1	2:1
% current or former smokers	>98%	80%–90%	90%–100%	100%
HRCT findings	Bronchial wall thickening, upper centrilobular nodules, GG	GG opacities mid to lower lung zones, reticulation	Diffuse nodules and cysts with upper and mid-lung predominance	Upper lobe emphysema with lower lobe fibrosis
Physiology	Restriction, reduced DLCO	Restriction, reduced VC, reduced DLCO	Variable, normal or reduced DLCO	Volumes normal, severely reduced DLCO
Pathology	Peribronchiolar pigmented macrophages	Uniform macrophage infiltration of alveolar spaces	LCs accumulate in and around bronchioles, patchy and focal	Upper lobe centrilobular emphysema, lower lobe UIP
Treatment	Smoking cessation	Corticosteroids	Smoking cessation, +/− immunosuppression	Smoking cessation with therapy similar to IPF
Outcome	Good	Good, rare progressive fibrosis	Median survival 12–13 years	5-year survival 25%–75% (with or without pHTN)

Abbreviations: CPFE = combined pulmonary fibrosis and emphysema; DIP = desquamative interstitial pneumonia; DLCO = diffusion capacity for carbon monoxide; F = female; GG = ground glass; HRCT = high-resolution computed tomography; IPF = idiopathic pulmonary fibrosis; LCs = Langerhans cells; M = male; pHTN = pulmonary hypertension; PLCH = pulmonary Langerhans cell histiocytosis; RBILD = respiratory-bronchiolitis-associated interstitial lung disease; UIP = usual interstitial pneumonia; VC = vital capacity.

cessation. This was the first description of the pathologic pattern of respiratory bronchiolitis (RB), a clinically silent histologic finding in the lungs of smokers. A follow-up study in 1980, looking at smokers over the age of 40, found similar bronchiolar abnormalities with coexistent emphysema (15). In 1983, Wright et al. found significant differences in the small airways between lifelong non-smokers and both current and former smokers (16). These changes were the same in current and ex-smokers despite an improvement in physiology after tobacco cessation. These findings were the first to suggest that smoking-induced small airway changes might persist well after smoking cessation.

In 1987, Myers et al. described a series of active smokers with clinicoradiographic evidence of interstitial lung disease (ILD) who were found to have RB as the sole pathologic pattern on surgical lung biopsy (SLB) (17). They speculated that this RB-associated ILD might be on a clinical spectrum with desquamative interstitial pneumonitis (DIP), a more diffuse and symptomatic smoking-related lung disease. Eighteen additional cases were subsequently reported by Yousem and the term 'respiratory bronchiolitis-interstitial lung disease' (RB-ILD) was proposed to distinguish the clinical disease from the histologic finding seen in asymptomatic smokers (18).

PATHOGENESIS AND RELATIONSHIP TO SMOKING

The accumulation of macrophages in RB may be related to the oxidative stress response as mice rendered resistant to oxidative stress and p53-dependent apoptosis are protected against emphysema but accumulate airway macrophages when exposed to cigarette smoke in a pattern similar to RB (19). The best evidence for a relationship with smoking was reported by Fraig in 2002. In 156 cases, RB was found in all 83 of the current smokers and 24 of 49 ex-smokers. Only two subjects with RB had no discernable tobacco history (20). These findings have been supported by a number of other studies (18,20–26). The histologic changes appear to resolve in some patients, although this likely takes years (the increased numbers of macrophages with smoking-related inclusions seen on bronchoalveolar [BAL] in active smokers takes 3 years to fall to non-smoker levels) (27). While smoking appears to be the dominant

cause of histologic RB, similar findings have been described in asbestos and non-asbestos mineral dust exposures, as well as rheumatoid arthritis (20,22).

CLINICAL FEATURES

Based on clinical data from 245 patients, the average age is 49 with a large range (21–83) (17,18,20–26,28). Males constitute 59% of subjects, and symptoms have an insidious onset. The most common symptom, progressive dyspnoea, is seen in 67%–100% of patients. Cough is seen 30%–80% of the time, and is most often productive of sputum. Infrequently, chest pain and wheeze are present (17,18,21,22,24–26,28).

CHEST IMAGING

A variety of abnormal plain chest radiographic findings can be seen. The most common include airway wall thickening in central and peripheral airways, diffuse ground-glass opacities and emphysema (24). Additional findings include low lung volumes, bibasilar bands and atelectasis, and reticulonodular densities (17,18,22,26,28). Up to 15% of patients may have a normal plain chest radiograph (24). In contrast, high-resolution computed tomographic (HRCT) scanning is universally abnormal (Figure 17.1). The most common findings are bronchial wall thickening in central and peripheral airways in 90% of patients, mid and upper lung zone centrilobular nodules in 70%, and upper-zone ground-glass opacities in 67%. About half the patients will have centrilobular emphysema (23,24,29). More rarely, reticular changes and increased intralobular septa have been reported (22,26,28). The HRCT changes correlate with pathologic findings. Centrilobular nodularity equates to macrophage accumulation and chronic inflammation of the respiratory bronchioles, and the ground-glass opacification equates to macrophage accumulation in the alveolar ducts and spaces (23,24).

PHYSIOLOGY

The physiologic abnormalities are variable and generally mild. The most common is a mild-to-moderate reduction in diffusion capacity for carbon monoxide (DLCO) (17,18,22,24–26). The severity of the DLCO reduction appears to correlate with the extent of centrilobular nodularity

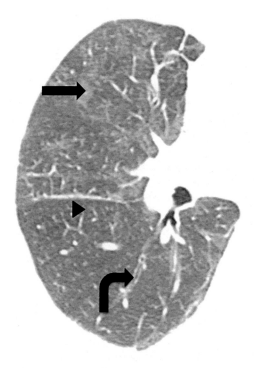

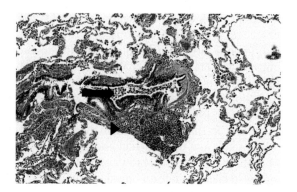

Figure 17.2 Pathology in respiratory bronchiolitis. Respiratory bronchiolitis is characterized by pigmented macrophages in the bronchiolar duct, alveolar space and peribronchiolar space (*arrow*). There are variable numbers of lymphocytes and histiocytes in the peribronchiolar and submucosal spaces (*arrowhead*) with occasional mild peribronchiolar fibrosis.

Figure 17.1 HRCT in respiratory bronchiolitis. HRCT scans in respiratory bronchiolitis are universally abnormal and show upper-zone ground-glass abnormalities (*arrow*), mid- and upper-zone centrilobular nodularity (*arrowhead*) and bronchial wall thickening in central and peripheral airways (*curved arrow*).

and ground-glass abnormality on HRCT (23). Both restrictive and obstructive physiologic abnormalities occur with restriction (31%–66%) being more common than obstruction (24%–47%) (17,18,22–26).

PATHOLOGY

Histopathologic findings are patchy and airway centred, predominately around the bronchiole (20,30). The lung tissue distal to the involved airways is normal unless there is superimposed emphysema. The defining characteristic is the presence of pigmented macrophages in the bronchiolar duct, alveolar space and peribronchiolar space (Figure 17.2). The macrophages have a finely granular, golden-brown cytoplasm with inclusions that stain with both periodic acid-Schiff and Prussian blue (30). These inclusions are thought to be components of cigarette smoke. Variable numbers of lymphocytes and histiocytes are seen in

the peribronchiolar and submucosal spaces with occasional mild peribronchiolar fibrosis. This inflammation and fibrosis can involve contiguous alveolar septa and is often accompanied by hyperplasia of type II pneumocytes, goblet cell hyperplasia and metaplastic cuboidal epithelium (17,31). If fibroblast foci, granulomas or Langerhans cells are present, one should consider an alternative diagnosis. Though early studies sought to separate the simple finding of pathologic RB from the clinical syndrome of RB-ILD by the extent of the histologic findings, later studies have confirmed that the histologic pattern is indistinguishable between the two (18,22,29,32).

DIAGNOSIS

The definitive diagnosis of RB-ILD requires a clinical syndrome of ILD – that is, the presence of respiratory symptoms with clinically significant pulmonary physiologic and chest imaging abnormalities in combination with the histologic pattern of RB on SLB (33). In the absence of any clinical signs or symptoms, the histologic pattern of RB simply suggests that the patient is or was a smoker. Given that the symptoms, clinical signs and physiologic abnormalities are non-specific, the HRCT pattern helps to support the diagnosis when pathology is not available. The HRCT findings can overlap with findings in DIP and hypersensitivity pneumonitis (HP), but the extent and distribution of ground-glass abnormalities seen in DIP (see below) and the general lack of smoking history for HP aid in these distinctions (34).

TREATMENT AND OUTCOME

There are only limited data on therapy. Smoking cessation appears to be the most important intervention (16,20,25,26). A significant reduction in symptoms, decreased ground-glass opacity and centrilobular nodularity, as well as improvements in DLCO and PaO2 have all been described in response to smoking cessation, although this is clearly not seen in all patients (23–25). The use of corticosteroids with or without other agents has been reported to be effective in improving symptoms, physiology and radiologic findings in some patients (17,18,21–23,26,31). However, these results are not universal, and lack of clinical improvement or even worsening in the face of smoking cessation with or without corticosteroids is routinely seen (22,25,26). Nonetheless, death from progressive RB-ILD appears to be extremely rare. In a study looking at long-term outcome, the median survival could not be calculated due to the prolonged survival. Seventy-five percent of patients are expected to survive 7 years or more (25). There is an association between RB-ILD and lung cancer (17% of patients in one series developed lung cancer), but this may reflect the shared risk factor of tobacco use (35,36). The pathologic pattern of RB is incidentally found in up to 37% of those undergoing surgical lung resection for lung carcinoma (36).

DESQUAMATIVE INTERSTITIAL PNEUMONIA

HISTORY

In 1965 Liebow described the clinical, radiographic and SLB findings in 18 patients with a clinical syndrome of ILD and a histologic pattern on surgical lung biopsy characterized by 'massive proliferation and desquamation of large alveolar cells, by slight thickening of the walls of distal airspaces, by the absence of necrosis and by minimal loss of tissue' (37). Termed DIP because the accumulated 'large alveolar cells' were thought

to be desquamated pneumocytes, it was felt that the distinctive pathologic features and response to therapy warranted a separation between it and the other interstitial pneumonias. In a follow-up study, Gaensler and colleagues described an additional 12 cases with long-term follow-up (38). They noted a more benign course when compared to the other fibrosing interstitial pneumonias and documented a brief remission with steroid treatment. Subsequent studies determined that the 'large alveolar cells' were, in fact, macrophages (39,40), and these cells were thought to be a nonspecific response to injury and the precursor lesion to the usual interstitial pneumonia (UIP) pathologic pattern. However, it is now widely accepted that UIP and DIP are separate entities (26,30,41–43).

RELATIONSHIP TO SMOKING

Early studies focused on a potential virologic aetiology due to the rare intranuclear inclusion bodies seen histologically (37,38). Subsequent investigation revealed that 80%–90% of patients are current or former smokers (18,26,29,44) (the disease has been reported in an 8-year-old child exposed solely to second-hand smoke [45]). While smoking is recognized as the dominant association, numerous case reports describe Cytomegalovirus and hepatitis C infection, exposures to aluminium, mycotoxins, nitrofurantoin, marijuana smoke, waterproofing spray and inorganic particulates (46,47,49–52,54,55). Additionally, the presence of systemic lupus erythematosus, systemic sclerosis, rheumatoid arthritis, myelodysplastic syndrome and monomyelocytic leukaemia have been associated with DIP (48,53,56–58).

CLINICAL FEATURES

Patients are generally young with an average age at presentation between the late 30s to mid-40s, and women and men are equally represented. Most complain of the insidious onset of dyspnoea with half describing a dry cough. A minority describe a systemic illness with weight loss and lethargy. Physical examination ranges from normal to auscultatory findings of crackles. Finger clubbing is seen in less than half. The occurrence of pneumothorax at some point during the course of illness has been reported in up to 25% (18,26,37,38).

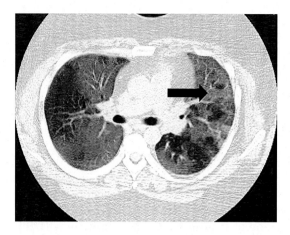

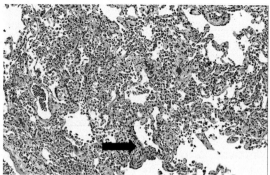

Figure 17.4 Pathology in desquamative interstitial pneumonia (DIP). DIP has a uniform and evenly distributed cellular infiltrate of pigmented macrophages within the alveolar spaces (*arrow*). This is accompanied by diffuse and uniform septal thickening consisting predominately of mononuclear cells with occasional eosinophils. Alveolar architecture is maintained and significant fibrosis or honeycombing is rare.

Figure 17.3 HRCT in desquamative interstitial pneumonia (DIP). HRCT findings in DIP consist of ground-glass opacities in the mid and lower lung zones with a peripheral distribution (*arrow*). Fibrotic features are seen in just over half of the patients; nodules, emphysema and foci of consolidation are rare.

CHEST IMAGING

Plain chest radiographs commonly show bibasilar ground-glass and/or interstitial infiltrates but are normal in up to a quarter of patients (18,26,37,38). The predominant HRCT findings are ground-glass opacities in the mid- and lower lung zones with a peripheral distribution (Figure 17.3). Fibrotic features, represented by reticular lines with or without architectural distortion, are seen in just over half of the patients. These also have a peripheral and basilar location. Other findings such as nodules, emphysema and foci of consolidation are rare (29,59).

PHYSIOLOGY

Pulmonary physiology is variable. Most have a restrictive defect with a total lung capacity (TLC) in the lower range of normal predicted value and a mildly reduced forced vital capacity (FVC). DLCO is impaired in almost all patients, and exercise-induced desaturation is common. Airflow obstruction is rare (18,26,37,38,44).

PATHOLOGY

The distinguishing histologic feature is a uniform cellular infiltrate of pigmented macrophages within the alveolar spaces (Figure 17.4) (30,59,60). These macrophages have golden-brown cytoplasms, fine black particles and stain with periodic acid-Schiff and Prussian blue in a manner similar to macrophages in RB. This infiltrate is evenly distributed throughout the involved area, leading to an early description of 'monotonous uniformity' (37). It is this uniformity of findings that helps distinguish DIP from RB and its patchy bronchiolocentric distribution (30). The alveolar space findings are accompanied by diffuse and uniform septal thickening consisting predominately of mononuclear cells with occasional eosinophils, and lymphoid nodules are common (54). The septal thickening is accompanied by comparatively minor collagen deposition and hyperplasia of type 2 pneumocytes. The alveolar architecture is maintained, and significant fibrosis or honeycombing is rare.

A focal DIP-like reaction can occasionally be seen in the SLBs of smokers diagnosed with other ILDs such as IPF, RB-ILD, nonspecific interstitial pneumonia (NSIP), eosinophilic pneumonia, chronic pulmonary haemorrhage, veno-occlusive disease, rheumatoid nodules, hamartomas and eosinophilic granulomas (61,62). Also, lung cancers can show a 'DIP-pattern of growth' with dis-cohesive bland appearing tumour cells simulating alveolar macrophages and filling the alveolar space (63).

DIAGNOSIS

Similar to RB-ILD, the definitive diagnosis of DIP requires a clinical syndrome of ILD in the setting of a DIP pattern on surgical pathology. As a DIP-like reaction may be seen in other diffuse lung diseases, the possibility of a sampling error must be considered. When pathology is not available, a confident diagnosis rests on a suggestive clinical syndrome in younger persons with characteristic HRCT findings. Active smoking supports the diagnosis, but up to 20% of these patients are non-smokers.

TREATMENT AND OUTCOME

Smoking cessation is critical and should be encouraged in all active smokers with DIP. In the initial descriptions of DIP, the majority of patients showed stabilization or improvement with corticosteroid treatment (37). In Gaensler's subsequent study, corticosteroids resulted in marked improvement in the majority of patients, with responses that were 'striking and immediate'. However, when the steroid dose was reduced or discontinued, all patients relapsed (38). Current expert opinion favors a 2-month trial of moderate doses (up to 40–60 mg) of prednisone followed by a slow taper over another 2 months. A steroid-sparing agent should be considered if the clinical response is inadequate or in the face of unacceptable corticosteroid side effects (64). Prognosis is good. A 10-year survival of up to 100% has been reported with a mean survival of 12 years from the date of diagnosis (44,65,66). However, a subset of patients may develop progressive fibrosis with honeycombing and an associated shorter lifespan (38,67). A percentage of patients will go on to develop lung cancer (29% in one series with a mean follow-up of 5 months), likely reflecting the shared risk factor of tobacco exposure (67).

PULMONARY LANGERHANS CELL HISTIOCYTOSIS

HISTORY

In 1950, Lichtenstein coined the term 'Histiocytosis X' to describe a group of disorders of varying clinical features and prognoses whose common feature was tissue infiltration with histiocytes (68). He described three specific diseases: Hand-Schüller-Christian, Letterer-Siwe and eosinophilic granuloma of bone. In 1978, the infiltrating histiocytes were found to be pathologically similar to the Langerhans cells (LCs) normally present in skin and other epithelia (69), and the new term 'Langerhans cell histiocytosis' (LCH) was offered as an alternative. In 1985, the Histiocyte Society was formed to study these diseases and to clarify a confusing nomenclature (70). The society divided the clinical syndromes into subgroups based on the site of involvement and extent of disease (71). Acute disseminated LCH (Letterer-Siwe) is a multifocal multisystem disease with a poor prognosis seen mainly in children under the age of two. Multifocal LCH (Hand–Schüller–Christian disease) is usually seen in children, carries a better prognosis and is often characterized by fever, lytic bone lesions and skin eruptions. Unifocal LCH (eosinophilic granuloma) can involve bone, skin, lungs or stomach. Though the lung can be involved in multisystem disease, the localized pulmonary form of the disease (pulmonary Langerhans cell histiocytosis [PLCH]) is the one most commonly encountered by pulmonologists. Its unique clinical picture warrants its consideration as a variant of LCH and separation from pulmonary involvement seen in childhood multisystem disease (71).

RELATIONSHIP TO SMOKING

The consistent risk factor associated with the development of PLCH is tobacco smoke. Ninety to 100% of patients are current or previous smokers (72–78), and there is an association with the amount of tobacco consumption. Smokers who develop PLCH have higher average daily tobacco consumption than smokers without PLCH (75). Clinical and radiographic resolution has also been seen with tobacco cessation alone (79).

Langerhans cells (dendritic or antigen-presenting cells produced in the marrow and found in most tissues of the body) are normally present in the healthy lung and are sparsely distributed in the tracheobronchial epithelia (80). Their numbers significantly increase in the presence of tobacco smoke, cancer and chronic pulmonary inflammation (81,82). Though multi-organ LCH seems to display a clonal proliferation of LCs, PLCH appears to generally be a non-clonal reactive proliferation to tobacco smoke in which non-malignant clonal proliferations may arise (83). Though described associations other than smoking are rare, PLCH has been described in the setting of malignancy including Hodgkin lymphoma and lung carcinoma (84).

CLINICAL FEATURES

Early studies suggested a male predominance, likely reflecting differences in tobacco use (73,75,76), but as tobacco use by women has increased, the ratio appears closer to 1:1 (74,77). While described cases have been predominately in Caucasians, the racial distribution is not known (85). A clinico-epidemiologic study conducted in Japan described a similar age of onset, smoking relationship and male predominance (78).

Isolated pulmonary LCH has a younger age of onset than other ILDs, usually presenting in the third or fourth decade. Two-thirds of the patients present with cough or dyspnoea. Extrapulmonary symptoms are common and include malaise, fevers and weight loss, while 15%–30% of patients will have extrapulmonary manifestations with bone, skin and pituitary being the most common (72–74,76–78). Liver involvement, common among children, can be seen in adults and is frequently overlooked (86). Pneumothorax is seen in up to 25% of patients either at diagnosis or during the course of their illness, and it can be recurrent (87).

Pulmonary hypertension (PH) is relatively common and can be severe (88). It seems to be related to a direct pulmonary vascular dysfunction with areas of infiltration of pulmonary arteries by Langerhans cell granulomata as well as medial and subintimal wall thickening in areas outside of the pulmonary histiocytosis nodules (89). PH is reported in up to 90% of patients awaiting lung transplant (90).

CHEST IMAGING

The characteristic plain chest radiograph finding is multiple small-to-medium-sized nodules with either an upper or mid-zone predominance that spares the costophrenic angles (74,91). Micronodules up to 2 mm in size are seen in over 90% of patients with larger nodules and cysts seen in half of the patients (91). HRCT findings have been well described and consist of diffuse nodules and cysts with an upper and mid-lung zone predominance (Figure 17.5) (92,93). The nodules tend to be small

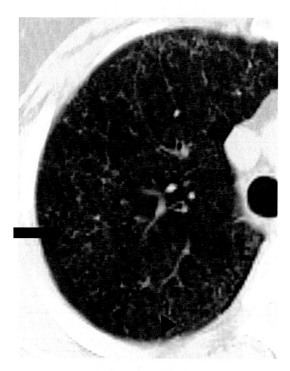

Figure 17.5 HRCT in pulmonary Langerhans cell histiocytosis (PLCH). HRCT findings in PLCH consist of diffuse cysts (*arrow*) and nodules (*arrowhead*) with upper and mid lung zone predominance. The nodules and cysts also tend to be small, usually less than 10 mm. Linear and ground-glass opacities are rare.

with the majority less than 10 mm in size. Cysts also tend to be small (<10 mm) and thin walled; larger cysts, confluent cysts and thick-walled cysts are less common. Linear and ground-glass opacities tend to be rare. Studies looking at evolution of CT findings with disease progression suggest that active disease is represented by the presence of nodular lesions, which regress or progress and can transform into cysts (92).

PHYSIOLOGY

The severity of physiologic impairment is variable. Normal physiology has been reported in up to 35% of patients, likely representing early diagnosis (73,74,77). The most common abnormality is a reduction in DLCO, which is seen in up to 90%. TLC and FVC can be mildly reduced, and obstruction with a reduced forced expiratory volume in 1 second (FEV1)/FVC ratio is rare in early and mild disease (72,73,76,77). Progression of disease is heralded by reductions in TLC, FVC and the FEV1/FVC ratio, and variable changes in residual volume are observed (72,76).

PATHOLOGY

In normal healthy lungs, LCs are sparse, while in PLCH these cells accumulate in and around the bronchioles in a patchy and focal fashion (Figure 17.6). They are different from other histiocytes in that they stain positively for the presence of CD1a antigen and S-100 protein and have pentalaminar Birbeck granules visible by electron microscopy (94). Macroscopic findings consist of palpable small subpleural nodules occasionally associated with cysts in an upper and mid-lung distribution with sparing of the costophrenic angles (95,96). The predominant microscopic finding is bronchiolocentric nodules, commonly forming a 'stellate' pattern (30). The nodules consist of a varying number of LCs, eosinophils, neutrophils, lymphocytes, fibroblasts and macrophages (often containing smoker's pigment), and can display necrosis or cavitation. The eosinophils vary in number, are occasionally the dominant cell type and are situated at the periphery of the nodule (96). A 'DIP-like' reaction with macrophages filling the airways can often be seen (74). Histologic

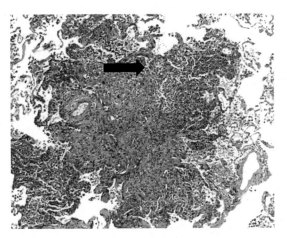

Figure 17.6 Pathology in pulmonary Langerhans cell histiocytosis (PLCH). Langerhans cells accumulate in and around the bronchioles in a patchy and focal fashion. This forms a nodule, usually with a stellate pattern, that consists of Langerhans cells, eosinophils, neutrophils, lymphocytes, fibroblasts and macrophages (*arrow*). These can have cavitation or necrosis.

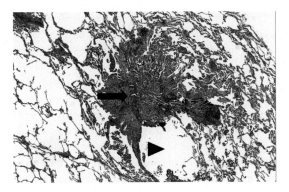

Figure 17.7 The stellate scar in pulmonary Langerhans cell histiocytosis (PLCH). The stellate scar is the final fibrotic stage of PLCH. These are seen around the bronchioles and are usually void of Langerhans cells (*arrow*). Cystic spaces are formed by traction of the surrounding normal airspaces by contraction of the scar (*arrowhead*).

progression is associated with fibroblast proliferation with collagen deposition and scarring, with stellate scars seen around the bronchioles (bronchiolocentric lesions). These scars are void of LCs and are presumed to be a final fibrotic stage (Figure 17.7) (30).

Mitogen-activated protein kinase (MAPK) pathway mutations, seen in up to 60% of patients with extrapulmonary LCH (97), have been identified in a subset of patients with PLCH. The V600E mutation of the *BRAF* gene (a missense substitution leading to constitutive activation of BRAF and downstream cellular protein kinases) has been described in 24%–35% of patients with PLCH, suggesting a clonal proliferation in a subset of these patients (98,99). Patients with *BRAF* V600E mutations are younger with a higher cumulative tobacco exposure (98,99). The role of this mutation in the clinical course of PLCH or the applicability of therapy with specific BRAF inhibitors is not known (85).

DIAGNOSIS

In the absence of alternative explanations, a young smoker with characteristic HRCT findings has a diagnosis of PLCH with a high degree of confidence. In the correct clinical setting, BAL findings of >5% LCs that stain positively for the presence of CD1a make a diagnosis of PLCH very likely (100,101). When the combination of the clinical and radiographic data provide less than a highly confident diagnosis, tissue biopsy may be required. As the lesions are focal in nature, the yield of transbronchial biopsy is low (in the range of 10%–40%), and a definitive diagnosis often requires a SLB (102). Tissue should be stained with antibodies for S-100 and CD1a (30). Extrapulmonary involvement in adults is rare and, in the absence of suggestive symptoms, routine screening for the presence of extrapulmonary disease is often not informative (103). Active disease is hypermetabolic on positive emission tomography (PET)/CT, an imaging modality that is increasingly being used for initial staging as well as determining response to therapy (104).

TREATMENT AND OUTCOME

Smoking cessation should be encouraged, as there have been documented cases of near-complete symptomatic and radiographic improvement in patients following tobacco cessation alone (79,105,106). Smoking cessation can also significantly lower the risk of lung function decline over time, although only 20% of patients in one study had sustained tobacco cessation over a 2-year period (107). In asymptomatic patients, additional therapy does not appear warranted. Patients with symptoms or significant physiologic derangement are often treated with corticosteroids alone, or in the case of multisystem disease, with corticosteroids combined with another immunosuppressive agent (77). Many immunosuppressive agents have been used including cyclophosphamide, vinblastine, chlorambucil, methotrexate, etoposide and cladribine (96,107). While there are accumulating data on the use of cladribine in patients with continued progression in spite of tobacco cessation and corticosteroid use (108–110), no strong data exist on the efficacy of any of these regimens. In those identified to have a *BRAF* mutation, there may be a role for MAPK pathway-targeted treatment (111). For subjects with pneumothoraces, surgical pleurodesis should be considered (87).

In patients with PLCH-associated PH, there are case reports and case series of improvements with the use of pulmonary vasodilator therapy (112–115). Survival after lung transplant is good, with a reported 57% 5-year survival, but PLCH recurs in about 20% of patients post-transplant (90).

Prognosis is variable. Fifty to sixty percent of patients will show improvement in symptoms with or without steroid therapy. The mortality rate has been estimated to be as high as 36% at 10 years (77), with a median survival of 12–13 years (73,77). Death usually results from respiratory failure, but patients also appear to be at increased risk of neoplasm, which is usually pulmonary or haematologic (73,77). Factors associated with a worsened survival include older age, reduced FEV1/FVC ratio, increased RV/TLC ratio, lower DLCO, and a higher World Health Organization functional class in those with PH (73,77,112).

IDIOPATHIC PULMONARY FIBROSIS AND COMBINED PULMONARY FIBROSIS AND EMPHYSEMA

Ever-smoking is a known risk factor for the development of IPF. Studies looking at environmental and occupational exposures in patients with IPF have found that when compared to never-smokers, ever-smokers have an increased risk of disease development (odds ratio ranging from 1.57 to 2.9) (116–118). A meta-analysis has provided additional support for a relationship (119), as have studies of subjects genetically at risk for the development of fibrosis (120). More recently, patients with IPF accompanied by severe breathlessness and a marked reduction in DLCO in spite of normal or near-normal lung volumes on pulmonary function testing have been described (121). HRCT scanning revealed a combination of upper-lobe emphysema and lower-lobe UIP patterns, and all patients were former or current smokers. This was an early description of 'combined pulmonary fibrosis and emphysema' (CPFE) (122–127), a syndrome reported almost exclusively in smokers. It has been estimated that it may account for 5%–10% of diffuse ILDs (123).

At least two-thirds of patients with CPFE are men with a primary complaint of breathlessness. Cough is less frequent. Clubbing is seen in up to half of patients (121,123–127). HRCT scans show predominantly upper-lobe centrilobular emphysema combined with lower-lobe UIP pattern fibrosis, although other chest imaging patterns (NSIP, DIP and RB-ILD) have been reported (123,127). In contrast to typical emphysema, near-normal lung volumes (80%–90% of predicted values) are seen, and air trapping is rare. Decreases in the

FEV1/FVC ratio are mild with a mean ratio of 0.70 (123,125). DLCO is markedly reduced (usually 30%–40% of predicted). The physiologic findings represent the additive effects of emphysema and IPF on gas transfer and their opposing effects on total lung volume and airflows (121). Pathology obtained from SLB or lung explants reveals upper lung zone centrilobular emphysema and lower lung zone UIP pattern fibrosis. Variable amounts of intra-alveolar pigmented macrophage deposition representing a smoker's 'DIP-like' reaction are present. Histologic patterns other than UIP have been reported, including DIP, organizing pneumonia and unclassifiable interstitial pneumonia (123). Therapy is similar to that for IPF (123). The risk of having PH is high (50%–90%), and the presence of echocardiographically proven PH decreases 5-year survival from 75% to 25% (126). These patients are at increased risk for lung cancer (128), which portends a poor prognosis (129,130). Degree of honeycombing, reductions in DLCO and the presence of a histopathologic UIP pattern have also been associated with a poorer outcome (131–133).

ACUTE EOSINOPHILIC PNEUMONIA

Acute eosinophilic pneumonia (AEP) is a rare syndrome characterized by fever, diffuse pulmonary infiltrates and pulmonary eosinophilia. Patients often develop fever, dyspnoea and cough 3–4 days before diagnosis (134). Chest x-ray and HRCT scans show diffuse airspace opacities with effusions present in up to 70% (135). Peripheral blood eosinophilia is less likely to be seen when AEP is caused by tobacco smoking. While diagnostic criteria are debated, other common causes of pulmonary eosinophilia must be excluded, including helminthic, fungal and bacterial infections, drugs, toxins, radiation exposure, Churg–Strauss vasculitis and Hodgkin disease (136). BAL eosinophilia in the range of 36%–54% is seen (134). Reported treatment regimens consist of varying doses of intravenous methylprednisolone that range from 240 mg to 1000 mg daily with an expected response of rapid improvement of the chest imaging abnormalities and resolution of respiratory failure. Prednisone tapers last from days to months, although recurrence has *not* been reported. While AEP has been associated with various inhaled exposures including World Trade Center dust (137), cocaine (138) and Scotchguard inhalation (139), the strongest association has been with smoking. Up to 97% of patients are active smokers, with new-onset smokers being over-represented (135,140,141). In a study of military personnel deployed in or near Iraq, all 18 cases of AEP identified were in current smokers, with 78% of cases noted in new-onset smokers (within the 2 months prior to diagnosis) (142).

SMOKING-RELATED INTERSTITIAL LUNG ABNORMALITIES

Smoking-related interstitial fibrosis (SRIF) was first described as an incidental finding in 45% of lobectomy specimens from current or past smokers (143). The lesion is found in areas of emphysematous as well as non-emphysematous lung and is characterized by varying degrees of collagen deposition in alveolar septa and minimal inflammation (Figure 17.8). None of the patients in this series had clinical evidence of ILD. Radiographic evidence of smoking-related interstitial changes has also been described (Figure 17.9). A study of 4,320 participants of the NHANES I study found a 40% increased risk of spirometric restriction in current smokers (144). Utilizing the Multi-Ethnic Study of Atherosclerosis (MESA) cohort, a follow-up investigation found a

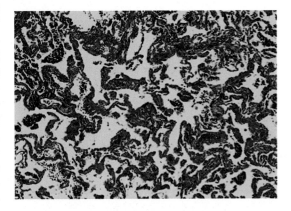

Figure 17.8 Pathology of smoking-related interstitial fibrosis (SRIF). Lung biopsy in a patient with SRIF shows mild interstitial fibrosis in deep lung parenchyma with a background of respiratory bronchiolitis. (From Katzenstein AL et al. *Hum Pathol.* 2010;41(3):316–25. With permission.)

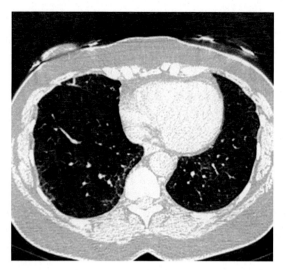

Figure 17.9 HRCT of early ILD in a smoker. This HRCT from a smoker shows a patchy basilar and peripheral predominant process consisting of ground glass abnormality, reticulation and traction bronchiectasis. (From Washko GR et al. *Acad Radiol.* 2010;17(1):48–53. With permission.)

correlation between pack-years smoked, spirometric restriction and the presence of high attenuation areas (HAAs) on quantitative HRCT, a finding correlated with ground glass, reticulation and atelectasis (145). A review of HRCT scans from patients enrolled in the COPDgene Study found chest imaging evidence of ILD in 5%–10% of scans and an association with smoking (146). In a follow-up study, the COPDgene investigators reviewed 2,416 HRCT scans and found that 8% had interstitial lung abnormalities (ILAs), and the presence of these abnormalities was associated with active smoking, greater exposure to tobacco smoke, a lesser amount of emphysema and a reduced total lung capacity (147). It is speculated that these changes may represent RB-ILD or the aforementioned SRIF. In a recent study, the presence of ILA was associated with a greater risk of all-cause mortality (148).

ANTI-GLOMERULAR BASEMENT MEMBRANE DISEASE

Anti-glomerular basement membrane (GBM) disease is a rare autoimmune disease characterized by circulating antibodies against type IV collagen.

While classically considered a pulmonary-renal syndrome, it presents with either isolated renal disease, renal disease with diffuse alveolar haemorrhage (DAH) or rarely with alveolar haemorrhage alone (149). There is a correlation between active cigarette smoking and both the development and relapse of DAH, with active smokers making up from 50% to 89% of patients (150–154). There is also speculation that smoking may play a more general role in precipitating haemoptysis in patients with a predisposition to haemorrhage, as heavy smoking appears associated with an increased risk of DAH in immunocompromised patients and in idiopathic pulmonary haemosiderosis (155–158).

RHEUMATOID ARTHRITIS–ASSOCIATED INTERSTITIAL LUNG DISEASE

Rheumatoid arthritis (RA) is common, affecting 1% of the US population (159). Smoking increases the risk of developing RA (160,161) and increases its severity in those with established disease (162); both consistent with the emerging data that the lungs are involved in the pathogenesis of RA (163,164). A significant number of these patients will develop interstitial lung disease (RA-ILD), with 1 in 10 patients dying from it (165). Though there are many risk factors for RA-ILD (166), smoking appears to be one of the strongest (167–169). In a cohort of 336 patients, smoking was the most consistent independent predictor of chest imaging and physiologic abnormalities suggestive of ILD (170).

CONCLUSION

Tobacco smoke is associated with a wide range of effects in the human lung. Beyond its known association with the development of lung cancer and emphysema, it is associated with the development of both incidental bronchiolar changes as well as a number of specific interstitial lung diseases. For example, RB as an incidental histologic finding in ever-smokers may persist without clinical impact for years, while RB-ILD is a clinically significant ILD disease with identical pathologic changes. The impact of smoking is not limited to its known associations with RB-ILD/DIP and PLCH, as it also appears to be associated with the development of lung fibrosis, eosinophilic pneumonia and alveolar haemorrhage in susceptible individuals. Overall, the impact of tobacco smoke is wide and almost universally detrimental.

REFERENCES

1. Kumra V, Markoff BA. Who's smoking now? The epidemiology of tobacco use in the United States and abroad. *Clin Chest Med.* 2000;21(1):1–9, vii.

2. Jamal A, Homa DM, O'Connor E, Babb SD, Caraballo RS, Singh T et al. Current cigarette smoking among adults—United States, 2005–2014. *MMWR Morb Mortal Wkly Rep.* 2015;64(44):1233–40.

3. Centers for Disease Control and Prevention. Tobacco product use among middle and high school students—United States, 2011 and 2012. *MMWR Morb Mortal Wkly Rep.* 2013;62(45):893–7.

4. World Health Organization (WHO). *WHO Report on the Global Tobacco Epidemic.* Geneva, Switzerland: WHO; 2015.

5. Pryor WA, Stone K. Oxidants in cigarette smoke. Radicals, hydrogen peroxide, peroxynitrate, and peroxynitrite. *Ann N Y Acad Sci.* 1993;686:12–27; discussion 27-18.

6. Smith CJ, Hansch C. The relative toxicity of compounds in mainstream cigarette smoke condensate. *Food Chem Toxicol.* 2000;38(7):637–46.

7. Wynder EL, Graham EA. Tobacco smoking as a possible etiologic factor in bronchiogenic carcinoma; A study of 684 proved cases. *J Am Med Assoc.* 1950;143(4):329–36.

8. Doll R, Hill AB. Smoking and carcinoma of the lung; preliminary report. *Br Med J.* 1950;2(4682):739–48.

9. Service USPH. *Smoking and Health: A Report of the Surgeon General.* Washington, DC: US Government Printing Office; 1964.

10. Bilello KS, Murin S, Matthay RA. Epidemiology, etiology, and prevention of lung cancer. *Clin Chest Med.* 2002;23(1):1–25.

11. Petty TL. The history of COPD. *Int J Chron Obstruct Pulmon Dis.* 2006;1(1):3–14.

12. World Health Organization (WHO). *WHO Report on the Global Tobacco Epidemic.* Geneva, Switzerland: WHO; 2008.

13. Centers for Disease Control and Prevention. State-specific smoking-attributable mortality and years of potential life lost—United States, 2000–2004. *MMWR Morb Mortal Wkly Rep.* 2009;58(2):29–33.

14. Niewoehner DE, Kleinerman J, Rice DB. Pathologic changes in the peripheral airways of young cigarette smokers. *N Engl J Med.* 1974;291(15):755–8.

15. Cosio MG, Hale KA, Niewoehner DE. Morphologic and morphometric effects of prolonged cigarette smoking on the small airways. *Am Rev Respir Dis.* 1980;122(2):265–71.

16. Wright JL, Lawson LM, Pare PD, Wiggs BJ, Kennedy S, Hogg JC. Morphology of peripheral airways in current smokers and ex-smokers. *Am Rev Respir Dis.* 1983;127(4):474–7.

17. Myers JL, Veal CF, Jr., Shin MS, Katzenstein AL. Respiratory bronchiolitis causing interstitial lung disease. A clinicopathologic study of six cases. *Am Rev Respir Dis.* 1987;135(4):880–4.

18. Yousem SA, Colby TV, Gaensler EA. Respiratory bronchiolitis-associated interstitial lung disease and its relationship to desquamative interstitial pneumonia. *Mayo Clin Proc.* 1989;64(11):1373–80.

19. Lunghi B, De Cunto G, Cavarra E, Fineschi S, Bartalesi B, Lungarella G et al. Smoking p66Shc knocked out mice develop respiratory bronchiolitis with fibrosis but not emphysema. *PLoS One.* 2015;10(3):e0119797.

20. Fraig M, Shreesha U, Savici D, Katzenstein AL. Respiratory bronchiolitis: A clinicopathologic study in current smokers, ex-smokers, and never-smokers. *Am J Surg Pathol.* 2002;26(5):647–53.

21. Craig PJ, Wells AU, Doffman S, Rassl D, Colby TV, Hansell DM et al. Desquamative interstitial pneumonia, respiratory bronchiolitis and their relationship to smoking. *Histopathology.* 2004;45(3):275–82.

22. Moon J, du Bois RM, Colby TV, Hansell DM, Nicholson AG. Clinical significance of respiratory bronchiolitis on open lung biopsy and

its relationship to smoking related interstitial lung disease. *Thorax.* 1999;54(11):1009–14.

23. Nakanishi M, Demura Y, Mizuno S, Ameshima S, Chiba Y, Miyamori I et al. Changes in HRCT findings in patients with respiratory bronchiolitis-associated interstitial lung disease after smoking cessation. *Eur Respir J.* 2007;29(3):453–61.

24. Park JS, Brown KK, Tuder RM, Hale VA, King TE Jr, Lynch DA. Respiratory bronchiolitis-associated interstitial lung disease: Radiologic features with clinical and pathologic correlation. *J Comput Assist Tomogr.* 2002;26(1):13–20.

25. Portnoy J, Veraldi KL, Schwarz MI, Cool CD, Curran-Everett D, Cherniack RM et al. Respiratory bronchiolitis-interstitial lung disease: Long-term outcome. *Chest.* 2007;131(3):664–71.

26. Ryu JH, Myers JL, Capizzi SA, Douglas WW, Vassallo R, Decker PA. Desquamative interstitial pneumonia and respiratory bronchiolitis-associated interstitial lung disease. *Chest.* 2005;127(1):178–84.

27. Agius RM, Rutman A, Knight RK, Cole PJ. Human pulmonary alveolar macrophages with smokers' inclusions: Their relation to the cessation of cigarette smoking. *Br J Exp Pathol.* 1986;67(3):407–13.

28. Holt RM, Schmidt RA, Godwin JD, Raghu G. High resolution CT in respiratory bronchiolitis-associated interstitial lung disease. *J Comput Assist Tomogr.* 1993;17(1):46–50.

29. Heyneman LE, Ward S, Lynch DA, Remy-Jardin M, Johkoh T, Muller NL. Respiratory bronchiolitis, respiratory bronchiolitis-associated interstitial lung disease, and desquamative interstitial pneumonia: different entities or part of the spectrum of the same disease process? *AJR Am J Roentgenol.* 1999;173(6):1617–22.

30. Aubry MC, Wright JL, Myers JL. The pathology of smoking-related lung diseases. *Clin Chest Med.* 2000;21(1):11–35, vii.

31. King TE Jr. Respiratory bronchiolitis-associated interstitial lung disease. *Clin Chest Med.* 1993;14(4):693–8.

32. Cottin V, Streichenberger N, Gamondes JP, Thevenet F, Loire R, Cordier JF. Respiratory bronchiolitis in smokers with spontaneous pneumothorax. *Eur Respir J.* 1998;12(3):702–4.

33. Davies G, Wells AU, du Bois RM. Respiratory bronchiolitis associated with interstitial lung disease and desquamative interstitial pneumonia. *Clin Chest Med.* 2004;25(4):717–26.

34. Wells AU, Nicholson AG, Hansell DM, du Bois RM. Respiratory bronchiolitis-associated interstitial lung disease. *Semin Respir Crit Care Med.* 2003;24(5):585–94.

35. Scheidl SJ, Kusej M, Flick H, Stacher E, Matzi V, Kovacs G et al. Clinical manifestations of respiratory bronchiolitis as an incidental finding in surgical lung biopsies: A retrospective analysis of a large Austrian Registry. *Respiration.* 2016;91(1):26–33.

36. Yamada Y, Terada J, Tatsumi K, Kono C, Tanno M, Takemura T et al. Respiratory bronchiolitis and lung carcinoma. *Respir Investig.* 2013;51(3):184–90.

37. Liebow AA, Steer A, Billingsley JG. Desquamative interstitial pneumonia. *Am J Med.* 1965;39:369–404.

38. Gaensler EA, Goff AM, Prowse CM. Desquamative interstitial pneumonia. *N Engl J Med.* 1966;274(3):113–28.

39. Farr GH, Harley RA, Hennigar GR. Desquamative interstitial pneumonia. An electron microscopic study. *Am J Pathol.* 1970;60(3):347–70.

40. Valdivia E, Hensley G, Leory EP, Wu J, Jaeschke W. Morphology and pathogenesis of desquamative interstitial pneumonitis. *Thorax.* 1977;32(1):7–18.

41. Akira M, Yamamoto S, Hara H, Sakatani M, Ueda E. Serial computed tomographic evaluation in desquamative interstitial pneumonia. *Thorax.* 1997;52(4):333–7.

42. Nagai S, Kitaichi M, Izumi T. Classification and recent advances in idiopathic interstitial pneumonia. *Curr Opin Pulm Med.* 1998;4(5):256–60.

43. Scadding JG, Hinson KF. Diffuse fibrosing alveolitis (diffuse interstitial fibrosis of the lungs). Correlation of histology at biopsy with prognosis. *Thorax.* 1967;22(4):291–304.

44. Carrington CB, Gaensler EA, Coutu RE, FitzGerald MX, Gupta RG. Natural history and treated course of usual and desquamative interstitial pneumonia. *N Engl J Med.* 1978;298(15):801–9.

45. Ischander M, Fan LL, Farahmand V, Langston C, Yazdani S. Desquamative interstitial pneumonia in a child related to cigarette smoke. *Pediatr Pulmonol.* 2014;49(3):E56–58.

46. Abraham JL, Hertzberg MA. Inorganic particulates associated with desquamative interstitial pneumonia. *Chest.* 1981;80(1 Suppl):67–70.

47. Bone RC, Wolfe J, Sobonya RE, Kerby GR, Stechschulte D, Ruth WE et al. Desquamative interstitial pneumonia following long-term nitrofurantoin therapy. *Am J Med.* 1976;60(5):697–701.

48. Goldstein JD, Godleski JJ, Herman PG. Desquamative interstitial pneumonitis associated with monomyelocytic leukemia. *Chest.* 1982;81(3):321–5.

49. Herbert A, Sterling G, Abraham J, Corrin B. Desquamative interstitial pneumonia in an aluminum welder. *Hum Pathol.* 1982;13(8):694–9.

50. Iskandar SB, McKinney LA, Shah L, Roy TM, Byrd RP Jr. Desquamative interstitial pneumonia and hepatitis C virus infection: A rare association. *South Med J.* 2004;97(9):890–3.

51. Lougheed MD, Roos JO, Waddell WR, Munt PW. Desquamative interstitial pneumonitis and diffuse alveolar damage in textile workers. Potential role of mycotoxins. *Chest.* 1995;108(5):1196–200.

52. Schroten H, Manz S, Kohler H, Wolf U, Brockmann M, Riedel F. Fatal desquamative interstitial pneumonia associated with proven CMV infection in an 8-month-old boy. *Pediatr Pulmonol.* 1998;25(5):345–7.

53. Farris AB 3rd, Hasserjian RP, Zukerberg LR, Amrein PC, Greene RE, Mark EJ et al. Diffuse cellular and fibrosing interstitial pneumonitis with desquamative interstitial pneumonitis-like features associated with myeloid neoplasia. *Am J Surg Pathol.* 2009;33(10):1485–93.

54. Tazelaar HD, Wright JL, Churg A. Desquamative interstitial pneumonia. *Histopathology.* 2011;58(4):509–16.

55. Nakazawa A, Hagiwara E, Harada S, Yoshida M, Baba T, Okudela K et al. Surgically proven desquamative interstitial pneumonia induced by waterproofing spray. *Intern Med.* 2014;53(18):2107–10.

56. Esmaeilbeigi F, Juvet S, Hwang D, Mittoo S. Desquamative interstitial pneumonitis in a patient with systemic lupus erythematosus. *Can Respir J.* 2012;19(1):50–2.

57. Swartz JS, Chatterjee S, Parambil JG. Desquamative interstitial pneumonia as the initial manifestation of systemic sclerosis. *J Clin Rheumatol.* 2010;16(6):284–6.

58. Ishii H, Iwata A, Sakamoto N, Mizunoe S, Mukae H, Kadota J. Desquamative interstitial pneumonia (DIP) in a patient with rheumatoid arthritis: Is DIP associated with autoimmune disorders? *Intern Med.* 2009;48(10):827–30.

59. Singh G, Katyal SL, Whiteside TL, Stachura I. Desquamative interstitial pneumonitis. The intra-alveolar cells are macrophages. *Chest.* 1981;79(1):128.

60. Fromm GB, Dunn LJ, Harris JO. Desquamative interstitial pneumonitis. Characterization of free intraalveolar cells. *Chest.* 1980;77(4):552–4.

61. American Thoracic Society/European Respiratory Society International Multidisciplinary Consensus Classification of the Idiopathic Interstitial Pneumonias. This joint statement of the American Thoracic Society (ATS), and the European Respiratory Society (ERS) was adopted by the ATS board of directors, June 2001 and by the ERS Executive Committee, June 2001. *Am J Respir Crit Care Med.* 2002;165(2):277–304.

62. Bedrossian CW, Kuhn C 3rd, Luna MA, Conklin RH, Byrd RB, Kaplan PD. Desquamative interstitial pneumonia-like reaction accompanying pulmonary lesions. *Chest.* 1977;72(2):166–9.

63. Raparia K, Ketterer J, Dalurzo ML, Chang YH, Colby TV, Leslie KO. Lung tumors masquerading as desquamative interstitial pneumonia (DIP): Report of 7 cases and review of the literature. *Am J Surg Pathol.* 2014;38(7):921–4.

64. Elkin SL, Nicholson AG, du Bois RM. Desquamative interstitial pneumonia and respiratory bronchiolitis-associated interstitial lung disease. *Semin Respir Crit Care Med.* 2001;22(4):387–98.

65. Nicholson AG, Colby TV, du Bois RM, Hansell DM, Wells AU. The prognostic significance of the histologic pattern of

interstitial pneumonia in patients presenting with the clinical entity of cryptogenic fibrosing alveolitis. *Am J Respir Crit Care Med.* 2000;162(6):2213–7.

66. Travis WD, Matsui K, Moss J, Ferrans VJ. Idiopathic nonspecific interstitial pneumonia: Prognostic significance of cellular and fibrosing patterns: Survival comparison with usual interstitial pneumonia and desquamative interstitial pneumonia. *Am J Surg Pathol.* 2000;24(1):19–33.

67. Kawabata Y, Takemura T, Hebisawa A, Sugita Y, Ogura T, Nagai S et al. Desquamative interstitial pneumonia may progress to lung fibrosis as characterized radiologically. *Respirology.* 2012;17(8):1214–21.

68. Lichtenstein L. Histiocytosis X; integration of eosinophilic granuloma of bone, Letterer-Siwe disease, and Schuller-Christian disease as related manifestations of a single nosologic entity. *AMA Arch Pathol.* 1953;56(1):84–102.

69. Nezelof C, Basset F, Rousseau MF. Histiocytosis X histogenetic arguments for a Langerhans cell origin. *Biomedicine.* 1973;18(5):365–71.

70. Histiocytosis syndromes in children. Writing Group of the Histiocyte Society. *Lancet.* 1987;1(8526):208–9.

71. Favara BE, Feller AC, Pauli M, Jaffe ES, Weiss LM, Arico M et al. Contemporary classification of histiocytic disorders. The WHO Committee on Histiocytic/Reticulum Cell Proliferations. Reclassification Working Group of the Histiocyte Society. *Med Pediatr Oncol.* 1997;29(3):157–66.

72. Crausman RS, Jennings CA, Tuder RM, Ackerson LM, Irvin CG, King TE Jr. Pulmonary histiocytosis X: Pulmonary function and exercise pathophysiology. *Am J Respir Crit Care Med.* 1996;153(1):426–35.

73. Delobbe A, Durieu J, Duhamel A, Wallaert B. Determinants of survival in pulmonary Langerhans' cell granulomatosis (histiocytosis X). Groupe d'Etude en Pathologie Interstitielle de la Societe de Pathologie Thoracique du Nord. *Eur Respir J.* 1996;9(10):2002–6.

74. Friedman PJ, Liebow AA, Sokoloff J. Eosinophilic granuloma of lung. Clinical aspects of primary histiocytosis in the adult. *Medicine (Baltimore).* 1981;60(6):385–96.

75. Hance AJ, Basset F, Saumon G, Danel C, Valeyre D, Battesti JP et al. Smoking and interstitial lung disease. The effect of cigarette smoking on the incidence of pulmonary histiocytosis X and sarcoidosis. *Ann N Y Acad Sci.* 1986;465:643–56.

76. Schonfeld N, Frank W, Wenig S, Uhrmeister P, Allica E, Preussler H et al. Clinical and radiologic features, lung function and therapeutic results in pulmonary histiocytosis X. *Respiration.* 1993;60(1):38–44.

77. Vassallo R, Ryu JH, Schroeder DR, Decker PA, Limper AH. Clinical outcomes of pulmonary Langerhans'-cell histiocytosis in adults. *N Engl J Med.* 2002;346(7):484–90.

78. Watanabe R, Tatsumi K, Hashimoto S, Tamakoshi A, Kuriyama T. Clinico-epidemiological features of pulmonary histiocytosis X. *Intern Med.* 2001;40(10):998–1003.

79. Mogulkoc N, Veral A, Bishop PW, Bayindir U, Pickering CA, Egan JJ. Pulmonary Langerhans' cell histiocytosis: Radiologic resolution following smoking cessation. *Chest.* 1999;115(5):1452–5.

80. Mellman I, Steinman RM. Dendritic cells: Specialized and regulated antigen processing machines. *Cell.* 2001;106(3):255–8.

81. Soler P, Moreau A, Basset F, Hance AJ. Cigarette smoking-induced changes in the number and differentiated state of pulmonary dendritic cells/Langerhans cells. *Am Rev Respir Dis.* 1989;139(5):1112–7.

82. Tazi A, Bouchonnet F, Grandsaigne M, Boumsell L, Hance AJ, Soler P. Evidence that granulocyte macrophage-colony-stimulating factor regulates the distribution and differentiated state of dendritic cells/Langerhans cells in human lung and lung cancers. *J Clin Invest.* 1993;91(2):566–76.

83. Yousem SA, Colby TV, Chen YY, Chen WG, Weiss LM. Pulmonary Langerhans' cell histiocytosis: Molecular analysis of clonality. *Am J Surg Pathol.* 2001;25(5):630–6.

84. Egeler RM, Neglia JP, Puccetti DM, Brennan CA, Nesbit ME. Association of Langerhans cell histiocytosis with malignant neoplasms. *Cancer.* 1993;71(3):865–73.

85. Tazi A. Adult pulmonary Langerhans' cell histiocytosis. *Eur Respir J.* 2006;27(6):1272–85.

86. Araujo B, Costa F, Lopes J, Castro R. Adult Langerhans cell histiocytosis with hepatic and pulmonary involvement. *Case Rep Radiol.* 2015;2015:536328.

87. Mendez JL, Nadrous HF, Vassallo R, Decker PA, Ryu JH. Pneumothorax in pulmonary Langerhans cell histiocytosis. *Chest.* 2004;125(3):1028–32.

88. Fartoukh M, Humbert M, Capron F, Maitre S, Parent F, Le Gall C et al. Severe pulmonary hypertension in histiocytosis X. *Am J Respir Crit Care Med.* 2000;161(1):216–23.

89. Travis WD, Borok Z, Roum JH, Zhang J, Feuerstein I, Ferrans VJ et al. Pulmonary Langerhans cell granulomatosis (histiocytosis X). A clinicopathologic study of 48 cases. *Am J Surg Pathol.* 1993;17(10):971–86.

90. Dauriat G, Mal H, Thabut G, Mornex JF, Bertocchi M, Tronc F et al. Lung transplantation for pulmonary Langerhans' cell histiocytosis: A multicenter analysis. *Transplantation.* 2006;81(5):746–50.

91. Lacronique J, Roth C, Battesti JP, Basset F, Chretien J. Chest radiological features of pulmonary histiocytosis X: A report based on 50 adult cases. *Thorax.* 1982;37(2):104–9.

92. Brauner MW, Grenier P, Mouelhi MM, Mompoint D, Lenoir S. Pulmonary histiocytosis X: Evaluation with high-resolution CT. *Radiology.* 1989;172(1):255–8.

93. Brauner MW, Grenier P, Tijani K, Battesti JP, Valeyre D. Pulmonary Langerhans cell histiocytosis: Evolution of lesions on CT scans. *Radiology.* 1997;204(2):497–502.

94. Gasent Blesa JM, Alberola Candel V, Solano Vercet C, Laforga Canales J, Semler C, Perez Antoli MR et al. Langerhans cell histiocytosis. *Clin Transl Oncol.* 2008;10(11):688–96.

95. Roden AC, Yi ES. Pulmonary Langerhans cell histiocytosis: An update from the pathologists' perspective. *Arch Pathol Lab Med.* 2016;140(3):230–40.

96. Basset F, Corrin B, Spencer H, Lacronique J, Roth C, Soler P et al. Pulmonary histiocytosis X. *Am Rev Respir Dis.* 1978;118(5):811–20.

97. Badalian-Very G, Vergilio JA, Degar BA, MacConaill LE, Brandner B, Calicchio ML et al. Recurrent BRAF mutations in Langerhans cell histiocytosis. *Blood.* 2010;116(11):1919–23.

98. Roden AC, Hu X, Kip S, Parrilla Castellar ER, Rumilla KM, Vrana JA et al. BRAF V600E expression in Langerhans cell histiocytosis: Clinical and immunohistochemical study on 25 pulmonary and 54 extrapulmonary cases. *Am J Surg Pathol.* 2014;38(4):548–51.

99. Kamionek M, Ahmadi Moghaddam P, Sakhdari A, Kovach AE, Welch M, Meng X et al. Mutually exclusive ERK pathway mutations are present in different stages of multifocal pulmonary Langerhans cell histiocytosis supporting clonal nature of the disease. *Histopathology.* 2016;69(3):499–509.

100. Auerswald U, Barth J, Magnussen H. Value of CD-1-positive cells in bronchoalveolar lavage fluid for the diagnosis of pulmonary histiocytosis X. *Lung.* 1991;169(6):305–9.

101. Takizawa Y, Taniuchi N, Ghazizadeh M, Enomoto T, Sato M, Jin E et al. Bronchoalveolar lavage fluid analysis provides diagnostic information on pulmonary Langerhans cell histiocytosis. *J Nippon Med Sch.* 2009;76(2):84–92.

102. Vassallo R, Ryu JH, Colby TV, Hartman T, Limper AH. Pulmonary Langerhans'-cell histiocytosis. *N Engl J Med.* 2000;342(26):1969–78.

103. Tazi A, de Margerie-Mellon C, Vercellino L, Naccache JM, Fry S, Dominique S et al. Extrathoracic investigation in adult patients with isolated pulmonary Langerhans cell histiocytosis. *Orphanet J Rare Dis.* 2016;11:11.

104. Hansen NJ, Hankins JH. Pulmonary Langerhans cell histiocytosis: PET/CT for initial workup and treatment response evaluation. *Clin Nucl Med.* 2015;40(2):153–5.

105. Chong SG, Samaha M, Samaha G, Casserly B. Rapid resolution of pulmonary Langerhans cell histiocytosis. *BMJ Case Rep.* 2013.

106. Routy B, Hoang J, Gruber J. Pulmonary Langerhans cell histiocytosis with lytic bone involvement in an adult smoker: Regression following smoking cessation. *Case Rep Hematol.* 2015;2015:201536.

107. Tazi A, de Margerie C, Naccache JM, Fry S, Dominique S, Jouneau S et al. The natural history of adult pulmonary Langerhans cell histiocytosis: A prospective multicentre study. *Orphanet J Rare Dis.* 2015;10:30.

108. Grobost V, Khouatra C, Lazor R, Cordier JF, Cottin V. Effectiveness of cladribine therapy in patients with pulmonary Langerhans cell histiocytosis. *Orphanet J Rare Dis.* 2014;9:191.

109. Lorillon G, Bergeron A, Detourmignies L, Jouneau S, Wallaert B, Frija J et al. Cladribine is effective against cystic pulmonary Langerhans cell histiocytosis. *Am J Respir Crit Care Med.* 2012;186(9):930–2.

110. Lazor R, Etienne-Mastroianni B, Khouatra C, Tazi A, Cottin V, Cordier JF. Progressive diffuse pulmonary Langerhans cell histiocytosis improved by cladribine chemotherapy. *Thorax.* 2009;64(3):274–5.

111. Haroche J, Cohen-Aubart F, Emile JF, Arnaud L, Maksud P, Charlotte F et al. Dramatic efficacy of vemurafenib in both multisystemic and refractory Erdheim-Chester disease and Langerhans cell histiocytosis harboring the BRAF V600E mutation. *Blood.* 2013;121(9):1495–500.

112. Le Pavec J, Lorillon G, Jais X, Tcherakian C, Feuillet S, Dorfmuller P et al. Pulmonary Langerhans cell histiocytosis-associated pulmonary hypertension: Clinical characteristics and impact of pulmonary arterial hypertension therapies. *Chest.* 2012;142(5):1150–7.

113. Yoshida T, Konno S, Tsujino I, Sato T, Ohira H, Chen F et al. Severe pulmonary hypertension in adult pulmonary Langerhans cell histiocytosis: The effect of sildenafil as a bridge to lung transplantation. *Intern Med.* 2014;53(17):1985–90.

114. Fukuda Y, Miura S, Fujimi K, Yano M, Nishikawa H, Yanagisawa J et al. Effects of treatment with a combination of cardiac rehabilitation and bosentan in patients with pulmonary Langerhans cell histiocytosis associated with pulmonary hypertension. *Eur J Prev Cardiol.* 2014;21(12):1481–3.

115. Held M, Schnabel P, Warth A, Jany B. Pulmonary hypertension in pulmonary Langerhans cell granulomatosis. *Case Rep Med.* 2012;2012:378467.

116. Iwai K, Mori T, Yamada N, Yamaguchi M, Hosoda Y. Idiopathic pulmonary fibrosis. Epidemiologic approaches to occupational exposure. *Am J Respir Crit Care Med.* 1994;150(3):670–5.

117. Hubbard R, Lewis S, Richards K, Johnston I, Britton J. Occupational exposure to metal or wood dust and aetiology of cryptogenic fibrosing alveolitis. *Lancet.* 1996;347(8997):284–9.

118. Baumgartner KB, Samet JM, Stidley CA, Colby TV, Waldron JA. Cigarette smoking: A risk factor for idiopathic pulmonary fibrosis. *Am J Respir Crit Care Med.* 1997;155(1):242–8.

119. Taskar VS, Coultas DB. Is idiopathic pulmonary fibrosis an environmental disease? *Proc Am Thorac Soc.* 2006;3(4):293–8.

120. Steele MP, Speer MC, Loyd JE, Brown KK, Herron A, Slifer SH et al. Clinical and pathologic features of familial interstitial pneumonia. *Am J Respir Crit Care Med.* 2005;172(9):1146–52.

121. Wiggins J, Strickland B, Turner-Warwick M. Combined cryptogenic fibrosing alveolitis and emphysema: The value of high resolution computed tomography in assessment. *Respir Med.* 1990;84(5):365–9.

122. Cottin V, Cordier JF. The syndrome of combined pulmonary fibrosis and emphysema. *Chest.* 2009;136(1):1–2.

123. Cottin V, Nunes H, Brillet PY, Delaval P, Devouassoux G, Tillie-Leblond I et al. Combined pulmonary fibrosis and emphysema: A distinct underrecognised entity. *Eur Respir J.* 2005;26(4):586–93.

124. Grubstein A, Bendayan D, Schactman I, Cohen M, Shitrit D, Kramer MR. Concomitant upper-lobe bullous emphysema, lower-lobe interstitial fibrosis and pulmonary hypertension in heavy smokers: Report of eight cases and review of the literature. *Respir Med.* 2005;99(8):948–54.

125. Jankowich MD, Polsky M, Klein M, Rounds S. Heterogeneity in combined pulmonary fibrosis and emphysema. *Respiration.* 2008;75(4):411–7.

126. Mejia M, Carrillo G, Rojas-Serrano J, Estrada A, Suarez T, Alonso D et al. Idiopathic pulmonary fibrosis and emphysema: Decreased survival associated with severe pulmonary arterial hypertension. *Chest.* 2009;136(1):10–5.

127. Rogliani P, Mura M, Mattia P, Ferlosio A, Farinelli G, Mariotta S et al. HRCT and histopathological evaluation of fibrosis and tissue destruction in IPF associated with pulmonary emphysema. *Respir Med.* 2008;102(12):1753–61.

128. Kwak N, Park CM, Lee J, Park YS, Lee SM, Yim JJ et al. Lung cancer risk among patients with combined pulmonary fibrosis and emphysema. *Respir Med.* 2014;108(3):524–30.

129. Mimae T, Suzuki K, Tsuboi M, Nagai K, Ikeda N, Mitsudomi T et al. Surgical outcomes of lung cancer in patients with combined pulmonary fibrosis and emphysema. *Ann Surg Oncol.* 2015;22(Suppl 3):S1371–9.

130. Kumagai S, Marumo S, Yamanashi K, Tokuno J, Ueda Y, Shoji T et al. Prognostic significance of combined pulmonary fibrosis and emphysema in patients with resected non-small-cell lung cancer: A retrospective cohort study. *Eur J Cardiothorac Surg.* 2014;46(6):e113–9.

131. Kim YS, Jin GY, Chae KJ, Han YM, Chon SB, Lee YS et al. Visually stratified CT honeycombing as a survival predictor in combined pulmonary fibrosis and emphysema. *Br J Radiol.* 2015;88(1055):20150545.

132. Sugino K, Nakamura Y, Ito T, Isshiki T, Sakamoto S, Homma S. Comparison of clinical characteristics and outcomes between combined pulmonary fibrosis and emphysema associated with usual interstitial pneumonia pattern and non-usual interstitial pneumonia. *Sarcoidosis Vasc Diffuse Lung Dis.* 2015;32(2):129–37.

133. Girard N, Marchand-Adam S, Naccache JM, Borie R, Urban T, Jouneau S et al. Lung cancer in combined pulmonary fibrosis and emphysema: A series of 47 Western patients. *J Thorac Oncol.* 2014;9(8):1162–70.

134. Janz DR, O'Neal HR Jr., Ely EW. Acute eosinophilic pneumonia: A case report and review of the literature. *Crit Care Med.* 2009;37(4):1470–4.

135. Philit F, Etienne-Mastroianni B, Parrot A, Guerin C, Robert D, Cordier JF. Idiopathic acute eosinophilic pneumonia: A study of 22 patients. *Am J Respir Crit Care Med.* 2002;166(9):1235–9.

136. Hayakawa H, Sato A, Toyoshima M, Imokawa S, Taniguchi M. A clinical study of idiopathic eosinophilic pneumonia. *Chest.* 1994;105(5):1462–6.

137. Rom WN, Weiden M, Garcia R, Yie TA, Vathesatogkit P, Tse DB et al. Acute eosinophilic pneumonia in a New York City firefighter exposed to World Trade Center dust. *Am J Respir Crit Care Med.* 2002;166(6):797–800.

138. Oh PI, Balter MS. Cocaine induced eosinophilic lung disease. *Thorax.* 1992;47(6):478–9.

139. Kelly KJ, Ruffing R. Acute eosinophilic pneumonia following intentional inhalation of Scotchguard. *Ann Allergy.* 1993;71(4):358–61.

140. Pope-Harman AL, Davis WB, Allen ED, Christoforidis AJ, Allen JN. Acute eosinophilic pneumonia. A summary of 15 cases and review of the literature. *Medicine (Baltimore).* 1996;75(6):334–42.

141. Uchiyama H, Suda T, Nakamura Y, Shirai M, Gemma H, Shirai T et al. Alterations in smoking habits are associated with acute eosinophilic pneumonia. *Chest.* 2008;133(5):1174–80.

142. Shorr AF, Scoville SL, Cersovsky SB, Shanks GD, Ockenhouse CF, Smoak BL et al. Acute eosinophilic pneumonia among US Military personnel deployed in or near Iraq. *JAMA.* 2004;292(24):2997–3005.

143. Katzenstein AL, Mukhopadhyay S, Zanardi C, Dexter E. Clinically occult interstitial fibrosis in smokers: Classification and significance of a surprisingly common finding in lobectomy specimens. *Hum Pathol.* 2010;41(3):316–25.

144. Mannino DM, Holguin F, Pavlin BI, Ferdinands JM. Risk factors for prevalence of and mortality related to restriction on spirometry: Findings from the First National Health and Nutrition Examination Survey and follow-up. *Int J Tuberc Lung Dis.* 2005;9(6):613–21.

145. Lederer DJ, Enright PL, Kawut SM, Hoffman EA, Hunninghake G, van Beek EJ et al. Cigarette smoking is associated with subclinical parenchymal lung disease: The multi-ethnic study of atherosclerosis (MESA)-lung study. *Am J Respir Crit Care Med.* 2009;180(5):407–14.

146. Washko GR, Lynch DA, Matsuoka S, Ross JC, Umeoka S, Diaz A et al. Identification of early interstitial lung disease in smokers from the COPDGene Study. *Acad Radiol.* 2010;17(1):48–53.

147. Washko GR, Hunninghake GM, Fernandez IE, Nishino M, Okajima Y, Yamashiro T et al. Lung volumes and emphysema in smokers with interstitial lung abnormalities. *N Engl J Med.* 2011;364(10):897–906.

148. Putman RK, Hatabu H, Araki T, Gudmundsson G, Gao W, Nishino M et al. Association between interstitial lung abnormalities and all-cause mortality. *JAMA.* 2016;315(7):672–81.

149. Pusey CD. Anti-glomerular basement membrane disease. *Kidney Int.* 2003;64(4):1535–50.

150. Donaghy M, Rees AJ. Cigarette smoking and lung haemorrhage in glomerulonephritis caused by autoantibodies to glomerular basement membrane. *Lancet.* 1983;2(8364):1390–3.

151. Herody M, Bobrie G, Gouarin C, Grunfeld JP, Noel LH. Anti-GBM disease: Predictive value of clinical, histological and serological data. *Clin Nephrol.* 1993;40(5):249–55.

152. Klasa RJ, Abboud RT, Ballon HS, Grossman L. Goodpasture's syndrome: Recurrence after a five-year remission. Case report and review of the literature. *Am J Med.* 1988;84(4):751–5.

153. Lazor R, Bigay-Game L, Cottin V, Cadranel J, Decaux O, Fellrath JM et al. Alveolar hemorrhage in anti-basement membrane antibody disease: A series of 28 cases. *Medicine (Baltimore).* 2007;86(3):181–93.

154. Levy JB, Lachmann RH, Pusey CD. Recurrent Goodpasture's disease. *Am J Kidney Dis.* 1996;27(4):573–8.

155. De Lassence A, Fleury-Feith J, Escudier E, Beaune J, Bernaudin JF, Cordonnier C. Alveolar hemorrhage. Diagnostic criteria and results in 194 immunocompromised hosts. *Am J Respir Crit Care Med.* 1995; 151(1):157–63.

156. Leaker B, Walker RG, Becker GJ, Kincaid-Smith P. Cigarette smoking and lung haemorrhage in anti-glomerular-basement-membrane nephritis. *Lancet.* 1984;2(8410):1039.

157. Lowry R, Buick B, Riley M. Idiopathic pulmonary haemosiderosis and smoking. *Ulster Med J.* 1993;62(1):116–8.

158. Montana E, Etzel RA, Allan T, Horgan TE, Dearborn DG. Environmental risk factors associated with pediatric idiopathic pulmonary hemorrhage and hemosiderosis in a Cleveland community. *Pediatrics.* 1997;99(1):E5.

159. Scott DL, Wolfe F, Huizinga TW. Rheumatoid arthritis. *Lancet.* 2010;376 (9746):1094–108.

160. Ruiz-Esquide V, Sanmarti R. Tobacco and other environmental risk factors in rheumatoid arthritis. *Reumatol Clin.* 2012;8(6):342–50.

161. Stolt P, Bengtsson C, Nordmark B, Lindblad S, Lundberg I, Klareskog L et al. Quantification of the influence of cigarette smoking on rheumatoid arthritis: Results from a population based case-control study, using incident cases. *Ann Rheum Dis.* 2003;62(9):835–41.

162. Manfredsdottir VF, Vikingsdottir T, Jonsson T, Geirsson AJ, Kjartansson O, Heimisdottir M et al. The effects of tobacco smoking and rheumatoid factor seropositivity on disease activity and joint damage in early rheumatoid arthritis. *Rheumatology (Oxford).* 2006;45(6):734–40.

163. Klareskog L, Stolt P, Lundberg K, Kallberg H, Bengtsson C, Grunewald J et al. A new model for an etiology of rheumatoid arthritis: Smoking may trigger HLA-DR (shared epitope)-restricted immune reactions to autoantigens modified by citrullination. *Arthritis Rheum.* 2006;54(1):38–46.

164. Makrygiannakis D, Hermansson M, Ulfgren AK, Nicholas AP, Zendman AJ, Eklund A et al. Smoking increases peptidylarginine deiminase 2 enzyme expression in human lungs and increases citrullination in BAL cells. *Ann Rheum Dis.* 2008;67(10):1488–92.

165. Olson AL, Swigris JJ, Sprunger DB, Fischer A, Fernandez-Perez ER, Solomon J et al. Rheumatoid arthritis-interstitial lung disease-associated mortality. *Am J Respir Crit Care Med.* 2011;183(3):372–8.

166. Solomon JJ, Brown KK. Rheumatoid arthritis-associated interstitial lung disease. *Open Access Rheumatol.* 2012;4:21–31.

167. Gochuico BR, Avila NA, Chow CK, Novero LJ, Wu HP, Ren P et al. Progressive preclinical interstitial lung disease in rheumatoid arthritis. *Arch Intern Med.* 2008;168(2):159–66.

168. Jurik AG, Davidsen D, Graudal H. Prevalence of pulmonary involvement in rheumatoid arthritis and its relationship to some characteristics of the patients. A radiological and clinical study. *Scand J Rheumatol.* 1982;11(4):217–24.

169. Banks J, Banks C, Cheong B, Umachandran V, Smith AP, Jessop JD et al. An epidemiological and clinical investigation of pulmonary function and respiratory symptoms in patients with rheumatoid arthritis. *Q J Med.* 1992;85(307–308):795–806.

170. Saag KG, Kolluri S, Koehnke RK, Georgou TA, Rachow JW, Hunninghake GW et al. Rheumatoid arthritis lung disease. Determinants of radiographic and physiologic abnormalities. *Arthritis Rheum.* 1996;39(10):1711–9.

18

Drug-induced and iatrogenic interstitial lung disease

PHILIPPE CAMUS AND PHILIPPE BONNIAUD

INTRODUCTION

Therapeutic drugs can specifically injure distinct subsets of the respiratory system including the lung parenchyma, pulmonary vasculature, larynx, tracheobronchial tree, pleural membrane, lymphatics, mediastinum, ventilatory muscles and nerves, chest wall, heart and haemoglobin. This damage can cause a variety of lung diseases including drug-induced interstitial lung disease (DI-ILD), pulmonary embolism, pulmonary hypertension or veno-occlusive disease, obstruction to airflow, asphyxia, pleural effusion, chylothorax, chest pain, respiratory depression, apnoea, chest wall rigidity, lung restriction, acute left ventricular failure, dysrhythmias or methaemoglobinemia, respectively (1).

Any of these clinical patterns may present acutely and can be life threatening (1,2). The suspicion that a drug may be at the origin of a respiratory adverse event (RAE) requires emergency management which includes securing the airway, providing adequate oxygenation and maintaining circulation. Rapid evaluation of drug causality is needed with immediate discussion of drug withdrawal in sight. Despite increasing popularity and recognition of drug-induced RAE, drug incidences are still prevalent with 5% of RAE being fatal, sometimes in otherwise healthy people. Ways to minimize drug incidences include avoiding non-essential exposure to drugs, accurate dosing, a short as possible treatment duration, quick access to updated information (1), compliance with existing guidelines (e.g. with amiodarone, which are largely not followed) (3), careful patient monitoring during treatment with pneumotoxic drugs,

311

early and reliable detection of DI-ILD and prompt stoppage of the drug once DI-ILD is suspected.

Drugs may cause almost any of the known clinical, imaging and pathologic patterns of ILD (1,4,5) including cellular interstitial pneumonia (NSIP-c), eosinophilic pneumonia, pulmonary granulomas, diffuse alveolar damage (DAD) and even rare patterns as Langerhans cell histiocytosis/granulomatosis, pulmonary alveolar proteinosis and desquamative and giant cell interstitial pneumonia (1). In most DI-ILD cases, the lung interstitium is predominantly involved. However, with some drugs or in some patients with severe or pre-existing ILD, alveolar filling with edematous fluid, fresh blood, inflammatory cells or amorphous material can be present (1,6–8). Since workup for the drug aetiology is similar in ILD with or without an alveolar component and because management issues are similar, both interstitial and alveolar drug reactions will be covered in this chapter. A few systemic drug reactions and adverse effects targeting the pulmonary circulation will also be discussed, as they may produce or mimic ILD (9,10).

Drugs account for approximately 90% of all iatrogenic RAE, as opposed to procedures which account for the remainder (1). ILD represents approximately two-thirds of all adverse reactions due to drugs (1). By 1973, 120 drugs had been identified as capable of causing lung injury (11). There were 455 such drugs in 2010 and 1,300 at the time of writing for a total of over 220 distinct patterns of involvement (1). Hence, the field of drug-induced respiratory adverse event (RAE) has become complex and difficult to summarize. Several drug-induced pneumonitides (e.g. amiodarone, bleomycin, cyclophosphamide, methotrexate, nitrosoureas, busulphan, nitrofurantoin, mTOR inhibitors and immune checkpoint inhibitors) have such a distinctive ILD profile on imaging and pathology, that a separate chapter to cover each of them adequately is ideally needed. This chapter will not cover RAE located outside the lung parenchyma such as drug-induced angio-oedema, pleural pathology or pulmonary hypertension (1).

Any route of administration of drugs may expose to the risk of developing ILD including the topical dermatologic, gynaecologic and urologic ones. Classic drugs which have been known for decades to cause ILD include chemotherapy drugs and related agents (bleomycin, cyclophosphamide, methotrexate, nitrosoureas), nitrofurantoin, anti-rheumatic drugs including non-steroidal anti-inflammatory

drugs (NSAIDs), blood transfusions and chest radiation therapy (1). While these agents still cause ILD in a number of patients, not many of them except amiodarone and nitrofurantoin currently reach the stage of publication in top-ranking journals. Thus, there is the risk that some harmful drugs may fall into oblivion and get unnoticed in the clinic. In the past three decades, many novel drugs such as amiodarone, statins, biologic agents including cytokines, small molecular weight agents (e.g. mTOR-, VEGF and EGF-receptor tyrosine kinase inhibitors), pulmonary vasodilators; imatinib, ponatinib, dasatinib, monoclonal antibodies (e.g. antiplatelet agents), TNF-α inhibitors, and ICPI (PD1, PDL1 and CTLA4 inhibitors) (1) have been shown to cause ILD in a significant fraction (3-to-35%) of the patients on the medication (12,13). Thus, examination of the drug aetiology in any ILD case is warranted. Importantly, cigarette or cannabis smoking and electronic nicotine delivery systems may also cause variegated patterns of ILD (1,14,15).

Assessment of drug causality is critical (16) because undue maintenance of the causal drug may lead to progression and further deterioration of the ILD, transition to severe acute respiratory distress syndrome (ARDS) and sometimes death. Conversely, unjustified discontinuation of a critically needed drug may cause the underlying inflammatory or neoplastic condition to progress, flare up or relapse, which can also be life threatening. In addition, once exonerated, retreatment with the drug may fail despite earlier efficacy. Rheumatic and bowel disease-modifying drugs in rheumatoid arthritis and inflammatory bowel disease, respectively, and targeted agents or immune checkpoint inhibitors (ICPI) in neoplastic conditions typify these difficulties. In those patients exposed to more than one drug capable of causing lung damage in concomitance, accurate identification of the causal compound can be challenging. Each drug has to be considered separately as the possible cause for the ILD (1).

Aside from therapeutic drugs, consideration should be given to (1) substances of abuse (17,18), slimming agents including the daunting 2,4-dinitrophenol; hyaluronic acid dermal fillers; sclerosing venous agents; herbal therapy; bone cement; inhaled drugs; inhalants, gases, fumes and vapours; untested, fake, overdosed or counterfeit drugs and chemicals; herbicides; ayurvedic medicine; substances available on the Internet (19); excipients or vehicle, synthol; drugs manufactured in the home which may also cause thermal injury or explosion-related trauma (20); so-called household disinfectants (21); and procedures such as cryoablation for atrial fibrillation (22). Though more difficult to track at history taking especially in the obtunded patient, all the latter substances raise causality issues similar to those of drugs. Information on RAE resulting from exposure to drugs and the aforementioned agents is now available at www.pneumotox.com (Pneumotox), a dedicated website which also addresses drug-induced cardiotoxicity and iatrogenic systemic conditions that may mimic idiopathic disease and manifest with pulmonary infiltrates, pulmonary oedema or diffuse alveolar haemorrhage (1).

DIAGNOSIS OF DRUG-INDUCED ILD

Diagnosis of DI-ILD (16,23) rests on the critical and uncompromising evaluation of the following:

- Current and, if available, pretherapy imaging including HRCT and pulmonary physiology are necessary.
- Timing of exposure to the drug or drugs (drug singularity or singleton is unusual) versus onset/progression of dyspnoea and pulmonary infiltrates with examination of the separate role of each drug should be taken in isolation, e.g. aside from antineoplastic drugs, patients with lung cancer may be exposed to several drugs due to their comorbidities (24). In patients who develop pulmonary infiltrates and pulmonary dysfunction and have received several lines of anti-neoplastic chemotherapy, identification of the culprit drug can prove nearly impossible (25).
- Exclusion of an infection since corticosteroids, anti-metabolites, immunosuppressive drugs, TNF-α inhibitors and rituximab increase the risk of developing pulmonary infections with bacteria, viruses, *Legionella pneumophila*, *Pneumocystis jiroveci*, Mycobacteriae or fungi (26,27). The infectious risk may not be adequately prevented by prophylactic antibiotic therapy (28). Viral pneumonia and DI-ILD may be difficult to separate on imaging (29,30).

- Exclusion of respiratory involvement from the underlying neoplastic or inflammatory-autoimmune condition for which the drug was being given (31), chronic aspiration (32) and idiopathic or incidental ILD (33).
- Adequacy of clinical, imaging, bronchoalveolar lavage (BAL) and pathologic (if available) pattern of involvement with the drug under consideration (1):
  - Clinically, in addition to non-productive cough, dyspnoea, crackles, chest pain, malaise and fever, changes suggestive of exposure to drugs may include concomitant adverse effects from the drug in extra-pulmonary organs (e.g. amiodarone and thyroid or the liver, drug-induced systemic reactions such as drug reaction with eosinophilia and systemic symptoms [DRESS] syndrome or vasculitis), muscle cramps (statins), finger skin burns (crack cocaine), the meth-mouth (methamphetamine) and ecchymotic skin changes in earlobes or elsewhere in the skin (levamisole-cocaine, propylthiouracil) (1).
  - On imaging (34–36), DI-ILD may express itself in the form of ground-glass opacities, alveolar opacification, opacities with a recognizable lobar or segmental anatomical distribution, wandering opacities, fixed consolidation, disseminated micronodules, septal lines, inter- or intra-lobular thickening, tree-in-bud, tree-in-bloom, nodules or masses, bilateral lymphadenopathy and sometimes an associated pleural effusion is present (1). Rarely, ILD presents only subclinically with normal imaging and evidence for ILD on pathology. Underlying emphysema may alter the expression of drug-induced ILD on imaging, a common situation in the patient with amiodarone pulmonary toxicity.
  - A few ILD display imaging features that may immediately suggest the drug aetiology (1). These include
    - Lung densities with high Hounsfield units/attenuation numbers due to iodine fortification of the amiodarone molecule in amiodarone pulmonary toxicity or in amiodarone lung, cement or metallic mercury embolism, barium aspiration, talcosis from drug abuse, and diffuse pulmonary calcification (1)

- Lung densities with low attenuation numbers consistent with exogenous lipoid- or sometimes hydrocarbon pneumonia ('fire eater's lung')
- Distribution of pulmonary opacities within the radiation portals in radiation-induced lung injury and in radiation recall, subpleurally in eosinophilic pneumonia, along the upper pleural surface with wedges encroaching the lung in pleuro-parenchymal fibroelastosis (37,38), or in the form of pleural thickening with associated ILD in ergoline-induced pleuro-pulmonary changes (1,39)
- Fleeting opacities of radiation- and DI organizing pneumonia (1)

- The BAL has a significant contributory role in the workup of most drug-induced ILD (1). The test may disclose a high lymphocyte, eosinophil or neutrophil count which may point to drug-induced cellular or granulomatous interstitial pneumonia, eosinophilic pneumonia or ARDS, respectively (40). Foam cells characterize both exposure to amiodarone and amiodarone pulmonary toxicity (41). The BAL is instrumental in establishing a diagnosis of diffuse alveolar haemorrhage (DAH). In rare cases, lipids at the air–fluid interface at gross examination point to exogenous lipoid pneumonia that may be confirmed with vacuolated lipid-laden macrophages on cytology (1). Importantly, the BAL also helps exclude an infection notably with *Pneumocystis* in the setting of systemic inflammatory conditions or oncology and chronic steroid dosing (27)

- Other laboratory tests include coagulation studies in patients with DAH and anti-nuclear and anti-neutrophil cytoplasmic antibodies (ANCA) when drug-induced *lupus* or ANCA-related vasculitis is suspected with hydralazine, minocycline, propylthiouracil (MPO-ANCA) or levamisole-adulterated cocaine (dual MPO- and PR3-ANCA) (1,9). Other biomarkers include KL6 which, although increased in DI-ILD, is not specific for a drug aetiology and may also increase under the influence of treatment in patients with no demonstrable

adverse effect (42). Other biomarkers examined in a limited number of studies include exhaled nitric oxide in radiation-induced lung injury, NLRP3 inflammasome, TGF-ß, thrombomodulin, IP-10, MCP-1, eotaxin, IL-6, TIMP-1 and HSP42. As regards drug-induced ILD, no biomarker including the suboptimally reliable *in vitro* lymphocyte transformation test (43) has yet gained acceptance.

- NT-proBNP may help separate amiodarone pulmonary toxicity from left ventricular failure, though both conditions may coexist in the same patient. NT-proBNP and troponin are increasingly used in an attempt to detect drug-induced cardiotoxicity at an earlier stage than is possible clinically (44).

- Measurement of serum concentration of drugs, metabolites and chemicals is indicated in suspected adverse reactions from amiodarone, aspirin-, mTOR inhibitors, opioids, 2-4-DNP and paraquat (1).

- Lung pathology (1,4,5,45). Changes in lung tissue are usually considered at best consistent with the diagnosis of drug-induced ILD (46,47). However, open lung biopsy and cryobiopsy are not without risk (48,49). Thus, pathology is seldom indicated to confirm the drug aetiology of ILD except when there is the real need to exclude another aetiology for the ILD. Pathological patterns consistent with the drug aetiology have also to be interpreted against the background of the underlying disease (46). Drug-induced ILD patterns include cellular or fibrotic NSIP, eosinophilic or organizing pneumonia, ILD with a granulomatous component, diffuse alveolar damage, alveolar haemorrhage, a reactive epithelium, pulmonary fibrosis and less often desquamative interstitial pneumonia, lymphoid hyperplasia, giant cell interstitial pneumonia or, when a history of active smoking is present, Langerhans cell histiocytosis or respiratory bronchiolitis-ILD (15,50). Changes which are almost pathognomonic for iatrogenic ILD can be occasionally found and include evidence of amiodarone pulmonary toxicity (45), metallic mercury, silicone, drug excipients, talc, Kayexalate, sevelamer crystals, evidence for pill aspiration and damage, exogenous lipids, calcific deposits, cyanoacrylate, polyacrylamide, cement, food debris or hyaluronic acid (see section XV in [1]). Special stains and x-ray diffractometry may be required to robustly confirm and label changes on microscopy and get to the exact cause (51,52).

- Improvement of signs and symptoms following drug discontinuance. The majority of DI-ILD are at least partly reversible upon drug withdrawal with or without corticosteroid therapy. Care must be taken to minimize the risks of drug withdrawal in terms of relapse of the underlying condition.
- Relapse upon rechallenge with the drug, when available. However, rechallenging patients may lead to fatal relapse of the drug condition; therefore, deliberate rechallenge is not generally recommended. For a few drugs including novel anti-neoplastic drugs, biologics and ICPI, gradual rechallenge can be discussed to induce tolerance, enabling continuation of treatment with a vital drug (53).

EPIDEMIOLOGY OF DRUG-INDUCED ILD

Since 1882, 26,600 papers on iatrogenic RAE have been published (1), representing a significant 0.1% of all literature docked in PubMed. An increase in RAE reports was noted in recent years, owing to the licensing of many novel targeted drugs having ILD and RAE as adverse effects. Evidence for drug causality in the literature is wide ranging, with recent issues concerning low impact factor open-access journals, meta-analyses of suboptimal quality (54), 'big data' (not all of which seem to be fueled or reviewed adequately), heterogenous incidence among different countries for reasons owing to terminology and use of pathology descriptors from radiological data which are notoriously inaccurate (55) and blur the analysis of drug-induced ILD (55). All papers are carefully reviewed before entering Pneumotox (1).

No age range is immune to the development of DI-RAE, from the newborn to the elderly with polypharmacy. Drugs should be a significant consideration in any patient with ILD, accounting for

2%–5% of all ILD cases, 10%–30% of pulmonary infiltrates and eosinophilia (PIE), 10%–14% of ARDS, 11%–18% of alveolar haemorrhage and 28% of organizing pneumonia cases. As for specific drugs, the prevalence of adverse pulmonary reactions is 0.11% for nitrofurantoin, 1.2% for blood transfusions, 1%–6.3% for amiodarone, 8.3% for fludarabine and 11%–15% for bleomycin, depending on which tools are used for diagnosis (signs and symptoms versus imaging and HRCT). Up to 50% incidence has been noted in some experimental chemotherapy regimens, leading to early termination. In-hospital DI-ILD mortality can be as high as 37% (56) and 28% for amiodarone or bleomycin, respectively. Risk factors for developing drug-induced ILD include a younger or an advancing age, being a smoker, combination of chemotherapy drugs and chest radiation or co-administration of high fractional oxygen with pneumotoxic drugs such as amiodarone, bleomycin or chemotherapy.

Ethnicity as a risk factor for DI-ILD has not been convincingly demonstrated. Potential risk factors do include the individual propensity of drugs towards pneumotoxicity, which is highest for bleomycin and amiodarone, drug dosage/schedule, possibly slow – as opposed to bolus – infusion, current renal failure and prior exposure to bleomycin or amiodarone which must be computed and may recall earlier sub-clinical toxicity.

PATTERNS OF IATROGENIC INTERSTITIAL LUNG DISEASE

Drug-induced ILD may present as dense diffuse pulmonary infiltrates and acute respiratory failure requiring emergency management, or in the form of subacute or chronic ILD. Both may mimic idiopathic ILD or ILD of other causes.

DRUG-INDUCED ILD WITH ACUTE RESPIRATORY FAILURE

DI-ILD in the form of pulmonary infiltrates and acute respiratory failure may fit the definition for ARDS, a combination of diffuse pulmonary infiltrates and hypoxemia of mild, moderate or high severity with PaO_2/FIO_2 thresholds of <300, <200 and <100, respectively. Drugs account for 10%–14% of all causes of ARDS. Thus, an accurate drug and smoking history taking is required for any ARDS case in adults (57) and in children (58), particularly when none of the classic contributing factors for ARDS are present (59). Over 200 drugs have been associated with ARDS, the most commonly cited being chemotherapy agents mostly bleomycin, busulphan, and nitrosoureas, amiodarone, crack cocaine, the class of mTOR inhibitors, methotrexate, rituximab, statins, transfusion of blood products and recently ICPI (1). ARDS may develop in conjunction with therapy with the drug or a combination of chemo drugs in the form of diffuse pulmonary opacities, air bronchograms and reduced lung volumes.

Steps for the workup of suspected drug-induced ARDS include the following:

1. Evaluate severity, decision for ICU admission and supportive care.
2. Collect a complete history of exposure to drugs, substances of abuse, chemicals and environmental agents from the patient, relatives or healthcare professionals (list available at [1]).
3. Obtain a laboratory panel including coagulation studies (60), autoantibodies including ANAs and ANCAs (9), salicylate, opiate- and anticoagulant screen (60), keeping in mind that novel street drugs may escape routine detection.
4. Discuss and undertake BAL, a well-founded examination for diagnosing DI-ILD and ruling out other causes including *Pneumocystis* by direct staining, immunofluorescence and nested polymerase chain reaction. In the borderline patient, BAL is best performed in or close to an ICU as mechanical ventilation may be necessary immediately subsequent to the procedure.
5. Discuss and implement drug discontinuance with evaluation of the attending risks.
6. Discuss routine antibiotics, the merit of which remains unclear, and whether corticosteroid therapy, usually intravenous is indicated. Mechanical ventilation may be indicated and an increasing number of acute drug-induced and toxic ILD cases have been placed under extracorporeal membrane oxygenation (ECMO) (19). Overall mortality of drug-induced ARDS is around 20%. On the basis of drug, imaging, laboratory investigation and BAL, drug-induced ARDS can be subsumed into the following.

ACUTE CELLULAR INTERSTITIAL PNEUMONITIS OR NON-SPECIFIC INTERSTITIAL PNEUMONIA

Prototypical drugs include chrysotherapy (now fallen into disfavour), the mTOR inhibitors sirolimus and everolimus, hydroxyurea, ibrutinib, idelalisib, ICPI, imatinib and nilutamide, among a total of over 120 drugs (1). Onset is subacute to rapid. Clinically, the condition is with dry cough, dyspnoea, fever and malaise and it can rapidly and unexpectedly accelerate into an *acme* with acute respiratory failure particularly if the drug is inadvertently continued. Incidence of methotrexate lung, once the most common causal agent for this pattern, seems on the decrease (61). Whether TNF-α inhibitors or leflunomide also induce this pattern is unclear (62,63). On chest imaging, areas of ground-glass, confluence, opacification and consolidation predominate in the lower zones from where they may extend rather than migrate.

HRCT imaging may disclose mosaic attenuation, diffuse haze, ground-glass, micronodules, disseminated inter- and/or intra-lobular septal thickening, crazy-paving and in severe cases a diffuse white-out (34). The BAL in acute cellular interstitial pneumonia may disclose marked lymphocytosis or a mixed pattern of lymphocytes and neutrophils with an admixture of eosinophils (64). Timing into the disease, being on corticosteroid therapy and the presence of underlying rheumatoid lung are likely to influence the cellular pattern in BAL (64). Most patients with acute cellular ILD being hypoxemic, the lung biopsy is not often considered a safe option and the diagnosis is more often suspected than proved once infection has been ruled out (65). The advent of cryobiopsy may change how such patients are approached 66).

Reliable exclusion of *Pneumocystis* or viral pneumonia can be challenging (29,30,67). The notion of an epidemic context especially for *Myxovirus influenzae*, the degree of immunosuppression, timing from cell or organ transplantation, the levels of neutrophils, immunoglobulins and blood CD4$^+$ which can all decrease severely with some drugs (1), cultures of BAL or of fine-needle aspirate and nucleic acid-targeted molecular techniques can be helpful to the diagnosis. Often, patients are given a course of trimethoprim-sulphamethoxazole, antibiotics and anti-viral agents to be removed once an infectious cause has been confidently ruled out, and intravenous corticosteroid therapy pending the results of BAL. Although no randomized study is available and will likely ever be to confirm this, corticosteroids appear efficacious in drug-induced cellular interstitial pneumonia, as drug withdrawal may not suffice. There is no evidence for increased efficacy of the now often quoted bolus doses of 1 g methylprednisolone daily over more conventional 120–240 mg dosages. Duration of treatment with corticosteroids is adjusted to the clinical response with lack of response in a few days prompting investigation for an alternative aetiology.

ACUTE ILD WITH A GRANULOMATOUS COMPONENT IS A VARIANT OF DRUG-INDUCED ACUTE NSIP

The diagnosis of granulomatous ILD requires tissue confirmation. The condition has a mild course except following topical BCG therapy in the urinary bladder and treatments with interferon, methotrexate, etanercept and mTOR inhibitors, the ILD of which can present acutely with respiratory failure and ARDS. It is essential to rule out an infection mainly due to *Mycobacterium bovis* (BCG) or *M. tuberculosis* in patients on BCG therapy, corticosteroids and/or TNF-α antagonists.

ACUTE EOSINOPHILIC PNEUMONIA

Acute eosinophilic pneumonia (AEP) also is quite a distinctive pattern of drug-induced ILD and ARDS (1,68). Patients present with diffuse pulmonary infiltrates, acute respiratory failure, BAL and often peripheral eosinophilia, and bilateral pleural effusion. A parasitic infestation must be carefully ruled out. Several drugs capable of inducing classic eosinophilic pneumonia can also produce AEP (1) particularly if the drug has been inadvertently continued. The drug list includes antibiotics (e.g. daptomycin, minocycline), NSAIDs, tobacco or cannabis smoking and insufflated drugs of abuse (1). In AEP, it is critically important to look for systemic involvement in the form of skin rash, extrapulmonary dysfunction, ANCAs and *herpes virus* reactivation which may point to the possibility of eosinophilic granulomatosis and polyangiitis or to the DRES syndrome (DRESS), respectively (1).

Drug withdrawal is required, but may not suffice. Corticosteroid therapy is effective in AEP and will quickly control all signs and symptoms of the condition. No relapse will take place unless steroids are removed too boldly or the patient re-exposes himself or herself to the causal agent.

DIFFUSE ALVEOLAR DAMAGE

Diffuse alveolar damage (DAD) is a typical pathological diagnosis underlying the clinical-imaging features of ARDS (5). DAD typically complicates treatments with anti-neoplastic drugs, particularly when multiagents are given intravenously (hence the name 'chemotherapy lung'), and associations are made of chemotherapy agents and oxygen or radiation therapy. DAD is a typical feature of exacerbation in idiopathic pulmonary fibrosis (IPF), the former being also a possible complication of drugs. Causal agents include amiodarone, everolimus, nitrofurantoin, salicylate, sertraline, sirolimus and the anti-neoplastic agents bleomycin, bortezomib, busulphan, cetuximab, cyclophosphamide, docetaxel, erlotinib, etoposide, gefitinib, gemcitabine, melphalan, mitomycin C, nitrosoureas, oxaliplatin, paclitaxel and haemotherapy among 220 drugs that can cause this pattern (1). DAD manifests with dyspnoea and hypoxaemia and, on imaging with diffuse haze and/or ground-glass opacification and/or consolidation, low lung volumes (34,36). Additional features on HRCT include inter- or intralobular thickening, ground-glass and in advanced or severe cases diffuse white-out (36). BAL has an exclusionary role for an infection and may disclose an increase in neutrophils and in severe cases, haemosiderin-laden macrophages and reactive epithelial cells can be present (40,69).

The recent fashion of diagnosing DAD on imaging (DAD *sine* pathology) cannot be used as a substitute for actual DAD, otherwise that would be at the expense of semantic accuracy. Not all suspected DAD cases will receive tissue confirmation as lung biopsy has a significant attrition rate in these patients (70). Further, DAD is not specific for the drug aetiology, and DI-DAD has limited therapeutic options beyond corticosteroid therapy. Except with amiodarone, histopathology may not separate drug-induced DAD from DAD of other causes well (46). On pathology in DAD, there is the combination of interstitial oedema, alveolar fibrin, hyaline membranes, resolving organizing alveolar damage, with chemo or radiation a reactive alveolar epithelium, and with amiodarone phospholipidotic changes.

Drug causality assessment is guided by a negative workup for an infection and a definite exposure versus symptom relationship. Overall, mortality in drug-induced DAD can reach 45%. Monitoring patients for the development of incipient or impending DAD from bleomycin may rely on imaging and pulmonary physiology with the diffusing capacity for CO falling by up to 40% without overt toxicity developing. Recently, 18F-PET imaging has been used to detect bleomycin-induced pneumonitis at an early stage (71). A balance between appropriate bleomycin dosage and dose for efficacy and early detection of bleomycin pulmonary toxicity has yet to be defined and agreed upon.

PULMONARY OEDEMA

This pattern of drug-induced injury is suspected when respiratory failure develops quickly to very quickly (sometimes within seconds, then called 'flash pulmonary oedema') following usually intravenous administration of the drug (1,72). Orally administered drugs may also cause pulmonary oedema (73). Drug-induced pulmonary oedema results from abrupt loss of fluid and proteins, and hence the high protein content of oedema fluid, e.g. in severe heroin pulmonary oedema cases, which can be collected in the plume at the mouth. Approximately 200 drugs may cause acute pulmonary oedema (1), including chemo agents, hydrochlorothiazide, gemcitabine, heroin, blood transfusions, intravenous beta-agonists near term, radiocontrast media, stem cell mobilization and several drug overdoses.

With blood transfusion, notification to the office for blood transfusion safety or blood bank is mandatory to possibly identify the antibody-bearing donor in the donor pool, usually a multiparous female, who should be removed from the pool thus preventing the development of further cases (72,74). Severe DI pulmonary oedema can be accompanied by some degree of alveolar haemorrhage (75). There may be a *continuum* from non-cardiac permeability pulmonary oedema to DAD with some patients in the low range of severity

having mild transient and reversible pulmonary infiltrates while others develop full-blown pulmonary oedema and yet others evolve to DAD and ARDS (6). Other drug-induced pulmonary oedema includes acute drug-induced left ventricular failure following therapy with anthracycline, trastuzumab or novel antineoplastic drugs (see sections II and XII in [1]), and pulmonary oedema of the acute vasoconstrictive type following the administration of the vasopressors epinephrine or derivatives (1).

BLAND DIFFUSE ALVEOLAR HAEMORRHAGE

This is a typical adverse reaction from most anticoagulants, antiplatelets, amiodarone, drugs of abuse (cocaine, cannabis, cannabis oil, levamisole), rodenticides of the vitamin K antagonist type, thrombolytic agents and mTOR inhibitors, among 130 specific drugs which can cause diffuse alveolar haemorrhage (DAH) (1). Haemoptysis, an increase in carbon monoxide diffusion and acute anaemia are not completely reliable findings. DAH is diagnosed by BAL, which shows a blood-stained return that is bloodier with subsequent aliquots. Prognosis is guarded as beyond a certain amount of blood or time, clotting in the airways or deep lung may take place impeding clearance of extravasated blood, and respiratory failure can be irreversible. Withdrawal of the anti-coagulant and prompt administration of vitamin K, prothrombin complex, protamine, specific antidote for the new oral anticoagulant or haemodialysis are indicated (60,76). Less often, DAH reflects hydralazine, penicillamine, propylthiouracil, TNF-α antagonist-induced ANCA-related disease and there is the suggestion that a few drugs and inhalants may trigger anti-GBM disease (1). Snorted cocaine in abusers (1,77) and fluid silicone in the context of plastic surgery or following injection by laypeople (10) are notable causes for sometimes severe or fatal DAH.

ACUTE AMIODARONE PULMONARY TOXICITY

Acute amiodarone pulmonary toxicity (APT) and ARDS following cardiothoracic surgery is a classic probably underappreciated complication which can be life threatening. A recent study summarized seven case series comprising 43 acute perioperative

APT cases giving a prevalence of 15% and 10 individual case reports (78). The complication developed mostly in men exposed to amiodarone chronically (up to 8 years) or only perioperatively (shortest time on the drug was 5 days). A history of exposure to high concentrations of oxygen was found in every patient. Onset of symptoms was from 2 hours to 2 weeks postsurgery and mortality rate was approximately 10%. The diagnosis of amiodarone pulmonary toxicity should be entertained in any postoperative ARDS patients with a recent or remote history of exposure to amiodarone. Foam cells can be present in lung despite only a few days on the drug (79,80). Early drug withdrawal and corticosteroid therapy are indicated. There is evidence that some cases are not appropriately labelled, with the risk of continued exposure to the drug and death. Systematic prophylactic amiodarone post-thoracic surgery should be avoided (81).

ACUTE FIBRINOUS AND ORGANIZING PNEUMONIA

Acute fibrinous and organizing pneumonia (AFOP) is defined solely on pathology, hence it is rarely documented, on the basis of fibrin balls in alveolar spaces (82). AFOP may be at the crossroads of organizing alveolar damage and organizing pneumonia. AFOP can be an incidental finding on a lung biopsy, or be diffuse across the lung accounting for diffuse shadowing, the white lung and an ARDS picture. Amiodarone, bleomycin, chemo agents and statins are the currently recorded culprits (1). Corticosteroids are indicated.

ACCELERATED PULMONARY FIBROSIS

This pattern is associated with about 20 drugs and can lead to death within a few weeks, even if no lung involvement was present prior to initiation of the drug (1). TNF-α inhibitors have been recently associated with this pattern in abundant case reports, but the nature of the association of drugs, rheumatoid arthritis, rheumatoid lung and accelerated ILD remains unclear at this time. Recent epidemiologic surveys did not confirm an increase in risk of developing ILD with TNF inhibitors (83) and indicate that overall mortality from ILD has not increased since the advent of this category of drugs (84). Reporting bias cannot be excluded

(62). Acute exacerbation of IPF can follow exposure to amiodarone or chemotherapeutic agents in patients treated for dysrhythmia, lung or colorectal carcinoma (1). Not all such exacerbations will reverse with corticosteroid therapy and patients who survive the episode may be left with severe chronic respiratory failure (see below under 'Drug-induced pulmonary fibrosis').

CHEMICAL PNEUMONITIS

This is a generic term referring to pulmonary infiltrates and in some cases ARDS and fatalities developing after exposure to paraffin, naphtha, kerosene, white spirit, Kerdane, diesel fuel, medicated vapour, chlorinated fumes, organic or metal fumes, fumes of heated mercury, anhydrous ammonia, chlorine (dichlorine), nitrogen dioxide, bromine, perfluorocarbons, household disinfectants, paraquat, waterproofing spray or insecticides (1). Sometimes, chemical pneumonitis occurred in microepidemics or epidemics (21). Corticosteroids have met with success in some cases. Sadly, warfare agents may still cause this sort of damage. Diffuse pulmonary infiltrates, DAH and ARDS have been described following inhalation of vaping drugs, cannabis oil, opiates or incense through shisha or other devices (18). In some, pathology was available (18).

SUBACUTE/CHRONIC INTERSTITIAL LUNG DISEASE

All of the patterns in the previous section (except maybe DAD) may exist in an attenuated form. Subacute ILD has been reported following variable time on the medication in the form of pulmonary infiltrates with a non-specific interstitial pneumonia pathology pattern. Often, however, histopathology is unknown and diagnosis is established on reversal upon stopping the drug (65) with or without corticosteroid therapy. Typical drugs and causal agents include BCG therapy, gold, hydrochlorothiazide, hydroxyurea, ibrutinib, idelalisib, the ICPI ipilimumab, nivolumab and pembrolizumab, infliximab, interferon alpha/beta, leflunomide, lenalidomide, methotrexate, mTOR inhibitors, nilutamide, mesalazine, nilotinib, paraquat, phenytoin, pirfenidone, propylthiouracil, statins, rituximab, sunitinib, TNF-α antagonists, EGFR tyrosine kinase inhibitors or chest radiation therapy, among 270 drugs or agents (1).

Regarding EGFR-TKI a surprising 13-fold increased incidence was reported in Japan compared to the West. BAL discloses lymphocytosis or a mixed pattern (1). Stopping the drug as the sole measure may lead to resolution of the pulmonary opacities. Corticosteroid therapy is not indicated in every patient, depending on drug and severity. Although drug withdrawal in isolation enables better analysis of drug causality, steroid therapy may hasten the healing phase and may enable retreatment with the drug, for instance ICPI, when indicated.

Typical subacute eosinophilic pneumonia is a possible complication of treatments with ACEI, NSAIDs, antibiotics or antidepressants (175 drugs can produce the syndrome) (1). Only half the patients display the characteristic distribution of pulmonary opacities in the upper lung fields subpleurally. Elevated eosinophil counts in blood and BAL can secure the diagnosis, obviating the need for biopsy, which was performed in only 5% of all drug-induced eosinophilic pneumonia cases in the literature. Stopping the drug enables resolution of the condition, which will usually relapse on re-exposure to the drug. Rarely patients on leukotriene receptor antagonists develop eosinophilic granulomatosis and angiitis (formerly known as the Churg–Strauss syndrome) (1). A search for parasitic infiltration is warranted in any patient with eosinophilic pneumonia.

Typical organizing pneumonia (OP) in the form of migratory foci of consolidation, a mass or masses with pathology confirmation has been reported during treatments with amiodarone, bleomycin, antineoplastic chemotherapy, ß-blockers, bleomycin, interferon alpha or beta, mTOR inhibitors, methotrexate, nilutamide, nitrofurantoin, oxaliplatin-based regimens, rituximab, rituximab, statins, trastuzumab and radiation therapy to the breast among 100 causal drugs or agents (1). The recent trend in some countries consisting in defining OP solely on imaging is not fitting the concept that OP should be a pathologically diagnosed condition. In each case, a careful discussion of other possible causes for OP is necessary, including connective tissue disease, inflammatory bowel disease or an infection. Since organizing pneumonia can also occur idiopathically, causality assessment can be challenging. In the typical drug-induced OP patient, pulmonary opacities may relapse despite sequential courses of corticosteroid therapy until the drug is eventually stopped. For those OP cases which relapse once or twice after stopping the drug, causality remains uncertain.

DRUG-INDUCED PULMONARY FIBROSIS

Published international IPF guidelines mention the requirement that 'other known causes of interstitial lung disease (e.g. domestic and occupational environmental exposures, connective tissue disease, and drug toxicity) should be excluded' (85). This statement is a real challenge to the practitioner because many IPF patients receive or have been exposed to a drug or drugs that have been associated with pulmonary fibrosis (1). The topic of drug-induced pulmonary fibrosis can be separated along several lines. There is ample clinical and experimental evidence supporting alkylating agent (bleomycin, BCNU, hydroxyurea, melphalan) nitrofurantoin, and amiodarone-induced pulmonary fibrosis (1). Regarding pathology, amiodarone, azathioprine, flecainide, gefitinib, ifosfamide, melphalan, nitrofurantoin, rituximab and radiation therapy have all been associated with lung fibrosis with honeycombing simulating IPF (1). Amiodarone, bleomycin, busulphan, cocaine, cyclophosphamide, docetaxel, ifosfamide, melphalan, nitrofurantoin, nitrosoureas, paclitaxel, paraffin, paraquat, propythiouracil and radiation therapy have been associated with the fibrotic non-specific interstitial pneumonia, a condition that is without honeycombing (1). Similar to idiopathic desquamative interstitial pneumonia (DIP), nitrofurantoin, tobacco smoking and possibly amiodarone can cause a DIP pattern. DIP can be associated clinically, pathologically and on imaging with pulmonary fibrosis as a complication. IPF patients on amiodarone, nitrofurantoin, statins, antineoplastic chemotherapy or ICPI may deteriorate due to drug-induced ILD superimposed on their underlying IPF. Timely discontinuation of the drug and corticosteroid therapy may confirm that. Adalimumab, amiodarone, bleomycin, certolizumab, antineoplastic chemotherapy, erlotinib, etanercept, the FOLFOX regimen, infliximab, interferon gamma, medroxyprogesterone, methotrexate, mitomycin C, paclitaxel, paraquat, pemetrexed, penicillamine, radiation therapy, infusional 131I or 90Y radioactivity and TNF-α inhibitors have been temporally associated with accelerated sometimes fatal pulmonary fibrosis. Finally, exposure to cyclophosphamide or nitrosoureas has been associated with the development of pleuroparenchymal fibroelastosis (a rare interstitial [pleuro-]-pneumonia) later in life (37,86).

Practically, drug removal in the typical IPF patient rarely produces any measurable changes.

DRUG-INDUCED ILD: SPECIFIC DRUGS

For each of the 1,300 drugs, abused substances, chemicals or procedures of interest, patterns of involvement and references are listed in Pneumotox (1). The following are examples of some of the more important drugs to consider in DI-ILD:

Abused substances (including cocaine and heroin): There has been a steep increase in the number of published cases in recent years. These may cause a multitude of airway and parenchymal problems including thermal injury, eosinophilic pneumonia and ARDS. Patient history taking can be difficult. Exposure should be systematically examined using appropriate drug screen. Novel synthetic opioids can be difficult to detect with routine drug screens.

Alkylating agents busulphan, nitrosoureas: Can cause pulmonary infiltrates, DAD, DAH, ARDS and/or irreversible pulmonary fibrosis. Prognosis is guarded. May explain post-stem cell transplantation pulmonary dysfunction and ILD (25).

Amiodarone: Has been described in 970 papers in the literature since 1976. Thousands of published cases. Comorbidities common. Varied patterns on imaging described (87). Pathology distinctive (45). Guidelines for monitoring patients on the drug exist, but are implemented suboptimally. Drug withdrawal and corticosteroid therapy for a few months are indicated. Shorter duration of corticosteroid therapy may expose to the risk of relapse. When extensive and severe, prognosis of amiodarone pulmonary toxicity is guarded. Post-operative amiodarone pulmonary toxicity may occasion the ARDS picture despite only a few days on the medication (78).

Antibiotics: Prone to causing eosinophilic pneumonia, sometimes severe, notably minocycline and daptomycin (1).

Anti-coagulants: Nearly all have been associated with DAH, sometimes fatal (1). Coagulation studies are indicated. Antidotes and renal replacement therapy may be needed. Watchful monitoring of the literature on antidotes is warranted (88).

Anti-thyroid drugs: May cause ANCA positivity and immune-mediated vasculitis with DAH and glomerulopathy (1).

BCG therapy: Can cause miliary opacities or 'white-out' post-infusion in the urinary bladder (1). Separating infection with *M. bovis* in BCG from hypersensitivity pneumonitis is essential as treatment differs radically.

Bleomycin: Can cause pneumonitis, DAD, ARDS or severe chronic pulmonary fibrosis (dose-related; oxygen may aggravate). Rare eosinophilic pneumonia described. Early detection encouraged, not at the expense of toxicity, though. Corticosteroid therapy may be effective. Transplantation recently described as a rescue.

Catheter ablation for atrial fibrillation: May cause pulmonary vein stenosis with pulmonary infiltrates corresponding to congestion, bleeding and infarction in the lobe or lobes upstream pulmonary vein damage (1).

Cement: Bone cement can embolize in the pulmonary circulation causing chest pain, acute pulmonary hypertension and mimicking ILD (1).

Chemotherapy: Can cause a constellation of RAE, among which several ILD subtypes (1). Disease progression and infection are other diagnostic considerations.

Cocaine: May occasion pulmonary infiltrates, eosinophilic pneumonia, ARDS and airway injury (1).

Daptomycin: Like other antibiotics, prone to inducing eosinophilic pneumonia, sometimes severe (1).

E-cigarette: ILD is a slowly emerging issue (1).

Etanercept: In addition to complications similar to TNF antagonists, may cause granulomatous ILD and/or a sarcoid-like pattern in the chest and/or in extrapulmonary sites (1).

FOLFOX regimen: A significant cause for ILD or ARDS in metastatic colorectal carcinoma patients (1).

Hemato-oncology drugs: ATRA, arsenic trioxide, bortezomib, fludarabine, hydroxyurea, ibrutinib, idelalisib, lenalidomide, thalidomide can all cause ILD or ARDS (1). Infection and underlying disease are significant diagnostic considerations.

Herbal remedies: There are many case reports from Asia and Japan. Causality is often problematic (1).

Immune checkpoint inhibitors (e.g. ipilimumab, nivolumab, pembrolizumab): These are very effective drugs in several solid tumours including melanoma and lung cancer. This category of drugs can cause varied ILD, presumably because of breakage of immune tolerance *vis-à-vis* normal tissues. Depending on severity, drug may have to be suspended and corticosteroid therapy initiated. Re-administration of the drug may not lead to relapse in every patient, thus enabling continued treatment of the underlying neoplastic condition.

Internet: Inhaled or smoked drugs purchased on the Internet can cause acute ILD, eosinophilic pneumonia or ARDS. Should be scrutinized in any patient with unexplained ILD.

mTOR inhibitors: May all cause variegated patterns of ILD including organizing pneumonia, DAD, DAH as well as non-ILD patterns. Prevalence up to 36% of the patient population.

Nitrofurantoin: 350 papers in the literature. Thousands of nitrofurantoin lung toxicity cases since 1962. Early pulmonary reaction is within a few days into treatment with chest pain, blunting of costophrenic angles, fever, dyspnoea and eosinophilia. Resolves upon stopping the drug. Subacute-chronic nitrofurantoin lung follows medium- to long-term treatments with the drug. Resembles pulmonary fibrosis, usually without the presence of honeycombing (89). May improve upon drug withdrawal and with corticosteroid therapy. However, resolution will not occur in every patient, and often is incomplete leaving a pulmonary fibrosis behind (89). OP cases and cases of ILD with autoimmune features (ANA) described with the drug (1).

Oil: Paraffin to combat constipation, lamp oil, lubricating sprays may cause exogenous lipoid pneumonia, a common condition (90). Frustrating when diagnosis is established on a lung biopsy specimen, indicating the condition was not diagnosed at history taking.

Paraquat: Now banned from many Western countries. Still prevalent as a pneumotoxin in the developing world where it can cause ARDS or acute pulmonary fibrosis and death (1).

Rituximab: May cause pulmonary infiltrates of different types and severity including ARDS mostly during treatment of haematologic malignancies. Adds extra-pulmonary toxicity when used on top of that of conventional chemotherapy regimens for lymphoma (1).

Statins: These may cause migratory areas of consolidation consistent with OP, responding to drug stoppage (1).

TNF-alpha antagonists: May expose to the risk of bacterial infections and tuberculosis. Pre-therapy workup and follow-up for latent tuberculosis infection indicated. May occasion acute ILD or lung fibrosis. Other drugs and underlying exacerbation of previously diagnosed rheumatoid ILD should be considered (1).

CONCLUSION

Drugs are a significant diagnostic consideration in ILD, no matter what the pattern and severity of disease. When questions arise at the bedside, Pneumotox should be consulted to check whether the patterns have been described with the given drug and check an updated literature list. The risk associated with drug discontinuance should be taken into account to avoid further domino adverse reactions, and inappropriate change to less well-tolerated drugs to treat the underlying condition.

In drug toxicology, it is essential to investigate whether an antidote is available. Although this is more true in poisonings compared to ILD (91–94) reversal provided by atropine, beta receptor agonists, methylene blue, chelation therapy, protamine, naloxone, vitamin K, factor VIIa, tranexamic acid, lipid therapy/fat emulsion, icatibant, prothrombin complex, the coming specific antidotes for novel anticoagulants (88) and renal replacement therapy should not be overlooked.

REFERENCES

1. Pneumotox II (V2.0). Producer: Ph Camus, 2012. http://www.pneumotox.com. Accessed 1 April 2017. Last update: April 1, 2017.

2. Shanholtz C. Acute life-threatening toxicity of cancer treatment. *Crit Care Clin.* 2001;17:483–502.

3. Camus P, Colby TV, Rosenow ECl. Amiodarone pulmonary toxicity. Drug-induced and iatrogenic lung disease, 2010. Oxford University Press, London, Chapter 23.

4. Myers JL. Diagnosis of drug reactions in the lung. *Monographs Pathol.* 1993;0:32–53.

5. Myers JL, Limper AH, Swensen SJ. Drug-induced lung disease: A pragmatic classification incorporating HRCT appearances. *Semin Respir Crit Care Med.* 2003;24:445–54.

6. Briasoulis E, Pavlidis N. Noncardiogenic pulmonary edema: An unusual and serious complication of anticancer therapy. *Oncologist.* 2001;6:153–61.

7. Gajic O, Gropper MA, Hubmayr RD. Pulmonary edema after transfusion: How to differentiate transfusion-associated circulatory overload from transfusion-related acute lung injury. *Crit Care Med.* 2006;34:S109–13.

8. Lara AR, Schwarz MI. Diffuse alveolar hemorrhage. *Chest.* 2010;137:1164–71.

9. Pendergraft WF 3rd, Niles JL. Trojan horses: Drug culprits associated with antineutrophil cytoplasmic autoantibody (ANCA) vasculitis. *Curr Opin Rheumatol.* 2014;26:42–9.

10. Schmid A, Tzur A, Leshko L, Krieger BP. Silicone embolism syndrome. A case report, review of the literature, and comparison with fat embolism syndrome. *Chest.* 2005;127:2276–81.

11. Stauffer J. Medical Staff Conference: Drug-induced lung disease: The price of progress. *Calif Med.* 1973;119:48–55.

12. Baas MC, Struijk GH, Moes DJ, van den Berk IA, Jonkers RE, de Fijter JW et al. Interstitial pneumonitis caused by everolimus: A case-cohort study in renal transplant recipients. *Transpl Int.* 2014;27:428–36.

13. Nishino M, Ramaiya NH, Awad MM, Sholl LM, Maattala JA, Taibi M et al. PD-1 inhibitor-related pneumonitis in advanced cancer patients: Radiographic patterns and clinical course. *Clin Cancer Res.* 2016;22:6051–60.

14. Walsh SL, Nair A, Desai SR. Interstitial lung disease related to smoking: Imaging considerations. *Curr Opin Pulm Med.* 2015;21:407–16.

15. Franks TJ, Galvin JR. Smoking-related 'interstitial' lung disease. *Arch Pathol Lab Med.* 2015;139:974–977.

16. Naranjo CA, Busto U, Sellers EM, Sandor P, Ruiz I, Roberts EA. A method for estimating the probability of adverse drug reactions. *Clin Pharmacol Ther.* 1981;30:239–45.

17. McMahon MJ, Bhatt NA, Stahlmann CG, Philip AI. Severe pneumonitis after inhalation of butane hash oil. *Ann Am Thorac Soc.* 2016;13:991–2.

18. He T, Oks M, Esposito M, Steinberg H, Makaryus M. Tree-in-Bloom: Severe acute lung injury induced by vaping cannabis oil. *Ann Am Thorac Soc.* 2017;14:468–70.

19. Alhadi S, Tiwari A, Vohra R, Gerona R, Acharya J, Bilello K. High times, low sats: Diffuse pulmonary infiltrates associated with chronic synthetic cannabinoid use. *J Med Toxicol.* 2013;9:199–206.

20. Lineberry TW, Bostwick JM. Methamphetamine abuse: A perfect storm of complications. *Mayo Clin Proc.* 2006;81:77–84.

21. Koo HJ, Do KH, Chae EJ, Kim HJ, Song JS, Jang SJ et al. Humidifier disinfectant-associated lung injury in adults: Prognostic factors in predicting short-term outcome. *Eur Radiol.* 2017;27:203–11.

22. Fender EA, Widmer RJ, Hodge DO, Cooper GM, Monahan KH, Peterson LA et al. Severe pulmonary vein stenosis resulting from ablation for atrial fibrillation: Presentation, management and clinical outcomes. *Circulation.* 2016;134:1812–21.

23. Hill AB. The environment and disease: Association or causation? *Proc Royal Soc Med.* 1965;58:295–300.

24. Leduc C, Antoni D, Charloux A, Falcoz PE, Quoix E. Comorbidities in the management of patients with lung cancer. *Eur Respir J.* 2017;49:pii: 1601721.

25. Scarlata S, Annibali O, Santangelo S, Tomarchio V, Ferraro S, Armiento D et al. Pulmonary complications and survival after autologous stem cell transplantation: Predictive role of pulmonary function and pneumotoxic medications. *Eur Respir J.* 2017;49(3):1601902.

26. Dixon WG, Abrahamowicz M, Beauchamp ME, Ray DW, Bernatsky S, Suissa S, Sylvestre MP. Immediate and delayed impact of oral glucocorticoid therapy on risk of serious infection in older patients with rheumatoid arthritis: A nested case-control analysis. *Ann Rheum Dis.* 2012;71:1128–33.

27. Caplan A, Fett N, Rosenbach M, Werth VP, Micheletti RG. Prevention and management of glucocorticoid-induced side effects: A comprehensive review: Infectious complications and vaccination recommendations. *J Am Acad Dermatol.* 2017;76:191–8.

28. Sichletidis L, Settas L, Spyratos D, Chloros D, Patakas D. Tuberculosis in patients receiving anti-TNF agents despite chemoprophylaxis. *Int J Tuberc Lung Dis.* 2006;10:1127–32.

29. Franquet T. High-resolution computed tomography (HRCT) of lung infections in non-AIDS immunocompromised patients. *Eur Radiol.* 2006;16:707–18.

30. Franquet T. Imaging of pulmonary viral pneumonia. *Radiology.* 2011;260:18–39.

31. Papiris SA, Manali ED, Kolilekas L, Kagouridis K, Maniati M, Filippatos G, Bouros D. Acute respiratory events in connective tissue disorders. *Respiration.* 2016;91:181–201.

32. Hu X, Lee JS, Pianosi PT, Ryu JH. Aspiration-related pulmonary syndromes. *Chest.* 2015;147:815–23.

33. Travis WD, Matsui K, Moss J, Ferrans VJ. Idiopathic nonspecific interstitial pneumonia: Prognostic significance of cellular and fibrosing patterns: Survival comparison with usual interstitial pneumonia and desquamative interstitial pneumonia. *Am J Surg Pathol.* 2000;24:19–33.

34. Rossi SE, Erasmus JJ, McAdams P, Sporn TA, Goodman PC. Pulmonary drug toxicity: Radiologic and pathologic manifestations. *Radiographics.* 2000;5:1245–59.

35. Ellis SJ, Cleverley JR, Müller NL. Drug-induced lung disease: High-resolution CT findings. *Am J Roentgenol.* 2000;175:1019–24.

36. Erasmus JJ, McAdams HP, Rossi SE. Drug-induced lung injury. *Semin Roentgenol.* 2002;37:72–81.

37. Camus P, von der Thusen J, Hansell DM, Colby TV. Pleuroparenchymal fibroelastosis: One more walk on the wild side of drugs? *Eur Respir J.* 2014;44:289–96.

38. Bonifazi M, Montero MA, Renzoni EA. Idiopathic pleuroparenchymal fibroelastosis. *Curr Pulmonol Rep.* 2017;6:9–15.

39. Pfitzenmeyer P, Foucher P, Dennewald G, Chevalon B, Debieuvre D, Bensa P et al. Pleuropulmonary changes induced by ergoline drugs. *Eur Respir J.* 1996;9:1013–9.

40. Costabel U, Uzaslan E, Guzman J. Bronchoalveolar lavage in drug-induced lung disease. *Clin Chest Med.* 2004;25:25–36.

41. Bedrossian CW, Warren CJ, Ohar J, Bhan R. Amiodarone pulmonary toxicity: Cytopathology, ultrastructure, and immunocytochemistry. *Ann Diagnost Pathol.* 1997;1:47–56.

42. Takamura A, Hirata S, Nagasawa H, Kameda H, Seto Y, Atsumi T et al. A retrospective study of serum KL-6 levels during treatment with biological disease-modifying antirheumatic drugs in rheumatoid arthritis patients: A report from the Ad Hoc Committee for Safety of Biological DMARDs of the Japan College of Rheumatology. *Mod Rheumatol.* 2013;23:297–303.

43. Matsuno O, Okubo T, Hiroshige S, Takenaka R, Ono E, Ueno T et al. Drug-induced lymphocyte stimulation test is not useful for the diagnosis of drug-induced pneumonia. *Tohoku J Exp Med.* 2007;212:49–53.

44. Duello KM, Louh IK, Burger CD. 48-Year-old woman with dyspnea, cough, and weight loss. *Mayo Clin Proc.* 2012;87:1124–7.

45. Myers JL, Kennedy JI, Plumb VJ. Amiodarone lung: Pathologic findings in clinically toxic patients. *Hum Pathol.* 1987;18:349–54.

46. Leslie KO, Gruden JF, Parish JM, Scholand MB. Transbronchial biopsy interpretation in the patient with diffuse parenchymal lung disease. *Arch Pathol Lab Med.* 2007;131:407–23.

47. Leslie KO. My approach to interstitial lung disease using clinical, radiological and histopathological patterns. *J Clin Pathol.* 2009;62:387–401.

48. Hutchinson JP, McKeever TM, Fogarty AW, Navaratnam V, Hubbard RB. Surgical lung biopsy for the diagnosis of interstitial lung disease in England: 1997–2008. *Eur Respir J.* 2016;48:1453–61.

49. Bango-Alvarez A, Ariza-Prota M, Torres-Rivas H, Fernandez-Fernandez L, Prieto A, Sanchez I et al. Transbronchial cryobiopsy in interstitial lung disease: Experience in 106 cases – How to do it. *ERJ Open Res.* 2017;3(1):00148-2016.

50. Madan R, Matalon S, Vivero M. Spectrum of smoking-related lung diseases: Imaging review and update. *J Thorac Imaging.* 2015;31:78–91.

51. Croft PR, Racz MI, Bloch JD, Palmer CH. Autopsy confirmation of severe pulmonary interstitial fibrosis secondary to Munchausen syndrome presenting as cystic fibrosis. *J Forensic Sci.* 2005;50:1194–8.

52. Lewin-Smith M, Kalasinsky V, Shilo K, Tomashefski J, Cropp A. Detection of silicone in lung tissue. *Arch Pathol Lab Med.* 2012;136:1179–80.

53. Bonamichi-Santos R, Castells M. Diagnoses and management of drug hypersensitivity and anaphylaxis in cancer and chronic inflammatory diseases: Reactions to taxanes and monoclonal antibodies. *Clin Rev Allergy Immunol.* 2016;22:6870–80.

54. Ioannidis JP. The mass production of redundant, misleading, and conflicted systematic reviews and meta-analyses. *Milbank Q.* 2016;94:485–514.

55. Cleverley JR, Screaton NJ, Hiorns MP, Flint JD, Müller NL. Drug-induced lung disease: High-resolution CT and histological findings. *Clin Radiol.* 2002;57:292–9.

56. Mankikian J, Favelle O, Guillon A, Guilleminault L, Cormier B, Jonville-Bera AP et al. Initial characteristics and outcome of hospitalized patients with amiodarone pulmonary toxicity. *Respir Med.* 2014;108:638–46.

57. Dhokarh R, Li G, Schmickl CN, Kashyap R, Assudani J, Limper AH, Gajic O. Drug associated acute lung injury: A population based cohort study. *Chest.* 2012;142:845–50.

58. Yanagisawa R, Takeuchi K, Kurata T, Sakashita K, Shimodaira S, Ishii E. Transfusion-related acute lung injury in an infant. *Pediatr Int.* 2016;58:543–4.

59. Gibelin A, Parrot A, Maitre B, Brun-Buisson C, Mekontso Dessap A, Fartoukh M, de Prost N. Acute respiratory distress syndrome mimickers lacking common risk factors of the Berlin definition. *Intensive Care Med.* 2016;42:164–72.

60. Samuelson BT, Cuker A, Siegal DM, Crowther M, Garcia DA. Laboratory assessment of the anticoagulant activity of direct oral anticoagulants (DOACs): A systematic review. *Chest.* 2017;151:127–38.

61. Conway R, Carey JJ. Methotrexate and lung disease in rheumatoid arthritis. *Panminerva Med.* 2017;59:33–46.

62. Dixon WG, Hyrich KL, Watson KD, Lunt M, Symmons DP. Influence of anti-TNF therapy on mortality in patients with rheumatoid arthritis-associated interstitial lung disease: Results from the British Society for Rheumatology Biologics Register. *Ann Rheum Dis.* 2010;69:1086–91.

63. Conway R, Low C, Coughlan RJ, O'Donnell MJ, Carey JJ. Leflunomide use and risk of lung disease in rheumatoid arthritis: A systematic literature review and meta-analysis of randomized controlled trials. *J Rheumatol.* 2016;43:855–60.

64. D'Elia T. Methotrexate-induced pneumonitis: Heterogeneity of bronchoalveolar lavage and differences between cancer and rheumatoid arthritis. *Inflamm Allergy Drug Targets.* 2014;13:25–33.

65. Greenberg A, Stammers K, Moonsie I, Jose RJ. Image of the month: All puffed out – A case of crack lung. *Clin Med (Lond).* 2017;17:186–7.

66. Colby TV, Tomassetti S, Cavazza A, Dubini A, Poletti V. Transbronchial cryobiopsy in diffuse lung disease: Update for the pathologist. *Arch Pathol Lab Med.* 2017;141(7):891–900.

67. Franquet T, Muller NL, Gimenez A, Guembe P, de La Torre J, Bague S. Spectrum of pulmonary aspergillosis: Histologic, clinical, and radiologic findings. *Radiographics.* 2001;21:825–37.

68. De Giacomi F, Decker PA, Vassallo R, Ryu JH. Acute eosinophilic pneumonia: Correlation of clinical characteristics with underlying cause. *Chest.* 2017;152(2):379–385.

69. Maldonado F, Patel RR, Iyer VN, Yi ES, Ryu JH. Are respiratory complications common causes of death in inflammatory myopathies? An autopsy study. *Respirology.* 2012;17:455–60.

70. Palakshappa JA, Meyer NJ. Which patients with ARDS benefit from lung biopsy? *Chest.* 2015;148:1073–82.

71. Falay O, Ozturk E, Bolukbasi Y, Gumus T, Ornek S, Ozbalak M et al. Use of fluorodeoxyglucose positron emission tomography for diagnosis of bleomycin-induced pneumonitis in Hodgkin lymphoma. *Leuk Lymphoma.* 2017;58:1114–22.

72. Alvarez P, Carrasco R, Romero-Dapueto C, Castillo RL. Transfusion-related acute lung injured (TRALI): Current concepts. *Open Respir Med J.* 2015;9:92–6.

73. Glisson JK, Vesa TS, Bowling MR. Current management of salicylate-induced pulmonary edema. *South Med J.* 2011;104:225–32.

74. Kopko PM, Marshall CS, MacKenzie MR, Holland PV, Popovsky MA. Transfusion-related acute lung injury. Report of a clinical look-back investigation. *JAMA.* 2002;287:1968–71.

75. Maldonado F, Parambil JG, Yi ES, Decker PA, Ryu JH. Haemosiderin-laden macrophages in the bronchoalveolar lavage fluid of patients with diffuse alveolar damage. *Eur Respir J.* 2009;33:1361–6.

76. Davis EM, Uhlmeyer EM, Schmidt DP, Schardt GL. Strategies for urgent reversal of target-specific oral anticoagulants. *Hosp Pract (1995).* 2014;42:105–25.

77. Dushay KM, Evans SK, Ghimire S, Liu J. Cocaine-induced diffuse alveolar hemorrhage: A case report and review of the literature. *R I Med J (2013).* 2016;99:34–6.

78. Teerakanok J, Tantrachoti P, Chariyawong P, Nugent K. Acute amiodarone pulmonary toxicity after surgical procedures. *Am J Med Sci.* 2016;352:646–51.

79. Kharabsheh S, Abendroth CS, Kozak M. Fatal pulmonary toxicity occurring within two weeks of initiation of amiodarone. *Am J Cardiol.* 2002;89:896–8.

80. Argyriou M, Hountis P, Antonopoulos N, Mathioudaki M. Acute fatal post-CABG low dose amiodarone lung toxicity. *Asian Cardiovasc Thorac Ann.* 2007;15:e66–8.

81. van Mieghem W, Coolen L, Malysse I, Lacquet LM, Deneffe GJD, Demedts MGP. Amiodarone and the development of ARDS after lung surgery. *Chest.* 1994;105:1642–5.

82. Beasley MB, Franks TJ, Galvin JR, Gochuico B, Travis WD. Acute fibrinous and organizing pneumonia. A histologic pattern of lung injury and possible variant of diffuse alveolar damage. *Arch Pathol Lab Med.* 2002;126:1064–70.

83. Herrinton LJ, Harrold LR, Liu L, Raebel MA, Taharka A, Winthrop KL et al. Association between anti-TNF-alpha therapy and interstitial lung disease. *Pharmacoepidemiol Drug Saf.* 2013;22:394–402.

84. Bongartz T, Nannini C, Medina-Velasquez YF, Achenbach SJ, Crowson CS, Ryu JH et al. Incidence and mortality of interstitial lung disease in rheumatoid arthritis: A population based study. *Arthritis Rheum.* 2010;62:1583–91.

85. Raghu G, Rochwerg B, Zhang Y, Garcia CA, Azuma A, Behr J et al. An official ATS/ERS/JRS/ALAT clinical practice guideline: Treatment of idiopathic pulmonary fibrosis. An Update of the 2011 Clinical Practice Guideline. *Am J Respir Crit Care Med.* 2015;192:e3–19.

86. Travis WD, Costabel U, Hansell DM, King TE Jr., Lynch DA, Nicholson AG et al. An official American Thoracic Society/European Respiratory Society statement: Update of the international multidisciplinary classification of the idiopathic interstitial pneumonias. *Am J Respir Crit Care Med.* 2013;188:733–48.

87. Van Cott TE, Yehle KS, Decrane SK, Thorlton JR. Amiodarone-induced pulmonary toxicity: Case study with syndrome analysis. *Heart Lung.* 2013;42:262–6.

88. Christos S, Naples R. Anticoagulation reversal and treatment strategies in major bleeding: Update 2016. *West J Emerg Med.* 2016;17:264–70.

89. Mendez JL, Nadrous HF, Hartman TE, Ryu JH. Chronic nitrofurantoin-induced lung disease. *Mayo Clin Proc.* 2005;80:1298–302.

90. Gondouin A, Manzoni P, Ranfaing E, Brun J, Cadranel J, Sadoun D et al. Exogenous lipid pneumonia: A retrospective multicentre study of 44 cases in France. *Eur Respir J.* 1996;9:1463–9.

91. White ML, Liebelt EL. Update on antidotes for pediatric poisoning. *Pediatr Emerg Care.* 2006;22:740–6.

92. Brooks DE, Levine M, O'Connor AD, French RN, Curry SC. Toxicology in the ICU: Part 2: Specific toxins. *Chest.* 2011;140:1072–85.

93. Levine M, Brooks DE, Truitt CA, Wolk BJ, Boyer EW, Ruha AM. Toxicology in the ICU: Part 1: General overview and approach to treatment. *Chest.* 2011;140:795–806.

94. Levine M, Ruha AM, Graeme K, Brooks DE, Canning J, Curry SC. Toxicology in the ICU: Part 3: Natural toxins. *Chest.* 2011;140:1357–1370.

19

Occupation-related ILD

TRACI ADAMS, ANNYCE S MAYER, CRAIG GLAZER AND LISA A MAIER

BACKGROUND

Numerous interstitial lung diseases (ILDs) are caused by exposure to agents in the workplace, termed here 'occupational ILDs' (Occ-ILDs). Occ-ILDs have similar clinical, radiographic and pathologic presentations as non-occupational ILDs (Table 19.1) (1). Distinguishing Occ-ILDs from non-occupational ILDs is important for several reasons. First, the Occ-ILDs are common, as discussed below (2,3). Additionally, the prognosis from Occ-ILD is different from that of the idiopathic interstitial pneumonias (IIPs). For example, both asbestosis and idiopathic pulmonary fibrosis (IPF) are characterized by a usual interstitial pneumonia (UIP) pattern on pathology, but the prognosis for asbestosis is far better (1). Finally, a diagnosis of Occ-ILD has implications for treatment and prevention. Minimizing or eliminating

exposure is a cornerstone of treatment of Occ-ILDs (4,5). Identification of an Occ-ILD also presents an opportunity for primary and secondary disease prevention among exposed co-workers and has implications for future employment of the patient as well as eligibility for compensation programmes (6,7).

A comprehensive review of Occ-ILDs is outside the scope of this clinically focused chapter. We review the clinical scenarios that should raise suspicion for Occ-ILD as well as the clinical, radiographic and pathologic features of the major causes of Occ-ILD, particularly asbestosis, silicosis, coal workers' pneumoconiosis (CWP) and chronic beryllium disease (CBD) (Table 19.2). Hypersensitivity pneumonitis (HP), a common Occ-ILD caused by exposure to bioaerosols and certain reactive chemicals, is covered in Chapter 11.

Table 19.1 Lung responses to injury

Pathologic pattern	Potential occupational causes of the pattern	Remaining differential
Usual interstitial pneumonia (UIP)	Asbestos, uranium mining, plutonium, mixed dust	IPF, Hermansky–Pudlak, chronic HP, familial IPF, medications, CTD
Non-specific interstitial pneumonia (NSIP)	Organic antigens	CTD, idiopathic NSIP, medication, infection, immunodeficiency
Desquamative interstitial pneumonitis (DIP)	Textile work, aluminium welding, inorganic particulates	Smoking-related, medications, CTD
Giant cell interstitial pneumonitis (GIP)	Hard metal lung disease	Idiopathic (rare), nitrofurantoin
Diffuse alveolar damage (DAD)	Irritant inhalational injury – NOx, SOx, cadmium, beryllium, chlorine, acid mists	Acute respiratory distress syndrome, acute interstitial pneumonia, CTD
Alveolar proteinosis	High-level silica exposure, aluminium dust, indium tin oxide (ITO), indium oxide and indium zinc oxide	Auto-immune, congenital, infection, malignancy, immunodeficiency particularly after bone marrow transplantation, medication
Organizing pneumonia (OP)	Spray-painting textiles – acramin-FWN; NOx; titanium dioxide nanoparticles	Cryptogenic, infection, radiation, medications, CTD, organizing DAD
Granulomatous lung disease	Beryllium, organic antigens, zirconium, aluminium, titanium, copper sulphate	Sarcoidosis, mycobacterial and fungal infections

Source: Data from Beckett WS. *N Engl J Med.* 2000;342:406–13; Coultas DB et al. *Am J Respir Crit Care Med.* 1994;150:967–72; Thomeer MJ et al. *Eur Respir J Suppl.* 2001;32:114s–8s; US Department of Health and Human Services. *Health Effects of Occupational Exposure to Respirable Crystalline Silica.* Cincinnati, OH: Department of Health and Human Services, National Institute for Occupational Safety and Health, Centers for Disease Control and Prevention; 2002; Becklake MR. *Chest.* 1991;100:248–54; Rutstein DD. *Arch Environ Health.* 1984;39:158.

SCIENTIFIC MECHANISMS

The pathogenesis of the Occ-ILDs varies by the type of exposure. Some exposures can provoke a non-specific inflammatory response; others can provoke an adaptive immune response (8). This difference in pathogenesis leads to several clinical features:

1. *Occ-ILDs due to a non-specific inflammatory response*: For some Occ-ILDs, particularly the classic pneumoconioses (asbestosis, silicosis and CWP), an injury that results in fibrosis occurs through a non-specific inflammatory response. Lung injury depends on both cumulative dose and the exposure's fibrogenic potential. These exposures cause lung injury via activation of the Nalp3 inflammasome following phagocytosis

of inhaled particles, which activates caspase-1, leading to the production of mature IL-1β (9). Persistent inflammation causes injury of type I epithelial cells and eventually fibrosis. Properties of the exposure effecting the toxicity include the size, solubility and charge; for fibres, the dimensions are also important (10,11). These Occ-ILDs have a linear dose–response relationship. Clinically this means that cumulative exposure is the most important determinant of disease progression (8,12).

2. *Occ-ILDs with immune sensitization*: Some exposures such as beryllium, cobalt and exposures that lead to HP depend more on the host adaptive immune response than on cumulative exposure. The most important determinant of disease for these exposures is whether a particular host activates an adaptive immune

Table 19.2 Characteristics that should increase suspicion for Occ-ILD

History	Exposure to agents known to cause Occ-ILD
	Productive cough (silicosis and CWP)
	Constitutional symptoms (CBD)
	Multiorgan involvement (CBD)
	No obvious cause of ILD
Physical exam	Raised subcutaneous nodules (CBD)
Pulmonary function testing	Obstructive or mixed pattern
Laboratory results	Positive BeLPT
	Asbestos bodies in sputum
Imaging	Slow progression on serial imaging
	Multicompartment involvement
	Upper lung zone predominance
Pathology	Foreign body identified on path such as silicotic nodules
Progression	Progression over decades

Source: Data from Beckett WS. N Engl J Med. 2000; 342:406–13.

response to the inhaled antigen, termed 'sensitization'; sensitized patients can progress to active inflammation and pulmonary fibrosis (13). Several factors influence which individuals are most likely to become sensitized. Some HLA haplotypes, such as HLA-DPB1 with a glutamic acid at position 69 of the β-chain, can facilitate the presentation of beryllium to T cells, which increases the hosts' probability of becoming sensitized to beryllium (BeS) (14). Because these Occ-ILDs depend on the host adaptive immune response, the dose–response relationship is not linear and even small doses can cause disease (15–17).

EPIDEMIOLOGY

The epidemiology of Occ-ILDs remains poorly characterized due to non-standardized diagnostic criteria, variable physician awareness, long latency period of many agents, limited large data sources

(e.g. from death certificates) and lack of standardized reporting (1). Despite these limitations, population-based studies and registries have demonstrated that occupational and environmental exposures are a common cause of ILD. One population-based study found that 14% of prevalent and 12% of incident cases of ILD were Occ-ILD (2). In European registries, Occ-ILD accounts for 4%–18% of prevalent and 13%–19% of incident cases of ILD (1,3). By comparison, these studies show 2%–13% of ILDs are caused by connective tissue disease (2,3).

Several studies have evaluated the prevalence of Occ-ILD among conditions labelled as an IIP. In one series, 25% of the biopsies referred for IPF were actually Occ-ILD (18). In another series, 40% of patients with a diagnosis of sarcoidosis were reclassified as CBD after evaluation with a BeLPT (19). From these data, it is clear that a significant percentage of ILDs is caused by exposure. In addition, some IIPs, such as IPF and sarcoidosis, may be exposure related, although studies are preliminary and associative and beyond the scope of this chapter.

HISTORY AND EXAMINATION

Given the prevalence of Occ-ILD, occupational causes should be considered in any patient presenting with ILD. This is particularly important when there is no obvious cause and before defining a disease as idiopathic (Table 19.2). The key to diagnosing an Occ-ILD is a thorough occupational history (Table 19.3).

Previously published questionnaires can also assist with obtaining a complete occupational history (1,20). A thorough occupational history allows clinicians to detect and quantify the amount of exposure and estimate the latency period, defined as the time between onset of exposure and disease (1,20,21). Common exposures associated with Occ-ILDs are described in Table 19.4, and additional features of the history and physical examination for the major Occ-ILDs are described below.

It is important to note that identification of an exposure is not sufficient to diagnosis an Occ-ILD. Additional investigations are needed to confirm the diagnosis and exclude other causes, including infection, connective tissue disease-associated ILD (CTD-ILD), vasculitis, and drug reactions.

Table 19.3 Components of a detailed occupational and environmental history

Work history outline	Work details for each job	Exposure for each job	Bystander exposure for each job and/or at home
Chronological list of all jobs	1. Employer 2. Job title 3. Years worked 4. Actual job tasks/activities 5. Any coworkers with similar symptoms or disease?	1. Job tasks/activities that caused vapours, dust, gas or fumes to be liberated into the air and/or settle on surfaces 2. If yes, was it visible? 3. Presence/absence of controls, e.g. enclosures, local exhaust ventilation, general ventilation, respiratory protection 4. Clean-up activities, e.g. compressed air, wet or dry methods 5. Temporal symptoms	1. Exposure estimate from the job tasks and activities performed around them by other workers 2. Were work clothes brought home to be laundered (spousal exposure) 3. Water damage, mould, high humidity, birds, hot tubs, humidifiers, standing and spraying water

Source: Data from Beckett WS. *N Engl J Med.* 2000;342:406–13; Registry AfTSaD. *Taking an Exposure History: Case Studies in Environmental Medicine.* Washington, DC: US Department of Health and Human Services; 2000; Burge P. *Occupational Disorders of the Lung.* Philadelphia, PA: WB Saunders; 2002:25–32.

1. *Occ-ILDs due to a non-specific inflammatory response*: Occ-ILDs due to a non-specific inflammatory response all feature long latency, with clinical disease appearing 10–40 years after exposure, although acute or accelerated disease can occur with heavy exposures (4,12). The presence of constitutional symptoms is rare, and if present this should raise concern for tuberculosis or malignancy. Disease progression is slow, and pulmonary symptoms do not worsen acutely with exposure to the agent or improve with exposure removal (1).

   Asbestosis: Patients with asbestosis typically present with slowly progressive dyspnoea on exertion, but cough is uncommon (22). Physician examination often reveals bibasilar dry crackles and clubbing, and in advanced disease cor pulmonale may occur (1). Suspicion should be particularly high among workers in at-risk industries (Table 19.4). The classic teaching is that at least 25 fibers/mL/year of exposure is required to develop asbestosis, although recent studies have demonstrated disease in some workers with lower cumulative exposure (10,23). Due to the dose–response relationship of asbestosis, the latency period is typically 10–40 years (12). Asbestosis is commonly associated with pleural plaques and/or pleural thickening and UIP on computed tomography (CT) in the presence of plaques should prompt the physician to question the patient for an exposure.

   Silicosis and CWP: Like asbestosis, patients with silicosis and CWP present with slowly progressive dyspnoea on exertion and bibasilar dry crackles on physical examination in workers in at-risk industries (Table 19.4) (1). Unlike asbestos, both silica and coal also cause chronic obstructive pulmonary disease so cough is much more common and can be either dry or productive (24). The latency period for simple silicosis and CWP is 10–40 years. Higher levels of silica exposure can lead to accelerated silicosis with a latency period of 5–10 years, and very high levels of exposure can lead to acute silicoproteinosis within a few months (4,24).

2. *Occ-ILDs with immune sensitization*: In this group, disease development depends on the development of an adaptive immune response and not cumulative exposure. As a result, the latency period can vary from as short as 2 months to as long as 40 years, and the disease

Table 19.4 Examples of workplaces with dust and fumes and specific exposures that can cause Occ-ILDs

Workplaces with dust and fumes	Specific exposure(s) causing Occ-ILD
Mining	Silica, coal dust, asbestos (vermiculite), talc
Foundry	Silica, mixed dust
Nuclear weapons/defense industry	Beryllium, zirconium, titanium
Aerospace	Beryllium, titanium
Dental prosthesis fabrication	Beryllium
Metal recycling	Beryllium, others
Electronics	Beryllium
Welding	Aluminium, iron[a]
Aluminium smelter, particularly pot room work	Beryllium (if present in the bauxite)
Hard metal production, grinding, diamond polishing	Cobalt-hard substance
Construction trades – sheet metal workers, insulators, shipbuilding and repair, work around others who were spraying or cutting asbestos	Asbestos
Boiler makers	Asbestos
Tin and barium production	Tin[a] and barium[a]
Organic antigens: mould/water damage, birds, hay, hot tubs and other standing or spraying water, decaying organic matter, musical instruments, bark stripping, etc.	Bioaerosols associated with HP
Isocyanates, epoxies, phthalic anhydride, etc.	Reactive chemicals associated with HP
World Trade Center	Unknown antigen, increased risk sarcoidosis, other unknown ILDs
Flat panel television manufacture	Indium-tin oxide
Military service	Asbestos (World War II–era ships and buildings), chipping aircraft carrier antiskid material (sarcoidosis), beryllium, Middle East deployment
High-level irritant exposures	NOx, SOx, ozone, beryllium, phosgene, certain thermal decomposition products, poorly water-soluble acid mists
Butter scents and flavorings	Diacetyl, 2,3 pentanedione

Source: Data from Beckett WS. N Engl J Med. 2000;342:406–13; Samuel G, Maier LA. Curr Opin Allergy Clin Immunol. 2008;8:126–34; Balmes JR, et al. Am J Resp Crit Care Med. 2014;190:e34–59; American Thoracic Society. Am J Resp Crit Care Med. 2004;170:691–715; Akira M, Morinaga K. Am J Ind Med. 2016;379:2008–18; Mayer A, Hamzeh N. Curr Opin Pulm Med. 2015;21:178–84.

[a] Siderosis (iron), stanosis (tin), baratosis (barium) are considered benign pneumoconioses.

can occur in patients with minimal apparent exposure (15–17). Furthermore, these Occ-ILDs may present with constitutional symptoms and occasionally multiorgan involvement, and symptoms may worsen acutely with antigen exposure and improve with antigen avoidance, although this is more typical for HP than CBD (1).

Chronic Beryllium Disease: In addition to pulmonary findings of bibasilar crackles, physical examination in CBD may reveal raised subcutaneous nodules in exposed skin surfaces resulting from penetration of beryllium dust through the skin (1). Industries associated with beryllium exposure are described in Table 19.4, but direct work with beryllium or its alloys is not required, as cases have been reported in security guards, short-term contract workers and others with bystander or dust-disturbing jobs with very low levels of exposure (1,25). Constitutional symptoms do occur and cough is frequently the initial pulmonary symptom.

INVESTIGATIONS

After taking a thorough occupational history, evaluation for Occ-ILD is similar to that of non-occupational ILD and includes laboratory testing, pulmonary function testing (PFT) and imaging (1).

PULMONARY FUNCTION TESTING

The presence of obstruction on PFTs in a non-smoking patient with ILD should increase suspicion for Occ-ILD (Table 19.2). Obstruction or mixed patterns can occur in Occ-ILD with various exposures, including silicosis, CWP, and CBD, but are uncommon in non-occupational variants with the exception of sarcoidosis or constrictive bronchiolitis (1,15,26). Restrictive PFTs and a reduction in diffusing capacity are common in advanced Occ-ILDs (1).

LABORATORY INVESTIGATIONS

In general, laboratory testing is not particularly helpful in the diagnosis of Occ-ILDs, other than for exclusion of other ILDs, such as CT-ILDs, infection and vasculitis (1). A notable exception is the beryllium lymphocyte proliferation test (BeLPT), which measures the delayed-type hypersensitivity response to beryllium. The test is performed on lymphocytes collected from either blood or bronchoalveolar lavage (BAL). Briefly, mononuclear cells are isolated and cultured with and without beryllium sulphate. The proliferative response is assessed by measuring the stimulation index, or the uptake of radiolabeled DNA precursors in the cells cultured with beryllium compared to those without. BeS is confirmed if a patient has two abnormal BeLPT, one abnormal and one borderline or three borderline BeLPTs. These criteria for BeS provide a sensitivity of 88% and a specificity of 96% (27). If a BeLPT is negative but suspicion remains high, BAL cells can be sent for BeLPT testing and a single

positive on BAL is considered adequate evidence for sensitization. A positive BeLPT supports a diagnosis of BeS, but does not demonstrate whether the sensitized individual has CBD (27).

Laboratory testing may be helpful to assess occupational exposure to asbestos if an occupational history is difficult to obtain (28). The presence of more than one asbestos body per millilitre of BAL measured by light microscopy in a qualified laboratory can identify patients with a high probability of exposure to asbestos dust (28).

RADIOLOGY

The high-resolution CT scan (HRCT) is a crucial part of the evaluation of occupational ILDs as in non-occupational disease. Chest radiographs interpreted according to International Labor Organization (ILO) guidelines may be useful for some compensation programmes and for assessment of Occ-ILD for workplace surveillance programmes.

The radiographic appearance of Occ-ILD overlaps with that of other types of ILD (Table 19.5).

Imaging features that should increase suspicion for an Occ-ILD include slow progression on serial imaging, upper lung zone predominance and multicompartment involvement, such as interstitial disease with either pleural or bronchiolar involvement (Table 19.2) (1).

Asbestosis

Asbestosis can present with imaging findings consistent with IPF, including thickened intralobular septal lines and intralobular core structures, honeycombing and basilar and subpleural predominance. HRCT findings that suggest a diagnosis of asbestosis rather than IPF include subpleural curvilinear lines that persist on prone imaging, subpleural dot-like opacities, parenchymal bands and pleural disease (29,30). Small studies show that 90% of patients with asbestosis will have pleural disease including pleural plaques on CT; however, the absence of pleural disease on HRCT or chest radiograph does not exclude asbestosis (1,29,31).

Silicosis and CWP

Silicosis and CWP present with upper lung zone predominant well-circumscribed nodules measuring less than 5 mm in diameter with a posterior and

Table 19.5 Radiographic and pathologic characteristics of Occ-ILDs

Occ-ILD	Exposure scenarios	Radiographic pattern	Pathologic pattern
Lower Lung Zone Predominant			
Asbestosis	Construction trades, building maintenance, mining, milling, production of asbestos products, shipbuilding and repair, automobile and railroad work, electrical wire insulation, as a contaminant in talc and vermiculite	Interlobular septal thickening, honeycombing, curvilinear subpleural lines, subpleural nodules, parenchymal bands; pleural disease in 90%	UIP
Palygorskites (attapulgite and sepiolite)	Fuller's earth, paint thickeners, drilling mud, asbestos substitute	Interlobular septal thickening	
Wollastonite	Mining and milling, asbestos substitute, ceramics	Interlobular septal thickening; may have associated pleural plaques	Mild fibrosis
Zeolites	Environmental exposure	Interlobular septal thickening; may have associated pleural plaques	Fibrosis; fibrous alveolitis
Kaolin	Kaolin mining, paper product manufacture, ceramics, refractory materials, ceramics, plastics	Mid-lower zone predominant with multiple nodules or masses; progressive massive fibrosis may occur; associated pleural disease is reported	Fibrosis; accumulation of inflammatory cells mostly macrophages, and epithelioid cells around fibre deposits
Rare earths (lanthanides)	Glass manufacturing, photoengraving, lens polishing, electronics, carbon arc lamp exposure	Interlobular septal thickening	
Cobalt	Hard metal production, grinding, use and maintenance of hard metal tools, diamond cutting and polishing	Mid-lower lung zone predominant, patchy lobular ground-glass opacities, consolidation, reticulation, centrilobular nodularity; honeycombing may occur	GIP

(Continued)

Table 19.5 (*Continued*) Radiographic and pathologic characteristics of Occ-ILDs

Occ-ILD	Exposure scenarios	Radiographic pattern	Pathologic pattern
Talc	Numerous uses: paint, paper, cosmetics, roofing products, rubber, dry lubricant, textile manufacture	Small centrilobular and subpleural nodules; may develop heterogeneous conglomerate masses with internal foci of high attenuation; may depend on degree of contamination with asbestos/silica	Granulomatous lung disease
Mica	Boiler and furnace lining, electronics industry, building materials, acoustic products, grinding	Mid-lower zone predominant interlobular septal thickening; honeycombing may occur	
Upper Lung Zone Predominant			
Beryllium	Nuclear weapons, electronics, aerospace, high-tech ceramics, metal recycling, dental prostheses, alloy machining, defense industries, automotive	Peribronchovascular nodularity, bronchial wall thickening, and ground-glass attenuation; hilar adenopathy in 20%–30%	Granulomatous lung disease
Crystalline silica	Hard rock mining, construction, road work, tunnelling, sandblasting, foundry work, granite/stone work, silica flour production/use, ceramics, glass manufacture	Well-circumscribed nodules measuring less than 5 mm in diameter in a posterior and central distribution; may develop progressive massive fibrosis; hilar adenopathy± calcification may occur	Silicotic nodules; alveolar proteinosis with high levels of exposure
Coal dust	Exposure to coal mine dust	Well-circumscribed nodules measuring less than 5 mm in diameter in a posterior and central distribution; may develop progressive massive fibrosis, emphysema	Coal macules
Silicon carbide (carborundum)	Abrasive, refractory materials, ceramics, metal matrix composites	Small nodules; may have pleural disease	Silicotic nodules; alveolar proteinosis with high levels of exposure

(*Continued*)

Table 19.5 (*Continued*) Radiographic and pathologic characteristics of Occ-ILDs

Occ-ILD	Exposure scenarios	Radiographic pattern	Pathologic pattern
Other carbon compounds (graphite, carbon black, oil shale)	Tyres, pigments, paints, pencils, foundry linings, mining, metallurgy, carbon electrodes, plastics	Small nodules; may develop progressive massive fibrosis	
Diatomaceous earth	Foundries, filter production, abrasives, dry lubricant; when heated above 450°C it converts to crystalline silica	Identical to silicosis	Acute/subacute inflammation
Aluminium	Abrasives, metals, alloys, explosives (pyro powder), building materials, glass manufacture, ceramics, welding	Poorly defined centrilobular nodules; may also have interlobular septal thickening with emphysema and bullae	Interstitial fibrosis, granulomatous disease, desquamative interstitial pneumonia, and pulmonary alveolar proteinosis
Iron (siderosis)	Iron welding, metal polishers	Ill-defined small centrilobular nodules; may have patchy ground-glass attenuation	Iron particles in macrophages aggregated along perivascular and peribronchial lymphatic vessels
Tin (stannosis)	Tin production: smelting and bagging	Upper zone predominant or diffuse nodules	
No Zonal Predominance			
Aluminium oxide	Aluminium oxide abrasive manufacture	Diffuse irregular interlobular septal thickening	Interstitial fibrosis, granulomatous disease, desquamative interstitial pneumonia, and pulmonary alveolar proteinosis
Nylon flock	Production of nylon flock (especially the random cut method)	Ground-glass attenuation and micronodules; interlobular septal thickening and consolidation may be seen	Lymphocytic bronchiolitis, peribronchiolitis with lymphoid hyperplasia, DIP, DAD, NSIP

(*Continued*)

Table 19.5 (Continued) Radiographic and pathologic characteristics of Occ-ILDs

Occ-ILD	Exposure scenarios	Radiographic pattern	Pathologic pattern
Nepheline	Nepheline mining, pottery, paint filler	Interlobular septal thickening, hilar adenopathy, atelectasis	
Titanium	Metal products, paints, aerospace, defense industry, electronics	Poorly described but likely interlobular septal thickening and nodularity; pleural disease may occur	Granulomatous lung disease
Zirconium	Foundry sands, refractory bricks, abrasives, optical lens polishing, ceramics, nuclear reactors	Diffuse nodules have been reported	Granulomatous lung disease
Barium (baritosis)	Inhalation of fine ground barium sulphate from paint, paper, textile, vinyl, rubber, and glass manufacture; medical diagnostics	Diffuse nodules	Alveolar filling with barium

Source: Data from Beckett WS. N Engl J Med. 2000;342:406–13; Samuel G, Maier LA. Curr Opin Allergy Clin Immunol. 2008;8:126–34; Balmes JR et al. Am J Resp Crit Care Med. 2014;190:e34–59; American Thoracic Society. Am J Resp Crit Care Med. 2004;170:691–715; Akira M, Morinaga K. Am J Ind Med. 2016;379:2008–18; Mayer A, Hamzeh N. Curr Opin Pulm Med. 2015;21:178–84; Tátrai E et al. J Appl Toxicol. 2004;24:147–54; Hull MJ, Abraham JL. Hum Pathol. 2002;33:819–25; Turcotte SE et al. Chest. 2013;143:1642–8; Chong S et al. Radiographics. 2006;26:59–77; Elmore AR, Cosmetic Ingredient Review Expert Panel. Int J Toxicol. 2003;22(Suppl 1):37–102.

central predominance. These nodules may coalesce leading to progressive massive fibrosis. HRCT findings may also include cicatricial emphysema and mild hilar adenopathy (usually not as large as seen in sarcoidosis), with 10% of patients having peripheral 'eggshell' calcification of the nodes. Rapid growth of masses or development of cavitation should prompt a search for alternative or secondary diagnoses such as tuberculosis or lung cancer (1).

Chronic beryllium disease

HRCT findings in CBD are similar to sarcoidosis, including peribronchovascular bilateral small nodules, bronchial wall thickening and ground-glass attenuation. Hilar lymphadenopathy is present in one-third of cases, but as with silicosis, to a lesser extent than in sarcoidosis. In advanced disease, honeycombing, conglomerate masses and emphysema can occur (1,27).

PATHOLOGY

Diagnosis of an Occ-ILD requires a history of exposure to an agent known to cause ILD (or in the case of CBD, an abnormal BeLPT as a surrogate of exposures), an appropriate latency period and clinical course, a radiographic and PFT pattern consistent with lung disease related to the exposure and exclusion of other causes of ILD.

1. *Occ-ILDs due to a non-specific inflammatory response*: Biopsy is usually not required for the classic pneumoconioses if there is a history of sufficient exposure, appropriate latency period, consistent clinical course and consistent radiographic imaging, and other causes of ILD have been excluded (1,27,29).

   Surgical lung biopsy should be considered when the imaging, presentation or radiographic imaging are not typical or when considering a possible Occ-ILD related to a novel or poorly characterized exposure (1). If a lung biopsy is obtained, clinicians must interpret pathologic findings in light of a patient's known exposure history, as pathologic findings in Occ-ILD may overlap with those seen in non-occupational ILD (Tables 19.1 and 19.5).

Asbestosis: Early pathologic findings in asbestosis include peribronchiolar fibrosis that extends into the alveolar walls. The peribronchiolar fibrosis correlates with the dot-like opacities on HRCT and the extension into alveolar walls leads to the curvilinear lines described above. However, as the disease progresses the pathology becomes similar to typical UIP. The presence of asbestos bodies on biopsy supports a diagnosis of asbestosis but absence of asbestos bodies does not exclude asbestosis (29).

Silicosis and CWP: Silicotic nodules are pathognomonic of silicosis. Initially the nodules are highly cellular, but in later stages they have an 'onion skin' appearance with little central cellularity. Dark pigment dust with birefringent particles may be present in the center of the nodules (1). CWP is characterized by coal dust macules containing coal dust-laden macrophages centered on respiratory bronchioles and focal emphysematous changes (32). Diffuse interstitial fibrosis with chronic inflammation may also be seen in silicosis and CWP (32,33).

2. *Occ-ILDs with immune sensitization*: In contrast to the pneumoconioses, biopsy is often required for diagnosis of Occ-ILDs due to immune sensitization. In CBD, transbronchial biopsy often provides sufficient tissue; open lung biopsy is rarely required. BAL lymphocytosis can also support a diagnosis of CBD in the setting of an abnormal BeLPT (27).

   Chronic beryllium disease: A diagnosis of CBD requires both evidence for beryllium sensitization and granulomatous lung disease on biopsy. The characteristic pathologic lesion in both CBD and sarcoidosis is the non-caseating granuloma, which consists of an aggregate of epithelioid histiocytes surrounded by lymphocytes and plasma cells (27). The clinician must rely on the occupational history and results of the BeLPT to distinguish these conditions (1,27).

GENERAL MANAGEMENT

Treatment of both Occ-ILD and non-occupational variants includes supportive and preventive care. Patients should receive pneumococcal vaccination, yearly influenza vaccines and oxygen supplementation to keep oxygen saturation $\geq$89%. For deconditioned patients, pulmonary rehabilitation can improve quality of life (1).

Specific to the management of Occ-ILD is the recommendation that patients be removed from exposure. This recommendation is based on the dose–response relationship of lung injury described for asbestosis and silicosis, with higher levels of cumulative exposure leading to worsening lung injury (4,5). For other agents, despite the lack of strong evidence, removal from the exposure is still advisable (1). Additionally, it is important to consider the possibility that other workers in the workplace may already have or also be at risk for the Occ-ILD, and exposure reduction may be needed for them as well (6,7). Finally, the clinician should provide a clearly written report defining the exposure, Occ-ILD diagnosis and causation that can be used to help the patient qualify for worker's compensation and other compensation programmes.

SPECIFIC ASPECTS OF MANAGEMENT

OCC-ILD DUE TO A NON-SPECIFIC INFLAMMATORY RESPONSE

There are no known effective pharmacologic therapies for the pneumoconioses (29,34). Patients with silicosis should be screened for tuberculosis with either the purified protein derivative skin test or interferon-gamma release assay (IGRA) and should be treated for latent tuberculosis infection if the PPD is $\geq$10 mm or IGRA is positive and active infection has been ruled out. Patients with silicosis who are diagnosed with active tuberculosis should receive therapy for 8 months rather than the standard of 6 months to reduce the risk of recurrence (1,34).

OCC-ILD DUE TO IMMUNE SENSITIZATION

The treatment approach for CBD is similar to that of sarcoidosis except that disease remission is unlikely in CBD. Early disease is often treated symptomatically with inhaled corticosteroids and short-acting bronchodilators. For patients with more significant respiratory impairment or severe symptoms or evidence of progressive decline in lung function, oral corticosteroids are considered first-line agents. Observational studies suggest that treatment with glucocorticoids leads to improved pulmonary function, radiographic abnormalities, symptoms and functional status. Relapse during the tapering of oral glucocorticoids is common. A steroid-sparing agent can be considered for those with significant side effects related to glucocorticoids. Lung transplantation has been performed for end-stage CBD (27).

PROGNOSIS AND LONG-TERM OUTLOOK

The prognosis of the Occ-ILDs depends on the pathogenesis of the condition.

OCC-ILD DUE TO A NON-SPECIFIC INFLAMMATORY RESPONSE

One of the distinguishing features of Occ-ILDs due to a non-specific inflammatory response is the slow clinical progression (Table 19.2) (1). This slow progression is considerably different from IPF, which has an average survival of about 3 years from diagnosis. Only 20%–40% of patients with asbestosis progress, and those that progress take an average of 5 years to increase one major ILO category. Higher levels of cumulative exposure and advanced disease at diagnosis are risk factors for progression (29,35). Silicosis similarly progresses slowly, taking an average of 12 years for end-stage fibrosis to develop in one study. HIV, smoking and tuberculosis increase the risk of progression of silicosis (33,34).

OCC-ILD DUE TO IMMUNE SENSITIZATION

The natural history of CBD is variable. The rate of progression from BeS to CBD is as high as 8.8% per year over a period of up to 20 years (27). Patients with CBD often experience a gradual decline, and cure is rare.

CURRENT AND FUTURE AREAS OF RESEARCH

New exposures in the workplace may introduce new Occ-ILDs. Indium tin oxide has recently been described in workers in the flat-panel display industry, primarily in Asia. Exposed workers may develop pulmonary alveolar proteinosis and fibrotic interstitial lung disease (36).

In addition to Occ-ILD cases due to new exposures, classic Occ-ILDs exposures have also been identified in new exposure scenarios. For example, denim sandblasting emerged as a new risk factor for silicosis in Turkey (37).

There is ongoing research on the medical treatment of Occ-ILDs. In CBD, a single randomized controlled trial of infliximab demonstrated improvement in those with abnormal DLCO at baseline, which was limited by small numbers. The two drugs, pirfenidone and nintedanib, which have been shown to slow the decline in forced vital capacity in patients with IPF have not yet been studied in Occ-ILDs. A number of treatments have been tried without convincing success in silicosis, and possible cell-based therapy has been proposed (44). To enhance the specificity of diagnosis and eliminate the need for biopsy, additional diagnostic assays are being evaluated such as cytokine assays to distinguish CBD from BeS. These rely on detection of cytokines produced during the Th1 immune response in patients with CBD (13,38). However, at this time, the best way to limit Occ-ILD impairment and diagnose disease continues to be considering these diseases in the differential diagnosis of idiopathic diseases and preventing severe disease by making the diagnosis early, removing the worker from ongoing exposure and implementing surveillance programmes to detect other workers with early disease.

REFERENCES

1. Beckett WS. Occupational respiratory diseases. *N Engl J Med.* 2000;342: 406–13.
2. Coultas DB, Zumwalt RE, Black WC, Sobonya RE. The epidemiology of interstitial lung diseases. *Am J Respir Crit Care Med.* 1994;150:967–72.
3. Thomeer MJ, Costabe U, Rizzato G, Poletti V, Demedts M. Comparison of registries of interstitial lung diseases in three European countries. *Eur Respir J Suppl.* 2001;32:114s–8s.
4. US Department of Health and Human Services. Health Effects of Occupational Exposure to Respirable Crystalline Silica. *Cincinnati, OH: Department of Health and Human Services, National Institute for Occupational Safety and Health, Centers for Disease Control and Prevention*; 2002.
5. Becklake MR. Asbestos and other fiber-related diseases of the lungs and pleura: Distribution and determinants in exposed populations. *Chest.* 1991;100:248–54.
6. Rutstein DD. The principle of the sentinel health event and its application to the occupational diseases. *Arch Environ Health.* 1984;39:158.
7. Aldrich TE, Leaverton PE. Sentinel event strategies in environmental health. *Annu Rev Public Health.* 1993;14:205–17.
8. Nemery B, Bast A, Behr J, Borm PJ, Bourke SJ, Camus PH et al. Interstitial lung disease induced by exogenous agents: Factors governing susceptibility. *Eur Respir J Suppl.* 2001;32:30s–42s.
9. Dostert C, Petrilli V, Van Bruggen R, Steele C, Mossman BT, Tschopp J. Innate immune activation through Nalp3 inflammasome sensing of asbestos and silica. *Science.* 2008;320:674–7.
10. Mossman BT, Churg A. Mechanisms in the pathogenesis of asbestosis and silicosis. *Am J Respir Crit Care Med.* 1998;157:1666–80.
11. Robledo R, Mossman B. Cellular and molecular mechanisms of asbestos-induced fibrosis. *J Cell Physiol.* 1999;180:158–66.
12. Epler GR, McLoud TC, Gaensler EA. Prevalence and incidence of benign asbestos pleural effusion in a working population. *JAMA.* 1982;247:617–22.
13. Samuel G, Maier LA. Immunology of chronic beryllium disease. *Curr Opin Allergy Clin Immunol.* 2008;8:126–34.
14. Maier LA, McGrath DS, Sato H, Lympany P, Welsh K, Du Bois R et al. Influence of MHC class II in susceptibility to beryllium sensitization and chronic beryllium disease. *J Immunol.* 2003;171:6910–8.

15. Newman LS, Maier L. Beryllium. In: Sullivan J, Krieger G, eds. *Clinical Environmental Health and Toxic Exposures*. Philadelphia, PA: Lippincott Williams and Wilkins; 2001:919–26.

16. Hardy HL. Beryllium poisoning: Lessons in control of man-made disease. *N Engl J Med*. 1965;273:1188–99.

17. Kreiss K, Mroz MM, Zhen B, Martyny JW, Newman LS. Epidemiology of beryllium sensitization and disease in nuclear workers. *Am Rev Respir Dis*. 1993;148:985–91.

18. Monso E, Tura JM, Marsal M, Morell F, Pujadas J, Morera J. Mineralogical micro-analysis of idiopathic pulmonary fibrosis. *Arch Environ Health*. 1990;45:185–8.

19. Muller-Quernheim J, Gaede KI, Fireman E, Zissel G. Diagnosis of chronic beryllium disease within cohorts of sarcoidosis patients. *Eur Respir J*. 2006;27:1190–5.

20. Registry AfTSaD. *Taking an Exposure History: Case Studies in Environmental Medicine*. Washington, DC: US Department of Health and Human Services; 2000.

21. Burge P. How to take an occupational exposure history relevant to lung disease. In: Hendrick D, Burge P, Beckett W et al., eds. *Occupational Disorders of the Lung*. Philadelphia, PA: WB Saunders; 2002:25–32.

22. Fraser RG, Pare JAP, Pare PD, Fraser RS, Genereux GP. Pleuropulmonary disease caused by inhalation of inorganic dust (pneumoconiosis). In: Fraser RG, Fraser RS, Genereux GP, eds. *Diagnosis of Diseases of the Chest*. Philadelphia, PA: WB Saunders; 1990:2346.

23. Green FH, Harley R, Vallyathan V, Althouse R, Fick G, Dement J et al. Exposure and mineralogical correlates of pulmonary fibrosis in chrysotile asbestos workers. *Occup Environ Med*. 1997;54:549–59.

24. Cohen RA, Patel A, Green FH. Lung disease caused by exposure to coal mine and silica dust. *Semin Respir Crit Care Med*. 2008;29:651–61.

25. Kreiss K, Mroz MM, Newman LS, Martyny J, Zhen B. Machining risk of beryllium disease and sensitization with median exposures below 2 $\mu g/m^3$. *Am J Industr Med*. 1996;30:16–25.

26. Kinsella M, Muller N, Vedal S, Staples C, Abboud RT, Chan-Yeung M. Emphysema in silicosis: A comparison of smokers with non-smokers using pulmonary function testing and computed tomography. *Am Rev Respir Dis*. 1990;141:1497–500.

27. Balmes JR, Abraham JL, Dweik RA, Fireman E, Fontenot AP, Maier LA et al. On behalf of the ATS Ad Hoc committee on beryllium sensitivity and chronic beryllium disease. An official American Thoracic Society statement: Diagnosis and management of beryllium sensitivity and chronic beryllium disease. *Am J Resp Crit Care Med*. 2014;190:e34–59.

28. Wolff H, Vehmas T, Oksa P, Rantanen J, Vainio H. Asbestos, asbestosis, and cancer, the Helsinki criteria for diagnosis and attribution 2014: Recommendations. *Scan J Work Environ Health*. 2015;41:5–15.

29. American Thoracic Society. Diagnosis and initial management of nonmalignant diseases related to asbestos. *Am J Resp Crit Care Med*. 2004;170:691–715.

30. Akira M, Morinaga K. The comparison of high-resolution computed tomography findings in asbestosis and idiopathic pulmonary fibrosis. *Am J Ind Med*. 2016;379:2008–18.

31. Copley SJ, Wells AU, Sivakumaran P, Rubens MB, Lee YC, Desai SR et al. Asbestosis and idiopathic pulmonary fibrosis: Comparison of thin-section CT features. *Radiology*. 2003;229:731–6.

32. Cohen RA, Petsonk EL, Rose C, Young B, Regier M, Najmuddin A et al. Lung pathology in US coal workers with rapidly progressive pneumoconiosis implicates silica and silicates. *Am J Resp Crit Care Med*. 2016;193:673–80.

33. Arakawa H, Fujimoto K, Honma K, Suganuma N, Morikubo H, Saito Y et al. Progression from near-normal to end-stage lungs in chronic interstitial pneumonia related to silica exposure: Long-term CT observations. *Am J Roentgenol*. 2008;191:1040–5.

34. Leung CC, Yu IT, Chen W. Silicosis. *Lancet* 2012;379:2008–18.

35. Oksa P, Huuskonen MS, Jarvisalo J, Klockars M, Zitting A, Suoranta H et al.

Follow-up of asbestosis patients and predictors for radiographic progression. *Int Arch Occup Environ Health.* 1998;71:465–71.

36. Omae K, Nakano M, Tanaka A, Hirata M, Hamaguchi T, Chonan T. Indium lung – Case reports and epidemiology. *Int Arch Occup Environ Health.* 2011;84:471–7.

37. Akgün M. Denim production and silicosis. *Curr Opin Pulm Med.* 2016;22:165–9.

38. Pott GB, Palmer BE, Sullivan AK, Silviera L, Maier LA, Newman LS et al. Frequency of beryllium-specific, TH1-type cytokine-expressing CD4+ T cells in patients with beryllium-induced disease. *J Allergy Clin Immunol.* 2005;115:1036–42.

39. Mayer A, Hamzeh N. Beryllium and other metal-induced lung disease. *Curr Opin Pulm Med.* 2015;21:178–84.

40. Tátrai E, Kováciková Z, Brózik M, Six E. Pulmonary toxicity of wollastonite *in vivo* and *in vitro. J Appl Toxicol.* 2004;24:147–54.

41. Hull MJ, Abraham JL. Aluminum welding fume-induced pneumoconiosis. *Hum Pathol.* 2002;33:819–25.

42. Turcotte SE, Chee A, Walsh R, Grant FC, Liss GM, Boag A et al. Flock Worker's lung disease: Natural history of cases and exposed workers in Kingston, Ontario. *Chest.* 2013;143:1642–8.

43. Chong S, Lee KS, Chung MJ, Han J, Kwon OJ, Kim TS. Pneumoconiosis: Comparison of imaging and pathologic findings. *Radiographics.* 2006;26:59–77.

44. Lopes-Pacheco M, Bandeira E, Morales MM. Cell-Based Therapy for Silicosis. *Stem Cells Int.* 2016;2016:5091838.

45. Elmore AR, Cosmetic Ingredient Review Expert Panel. Final report on the safety assessment of aluminum silicate, calcium silicate, magnesium aluminum silicate, magnesium silicate, magnesium trisilicate, sodium magnesium silicate, zirconium silicate, attapulgite, bentonite, fuller's earth, hectorite, kaolin, lithium magnesium silicate, lithium magnesium sodium silicate, montmorillonite, pyrophyllite, and zeolite. *Int J Toxicol.* 2003;22(Suppl 1):37–102.

20

Pulmonary vasculitis and alveolar haemorrhage syndromes

REBECCA C KEITH AND STEPHEN K FRANKEL

This chapter presents a general overview of the diffuse alveolar haemorrhage (DAH) syndromes and pulmonary vasculitis. The alveolar haemorrhage syndromes and pulmonary vasculitides are a complex group of potentially life-threatening conditions that require a thoughtful diagnostic approach and often require emergent therapeutic interventions. This chapter details the clinical approach to the diagnosis and management of these syndromes with a focus on clinically relevant pearls of wisdom. We advocate for a collaborative approach to these complex diseases and consideration of early referral to a tertiary care centre.

ALVEOLAR HAEMORRHAGE SYNDROMES

Alveolar haemorrhage syndromes are uniformly characterized by a disruption of the alveolar–capillary membrane and diffuse bleeding into the

Table 20.1 Aetiology of alveolar haemorrhage syndromes categorized by histopathology

Pulmonary capillaritis	Acute lung transplant rejection
	Anti-GBM disease (Goodpasture syndrome)
	Anti-phospholipid antibody syndrome
	Behçet syndrome
	Cryoglobulinemia
	Drugs and medications
	Granulomatosis with polyangiitis (Wegener granulomatosis)
	Haematopoietic stem cell transplantation
	Henoch–Schönlein purpura
	Isolated pauci-immune pulmonary capillaritis
	Microscopic polyangiitis
	Systemic lupus erythematosus
	Other connective tissue diseases
Bland pulmonary haemorrhage	Anti-GBM disease (Goodpasture syndrome)
	Disorders of the coagulation system
	Drugs and medications
	Idiopathic pulmonary haemosiderosis
	Inhalational exposures
	Mitral stenosis
	Obstructive sleep apnoea
	Pulmonary veno-occlusive disease
Diffuse alveolar damage	Acute exacerbation of idiopathic pulmonary fibrosis
	Acute idiopathic pneumonia
	Acute respiratory distress syndrome (ARDS)
	Drugs and medications
	Haematopoietic stem cell transplantation
Miscellaneous	Human immunodeficiency virus infection
	Lymphangioleiomyomatosis
	Pulmonary capillary haemangiomatosis

alveolar space. While haemoptysis often prompts an investigation of the possibility of DAH, this diagnosis should also be considered in any patient who presents with dyspnoea, hypoxaemia and a chest radiograph that demonstrates diffuse pulmonary infiltrates. Anaemia or haemoptysis are common but may not always be identified at the time of presentation. Diagnosis is usually made at the time of bronchoscopy when serial lung lavage reveals a progressive increase in blood content of sequentially retrieved bronchoalveolar lavage (BAL) aliquots, which verifies the presence of blood in the alveolar space. DAH is not a specific diagnosis but instead is a manifestation of an underlying disease process for which there is a broad differential diagnosis. Pulmonary histopathology can be used to classify the alveolar haemorrhage syndromes into one of three subgroups based on the histopathologic findings that are (a) pulmonary capillaritis, (b) bland pulmonary haemorrhage, or (c) diffuse alveolar damage (DAD) with haemorrhage (Table 20.1).

HISTORY AND EXAMINATION

DAH can occur at any age. The 'classic' presenting symptom of DAH is haemoptysis that can occur suddenly or develop over a period of days to weeks. However, haemoptysis can be absent in approximately 30% of patients at the time of presentation (1). A detailed history can identify additional symptoms such as fatigue, malaise, non-productive cough, chest discomfort, dyspnoea and/or exercise limitation. The past medical history may provide additional clues that help to determine the specific aetiology of the haemorrhage syndrome. A history of multiple extra-pulmonary symptoms or a known collagen vascular disease (CVD) suggests capillaritis secondary to a systemic auto-immune disease. A history of a heart murmur could suggest bland haemorrhage from mitral stenosis. A detailed medication history can identify medications such as hydralazine (2) or warfarin (3), which are known to be associated with alveolar haemorrhage. Pneumotox online (www.pneumotox.com) provides a valuable resource to help identify drugs that might be contributing to alveolar haemorrhage (4).

Physical examination findings are generally non-specific and include fever, tachycardia, tachypnea and hypoxaemia. Lung auscultation may elicit diffuse crackles (rales) or bronchial breath sounds. Extra-pulmonary exam findings can often provide the most helpful clues as to the aetiology of alveolar haemorrhage, as inflammatory arthritis, palpable purpura, iritis or mononeuritis multiplex can suggest the presence of an underlying auto-immune disorder. Still, additional diagnostic testing is often required to determine the aetiology of DAH.

INVESTIGATIONS

Initial laboratory testing should include a complete blood count, comprehensive metabolic profile, inflammatory markers, coagulation studies and a urinalysis with sediment examination. Blood counts may reveal an elevated white blood cell count or anaemia with a low or falling haematocrit. The platelet count may be elevated or can be low as in the case of idiopathic thrombocytopenic purpura, thrombotic thrombocytopenia purpura, haemolytic uremic syndrome or disseminated intravascular coagulation (5,6). Coagulation studies are needed to exclude a coagulopathy. An elevated erythrocyte sedimentation rate or C-reactive protein suggests systemic inflammation, but are non-specific. Renal function studies and urinalysis can identify evidence of glomerulonephritis that in turn focuses the differential on those entities that can present with a pulmonary-renal syndrome. An echocardiogram should also be performed to evaluate for evidence of mitral stenosis, left ventricular dysfunction or pulmonary hypertension.

Ultimately, bronchoscopy is the most effective way to confirm a suspected diagnosis of DAH. To properly perform this procedure, the bronchoscope is inserted into a 'wedge position' in one of the segmental or sub-segmental airways in an affected anatomic area (as may be identified on imaging). The right middle lobe or lingula often give the best return of fluid and may be good targets if involved. Three to five saline aliquots of 30–60 mL are serially instilled and removed into separate containers for a total lavage volume of 100 mL (7). DAH is identified when the returned aliquots are increasingly haemorrhagic (or at a minimum, do not significantly clear) in appearance with increasing red blood cell (RBC) counts upon laboratory testing (Figure 20.1).

Serologic studies can sometimes provide the best clues as to the aetiology of a haemorrhage syndrome if they can confirm a specific diagnosis without having to proceed to surgical lung biopsy (Table 20.2). However, in some cases, surgical lung biopsy (SLB) may ultimately be necessary to obtain a final diagnosis. For example, the presence of anti-glomerular basement membrane antibodies (anti-GBMs) can confirm a diagnosis of Goodpasture syndrome (8), or a positive ANA, in the right clinical context, may result in a diagnosis of systemic lupus erythematosus (SLE).

RADIOLOGY

DAH is radiographically characterized by a non-specific alveolar filling process. Chest radiography demonstrates patchy, diffuse, alveolar infiltrates that may include bilateral ground-glass opacities and/or areas of focal consolidation (9). Opacities can be migratory and change in both extent and pattern. Thoracic high-resolution computed tomography (HRCT) typically demonstrates diffuse, multilobar, ground-glass opacities. Septal thickening may also be present, and there may be areas of consolidation. Repeated episodes of DAH can lead to fibrosis or obstructive lung disease (10,11). Imaging studies of other affected target end organs can help both with diagnosis and with defining the extent of a given disease. For example, a computed tomogram of the sinuses may be helpful in the evaluation of sinus involvement that is commonly found in granulomatosis with polyangiitis (GPA).

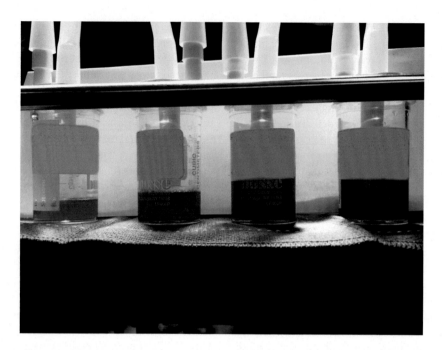

Figure 20.1 Diffuse alveolar haemorrhage can be identified by performing a bronchoalveolar lavage (BAL) that returns increasing numbers of red blood cells in retrieved BAL fluid aliquots. In order to obtain an accurate result, the bronchoscope is inserted into a 'wedge position' in one of the segmental or subsegmental airways. Choose an anatomic area that is among the most affected on imaging. If involved in the disease process, the right middle lobe or lingula often give the best return of fluid. Three to five saline aliquots of 30–60 mL each are serially instilled and removed and stored in separate containers for a total lavage volume of 100–300 mL (7). Diffuse alveolar haemorrhage is identified when the returned aliquots are increasingly haemorrhagic, or at a minimum, do not demonstrate any evidence of clearing. Serial red blood cell counts may be used if the result is not obvious on gross examination. (Image generously provided by Edward C Dempsey, MD, VA Eastern Colorado Health Care System, Denver, Colorado.)

PATHOLOGY

Pulmonary histopathology can be used to classify the alveolar haemorrhage syndromes into three broad categories that include pulmonary capillaritis, bland pulmonary haemorrhage and DAD with haemorrhage. Pulmonary capillaritis is characterized by RBCs filling the airspaces and a neutrophil-predominant inflammatory infiltrate invading the walls of the pulmonary capillaries, arterioles and venules as well as the adjacent interstitium and alveolar wall (12). As the disease process organizes, the capillaritis can resolve, leaving haemosiderin-laden macrophages and other injury patterns (e.g. organizing pneumonia) in its wake (12). Alveolar walls may become thickened with associated inflammatory infiltrates and reactive type II cells (12).

Similar to the pathologic findings of capillaritis, bland pulmonary haemorrhage is characterized by RBC-filled airspaces, the presence of haemosiderin-laden macrophages, oedema of the alveolar septal wall, and reactive type II hyperplasia (12). Unlike capillaritis, there is no evidence of inflammatory cell infiltration, necrosis or damage to the vessel wall (12,13). Partially treated or resolving capillaritis may have a similar appearance to bland haemorrhage, confounding the diagnosis (13).

DAD is initially characterized by hyaline membrane formation, capillary congestion, oedema of the alveolar walls, and microthombi (14). Following the acute phase of DAD, there is an organizing phase that consists of deposition of fibromixoid tissue within the alveolar spaces, type II cell hyperplasia and fibrinous organization of the airspace (14). In more pronounced cases of DAD, the damage to the alveolar-capillary unit is such that RBCs

Table 20.2 Laboratory testing in alveolar haemorrhage syndromes

Routine testing	Complete blood count with differential
	Metabolic profile
	Hepatic function panel
	Urinalysis with microscopic sediment examination
	Erythrocyte sedimentation rate
	C-reactive protein
	Prothrombin time/international normalized ratio (INR)
	Partial thromboplastin time
	Urine drug screening (cocaine)
Auto-immune serologies	Antinuclear antibodies (ANA)
	Anti-double-stranded DNA (anti-dsDNA)
	Complement levels (C3 and C4)
	Anti-glomerular basement membrane antibodies (GBM)
	Anti-neutrophil cytoplasmic antibodies (ANCA)
	Proteinase 3 antibodies (PR3)
	Myeloperoxidase antibodies (MPO)
	Rheumatoid factor (RF)
	Anti-cyclic citrullinated peptide antibodies (CCP)
	Dilute Russell viper venom time (dRVVT)
	Anticardiolipin antibodies
	Anti-ß-2-glycoprotein
	Lupus anti-coagulant

enter the airspaces creating a component of alveolar haemorrhage. However, in these cases, DAD remains the dominant pathologic finding, and the DAH is a secondary result of the injury.

DISORDERS ASSOCIATED WITH DAH

ANCA-ASSOCIATED SMALL-VESSEL VASCULITIS: MICROSCOPIC POLYANGIITIS

Microscopic polyangiitis (MPA) is a common aetiology of pulmonary renal syndrome in which patients present with both alveolar haemorrhage and glomerulonephritis. MPA disease onset peaks in the fifth and sixth decades of life, is male predominant and has an incidence of 2–10 cases per million (15,16). Eighty percent of patients with MPA have renal manifestations ranging from asymptomatic microscopic haematuria to renal failure requiring dialysis (17). MPA patients also commonly have profound constitutional symptoms including fatigue, malaise, anorexia and/or weight loss. In a large series of patients of MPA, pulmonary haemorrhage occurred in 47% of patients (18). Approximately two-thirds of patients will demonstrate positive serologies for anti-neutrophil cytoplasmic antibodies (ANCAs), and this will most commonly occur in a perinuclear staining pattern (p-ANCA), MPA frequently is associated with anti-myeloperoxidase (MPO) antibodies and is only rarely associated with anti-proteinase 3 (PR3) antibodies (17). MPA will be discussed in more detail in the following section on pulmonary vasculitis.

ANCA-ASSOCIATED SMALL-VESSEL VASCULITIS: GRANULOMATOSIS WITH POLYANGIITIS

Classically, patients with granulomatosis with polyangiitis (GPA) present with or develop a 'triad' of upper airway, pulmonary and renal involvement, and serologically, these patients are characterized by a cytoplasmic ANCA (c-ANCA) staining pattern directed at proteinase 3 (PR3). GPA is diagnosed more commonly between the ages of 45 and 60, but it can affect patients of almost any age and has an incidence of 2–14 per million (16,19). In one case series, 8% of patients with GPA presented with alveolar haemorrhage (20). GPA will be discussed in more detail in the following section on pulmonary vasculitis.

ISOLATED PAUCI-IMMUNE PULMONARY CAPILLARITIS

By definition, isolated pauci-immune pulmonary capillaritis is a lung limited, small-vessel vasculitis without clinical or serologic evidence of a systemic disease. Patients with isolated pauci-immune pulmonary capillaritis appear to have a better prognosis than those with systemic vasculitis (21).

SYSTEMIC LUPUS ERYTHEMATOSUS

Systemic lupus erythematosus (SLE) is the most common primary CVD associated with DAH. DAH occurs in 1%–5% of patients with SLE (22). The survival rate can be variable depending on the cohort studied and when the study was performed, ranging from a low of 8% in 1985 to up to 80% in a more recent cohort (23).

ANTI-PHOSPHOLIPID ANTIBODY SYNDROME

Anti-phospholipid antibody syndrome (APLS) is defined by the presence of vascular (arterial and venous) thromboses, pregnancy loss and positive serologies including lupus anti-coagulant, anti-cardiolipin antibody and/or anti-β_2 glycoprotein-I antibody (24). APLS can occur as an independent syndrome or as a secondary manifestation of SLE. DAH is an uncommon complication of APLS, carries a poor prognosis and is among the most challenging entities to manage because of the concurrent risk of bleeding and clotting. Often, these patients require anti-coagulation to prevent life-threatening thrombotic complications, such that reversing the anti-coagulation has its own inherent risk. The DAH in APLS, while complicated by anti-coagulation, is primarily due to small-vessel vasculitis, and aggressive therapy needs to be deployed to reverse the vasculitis including plasmapheresis and intravenous steroids (25,26). Transfer to a tertiary centre, if possible, is recommended.

ANTI-GLOMERULAR BASEMENT MEMBRANE ANTIBODY (GOODPASTURE) DISEASE (ANTI-GBM DISEASE)

Anti-GBM (glomerular basement membrane) disease may present as with pulmonary-renal syndrome, isolated glomerulonephritis or isolated DAH. Anti-GBM disease is characterized by serum autoantibodies to the collagen IV alpha-3 constituents of the basement membrane (27). Pulmonary haemorrhage occurs in approximately 50% of patients when antibodies react to the pulmonary basement membrane (27). It is a rare disease, occurring in one person per million (28). Isolated lung disease is uncommon but does occur (29). Diagnosis can be made by the identification of serum anti-GBM antibodies, but not all patients will have positive serologies. A renal biopsy is often performed to confirm the diagnosis.

IDIOPATHIC PULMONARY HAEMOSIDEROSIS

The classic presentation of idiopathic pulmonary haemosiderosis (IPH) includes haemoptysis, iron deficiency and diffuse pulmonary infiltrates. IPH is a diagnosis of exclusion and is made when bland alveolar haemorrhage is demonstrated and no compelling cause of the haemorrhage can be identified; SLB is generally required to make the diagnosis. IPH is a rare disease with an incidence of 0.2–1.3 cases per million with 80% of cases identified in children (22). Several cases have been associated with coeliac disease. Glucocorticoids are used to treat the acute phase of disease (30).

MANAGEMENT

In the acute phase, patients with DAH can be severely ill and require an advanced level of care. Supportive care with supplemental oxygen, or in more severe cases, endotracheal intubation and mechanical ventilation, may be required. If any evidence of coagulopathy is identified, it should be expeditiously reversed (except in cases of APLS in which a careful review of the risks and benefits needs to be performed). More specifically, treatment of DAH should be based on the underlying aetiology of the alveolar haemorrhage syndrome.

If a causative medication, exposure or substance is identified, then removal of the offending agent is key. In those patients in whom a capillaritis lesion is strongly suspected, treatment directed towards an underlying ANCA-associated vasculitis, anti-GBM disease and/or SLE should strongly be considered. It is often necessary to begin therapy based on a suspected or presumed diagnosis while awaiting confirmatory testing. Delays in proceeding with urgent therapeutic interventions for the treatment of vasculitis (i.e. corticosteroids and plasmapheresis as discussed in detail in the next section) can result in poor outcomes. In this scenario, empiric therapy is the preferred approach.

In the small subset of patients who do not respond to conventional therapy, a number of salvage therapies have been attempted and are reported in the literature. Activated Factor VII has been given both intravenously and intra-tracheally; at the case report level, this has been shown to control bleeding in some alveolar haemorrhage syndromes (30,31). Extracorporeal membrane oxygenation (ECMO) has also been used at the case report level in young adults (31,32). Concerns around the use of anti-coagulation to maintain the ECMO circuit have limited enthusiasm for attempting salvage therapy with ECMO, but consideration may be given to the use of lower levels of anti-coagulation than are typically used to maintain a patent circuit in these patients (32).

PULMONARY VASCULIDITIES

The vasculidities are a rare group of heterogenous diseases that are characterized and unified by the histopathologic presence of inflammation in and disruption of the blood vessel wall. More specifically, the term 'pulmonary vasculitis', narrows the spectrum of disease to those clinical entities that significantly target the pulmonary parenchyma and/or airways as part of the disease presentation, and commonly refers to the cases of ANCA-associated vasculitis (AAVs) of MPA, GPA (formerly known as Wegener granulomatosis) and eosinophilic granulomatosis with polyangiitis (EGPA) (formerly known as Churg-Strauss syndrome), as well as idiopathic pauci–immune pulmonary capillaritis, SLE, anti-GBM disease (Goodpasture syndrome), and APLS. Clinically, the pulmonary manifestations are varied and can include not only alveolar haemorrhage, as previously discussed, but also pulmonary nodules, cavitary lesions, radiographic infiltrates and airway disease.

ANCA-ASSOCIATED SMALL-VESSEL VASCULITIS: MICROSCOPIC POLYANGIITIS

Clinically, patients with microscopic polyangiitis (MPA) will commonly present with profound constitutional symptoms, such as fatigue, malaise, anorexia and/or weight loss (often preceding fulminant disease onset by weeks to months), and renal involvement that may range from an asymptomatic urinary sediment to rapidly progressive glomerulonephritis requiring dialysis (33). The 'classic' pulmonary manifestation of MPA is DAH that causes patients to present with dyspnoea, cough and haemoptysis. DAH will occur in roughly 30%–50% of patients with MPA. The combination of DAH plus glomerulonephritis defines the term 'pulmonary-renal syndrome'. MPA is one of the more common causes of pulmonary renal syndrome (along with GPA, SLE and anti-GBM disease). The peripheral nervous system, skin, gastrointestinal tract and musculoskeletal system represent additional target end organs that are frequently involved in MPA. Skin manifestations may include palpable purpura, livedo reticularis, urticaria, nodules or ulcers (34). Gastrointestinal involvement may present with abdominal pain, bowel ischemia or bleeding (35). The nervous system is involved in 30%–70% of patients, and neuropathy and mononeuritis multiplex are among the more common manifestations (23,36). The central nervous system may be affected, albeit uncommonly (23,37). Ear, nose and throat involvement is classically associated with GPA rather than MPA; however, involvement has been described in up to 30% of patients in at least one case series (15).

As is the case with all patients with vasculitis, the diagnosis of MPA rests upon the clinician determining whether or not the preponderance of the clinical, laboratory, radiographic and/or pathologic data, collectively, do or do not support a diagnosis of vasculitis. It is worth noting that the classification criteria (Chapel Hill Consensus Conference criteria and American College of Rheumatology criteria) are not intended to be used as diagnostic criteria and cannot be used in lieu of clinical judgment (38,39). Hence, the diagnostic approach to MPA generally requires both laboratory studies and imaging of the affected end organs. Renal function, urinalysis and urine sediment examination are critical to identifying glomerulonephritis. Inflammatory markers are commonly elevated, but are poorly specific. Approximately half to three-quarters of patients will demonstrate positive serologies for ANCA, again, most commonly occurring in a perinuclear staining pattern (p-ANCA) and frequently associated with anti-myeloperoxidase (MPO) antibodies (17). In those patients who develop DAH, radiographic imaging will typically reveal diffuse ground-glass infiltrates consistent with DAH (40).

Surgical biopsy of the kidney, skin or lung is often required to confirm a suspected diagnosis of MPA. Lung pathology is characterized by necrotizing vasculitis of the small vessels without evidence of immune deposits or granulomatous inflammation (41). Kidney biopsy most commonly reveals necrotizing, crescentic glomerulonephritis (42).

ANCA-ASSOCIATED SMALL-VESSEL VASCULITIS: GRANULOMATOSIS WITH POLYANGIITIS

As mentioned above, the classic 'triad' of GPA is a combination of upper airway, pulmonary and renal involvement. That said, GPA is a systemic disease that may present with constitutional, musculoskeletal, gastrointestinal, neurologic, cardiac, cutaneous or ophthalmologic manifestations as well as respiratory and renal disease.

As with most of the vasculitides, constitutional symptoms including fever, anorexia and weight loss are common. The upper respiratory tract (i.e. ear, nose and throat) is the most common organ system involved in GPA, affecting up to 90% of patients (43). Manifestations include saddle nose deformity, rhinitis, epistaxis, nasal crusting, septal perforation, chronic sinusitis, mastoiditis, otitis and hearing loss (43). Pulmonary involvement occurs in 50%–90% of patients and presents with cough, dyspnoea, chest discomfort, haemoptysis and/or abnormal chest imaging. Further evaluation may reveal alveolar haemorrhage, nodules, cavities and/or infiltrates (19). Airway involvement including tracheal, endobronchial and subglottic inflammation and/or stenosis can be found in up to 50%–60% of cases (44). Renal involvement, most notably glomerulonephritis, occurs in 40%–90% of

cases, and the peripheral nervous system is affected in one-third of patients (19). Cardiac involvement and central nervous system (CNS) involvement are less common, but by definition, represent severe, life-threatening disease. Cutaneous disease (classically purpuric skin lesions, but also including nodules, ulcers, etc.) are identified in 10%–20% of cases (19). The 5-year survival rate for patients with GPA is estimated to be 74%–91% (16).

ANCA-ASSOCIATED SMALL-VESSEL VASCULITIS: EOSINOPHILIC GRANULOMATOSIS WITH POLYANGIITIS (CHURG–STRAUSS SYNDROME)

EGPA is an ANCA-associated, systemic vasculitis characterized by allergic rhinitis, asthma and peripheral eosinophilia. Mean age of onset is 38–54 years (45) and the annual incidence of EGPA is 0.5–3.7 per million (16). The presence of asthma is nearly universal, and while patients commonly will have severe, steroid-dependent asthma for a number of years prior to diagnosis, the asthma of EGPA may be mild, moderate or severe, and asthma may be diagnosed many years before, or concurrent with the EGPA diagnosis. EGPA is a systemic disease that can affect any number of organ systems including sinuses, skin, heart, gastrointestinal tract, kidneys and nervous system. Up to 70% of patients develop neurologic manifestations such as peripheral neuropathy or mononeuritis multiplex (46). Renal manifestations (including rapidly progressive glomerulonephritis) can occur in 25% of patients (45). Skin involvement can resemble palpable purpura, erythema multiforme, livedo reticularis, petechiae or urticaria (45).

EGPA typically evolves over time, and the disease presentation may be thought of as having sequential phases. The prodromal or initial phases are typically characterized by asthma, allergic rhinitis (potentially complicated by nasal polyposis), chronic sinusitis and atopic disease (47). This phase may also include arthralgias, myalgias, malaise, fever and weight loss and can be difficult to distinguish from other allergic/atopic disease states. This phase is followed by an 'eosinophilic phase' that is characterized by peripheral eosinophilia and/or end-organ eosinophilic infiltration that may invade the heart, lungs or gastrointestinal tract (45). Finally, it is the 'vasculitic' phase, which is characterized by constitutional symptoms, organ dysfunction and histopathologic vasculitis on biopsy, that tends to lead the bedside clinician to the diagnosis (45).

Positive ANCA with a p-ANCA pattern and a positive enzyme-linked immunosorbent assay (ELISA) for MPO antibodies are common laboratory findings (one-third to one-half of patients), but these findings are not necessary for making a diagnosis (48). Interestingly, patients may be grouped into ANCA-positive EGPA, in which patients will more commonly have 'vasculitic' disease manifestations similar to those found in patients with GPA and MPA (i.e. renal, gastrointestinal and nervous system involvement), or ANCA-negative EGPA patients, who have more 'eosinophilic' disease manifestations such as asthma, eosinophilic pneumonia and cardiac involvement (49).

Lung imaging in EGPA can show diffuse ground-glass, non-specific infiltrates (often migratory) or nodules (45). Lung biopsy, when obtained, may show necrotizing vasculitis associated with tissue infiltration by eosinophils and extravascular granulomas (50). The 5-year survival is estimated at 60%–97%, and cardiac and CNS involvement are poor prognostic features (51). Indeed, up to half of deaths caused by EGPA are due to cardiac disease.

GENERAL APPROACH TO THE MANAGEMENT OF PULMONARY VASCULITIS

The management of AAV is based on the current European League Against Rheumatism (EULAR)/European Renal Association-European Dialysis and Transplant Association (ERA-EDTA) recommendations (16) and relies upon cytotoxic/immunosuppressive agents or biologic therapies as well as corticosteroids, which, while life saving, may all be associated with significant side effects or toxicity. As such, therapy is carefully titrated to the intensity of the disease. In this context, therapy may be divided into an induction of disease remission phase, in which more intensive therapy is deployed, and a maintenance of disease remission phase, in which therapy is de-escalated to that which is both necessary and sufficient to control the disease (16).

Patients are risk stratified based on whether the disease is limited or systemic, whether organ function is threatened or not, or whether the disease is life threatening or not. Special consideration is given to rapidly progressive renal failure, pulmonary haemorrhage, cardiac involvement and CNS involvement. Two clinical tools that are commonly used to help risk-stratify patients and determine the appropriate therapeutic regimen are the Five Factor Score (FFS) validated in MPA and EGPA (52) and the EUVAS classification system.

To assist with risk stratification and disease assessment, validated instruments, such as the Birmingham Vasculitis Activity Score (BVAS) allow for an objective, reproducible assessment of disease activity. The BVAS is validated for AAV, although it is more commonly used in a research setting rather than a clinical setting (53). The Vasculitis Damage Index (VDI) is a similar instrument that has been validated to reproducibly assess the non-reversible damage caused by a vasculitis (54).

DISEASE-SPECIFIC APPROACH TO MANAGEMENT

ANCA-ASSOCIATED VASCULITIS

The initial approach to remission induction in patients with early, generalized (non-organ threatening) or limited disease should include glucocorticoids and/or a moderate potency cytotoxic agent such as methotrexate, azathioprine or mycophenolate mofetil (MMF) (55–58). While limited disease usually refers to isolated upper airway disease (nasal, otic or sinus disease), other examples of limited disease might include isolated skin involvement or isolated non-cavitary pulmonary nodules (16).

Early generalized disease is defined by the presence of constitutional symptoms plus the presence of identifiable disease in one or more end organs in which the function of those organs is not immediately threatened. For example, renal involvement in which proteinuria and microscopic haematuria are found but renal function (serum creatinine <1.4 mg/dL) is preserved plus fatigue and malaise would be classified as early generalized disease. There are currently more data informing the use of methotrexate and cyclophosphamide (CYC) for induction therapy in early generalized disease than there are for other disease-modifying agents, and to date, these two agents are the preferred options for early generalized disease. However, alternative agents such as MMF and azathioprine have also been proposed for milder disease (16,56,59).

Therapy for patients with evidence of organ-threatening or life-threatening disease (generalized active disease or severe disease) has evolved greatly over time. Beginning in the early 1980s, patients with generalized active and severe disease were treated with glucocorticoids and CYC, and this regimen had been shown to be very effective compared with the poor outcomes associated with historical experience (60,61). Attempts to identify regimens that were equally (or more) effective and associated with less toxicity led investigators to study the use of intravenous (IV) CYC relative to oral CYC. While IV CYC was associated with a lower cumulative dose of drug to achieve remission and a lower rate of leukopenia, long-term relapse rates were also higher in the IV therapy group (62).

In 2010, a large randomized controlled trial (Rituximab versus Cyclophosphamide for ANCA Associated Vasculitis [RAVE]) identified that rituximab, a monoclonal antibody directed against CD20, was as efficacious as oral CYC in inducing remission in generalized active and severe ANCA-associated vasculitis (including patients with alveolar haemorrhage) and may be superior in relapsing disease (63). A second large randomized trial, published at the same time, found that rituximab was equivalent to CYC when used in conjunction with standard glucocorticoid therapy for ANCA-associated vasculitis with renal involvement (64). As such, rituximab, in conjunction with oral corticosteroids, now also represents standard first-line therapy for the treatment of generalized active and severe ANCA-associated vasculitis. Again, it should be emphasized that the treating clinician should be very familiar with the management of vasculitis including the dosing and administration of the medications, drug-specific monitoring required for each medication, and their potential side effects.

For patients with severe disease, as defined by renal failure (serum creatinine >5.7 mg/dL), DAH, or severe cardiac or CNS involvement, it is recommended that patients undergo prompt plasma exchange in conjunction with intravenous corticosteroids and the aforementioned immunosuppressive therapy (16,65). This recommendation is informed by the Methylprednisolone as Adjunctive Therapy for Severe Renal Vasculitis (MEPEX) study in which patients with severe renal impairment were randomized to plasma exchange or IV steroids in addition to oral steroids and cytotoxic therapy. The group that received plasma exchange in addition to corticosteroids and cytotoxic therapy had improved rates of dialysis-free survival. A case series evaluating this strategy in patients with DAH further suggested that this strategy was also effective in that severely affected patient population (65). That said, while the short-term results of the MEPEX trial were certainly encouraging, the long-term benefits of incorporating plasma exchange into the treatment regimen were less clear (66). As such, the efficacy of plasma exchange is being re-assessed in the current, ongoing PEXIVAS study (67).

REMISSION MAINTENANCE

Once patients achieve a clinical disease remission in which there is no further ongoing evidence of disease activity, the immunosuppressive regimen is then transitioned to a more moderate 'maintenance' regimen. For remission maintenance, EULAR/ERA-EDTA recommends a combination of either azathioprine, fixed schedule rituximab, methotrexate, leflunomide or MMF plus a low dose of oral corticosteroid that is eventually tapered to off (16,68–71). In general, azathioprine is the preferred first-line agent, although a case can also be made for methotrexate (72). Mycophenolate mofetil has its share of proponents for more mild disease, but a head-to-head clinical trial found azathioprine to be more effective at maintenance of disease remission than MMF (73). Fixed-dose rituximab, administered every 4 or 6 months, also has gained traction in recent years, and the currently enrolling RITAZAREM trial (An International, Open-label, Randomized Controlled Trial Comparing Rituximab with Azathioprine as Maintenance Therapy in Relapsing ANCA-associated Vasculitis) is actively comparing fixed schedule rituximab (1 g IV every 4 months) with oral azathioprine (2 mg/kg/day) to determine which of these two strategies is more effective and/or better tolerated.

Patients generally require at least 2 years of maintenance therapy after remission in order to avoid premature disease relapse. The optimal duration of maintenance therapy remains unknown, but the REMAIN study (Randomized Trial of Prolonged Remission-Maintenance Therapy in Systemic Vasculitis), which compares 2 years of maintenance therapy with 4 years of maintenance therapy, is currently undergoing data analysis and should help inform our understanding of the duration of therapy.

MONITORING AND LONGITUDINAL CARE

While much attention is focused on the pharmacologic agents used to induce and maintain disease remission in vasculitis, the bedside clinician also needs to address the comprehensive care needs and longitudinal monitoring of the vasculitis patient. Drug-specific monitoring with serial clinical and laboratory assessment should be employed for any patient maintained on an immunosuppressive or cytotoxic agent. *Pneumocystis jirovecii* (PJP) prophylaxis should be considered in any patient on moderate-to-high-dose immunosuppressive therapy. Careful attention to bone health, vaccination status, musculoskeletal conditioning, nutrition, sleep hygiene and co-morbid medical conditions can improve functionality and quality of life in the vasculitis patient.

Patients with vasculitis are at risk for disease relapse, and it is estimated that between one-third and two-thirds of patients will suffer one or more relapses of their disease, with relapse being more common in GPA than MPA or EGPA. As such, prospective monitoring for evidence of disease recurrence is important, and tools such as the BVAS and VDI, mentioned above, can be helpful in objectively documenting serial assessments. That said, disease recurrence is only one potential explanation for any new signs or symptoms in a patient with a history of vasculitis. Infection, drug toxicity and venous thromboembolic disease all need to be considered and excluded when a patient develops clinical deterioration. Indeed, infection (rather than disease recurrence) is the most common cause of death in patients with vasculitis (74). Also, the bedside clinician needs to recall that patients may still develop diseases and conditions unrelated to the underlying vasculitis or its therapy.

SLE AND APLS SYNDROME

As in AAV, the therapy for DAH in the context of SLE and APLS consists of aggressive and comprehensive supportive care, plasma exchange and immunosuppression that is similar to that for DAH secondary to ANCA-associated vasculitis. The role of plasma exchange in DAH in the context of SLE is less well defined but appears to be used in at least one-third of patients with DAH based upon a recent systematic review (75). Glucocorticoids and cCYC remain the mainstay of pharmacologic treatment for DAH secondary to SLE and APLS (23). Case reports have also suggested that rituximab in conjunction with intravenous immunoglobulin therapy may be a possible alternative therapy (76). In APLS, given the mechanism of action, rituximab has been gaining favour as a possible therapeutic agent as well. When anti-phospholipid antibody syndrome is catastrophic and patients have both thrombotic and haemorrhagic complications, anticoagulation should be maintained, as much as possible, due to the life-threatening risk of concomitant thrombosis, but this may not always be feasible.

ANTI-GBM DISEASE

The preferred therapy for anti-GBM disease is plasma exchange, glucocorticoids and CYC in the same doses as outlined for AAV (77,78). Again there have been several case reports of successful treatment with rituximab, and while rituximab has been gaining favour with clinicians, further clinical trials would be of great help in informing these complex treatment decisions (79).

Clinical case

A young adult male developed problematic sinus congestion characterized by worsening sinus pain, congestion and, ultimately, epistaxis. He also noted a frequent sensation of fluid in his ears. His physician prescribed multiple courses of antimicrobial therapy for presumed sinus infection, but his symptoms persisted. Several months later, the patient developed diffuse body aches, fever, progressive cough and haemoptysis. Blood testing revealed a positive PR3 and c-ANCA. Neither urinalysis with sediment examination nor renal function (serum creatinine) suggested renal involvement. A tissue biopsy of his nasal disease was consistent with vasculitis. As such, the patient was diagnosed with granulomatosis with polyangiitis based upon a compelling clinical phenotype, positive serology and a compatible biopsy. His disease was risk stratified as generalized active disease.

Therapy was initiated with oral glucocorticoids and an induction course of rituximab. Unfortunately, he developed an allergic reaction to rituximab with dyspnoea and hives, and his induction therapy was transitioned to CYC. Given the known potential side effects of CYC, the patient performed sperm banking and was monitored closely with serial complete blood counts and urinalysis.

After disease remission was induced, he was transitioned to azathioprine for maintenance therapy, which he tolerated well. He regularly used sinus irrigation with budesonide as well as mupirocin to control his sinus symptoms. Audiometry revealed conductive hearing loss and hearing aides were introduced. He remained on Bactrim for PJP prophylaxis and was vaccinated against influenza and pneumonia. Baseline laboratory testing, bone mineral density testing, an electrocardiogram and an echocardiogram were obtained, and he was followed regularly by a multidisciplinary team that included rheumatologists, pulmonologists and otolaryngologists.

At his 18-month visit he reported difficulty breathing while in the supine position. He felt like his breathing had become particularly audible at night and with exercise. This was associated with some dysphagia and ear fullness. Fiberoptic laryngoscopy revealed mild subglottic stenosis that was treated with CO_2 laser excision, balloon dilation and a Kenalog 40 injection. After therapy, he immediately felt that his breathing had improved, and the sensation of audible breathing was resolved. However, repeat imaging done at that time revealed an increase in the size of a cavitary lesion within the posterior aspect of the left upper lobe (Figure 20.2). His prednisone dose was accordingly increased. After carefully weighing the alternatives by which disease remission might be re-induced and the pros, cons, risks and benefits of each approach were

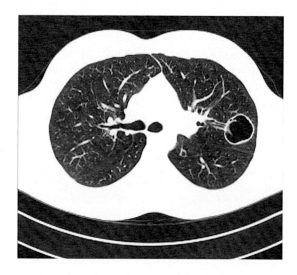

Figure 20.2 High resolution computed tomography image of the chest demonstrating an enlarging left upper lobe cavitary lesion.

discussed, the patient was carefully de-sensitized to rituximab with expert allergy/immunology oversight, and an induction course of rituximab was successfully administered. The azathioprine was continued at a lower dose, the prednisone was weaned to a low (but non-zero) dose and PJP prophylaxis was continued.

The patient's maintenance therapy consists of fixed-schedule rituximab infusions, azathioprine and low-dose prednisone. He returns to clinic every 3 months for a detailed clinical examination (including BVAS scoring), blood work, urinalysis and pulmonary physiology. He is followed collaboratively by rheumatology, allergy/immunology, otolaryngology and pulmonology consultants, and his prednisone is being weaned as tolerated.

REFERENCES

1. Zamora MR, Warner ML, Tuder R, Schwarz MI. Diffuse alveolar hemorrhage and systemic lupus erythematosus. Clinical presentation, histology, survival, and outcome. *Medicine*. 1997;76(3):192–202.
2. Kalra A, Yokogawa N, Raja H, Palaniswamy C, Desai P, Zanotti-Cavazzoni SL et al. Hydralazine-induced pulmonary-renal syndrome: A case report. *Am J Ther*. 2012;19(4):e136–8.

3. Uysal E, Cevik E, Solak S, Acar YA, Yalimol M. A life-threatening complication of warfarin therapy in ED: Diffuse alveolar hemorrhage. *Am J Emerg Med.* 2014;32(6):690e3–4.

4. Ph Bonniaud NB, A Fanton, C Camus, N Favrolt, M Guerriaud, L Jacquet. Pneumotox On Line www.pneumotox.com: Department of Pulmonary Medicine and Intensive Care, University Hospital Dijon France; 2016.

5. Martinez AJ, Maltby JD, Hurst DJ. Thrombotic thrombocytopenic purpura seen as pulmonary hemorrhage. *Arch Intern Med.* 1983;143(9):1818–20.

6. Robboy SJ, Minna JD, Colman RW, Birndorf NI, Lopas H. Pulmonary hemorrhage syndrome as a manifestation of disseminated intravascular coagulation: Analysis of ten cases. *Chest.* 1973;63(5):718–21.

7. Meyer KC, Raghu G, Baughman RP, Brown KK, Costabel U, du Bois RM et al. An official American Thoracic Society clinical practice guideline: The clinical utility of bronchoalveolar lavage cellular analysis in interstitial lung disease. *Am J Respir Crit Care Med.* 2012;185(9):1004–14.

8. Lazor R, Bigay-Game L, Cottin V, Cadranel J, Decaux O, Fellrath JM et al. Alveolar hemorrhage in anti-basement membrane antibody disease: A series of 28 cases. *Medicine.* 2007;86(3):181–93.

9. Cortese G, Nicali R, Placido R, Gariazzo G, Anro P. Radiological aspects of diffuse alveolar haemorrhage. *La Radiologia Medica.* 2008;113(1):16–28.

10. Buschman DL, Ballard R. Progressive massive fibrosis associated with idiopathic pulmonary hemosiderosis. *Chest.* 1993;104(1):293–5.

11. Schwarz MI, Mortenson RL, Colby TV, Waldron JA, Lynch DA, Hutt MP et al. Pulmonary capillaritis. The association with progressive irreversible airflow limitation and hyperinflation. *Am Rev Respir Dis.* 1993;148(2):507–11.

12. Colby TV, Fukuoka J, Ewaskow SP, Helmers R, Leslie KO. Pathologic approach to pulmonary hemorrhage. *Ann Diagn Pathol.* 2001; 5(5):309–19.

13. Travis WD, Colby TV, Lombard C, Carpenter HA. A clinicopathologic study of 34 cases of diffuse pulmonary hemorrhage with lung biopsy confirmation. *Am J Surg Pathol.* 1990;14(12):1112–25.

14. Kligerman SJ, Franks TJ, Galvin JR. From the radiologic pathology archives: Organization and fibrosis as a response to lung injury in diffuse alveolar damage, organizing pneumonia, and acute fibrinous and organizing pneumonia. *Radiographics.* 2013;33(7):1951–75.

15. Greco A, De Virgilio A, Rizzo MI, Gallo A, Magliulo G, Fusconi M et al. Microscopic polyangiitis: Advances in diagnostic and therapeutic approaches. *Autoimmun Rev.* 2015;14(9):837–44.

16. Yates M, Watts RA, Bajema IM, Cid MC, Crestani B, Hauser T et al. EULAR/ERA-EDTA recommendations for the management of ANCA-associated vasculitis. *Ann Rheum Dis.* 2016;75(9):1583–94.

17. Guillevin L, Durand-Gasselin B, Cevallos R, Gayraud M, Lhote F, Callard P et al. Microscopic polyangiitis: Clinical and laboratory findings in eighty-five patients. *Arthritis Rheum.* 1999;42(3):421–30.

18. Wilke L, Prince-Fiocco M, Fiocco GP. Microscopic polyangiitis: A large single-center series. *J Clin Rheumatol.* 2014;20(4):179–82.

19. Comarmond C, Cacoub P. Granulomatosis with polyangiitis (Wegener): Clinical aspects and treatment. *Autoimmun Rev.* 2014;13(11):1121–5.

20. Cordier JF, Valeyre D, Guillevin L, Loire R, Brechot JM. Pulmonary Wegener's granulomatosis. A clinical and imaging study of 77 cases. *Chest.* 1990;97(4):906–12.

21. Jennings CA, King TE, Jr., Tuder R, Cherniack RM, Schwarz MI. Diffuse alveolar hemorrhage with underlying isolated, pauci-immune pulmonary capillaritis. *Am J Respir Crit Care Med.* 1997;155(3):1101–9.

22. Khorashadi L, Wu CC, Betancourt SL, Carter BW. Idiopathic pulmonary haemosiderosis: Spectrum of thoracic imaging findings in the adult patient. *Clin Radiol.* 2015;70(5):459–65.

23. Andrade C, Mendonca T, Farinha F, Correia J, Marinho A, Almeida I et al.

Alveolar hemorrhage in systemic lupus erythematosus: A cohort review. *Lupus*. 2016;25(1):75–80.

24. Miyakis S, Lockshin MD, Atsumi T, Branch DW, Brey RL, Cervera R et al. International consensus statement on an update of the classification criteria for definite antiphospholipid syndrome (APS). *J Thromb Haemost*. 2006;4(2):295–306.

25. Cartin-Ceba R, Peikert T, Ashrani A, Keogh K, Wylam ME, Ytterberg S et al. Primary antiphospholipid syndrome-associated diffuse alveolar hemorrhage. *Arthr Care Res*. 2014;66(2):301–10.

26. Yachoui R, Sehgal R, Amlani B, Goldberg JW. Antiphospholipid antibodies-associated diffuse alveolar hemorrhage. *Semin Arthritis Rheum*. 2015;44(6):652–7.

27. Troxell ML, Houghton DC. Atypical anti-glomerular basement membrane disease. *Clin Kidney J*. 2016;9(2):211–21.

28. Pusey CD. Anti-glomerular basement membrane disease. *Kidney Int*. 2003;64(4):1535–50.

29. Lahmer T, Heemann U. Anti-glomerular basement membrane antibody disease: A rare autoimmune disorder affecting the kidney and the lung. *Autoimmun Rev*. 2012;12(2):169–73.

30. Xi-Yuan C, Jin-Ming S, Xiao-Jun H. Idiopathic pulmonary hemosiderosis in adults: Review of cases reported in the latest 15 years. *Clin Respir J*. 2015.

31. Yusuff H, Malagon I, Robson K, Parmar J, Hamilton P, Falter F. Extracorporeal membrane oxygenation for life-threatening ANCA-positive pulmonary capillaritis. A review of UK experience. *Heart Lung Vessels*. 2015;7(2):159–67.

32. Abrams D, Agerstrand CL, Biscotti M, Burkart KM, Bacchetta M, Brodie D. Extracorporeal membrane oxygenation in the management of diffuse alveolar hemorrhage. *ASAIO J*. 2015;61(2):216–8.

33. Rathi M, Pinto B, Dhooria A, Sagar V, Mittal T, Rajan R et al. Impact of renal involvement on survival in ANCA-associated vasculitis. *Int Urol Nephrol*. 2016;48(9):1477–82.

34. Chung SA, Seo P. Microscopic polyangiitis. *Rheum Dis Clin North Am*. 2010;36(3):545–58.

35. Pagnoux C, Mahr A, Cohen P, Guillevin L. Presentation and outcome of gastrointestinal involvement in systemic necrotizing vasculitides: Analysis of 62 patients with polyarteritis nodosa, microscopic polyangiitis, Wegener granulomatosis, Churg-Strauss syndrome, or rheumatoid arthritis-associated vasculitis. *Medicine*. 2005;84(2):115–28.

36. Hattori N, Mori K, Misu K, Koike H, Ichimura M, Sobue G. Mortality and morbidity in peripheral neuropathy associated Churg-Strauss syndrome and microscopic polyangiitis. *J Rheumatol*. 2002;29(7):1408–14.

37. Zhang W, Zhou G, Shi Q, Zhang X, Zeng XF, Zhang FC. Clinical analysis of nervous system involvement in ANCA-associated systemic vasculitides. *Clin Exp Rheumatol*. 2009;27(1 Suppl 52):S65–9.

38. Jennette JC, Falk RJ, Bacon PA, Basu N, Cid MC, Ferrario F et al. 2012 revised International Chapel Hill Consensus Conference nomenclature of vasculitides. *Arthritis Rheum*. 2013;65(1):1–11.

39. Fries JF, Hunder GG, Bloch DA, Michel BA, Arend WP, Calabrese LH et al. The American College of Rheumatology 1990 criteria for the classification of vasculitis. Summary. *Arthritis Rheum*. 1990;33(8):1135–6.

40. Comarmond C, Crestani B, Tazi A, Hervier B, Adam-Marchand S, Nunes H et al. Pulmonary fibrosis in antineutrophil cytoplasmic antibodies (ANCA)-associated vasculitis: A series of 49 patients and review of the literature. *Medicine*. 2014;93(24):340–9.

41. Villiger PM, Guillevin L. Microscopic polyangiitis: Clinical presentation. *Autoimmun Rev*. 2010;9(12):812–9.

42. Cordova-Sanchez BM, Mejia-Vilet JM, Morales-Buenrostro LE, Loyola-Rodriguez G, Uribe-Uribe NO, Correa-Rotter R. Clinical presentation and outcome prediction of clinical, serological, and histopathological classification schemes in ANCA-associated vasculitis with renal involvement. *Clin Rheumatol*. 2016;35(7):1805–16.

43. Lally L, Lebovics RS, Huang WT, Spiera RF. Effectiveness of rituximab for the

otolaryngologic manifestations of granulomatosis with polyangiitis (Wegener's). *Arthritis Care Res.* 2014;66(9):1403–9.

44. Martinez Del Pero M, Jayne D, Chaudhry A, Sivasothy P, Jani P. Long-term outcome of airway stenosis in granulomatosis with polyangiitis (Wegener granulomatosis): An observational study. *JAMA Otolaryngol Head Neck Surg.* 2014;140(11):1038–44.

45. Greco A, Rizzo MI, De Virgilio A, Gallo A, Fusconi M, Ruoppolo G et al. Churg-Strauss syndrome. *Autoimmun Rev.* 2015;14(4):341–8.

46. Santos-Pinheiro F, Li Y. Eosinophilic granulomatosis with polyangiitis (Churg-Strauss syndrome) presenting with polyneuropathy—A case series. *J Clin Neuromuscul Dis.* 2015;16(3):125–30.

47. Lanham JG, Elkon KB, Pusey CD, Hughes GR. Systemic vasculitis with asthma and eosinophilia: A clinical approach to the Churg-Strauss syndrome. *Medicine.* 1984;63(2):65–81.

48. Groh M, Pagnoux C, Baldini C, Bel E, Bottero P, Cottin V et al. Eosinophilic granulomatosis with polyangiitis (Churg-Strauss) (EGPA) Consensus Task Force recommendations for evaluation and management. *Eur J Intern Med.* 2015;26(7):545–53.

49. Sinico RA, Di Toma L, Maggiore U, Bottero P, Radice A, Tosoni C et al. Prevalence and clinical significance of antineutrophil cytoplasmic antibodies in Churg-Strauss syndrome. *Arthritis Rheum.* 2005;52(9):2926–35.

50. Katzenstein AL. Diagnostic features and differential diagnosis of Churg-Strauss syndrome in the lung. A review. *Am J Clin Pathol.* 2000;114(5):767–72.

51. Mukhtyar C, Flossmann O, Hellmich B, Bacon P, Cid M, Cohen-Tervaert JW et al. Outcomes from studies of antineutrophil cytoplasm antibody associated vasculitis: A systematic review by the European League Against Rheumatism systemic vasculitis task force. *Ann Rheum Dis.* 2008;67(7):1004–10.

52. Guillevin L, Lhote F, Gayraud M, Cohen P, Jarrousse B, Lortholary O et al. Prognostic factors in polyarteritis nodosa and Churg-Strauss syndrome. A prospective study in 342 patients. *Medicine.* 1996;75(1):17–28.

53. Mukhtyar C, Lee R, Brown D, Carruthers D, Dasgupta B, Dubey S et al. Modification and validation of the Birmingham Vasculitis Activity Score (version 3). *Ann Rheum Dis.* 2009;68(12):1827–32.

54. Exley AR, Bacon PA, Luqmani RA, Kitas GD, Gordon C, Savage CO et al. Development and initial validation of the Vasculitis Damage Index for the standardized clinical assessment of damage in the systemic vasculitides. *Arthritis Rheum.* 1997;40(2):371–80.

55. De Groot K, Rasmussen N, Bacon PA, Tervaert JW, Feighery C, Gregorini G et al. Randomized trial of cyclophosphamide versus methotrexate for induction of remission in early systemic antineutrophil cytoplasmic antibody-associated vasculitis. *Arthritis Rheum.* 2005;52(8):2461–9.

56. Faurschou M, Westman K, Rasmussen N, de Groot K, Flossmann O, Hoglund P et al. Brief report: Long-term outcome of a randomized clinical trial comparing methotrexate to cyclophosphamide for remission induction in early systemic antineutrophil cytoplasmic antibody-associated vasculitis. *Arthritis Rheum.* 2012;64(10):3472–7.

57. Hu W, Liu C, Xie H, Chen H, Liu Z, Li L. Mycophenolate mofetil versus cyclophosphamide for inducing remission of ANCA vasculitis with moderate renal involvement. *Nephrol Dial Transplant.* 2008;23(4):1307–12.

58. Han F, Liu G, Zhang X, Li X, He Q, He X et al. Effects of mycophenolate mofetil combined with corticosteroids for induction therapy of microscopic polyangiitis. *Am J Nephrol.* 2011;33(2):185–92.

59. Silva F, Specks U, Kalra S, Hogan MC, Leung N, Sethi S et al. Mycophenolate mofetil for induction and maintenance of remission in microscopic polyangiitis with mild to moderate renal involvement—A prospective, open-label pilot trial. *Clin J Am Soc Nephrol.* 2010;5(3):445–53.

60. Novack SN, Pearson CM. Cyclophosphamide therapy in Wegener's granulomatosis. *N Engl J Med.* 1971;284(17):938–42.

61. Fauci AS, Wolff SM. Wegener's granulomatosis: Studies in eighteen patients

and a review of the literature. *Medicine*. 1973;52(6):535–61.

62. Harper L, Morgan MD, Walsh M, Hoglund P, Westman K, Flossmann O et al. Pulse versus daily oral cyclophosphamide for induction of remission in ANCA-associated vasculitis: Long-term follow-up. *Ann Rheum Dis*. 2012;71(6):955–60.

63. Stone JH, Merkel PA, Spiera R, Seo P, Langford CA, Hoffman GS et al. Rituximab versus cyclophosphamide for ANCA-associated vasculitis. *N Engl J Med*. 2010;363(3):221–32.

64. Jones RB, Tervaert JW, Hauser T, Luqmani R, Morgan MD, Peh CA et al. Rituximab versus cyclophosphamide in ANCA-associated renal vasculitis. *N Engl J Med*. 2010;363(3):211–20.

65. Klemmer PJ, Chalermskulrat W, Reif MS, Hogan SL, Henke DC, Falk RJ. Plasmapheresis therapy for diffuse alveolar hemorrhage in patients with small-vessel vasculitis. *Am J Kidney Dis*. 2003;42(6):1149–53.

66. Walsh M, Casian A, Flossmann O, Westman K, Hoglund P, Pusey C et al. Long-term follow-up of patients with severe ANCA-associated vasculitis comparing plasma exchange to intravenous methylprednisolone treatment is unclear. *Kidney Int*. 2013;84(2):397–402.

67. Walsh M, Merkel PA, Peh CA, Szpirt W, Guillevin L, Pusey CD et al. Plasma exchange and glucocorticoid dosing in the treatment of anti-neutrophil cytoplasm antibody associated vasculitis (PEXIVAS): Protocol for a randomized controlled trial. *Trials*. 2013;14:73.

68. Jayne D, Rasmussen N, Andrassy K, Bacon P, Tervaert JW, Dadoniene J et al. A randomized trial of maintenance therapy for vasculitis associated with antineutrophil cytoplasmic autoantibodies. *N Engl J Med*. 2003;349(1):36–44.

69. Slot MC, Tervaert JW, Boomsma MM, Stegeman CA. Positive classic antineutrophil cytoplasmic antibody (C-ANCA) titer at switch to azathioprine therapy associated with relapse in proteinase 3-related vasculitis. *Arthritis Rheum*. 2004;51(2):269–73.

70. Langford CA, Talar-Williams C, Barron KS, Sneller MC. Use of a cyclophosphamide-induction methotrexate-maintenance regimen for the treatment of Wegener's granulomatosis: Extended follow-up and rate of relapse. *Am J Med*. 2003;114(6):463–9.

71. Guillevin L, Pagnoux C, Karras A, Khouatra C, Aumaitre O, Cohen P et al. Rituximab versus azathioprine for maintenance in ANCA-associated vasculitis. *N Engl J Med*. 2014;371(19):1771–80.

72. Puechal X, Pagnoux C, Perrodeau E, Hamidou M, Boffa JJ, Kyndt X et al. Long-term outcomes among participants in the WEGENT Trial of Remission-Maintenance Therapy for Granulomatosis With Polyangiitis (Wegener's) or Microscopic Polyangiitis. *Arthritis Rheumatol*. 2016;68(3):690–701.

73. Hiemstra TF, Walsh M, Mahr A, Savage CO, de Groot K, Harper L et al. Mycophenolate mofetil vs azathioprine for remission maintenance in antineutrophil cytoplasmic antibody-associated vasculitis: A randomized controlled trial. *JAMA*. 2010;304(21):2381–8.

74. Kronbichler A, Jayne DR, Mayer G. Frequency, risk factors and prophylaxis of infection in ANCA-associated vasculitis. *Eur J Clin Invest*. 2015;45(3):346–68.

75. Ednalino C, Yip J, Carsons SE. Systematic review of diffuse alveolar hemorrhage in systemic lupus erythematosus: Focus on outcome and therapy. *J Clin Rheumatol*. 2015;21(6):305–10.

76. Martis N, Blanchouin E, Lazdunski R, Lechtman S, Robert A, Hyvernat H et al. A therapeutic challenge: Catastrophic anti-phospholipid syndrome with diffuse alveolar haemorrhage. *Immunol Res*. 2015;62(2):222–4.

77. Levy JB, Turner AN, Rees AJ, Pusey CD. Long-term outcome of anti-glomerular basement membrane antibody disease treated with plasma exchange and immunosuppression. *Ann Intern Med*. 2001;134(11):1033–42.

78. Kaplan AA. The use of apheresis in immune renal disorders. *Ther Apher Dial*. 2003;7(2):165–72.

79. Syeda UA, Singer NG, Magrey M. Anti-glomerular basement membrane antibody disease treated with rituximab: A case-based review. *Semin Arthritis Rheum*. 2013;42(6):567–72.

21

Lymphangioleiomyomatosis and other cystic interstitial lung diseases

AMANDA T GOODWIN AND WILLIAM YC CHANG

BACKGROUND

The cystic interstitial lung diseases (ILDs) have varying aetiologies and clinical manifestations as shown in Table 21.1. They result from a variety of pathophysiological mechanisms, but impaired gas exchange, hypoxaemia, and respiratory failure are common features to all cystic ILDs. This chapter reviews these conditions, focussing on lymphangioleiomyomatosis (LAM).

TYPES OF CYSTIC ILDs

LYMPHANGIOLEIOMYOMATOSIS

In LAM, the lungs and lymphatics are infiltrated by LAM cells which are smooth muscle-like cells with inactivating mutations in the tuberous sclerosis genes, *TSC1* (chromosome 16) or *TSC2* (chromosome 9), which encode the proteins

hamartin and tuberin, respectively. Dysfunction of these proteins constitutively activates the serine–threonine kinase mammalian target of rapamycin (mTOR), causing inappropriate proliferation, migration and invasion of LAM cells (1). LAM has been postulated to represent a low-grade neoplasm originating from a single progenitor cell (2,3).

LAM exists in two forms: sporadic (S-LAM) and tuberous sclerosis complex-associated (TSC-LAM). In S-LAM, two somatic *TSC* mutations occur in the progenitor cell, which propagates these mutations to its descendants. Conversely, in TSC-LAM there is a germline *TSC* mutation, and a subsequent somatic mutation provides the 'second hit' required for uncontrolled mTOR activity (Figure 21.1). *TSC1* and *TSC2* mutations occur in TSC-LAM, whereas *TSC2* mutations cause most S-LAM cases (4).

LAM cells destroy the lung parenchyma by disrupting the balance of proteolytic enzymes, e.g. matrix metalloproteinases (MMPs), and their inhibitors (5–9). LAM cells obstruct lymphatic vessels, causing lymphangioleiomyomas, chylous

Table 21.1 Classification of cystic ILDs

Neoplastic	Lymphangioleiomyomatosis
	Non-Langerhans cell histiocytosis, e.g. Erdheim–Chester disease
	Primary and metastatic neoplasms
Congenital	Birt–Hogg–Dubé syndrome
	Proteus syndrome
	Neurofibromatosis
	Congenital airway malformation
Lymphoproliferative	Lymphocytic interstitial pneumonia
	Light-chain deposition disease
	Follicular bronchiolitis
	Amyloidosis
Infectious	See Table 21.2
ILD associated	Desquamative interstitial pneumonia
	Hypersensitivity pneumonitis
Smoking related	Pulmonary Langerhans cell histiocytosis
	Desquamative interstitial pneumonia
	Respiratory bronchiolitis
Cyst mimics	Emphysema
	Bronchiectasis
	Honeycombing
	Loculated pneumothorax

Source: Adapted from Gupta 2015 *Am J Respir Crit Care Med.* 191(12):1354–66. Copyright 2016, with permission from American Thoracic Society.

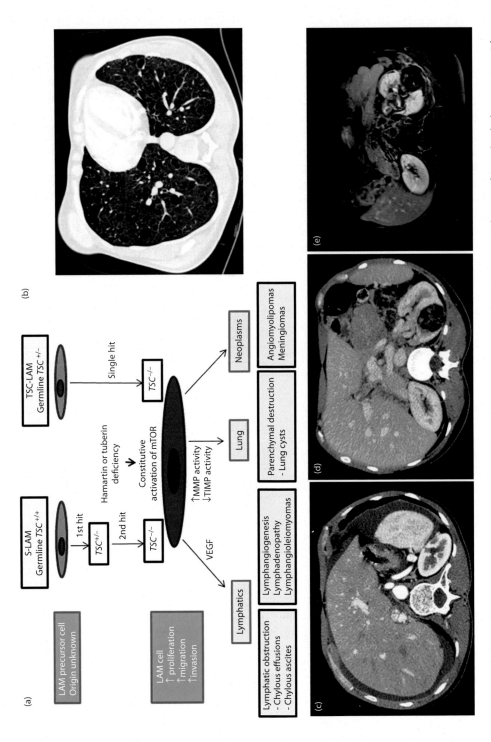

Figure 21.1 The pathophysiology and imaging features of LAM. **(a)** Pathophysiological mechanisms of LAM. **(b)** Multiple lung cysts with normal intervening lung parenchyma. **(c)** Chylous ascites in abdominal LAM involvement. **(d)** A large left renal angiomyolipoma shown on CT. **(e)** A large left renal angiomyolipoma shown on MRI. (Abbreviations: LAM = lymphangioleiomyomatosis; MMP = matrix metalloproteinase; mTOR = mammalian target of rapamycin; TIMP = tissue inhibitor of metalloproteinases; TSC = tuberous sclerosis complex; VEGF = vascular endothelial growth factor.)

pleural effusions and ascites (10). Vascular endo-thelial growth factors (VEGFs) stimulate lymphangiogenesis (11,12). Oestrogens may drive the pathogenesis of LAM (13–17), although the exact mechanisms are unknown.

PULMONARY LANGERHANS CELL HISTIOCYTOSIS

Langerhans cell histiocytosis (LCH) is characterized by the abnormal proliferation and infiltration of tissues by Langerhans cells (LCs). The isolated pulmonary variant of LCH (PLCH) is also known as histiocytosis X and Langerhans cell granulomatosis.

LCs are of monocyte–macrophage lineage and present antigens to T lymphocytes to stimulate an immune response (18). In the lung, the activation and persistence of LCs, and recruitment of other immune cells, generate nodules (1). Subsequent MMP production mediates bronchiolar destruction and cystic change (1,19).

PLCH is strongly associated with smoking. Abnormal LC activity may occur secondary to the recognition of tobacco components as foreign antigens (20), immunomodulatory cytokine production (1,21–24) or smoking-induced epithelial stress in susceptible individuals (18,25,26).

A mutation in the proto-oncogene *BRAF* (BRAF V600E) is present in some PLCH patients, suggesting clonal proliferation of LCs in some individuals (27). The same mutation has also been found in other forms of LCH (28–31), implying a common mechanism between diffuse and localized variants.

BIRT–HOGG–DUBÉ SYNDROME

Birt–Hogg–Dubé syndrome (BHDS) is an autosomal dominant disorder caused by folliculin gene mutations (*FLCN*, 17p11.2) (32). *FLCN* is a tumour suppressor gene, and mutations cause dysregulated mTOR signalling and abnormal cell growth, resulting in hair follicle tumours, renal neoplasms and pulmonary cysts (33–35).

LYMPHOCYTIC INTERSTITIAL PNEUMONIA

Lymphocytic interstitial pneumonia (LIP) is characterized by lymphocytic infiltration of the lung parenchyma and alveoli (35). Ischaemia secondary to vascular obstruction, post-obstructive bronchial

ectasia and bronchiolar compression cause cyst formation (35,36).

LIGHT-CHAIN DEPOSITION DISEASE

Light-chain deposition disease (LCDD) is a lymphoproliferative disorder characterized by immunoglobulin light-chain deposition in the tissues (35). Lung cysts occur with pulmonary involvement (37).

EPIDEMIOLOGY OF CYSTIC ILDS

LYMPHANGIOLEIOMYOMATOSIS

LAM occurs almost exclusively in women, although cases in men and children have been reported (38). LAM usually presents in the fourth decade (39,40). LAM is rare, affecting 3.4–7.8 per million women in Europe and the United States (41), and affects all ethnic groups (39).

PULMONARY LANGERHANS CELL HISTIOCYTOSIS

PLCH is rare, affecting 0.07–0.27 people per 100,000 population (42). PLCH usually affects those with a significant personal or second-hand smoking history, aged 20–40 years with an equal gender distribution (25,43).

BIRT–HOGG–DUBÉ SYNDROME

BHDS is a rare inherited condition that affects both genders equally (32).

LYMPHOCYTIC INTERSTITIAL PNEUMONIA

LIP presents in the fifth or sixth decade, with a female preponderence (44–46).

LIGHT-CHAIN DEPOSITION DISEASE

LCDD is rare, predominantly affecting females (47).

HISTORY AND EXAMINATION

GENERAL FEATURES

The clinical history and examination often indicate the likely diagnosis as shown in Table 21.2.

Table 21.2 Features of cystic ILDs

Clinical features	Disease
Pneumothorax	Lymphangioleiomyomatosis
	Langerhans cell histiocytosis
	Birt–Hogg–Dubé syndrome
Gradual-onset dyspnoea and cough (± pneumothoraces)	Desquamative interstitial pneumonia
	Lymphocytic interstitial pneumonia
	Hypersensitivity pneumonitis
Predominantly extra-pulmonary features	Light-chain deposition disease
	Amyloidosis
	Neurofibromatosis type 1
Infective symptoms	*Pneumocystis jirovecii* pneumonia
	Staphylococcal pneumonia
	Recurrent respiratory papillomatosis
	Fungal, e.g. coccidioidomycosis
	Parasitic, e.g. *Echinococcus granulosus*
Incidental finding of pulmonary cysts in an adult ± recurrent pneumonia	Bronchogenic cysts
	Pulmonary sequestration
	Congenital airway malformation

Source: Adapted from Ha D, Yadav R, Mazzone PJ. *Cleve Clin J Med.* 2015;82:115–127, with permission.

Key features include dyspnoea, pneumothoraces (particularly bilateral or recurrent), infective symptoms and extrapulmonary manifestations (48). Family and smoking histories are essential. Physical examination should assess for respiratory, skin and connective tissue diseases. Signs of pulmonary hypertension and cor pulmonale may occur in advanced disease (18).

Lymphangioleiomyomatosis

LAM commonly presents with dyspnoea and pneumothoraces (39,40). Other features include chylous pleural effusions, wheeze, cough, haemoptysis and chyloptysis (40). Half will have renal angiomyolipomas (AMLs) (49), and all patients should have abdominal imaging to look for these. AMLs may cause abdominal pain and renal impairment secondary to renal architectural distortion (50). Spontaneous bleeding may occur, particularly with large AMLs. Large and multiple AMLs are more common in TSC-LAM than S-LAM (50).

Abdominal swelling, nausea and urinary symptoms occur due to abdominal and pelvic lymphangioleiomyomas. Lymphangioleiomyomas have diurnal variation in size, causing variable symptoms throughout the day (51). Abdominopelvic lymphadenopathy is usually asymptomatic, but may be seen on imaging (39).

LAM carries an increased risk of meningiomas, which may present with neurological symptoms (52).

Respiratory examination in LAM is normal unless a pneumothorax or pleural effusion is present. Most patients have obstructive spirometry, but restrictive or mixed patterns can occur (39).

Fifteen percent of LAM patients have TSC (39), a genetic multiorgan condition that can also occur sporadically (53). All LAM patients should be assessed for features of TSC, including cutaneous features (subungual fibromas, facial angiofibromas, shagreen patches), epilepsy and AMLs. Women with TSC should be screened for LAM by HRCT at 18 years of age, repeated at 30–40 years if the first HRCT is negative (54).

Pulmonary Langerhans cell histiocytosis

PLCH presents with cough, dyspnoea and pneumothoraces (25); haemoptysis may also occur (25,43). Extra-pulmonary manifestations include fever, weight loss, diabetes insipidus, bone pain, abdominal pain from hepatic or splenic involvement, lymphadenopathy and skin involvement (25,26,43).

Physical examination is often normal, but may reveal inspiratory crackles. Spirometry is typically obstructive, but can follow any pattern (1), and the carbon monoxide transfer factor (TLCO) is commonly reduced (18,25,55).

Birt–Hogg–Dubé syndrome

BHDS is characterized by hair follicle tumours (fibrofolliculomas, trichodiscomas), renal tumours and pulmonary cysts. A quarter of patients with BHDS and lung cysts develop pneumothoraces, with significant recurrence rates (56). Renal cancers, which may be bilateral and multifocal, occur in over 20% of patients (57).

A personal or family history of pneumothoraces, skin lesions or renal tumours should prompt investigation for BHDS.

Lymphocytic interstitial pneumonia

LIP is associated with immune dysregulation, therefore the clinical assessment should evaluate for connective tissue diseases and immunodeficiency states (35,44). The incidence of pneumothorax is unknown (35). Spirometry commonly shows a restrictive defect and a reduced TLCO (44).

Light-chain deposition disease

LCDD typically affects the kidneys and is associated with lymphoproliferative disorders. The incidence of pneumothorax is unknown (35).

INVESTIGATIONS

The complexity of the cystic ILDs warrants a multidisciplinary approach, involving chest physicians, radiologists and pathologists. A stepwise least-invasive method is advocated, and it is often possible to make a diagnosis without tissue sampling (Table 21.3). Genetic testing may be indicated.

RADIOLOGY

High-resolution computed tomography (HRCT) is an essential diagnostic tool (Figure 21.2). An approach to image interpretation is presented here.

1. *Differentiate cysts from cyst mimics*: Cavities, malignant nodules and centrilobular emphysema can mimic lung cysts. A cyst is a round, thin-walled (<2–3 mm) area of parenchymal

lucency (58). In contrast, cavities are thick walled (>4 mm), and develop within consolidation, masses or nodules (59).

Cystic metastases may be thin walled, and should be considered in cases of extrapulmonary malignancy (59). Centrilobular emphysema can mimic cystic ILD, but does not usually have a well-defined wall (59). Honeycombing in pulmonary fibrosis and bronchiectasis can also be mistaken for cysts (58).

2. *Assess cyst features*: Cyst size, shape and distribution, and additional HRCT features, may indicate the diagnosis.

For multiple diffuse pulmonary cysts the differential diagnosis is LAM, PLCH, BHDS, LCDD. For scattered cysts with additional imaging features the differential diagnosis is LIP, desquamative interstitial pneumonia (DIP). For isolated or scattered cysts the differential diagnosis is early cystic ILD, pneumatocoele and malignancy. Isolated cysts are unusual in the cystic ILDs; therefore, alternatives should be considered.

Lymphangioleiomyomatosis

Cysts in LAM are round, thin walled and diffusely distributed, with normal intervening lung parenchyma. Cysts may involve the juxtaphrenic recesses and usually spare the apices (59,60).

Pulmonary Langerhans cell histiocytosis

Centrilobular nodules occur in early PLCH, which subsequently cavitate and coalesce to generate bizarrely shaped and unequal-sized cysts, predominantly occurring at the apices and sparing the bases (18,25,59,61,62). Ground-glass opacification is sometimes seen (18). The combination of nodules and cysts in a smoker allows a confident diagnosis of PLCH (59).

Birt–Hogg–Dubé syndrome

In BHDS, cysts are basal and sub-pleural, thin walled and often lentiform in shape (35).

Light-chain deposition disease

Features of LCDD vary from multiple diffusely distributed small cysts, to large cystic spaces alongside

Table 21.3 Diagnostic approach to cystic ILDs

Approach		LAM	PLCH	BHD	LIP	DIP	LCDD
1. History and examination	Clinical features	Female Pneumothorax Chylous effusions	Pneumothorax Smoking history	Pneumothorax	HIV, collagen vascular disorders	Smoker Dyspnoea, cough	Lymphoproliferative disorders
	Family history	TSC	No	Pneumothoraces, skin lesions, renal cancer	No	No	No
2. HRCT features	Cyst distribution	Diffuse, apices spared	Upper zone predominance, bases spared	Lower zone/ peripheral/ sub-pleural/ perivascular	Scattered, random, perivascular	Within ground-glass change	Diffuse
	Cyst characteristics	Round, thin-walled cysts	Bizarre/irregular shape, thin- and thick-walled cysts	Lentiform/ elliptical shape	Small, thin walled	Small cysts	Large, round
	Other HRCT features	Normal parenchyma between cysts	Nodules +/− cavities	–	Ground-glass opacities, nodules, interlobular septal thickening	Ground-glass opacification	Nodules abutting cyst walls
3. Biopsy	Histopathology	HMB-45 +ve LAM cells	Langerhans cells (S100- and CD1a +ve). Birbeck granules	Indistinguishable from emphysema	Lymphocytic infiltrate	Macrophages, chronic inflammation	Kappa light-chain deposition, lacks apple green birefringence
4. Other tests	Laboratory tests	Serum VEGF-D	–	–	Polyclonal dysproteinaemia	–	–
	Genetic tests	TSC1/TSC2 mutations	BRAF mutation	FLCN gene mutation	–	–	–
	Extrapulmonary features	Angiomyolipomas TSC features	Diabetes insipidus Skin lesions Lytic bone lesions	Fibrofolliculomas Renal tumours	Hepatospleno-megaly	–	Lymphoproliferative disorders, renal failure

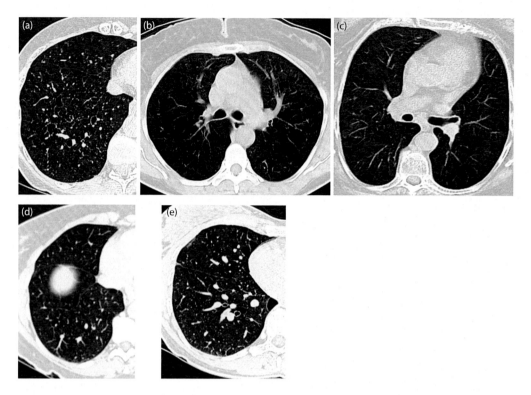

Figure 21.2 CT features of non-LAM cystic ILDs. **(a)** A case of PLCH, with nodules and irregularly shaped lung cysts. **(b)** Unequally sized lung cysts of PLCH. **(c)** A HRCT of LIP showing scattered cysts near vessels. Ground-glass change is also shown in the right lung. **(d)** Elliptically shaped cysts in BHDS. **(e)** Peripheral and sub-pleural cysts typical of BHDS.

reticulonodular opacities (35). Lung cysts in LCDD are uncommon relative to LAM and PLCH (48).

Lymphocytic interstitial pneumonia

The imaging features of LIP include ground-glass opacification, centrilobular nodules and cystic changes. Cysts occur in up to 80% of cases, may be bilateral or unilateral with a random distribution, and usually involve less than 10% of the lung parenchyma (35,46,63).

Desquamative Interstitial Pneumonia

Cysts may occur in DIP (64,65), as discussed elsewhere in this book.

HISTOPATHOLOGY

When clinical and HRCT features are not diagnostic, histological sampling via bronchoalveolar lavage (BAL), transbronchial biopsy (TBBx) or surgical lung biopsy (SLB) may be required. The

likely diagnostic yield from tissue sampling and the procedural risks should be carefully considered (35,66,67) (Table 21.4).

Lymphangioleiomyomatosis

LAM cells include myofibroblast-like, spindle-shaped and epithelioid-like forms that can be identified immunohistochemically by expression of

Table 21.4 Histological assessment of cystic ILDs

Condition	Diagnostic yield of BAL or TBBx	Consider SLB?
LAM	>60%	Yes
PLCH	30%–50%	Yes
BHDS	0%	No
DIP	Low	Yes
LIP	Low	Yes
LCDD	Low	Yes

Source: Adapted from Gupta 2015 *Am J Respir Crit Care Med.* 192(1):17–29. Copyright 2016, with permission from American Thoracic Society.

proteins including smooth muscle actin (SMA), vimentin and desmin (68,69). They have less cytoplasm and are less eosinophilic than smooth muscle cells (19). LAM cells react with the human melanoma black-45 (HMB45) monoclonal antibody, a key diagnostic feature (70). LAM cells may also express the progesterone and oestrogen receptors (19,68).

Pulmonary Langerhans cell histiocytosis

In PLCH, large numbers of LCs around the distal airways alongside variable numbers of eosinophils, lymphocytes and alveolar macrophages are seen histologically (18) (Table 21.5). LCs have pale, eosinophilic cytoplasm, indistinct cell borders and grooved nuclei with small nucleoli (1,26). Immunostaining for CD1a and CD207 and the presence of Birbeck granules on electron microscopy confirm the presence of LCs (26,71–73). PLCH lesions evolve from highly cellular nodules to paucicellular fibrotic areas (1). Venous and arterial structures often appear abnormal (74).

BAL is diagnostic if there are over 5% LCs on cell count (26,71–73). Due to the patchy nature of PLCH, TTBx has a low diagnostic yield and SLB is required if BAL is inconclusive (73,75).

Birt–Hogg–Dubé syndrome

BHDS is indistinguishable from emphysema histologically, therefore biopsy is not recommended.

Table 21.5 Diagnostic criteria for PLCH

Definitive	Presumptive
Based on clinico-pathological evidence with microscopic examination and at least one of the following immunological staining: Langerin (CD207) positivity CD1a positivity Birbeck granules	Based on clinico-radiological evidence, without biopsy: e.g. typical lesions on CT in a smoker

Source: Adapted from Girschikofsky et al. *Orphanet Journal of Rare Diseases* 2013;8:72–3, with permission.

Table 21.6 Diagnostic criteria for Birt–Hogg–Dubé syndrome

Major criteria	Minor criteria
≥5 adult onset fibrofolliculomas or trichodiscomas	Cysts: bilateral basally located lung cysts +/− spontaneous pneumothorax
FLCN mutation	Renal cancer: age <50 years, multifocal or bilateral, mixed chromophobe and oncocytic histology
	First-degree relative with BHDS

Source: Reprinted from *Lancet Oncol.*, 10(12), Menko et al., European BHD Consortium. Birt–Hogg–Dubé syndrome: Diagnosis and management, 1199–206. Copyright 2009, with permission from Elsevier.

The European BHD Consortium have proposed diagnostic criteria for BHDS (Table 21.6). Patients should fulfil one major or two minor criteria (32).

Lymphocytic interstitial pneumonia

BAL has a low diagnostic yield in LIP, but may show a lymphocytosis (35,44). SLB demonstrates dense polyclonal lymphocytic infiltration, which must be differentiated from the monoclonal infiltration of malignant lymphoproliferative disorders (35).

Light-chain deposition disease

LCDD is characterized by kappa light-chain deposition in the walls of the small airways, with associated airway dilatation (35). Electron microscopy shows granular deposits along the basement membrane (35,76). The serum free kappa/lambda light-chain ratio is increased (47). Both amyloidosis and LCDD most commonly affect the kidneys, and their distinction requires biopsy and Congo-red staining (48).

DIAGNOSTIC GUIDELINES FOR LAM

Guidelines for the diagnosis and management of LAM were published in 2010 (54) (Table 21.7). A complete workup to exclude other cystic ILDs is required in 'probable' and 'possible' LAM.

Table 21.7 European Respiratory Society diagnostic criteria for LAM

Definite LAM	Probable LAM	Possible LAM
Characteristic or compatible HRCT and biopsy typical for LAM	Characteristic HRCT and compatible clinical history	Characteristic or compatible HRCT
or	or	
Characteristic HRCT and any of:	Compatible HRCT and any of:	
Angiomyolipoma	Angiomyolipoma	
Chylous effusion	Chylous effusion	
Lymph node involvement		
Definite or probable TSC		

Source: Johnson SR et al. Eur Respir J. 2010;35:14–26.
Note: Characteristic HRCT: Multiple (>10) thin-walled cysts. No other pulmonary involvement.
Compatible HRCT: As above, but fewer cysts.

A serum VEGF-D concentration over 800 pg/mL is considered diagnostic of LAM and differentiates LAM from other cystic ILDs (77,78), but is not part of the current guidelines.

MANAGEMENT

GENERAL ASPECTS OF MANAGEMENT

Management of the cystic ILDs includes smoking cessation, pulmonary rehabilitation, influenza and pneumococcal vaccinations, and lung transplantation for end-stage disease. Bronchodilators are useful for airways obstruction (54).

The initial treatment for pneumothoraces is drainage, but they frequently recur. Further treatments, such as talc pleurodesis, mechanical pleurodesis or partial pleurectomy, should be considered (79) and do not preclude later consideration of lung transplantation.

LYMPHANGIOLEIOMYOMATOSIS

Patients should avoid exogenous oestrogens, such as hormone replacement therapy and some contraceptives (54). Progesterone may be considered in patients with rapidly declining lung function, but the benefits are inconsistent. Progesterone may increase the incidence of meningiomas (52,54) and brain magnetic resonance imaging (MRI) should be performed prior to starting treatment (52,54). There is insufficient evidence for other hormonal therapies in LAM (80).

Conservative treatment for chylous pleural effusions includes a fat-free diet supplemented with mid-chain triglycerides and aspiration, but they often recur (54). Pleurodesis or thoracic duct ligation may be required (81).

The mTOR inhibitors, sirolimus and everolimus, inhibit the proliferation of LAM cells, reducing the volume of cysts and AMLs (69,82–84). In the MILES study, sirolimus stabilized lung function and improved quality of life in patients with LAM (85). Sirolimus is recommended for patients with an FEV1 ≤70% predicted (1). The mTOR inhibitors are not curative, and lung function continues to decline when treatment is discontinued (85). Additionally, mTOR inhibitors have side effects, most commonly mucositis, gastrointestinal effects, hypercholesterolaemia, rashes and leg swelling (83,85). However, they may delay the need for lung transplantation.

AMLs may bleed, particularly when large, and ultrasound, MRI or computed tomography (CT) monitoring is recommended. Asymptomatic AMLs should be followed up annually if less than 4 cm diameter, or biannually if larger (50). Symptomatic AMLs can be treated with renal artery embolization or nephron-sparing surgery (50). Patients with TSC are susceptible to renal malignancies, which should be considered when a renal mass is found.

PULMONARY LANGERHANS CELL HISTIOCYTOSIS

Smoking cessation often results in stabilization or regression of PLCH (86,87), but corticosteroids or cytotoxic chemotherapy may be

Table 21.8 Management of PLCH

Step 1	Smoking cessation
Step 2	Asymptomatic or minimal symptoms → watchful waiting
	Symptomatic → corticosteroids
Step 3	Progressive disease despite corticosteroids → chemotherapy (e.g. cladribine)
Step 4	Severe respiratory failure or pulmonary hypertension → lung transplantation

Source: Adapted from Girschikofsky et al. *Orphanet J Rare Dis.* 2013;8:72–3.

required in progressive or disseminated disease (88) (Table 21.8).

BIRT–HOGG–DUBÉ SYNDROME

BHDS is associated with renal malignancies, and annual screening from age 20 years is recommended (32,89). MRI is more sensitive than ultrasound (32), and does not carry the radiation exposure of CT scanning, but may not be widely available. Therefore, we recommend initial CT imaging, and subsequent ultrasound surveillance.

LYMPHOCYTIC INTERSTITIAL PNEUMONIA

Corticosteroids may improve outcomes in LIP but the evidence is not conclusive (44).

LIGHT-CHAIN DEPOSITION DISEASE

The management of LCDD centres on treating underlying haematological conditions (35,47).

PROGNOSIS AND LONG-TERM OUTLOOK

LYMPHANGIOLEIOMYOMATOSIS

LAM has a 91% 10-year survival rate (40). Ten years post-diagnosis, 23% of LAM patients require oxygen and 55% have MRC grade 3 dyspnoea (40).

Weight loss, supplemental oxygen requirements and reversible airways obstruction are poor prognostic indicators (69). TSC-LAM usually causes less lung function impairment and follows a more indolent course than S-LAM (19,39).

Serum VEGF-D is emerging to be a reliable non-invasive prognostic biomarker, with higher levels indicating more severe disease and better response to sirolimus (90–92).

PULMONARY LANGERHANS CELL HISTIOCYTOSIS

Survival from diagnosis in PLCH is around 12 years (43), but the clinical course is variable (93). Poor prognostic indicators include older age, constitutional symptoms, numerous pulmonary cysts, decreased TLCO, severe lung function impairment, recurrent pneumothoraces, multisystem disease, continued smoking and pulmonary hypertension (18,82,94–96).

BIRT–HOGG–DUBÉ SYNDROME

Respiratory failure is unusual in BHDS. Renal malignancy is the primary threat to these patients.

LYMPHOCYTIC INTERSTITIAL PNEUMONIA

LIP has a variable prognosis, with a median survival of 5–11.5 years (36,44).

LIGHT-CHAIN DEPOSITION DISEASE

LCDD is progressive, and frequently causes respiratory failure (35).

CURRENT AND FUTURE AREAS OF RESEARCH

There are few clinical trials in the cystic ILDs, but these are imperative to establish new treatments and optimal regimens of existing drugs. Research into the molecular mechanisms underlying the cystic ILDs may reveal diagnostic and prognostic biomarkers that can be measured non-invasively. Methods of predicting disease course are lacking, but are needed to identify patients to prioritize for lung transplant.

Clinical cases

CASE 1

A 30-year-old woman has a pneumothorax. She smokes, but is otherwise fit and well. Her mother had a nephrectomy for a renal mass aged 50.

On examination the patient has skin lesions, which she describes as 'skin tags' that have increased in number. Her HRCT shows multiple thin-walled cysts in the lower lung zones. What is the diagnosis?

Answer: BHDS. *FLCN* gene mutation was confirmed. BHDS is underdiagnosed due to its variable presenting features. An alternative diagnosis in a young woman with lower zone lung cysts, skin lesions and a family history of renal tumours is TSC-LAM. PLCH should be considered in smokers, but predominantly affects the upper zones.

CASE 2

A 30-year-old woman with LAM attends for a routine review. Her lung function is stable and she does not require supplemental oxygen. She wants to start a family. How should you advise her?

Answer: The hormonal changes associated with pregnancy may accelerate lung function decline and increase the risk of pneumothorax (13,40,97). Those with poor lung function and pneumothoraces or chylous effusions prior to pregnancy are at the highest risk (54). However, women with LAM often have uncomplicated pregnancies. Each case should be considered individually, and the risks discussed with the patient.

CASE 3

A 32-year-old woman was diagnosed with LAM following her second pneumothorax. She frequently travels, and she is concerned about the risks of flying. How should you advise her?

Answer: The risks of air travel in LAM are higher than other cystic ILDs (98), but are low overall (99). Risks include in-flight pneumothorax and hypoxaemia. Patients should not fly with symptoms of a pneumothorax or within 1 month of a pneumothorax being treated (54). Her ability to tolerate a pneumothorax, based on lung function and oxygen saturations, should be considered. Supplemental in-flight oxygen may be indicated (98). Pleurectomy may be considered when the risk of recurrent pneumothoraces in unacceptable.

REFERENCES

1. Gupta N, Vassallo R, Wikenheiser-Brokamp KA, McCormack FX. Diffuse cystic lung disease: Part 1. *Am J Respir Crit Care Med.* 2015;191(12):1354–66.
2. Bittmann I, Rolf B, Amann G, Löhrs U. Recurrence of lymphangioleiomyomatosis after single lung transplantation: New insights into pathogenesis. *Hum Pathol.* 2003;34(1):95–8.
3. Karbowniczek M, Astrinidis A, Balsara BR, Testa JR, Lium JH, Colby TV et al. Recurrent lymphangioleiomyomatosis after transplantation: Genetic analyses reveal a metastatic mechanism. *Am J Respir Crit Care Med.* 2003;167(7):976–82.
4. Sato T, Seyama K, Fujii H, Maruyama H, Setoguchi Y, Iwakami S et al. Mutation analysis of the TSC1 and TSC2 genes in Japanese patients with pulmonary lymphangioleiomyomatosis. *J Hum Genet.* 2002;47(1):20–8.
5. Odajima N, Betsuyaku T, Nashuhara Y, Inoue H, Seyama K, Nishimura M. Matrix metalloproteinases in blood from patients with LAM. *Respir Med.* 2009;103:124–9.
6. Chang W, Cane J, Blakey JD, Kumaran M, Pointon KS, Johnson SR. Clinical utility of diagnostic guidelines and putative biomarkers in lymphangioleiomyomatosis. *Respir Res.* 2012;13:34.
7. Hayashi T, Fleming MV, Stetler-Stevenson EG, Liotta LA, Moss J, Ferrans VJ, Travis WD. Immunohistochemical study of matrix metalloproteinases (MMPs) and their tissue inhibitors (TIMPs) in pulmonary lymphangioleiomyomatosis (LAM). *Hum Pathol.* 1997;28(9):1071–78.
8. Matsui K, Takeda K, Yu ZX, Travis WD, Moss J, Ferrans VJ. Role for activation of matrix metalloproteinases in the

pathogenesis of pulmonary lymphangi-oleiomyomatosis. *Arch Pathol Lab Med.* 2000;124(2):267–75.

9. Zhe X, Yang Y, Jakkaraju S, Schuger L. Tissue inhibitor of metalloproteinase-3 downregulation in lymphangioleiomyo-matosis: Potential consequence of abnor-mal serum response factor expression. *Am J Respir Cell Mol Biol.* 2003;24(4): 504–11.

10. Glasgow CG, Steagall WK, Taveira-DaSilva A, Pacheco-Rodriguez G, Cai X, El-Chemaly S et al. Lymphangioleiomyomatosis (LAM): Molecular insights lead to targeted thera-pies. *Respir Med.* 2010;140:s45–58.

11. Kumasaka T, Seyama K, Mitani KS, Sato T, Souma S, Kondo T et al. Lymphangiogenesis in lymphangioleiomyomatosis: Its impli-cation in the progression of lymphan-gioleiomyomatosis. *Am J Surg Pathol.* 2004;28:1007–16.

12. Kumasaka T, Seyama K, Mitani K, Souma S, Kashiwagi S, Hebisawa A et al. Lymphangiogenesis-mediated shedding of lymphangioleiomyomatosis cell clusters as a mechanism for dissemination in lymphan-gioleiomyomatosis. *Am J Surg Pathol.* 2005;29:1356–66.

13. Yockey CC, Riepe RE, Ryan K. Pulmonary lymphangioleiomyomatosis complicated by pregnancy. *Kan Med.* 1986;87(10):277–8, 293.

14. Yano S. Exacerbation of pulmonary lymphangioleiomyomatosis by exogenous oestrogen used for infertility treatment. *Thorax.* 2002;57(12): 1085–6.

15. Oberstein EM, Fleming LE, Gómez-Marin O, Glassberg MK. Pulmonary lymphangioleio-myomatosis (LAM): Examining oral con-traceptive pills and the onset of disease. *J Womens Health (Larchmt).* 2003;12(1):81–5.

16. Wahedna I, Cooper S, Williams J, Paterson IC, Britton JR, Tattersfield AE. Relation of pulmonary lymphangio-leiomyomatosis to use of the oral contraceptive pill and fertil-ity in the UK: A national case control study. *Thorax.* 1994;49(9):910–4.

17. Johnson SR, Tattersfield AE. Decline in lung function in lymphangioleiomyoma-tosis. Relation to menopause and pro-gesterone. *Am J Respir Crit Care Med.* 1999;160(2):628–33.

18. Harari S, Caminati A. Chapter 10: Pulmonary Langerhans' cell histiocytosis. In: du Bois RM, Richeldi L, eds. *Interstitial Lung Diseases.* European Respiratory Society Journals Ltd, Sheffield, UK; 2009:155–75.

19. Clarke BE. Cystic lung disease. *J Clin Pathol.* 2013;66:904–8.

20. Yousem SA, Colby TV, Chen YY, Chen WG, Weiss LM. Pulmonary Langerhans' cell histiocytosis: Molecular analy-sis of clonality. *Am J Surg Pathol.* 2001;25(5):630–6.

21. Youkeles LH, Griazzanti JN, Liao Z, Chang CJ, Rosenstreich DL. Decreased tobacco-glycoprotein-induced lymphocyte prolif-eration *in vitro* in pulmonary eosinophilic granuloma. *Am J Respir Crit Care Med.* 1995;151(1):145–50.

22. Tazi A, Bonay M, Bergeron A, Grandsaigne M, Hance AJ, Soler P. Role of granulo-cyte-macrophage colony stimulating factor (GM-CSF) in the pathogenesis of adult pulmonary histiocytosis X. *Thorax.* 1996;51:611–14.

23. Asakura S, Colby TV, Limper AH. Tissue localisation of transforming growth factor-beta1 in pulmonary eosinophilic granuloma. *Am J Respir Crit Care Med.* 1996;154:1525–30.

24. Prasse A, Stahl M, Schulz G, Kayser G, Wang L, Ask K, et al. Essential role of osteopontin in smoking-related interstitial lung diseases. *Am J Pathol.* 2009;174:1683–91.

25. Elia D, Torre O, Cassandro R, Caminati A, Harari S. Pulmonary Langerhans cell his-tiocytosis: A comprehensive analysis of 40 patients and literature review. *Eur J Intern Med.* 2015;26:351–56.

26. Vassallo R, Ryu JH, Colby TV, Hartman T, Limper AH. Pulmonary Langerhans'-cell histiocytosis in adults. *N Engl J Med.* 2000;342:1969–78.

27. Roden AC, Hu X, Kip S, Parrilla Castellar ER, Rumilla KM, Vrana JA et al. BRAF V600E expression in Langerhans cell histiocytosis: Clinical and immunohisto-chemical study on 25 pulmonary and 54 extrapulmonary cases. *Am J Surg Pathol.* 2014;38(4):548–51.

28. Badalian-Very G, Vergilio JA, Degar BA, MacConaill LE, Brandner B, Calicchio

ML et al. Recurrent BRAF mutations in Langerhans cell histiocytosis. *Blood.* 2010;116(11):1919–23.

29. Satoh T, Smith A, Sarde A, Lu HC, Mian S, Trouillet C et al. B-RAF mutant alleles associated with Langerhans cell histiocytosis, a granulomatous pediatric disease. *PLoS One.* 2012;7(4): e33891.

30. Sahm F, Capper D, Preusser M, Meyer J, Stenzinger A, Lasitschka F et al. BRAFV600E mutant protein is expressed in calls of variable maturation in Langerhans cell histiocytosis. *Blood.* 2012;120(12):e28–34.

31. Hervier B, Haroche J, Arnaud L, Charlotte F, Donadieu I, Néel A et al. French Histiocytosis Study Group. Association of both Langerhans cell histiocytosis and Erdheim-Chester disease linked to the BRAFV600E mutation. *Blood.* 2014;124(7):1119–26.

32. Menko FH, van Steensel MA, Giraud S, Friis-Hansen L, Richard S, Ungari S et al. European BHD Consortium. Birt-Hogg-Dubé syndrome: Diagnosis and management. *Lancet Oncol.* 2009;10(12):1199–206.

33. Baba M, Hong SB, Sharma N, Warren MB, Nickerson ML, Iwamatsu A et al. Folliculin encoded by the BHD gene interacts with a binding protein, FNIP1, and AMPK, and is involved in AMPK and mTOR signalling. *Proc Natl Acad Sci USA.* 2006;103:15552–7.

34. Hartman TR, Nicolas E, Klein-Szanto A, Al-Saleem T, Cash TP, Simon MC, Henske EP. The role of the Birt-Hogg-Dubé protein in mTOR activation and renal tumorigenesis. *Oncogene.* 2009;28:1594–604.

35. Gupta N, Vassallo R, Wikenheiser-Brokamp KA, McCormack FX. Diffuse cystic lung disease: Part 2. *Am J Respir Crit Care Med.* 2015;192(1):17–29.

36. Swigris JJ, Berry GJ, Raffin TA, Kuschner WG. Lymphoid interstitial pneumonia: A narrative review. *Chest.* 2002;122:2150–64.

37. Colombat M, Caudroy S, Lagonette E, Mal H, Danel C, Stern M et al. Pathomechanisms of cyst formation in pulmonary light chain deposition disease. *Eur Respir J.* 2008;32:1399–403.

38. Aubrey MC, Myers JL, Ryu JH, Henske EP, Logginidou H, Jalal SM, Tazelaar HD. Pulmonary lymphangioleiomyomatosis in a man. *Am J Respir Crit Care Med.* 2000;162(2 Pt 1):749–52.

39. Ryu JH, Moss J, Beck GJ, Lee JC, Brown KK, Chapman JT et al. NHLBI LAM Registry Group. The NHLBI lymphangioleiomyomatosis registry: Characteristics of 230 patients at enrollment. *Am J Respir Crit Care Med.* 2006;173(1):105–11.

40. Johnson SR, Whale CI, Hubbard RB, Lewis SA, Tattersfield AE. Survival and disease progression in UK patients with lymphangioleiomyomatosis. *Thorax.* 2004;59:800–3.

41. Harknett EC, Chang WY, Byrnes S, Johnson J, Lazor R, Cohen MM et al. Use of variability in national and regional data to estimate the prevalence of lymphangioleiomyomatosis. *QJM.* 2011;104:971–9.

42. Watanabe R, Tatsumi K, Hashimoto S, Tamakoshi A, Kuriyama T; Respiratory Failure Research Group of Japan. Clinico-epidemiological features of pulmonary histiocytosis X. *Intern Med.* 2001;40(10):998–1003.

43. Vassallo R, Ryu JH, Schroeder DR, Decker PA, Limper AH. Clinical outcomes of pulmonary Langerhans cell histiocytosis in adults. *NEJM.* 2002;346(7):484–90.

44. Cha SI, Fessler MB, Cool CD, Schwarz MI, Brown KK. Lymphoid interstitial pneumonia: Clinical features, associations and prognosis. *Eur Respir J.* 2006;28:364–9.

45. Strimlan CV, Rosenow EC3rd, Weiland LH, Brown LR. Lymphocytic interstitial pneumonitis. Review of 13 cases. *Ann Intern Med.* 1978;88:616–21.

46. Johkoh T, Müller NL, Pickford HA, Hartman TE, Ichikado K, Akira M et al. Lymphocytic interstitial pneumonia: Thin-section CT findings in 22 patients. *Radiology.* 1999;212:567–72.

47. Hirschi S, Colombat M, Kessler R, Reynau-Gaubert M, Stern M, Chenard MP et al. Lung transplantation for advanced cystic lung disease due to nonamyloid kappa light chain deposits. *Ann Am Thorac Soc.* 2014;11:1025–31.

48. Ha D, Yadav R, Mazzone PJ. Cystic lung disease: Systematic, stepwise diagnosis. *Cleveland Clin J Med.* 2015;82(2):115–27.

49. Johnson SR. Lymphangioleiomyomatosis. *Eur Repir J.* 2006;27:1056–65.

50. Avila NA, Dwyer AJ, Rabel A, Moss J. Sporadic lymphangioleiomyomatosis and tuberous sclerosis complex with lymphangioleiomyomatosis: Comparison of CT features. *Radiology.* 2007;242(1):277–85.

51. Avila NA, Bechtle J, Dwyer AJ, Ferrans VJ, Moss J. Lymphangioleiomyomatosis: CT of diurnal variation of lymphangioleiomyomatosis. *Radiology.* 2001;221(2):415–21.

52. Moss J, DeCastro R, Patronas NJ, Taveira-DaSilva A. Meningiomas in lymphangioleiomyomatosis. *JAMA.* 2001;286(15):1879–81.

53. Roach ES, DiMario FJ, Kandt RS, Northrup H. Tuberous Sclerosis Consensus Conference: Recommendations for diagnostic evaluation. National Tuberous Sclerosis Association. *J Chil Neurol.* 1999;19(4):401–7.

54. Johnson SR, Cordier JF, Lazor R, Cottin V, Costabel U, Harari S et al. Review Panel of the ERS LAM Task Force. European Respiratory Society guidelines for the diagnosis and management of lymphangioleiomyomatosis. *Eur Respir J.* 2010;35:14–26.

55. Crausman RS, Jennings CA, Tuder RM, Ackerson LM, Irvin CG, King TE Jr. Pulmonary histiocytosis X: Pulmonary function and exercise pathophysiology. *Am J Respir Crit Care Med.* 1996;153:426–35.

56. Toro JR, Paulter SE, Stewart L, Glenn GM, Weinreich M, Toure O et al. Lung cysts, spontaneous pneumothorax, and genetic associations in 89 families with Birt-Hogg-Dubé syndrome. *Am J Respir Crit Care Med.* 2007;175:1044–53.

57. Pavlovich CP, Grubb RL III, Hurley K, Glenn GM, Toro J, Schmidt LS et al. Evaluation and management of renal tumors in the Birt-Hogg-Dubé syndrome. *J Urol.* 2005;173:1482–86.

58. Hansell DM, Bankier AA, MacMahon H, McLoud TC, Müller NL, Remy J. Fleischner Society: Glossary of terms for thoracic imaging. *Radiology.* 2008;246:697–722.

59. Beddy P, Babr J, Devaraj A. A practical approach to cystic lung disease on HRCT. *Insights Imaging.* 2011;2:1–7.

60. Koyama M, Johkoh T, Honda O, Tsubamoto M, Kozuka T, Tomiyama N et al. Chronic cystic lung disease: Diagnostic accuracy of high-resolution CT in 92 patients. *AJR Am J Roentgenol.* 2003;180:827–35.

61. Colby TV, Lombard C. Histiocytosis X in the lung. *Hum Pathol.* 1983;14:847–56.

62. Caminati A, Harari S. Smoking-related interstitial pneumonias and pulmonary Langerhans cell histiocytosis. *Proc Am Thorac Soc.* 2006;3:299–306.

63. Honda O, Johkoh T, Ichikado K, Tomiyama N, Maeda M, Mihara N et al. Differential diagnosis of lymphocytic interstitial pneumonia and malignant lymphoma on high-resolution CT. *AJR Am J Roentgenol.* 1999;173:71–4.

64. Akira M, Yamamoto S, Hara H, Sakatani M, Ueda E. Serial computed tomographic evaluation in desquamative interstitial pneumonia. *Thorax.* 1997;52:333–7.

65. Hartman TE, Primack SL, Swensen SJ, Hansell D, McGuinness G, Müller NL. Desquamative interstitial pneumonia: Thin-section CT findings in 22 patients. *Radiology.* 1993;187:787–90.

66. Harari S, Torre O, Cassandro R, Taveira-DaSilva AM, Moss J. Bronchoscopic diagnosis of Langerhans cell histiocytosis and lymphangioleiomyomatosis. *Respir Med.* 2012;106:1286–92.

67. Meraj R, Wikenheiser-Brokamp KA, Young LR, Byrnes S, McCormack FX. Utility of transbronchial biopsy in the diagnosis of lymphangioleiomyomatosis. *Front Med.* 2012;6:395–405.

68. Gao L, Yue MM, Davis J, Hyjek E, Schuger L. In pulmonary lymphangioleiomyomatosis expression of progesterone receptor is frequently higher than that of estrogen receptor. *Virchows Arch.* 2014;464:495–503.

69. Harari S, Torre O, Cassandro R, Moss J. The changing face of a rare disease: Lymphangioleiomyomatosis. *Eur Respir J.* 2015;46:1471–85.

70. Matsumoto Y, Horiba K, Usuki J, Chu SC, Ferrans VJ, Moss J. Markers of cell proliferation and expression of melanosomal antigen in lymphangioleiomyomatosis. *Am J Respir Cell Mol Biol.* 1999;21:327–36.

71. Chollet S, Soler P, Dournovo P, Richard MS, Ferrans VJ, Basset F. Diagnosis of pulmonary histiocytosis X by immunodetection of Langerhans' cells in bronchoalveolar lavage fluid. *Am J Pathol.* 1984;115:225–32.

72. Auerswald U, Barth J, Magnussen H. Value of CD1-positive cells in bronchoalveolar lavage fluid for the diagnosis of pulmonary histiocytosis X. *Lung.* 1991;169:305–9.

73. Girschikofsky M, Arico M, Castillo D, Chu A, Doberauer C, Fichter J et al. Management of adult patients with Langerhans cell histiocytosis: Recommendations from an expert panel on behalf of Euro-Histio-Net. *Orphanet J Rare Dis.* 2013;8:72–3.

74. Travis WD, Borok Z, Roum JH, Zhang J, Feuerstein I, Ferrans VJ, Crystal RG. Pulmonary Langerhans cell granulomatosis (histiocytosis X): A clinicopathologic study of 48 cases. *Am J Surg Pathol.* 1993;17:971–86.

75. Housini I, Tomashefski JF Jr, Cohen A, Crass J, Kleinerman J. Transbronchial biopsy in patients with pulmonary eosinophilic granuloma: Comparison with findings on open lung biopsy. *Arch Pathol Lab Med.* 1994;118:523–30.

76. Randall RE, Williamson WC Jr, Mullinax F, Tung MY, Still WJ. Manifestations of systemic light chain deposition. *Am J Med.* 1976;60:293–9.

77. Young LR, Inoue Y, McCormack FX. Diagnostic potential of serum VEGF-D for lymphangioleiomyomatosis. *N Engl J Med.* 2008;358:199–200.

78. Young LR, Vandyke R, Gulleman PM, Inoue Y, Brown KK, Schmidt LS et al. Serum vascular endothelial growth factor-D prospectively distinguishes lymphangioleiomyomatosis from other diseases. *Chest.* 2010;138:674–81.

79. Mendez JL, Nadrous HF, Vassallo R, Decker PA, Ryu JH. Pneumothorax in pulmonary Langerhans cell histiocytosis. *Chest.* 2004;125(3):1028–32.

80. Harari S, Cassandro R, Chiodini I, Taveira-DaSilva AM, Moss J. Effect of a gonadotrophin-releasing hormone analogue in lung function in lymphangioleiomyomatosis. *Chest.* 2008;133(2):448–54.

81. Ryu JH, Doerr CH, Fisher SD, Olson EJ, Sahn SA. Chylothorax in lymphangioleiomyomatosis. *Chest.* 2003;123(2):623–7.

82. Argula RG, Kokosi M, Lo P, Kim HJ, Ravenel JG, Meyer C et al; MILES Study Investigators. A novel quantitative computed tomographic analysis suggests how sirolimus stabilizes progressive air trapping in lymphangioleiomyomatosis. *Ann Am Thorac Soc.* 2016;13(3):342–9.

83. Bissler JJ, Kingswood JC, Radzikowska E, Zonnenberg BA, Frost M, Belousova E et al. Everolimus for angiomyolipoma associated with tuberous sclerosis complex or sporadic lymphangioleiomyomatosis (EXIST-2): A multicentre, randomised, double-blind, placebo-controlled trial. *Lancet.* 2013;381:817–24.

84. Taveria-DaSilva AM, Hathaway O, Stylianou M, Moss J. Changes in lung function and chylous effusions in patients with lymphangioleiomyomatosis treated with sirolimus. *Ann Intern Med.* 2011;154:797–805.

85. McCormack FX, Inoue Y, Moss J, Singer LG, Strange C, Nakata K et al. National Institutes of Health Rare Lung Diseases Consortium; MILES Trial Group. Efficacy and safety of sirolimus in lymphangioleiomyomatosis. *N Eng J Med.* 2011;364(17):1595–606.

86. Schönfeld N, Dirks K, Costabel U, Loddenkemper R; Wissenschaftliche Arbeitsgemeinschaft für die Therapie von Lungenkrankheiten. A prospective clinical multicentre study on adult pulmonary Langerhans' cell histiocytosis. *Sarcoidosis Vasc Diffuse Lung Dis.* 2012;29(2):132–8.

87. Mogulkoc N, Veral A, Bishop PW, Bayindir U, Pickering CA, Egan JJ. Pulmonary Langerhans' cell histiocytosis: Radiologic resolution following smoking cessation. *Chest.* 1999;115:1452–55.

88. Howarth DM, Gilchrist GS, Mullan BP, Wiseman GA, Edmonson JH, Schomberg PJ. Langerhans cell histiocytosis. Diagnosis, natural history, management, and outcome. *Cancer.* 1999;85:2278–90.

89. Stamatakis L, Metwalli AR, Middelton LA, Marston Linehan W. Diagnosis and

management of BHD-associated kidney cancer. *Fam Cancer.* 2013;12(3):397–402.

90. Young LR, Lee H, Inoue Y, Moss J, Singer LG, Strange C et al. MILES Trial Group. Serum VEGF-D concentration as a biomarker of lymphangioleiomyomatosis severity and treatment response: A prospective analysis of the Multicenter International Lymphangioleiomyomatosis Efficacy of Sirolimus (MILES) trial. *Lancet Respir Med.* 2013;1(6):445–52.

91. Seyama K, Kumasaka T, Souma S, Sato T, Kurihara M, Mitani K et al. Vascular endothelial growth factor-D is increased in serum of patients with lymphangioleiomyomatosis. *Lymphat Res Biol.* 2006;4(3):143–52.

92. Glasgow CG, Avila NA, Lin JP, Stylianou MP, Moss J. Serum vascular endothelial growth factor-D levels in patients with lymphangioleiomyomatosis reflect lymphatic involvement. *Chest.* 2009;135(5):1293–300.

93. Tazi A, Marc K, Dominique S, de Bazelaire C, Crestani B, Chinet T et al. Serial computed tomography and lung function testing in pulmonary Langerhans'

cell histiocytosis. *Eur Respir J.* 2012;40:905–12.

94. Fartoukh M, Humbert M, Capron F, Maître S, Parent F, Le Gall C et al. Severe pulmonary hypertension in histiocytosis X. *Am J Respir Crit Care Med.* 2000;161:216–23.

95. Harari S, Simonneau G, De Juli E, Brenot F, Cerrina J, Colombo P et al. Prognostic value of pulmonary hypertension in patients with chronic interstitial lung disease referred for lung or heart-lung transplantation. *J Heart Lung Transplant.* 1997;16:460–3.

96. Delobbe A, Durieu J, Duhamel A, Wallaert B. Determinants of survival in pulmonary Langerhans' cell granulomatosis (histiocytosis X). *Eur Respir J.* 1996;9:2002–6.

97. Cohen MM, Freyer AM, Johnson SR. Pregnancy experiences among women with lymphangioleiomyomatosis. *Respir Med.* 2009;103(5):766–72.

98. Pollock-BarZiv S, Cohen MM, Downey GP, Johnson SR, Sullivan E, McCormack FX. Air travel in women with lymphangioleiomyomatosis. *Thorax.* 2007;62(2):176–80.

99. Hu X, Cowl CT, Bagir M, Ryu JH. Air travel and pneumothorax. *Chest.* 2014;145(4):688–94.

22

Pulmonary alveolar proteinosis

CLIFF MORGAN

INTRODUCTION

Pulmonary alveolar proteinosis (PAP) is a rare condition with occurrence at around 1–7 per million of population. This means that even busy interstitial lung disease (ILD) specialists have little clinical exposure to it during a typical working lifetime. Therefore, all the usual issues of rare disease management apply but in the challenging context of an opportunity to radically improve the health and prognosis of most of the patients if they receive the right treatment at the right time. Conversely, if diagnosis is delayed and treatment is not optimal patients can fare much worse. PAP is a syndrome and not a specific and consistent disease entity so optimal treatment also depends on accurate assessment of which variant the patient actually has. Some of the key elements of PAP are summarized as follows:

- Rare – around 1–7 per million of population (estimates vary in the published literature and there may be some under-reporting)
- Typically presents in adults between 20 and 50 years but all ages can be affected and with a slight predilection for males
- Range of severity
  - Mild and may spontaneously resolve in a small percentage of cases
  - Moderately severe with serious symptoms and significant treatment requirements
  - Severe and difficult to treat
- Syndrome; common phenotype with
  - Excess alveolar accumulation of surfactant lipoproteins and dysfunctional macrophages
  - Associated gas exchange defect causing progressive hypoxaemia
  - Typical radiological image appearance and histology
- Various pathophysiological mechanisms

- Anti-GM-CSF antibody-mediated neutralization of GM-CSF expression leading to alveolar macrophage dysfunction ('Auto-Immune PAP' or aPAP – around 90% of the cases)
- Hereditary or mutation-based defect in surfactant or macrophage control pathways
- Secondary PAP – where there is usually an obvious and severe disease, typically a haematological malignancy that is provoking the PAP in some way

- Whole lung lavage (WLL) may have a place in all forms of PAP but the comprehensive treatment of an individual patient depends on which variant the patient has.

HISTORY OF PAP

PAP was described for the first time in 1957 and effective treatment by WLL was first described soon after in 1963. The review articles by Seymour (1) and Trapnell (2) cover the history of PAP and the interesting developments over the past few decades. The refinements in treatment were perhaps to be expected but the leaps in understanding the pathophysiology that came from a mixture of serendipity and hard graft were much better than could have been expected for such a rare disease. Not so surprising perhaps if the combined talent drawn to

the investigation and treatment of this interesting condition is considered. PAP is not a single disease entity but rather a syndrome with certain features in common and some important variances. This element of PAP makes it all the more important that patients are investigated and treated appropriately and preferably in a centre with a track record in treating the syndrome. PAP is rare with an estimated incidence of less than 7 per million, another reason to concentrate experience in a relatively small number of centres to ensure better understanding and more consistent care.

THE NATURE OF PAP

The common factor in all variants of PAP is the phenotype, i.e. the progressive massive accumulation of dysfunctional, foamy macrophages and effete surfactant lipoproteins within the alveolar space. This causes a steadily worsening gas exchange defect through a mixture of impaired oxygen diffusion and eventually shunt (Figure 22.1). The lung architecture is typically preserved but lung biopsy reveals alveolar spaces filled with proteinaceous material (Figure 22.2) which stains pink in periodic acid-Schiff preparations. This alveolar filling effect also explains the typical radiological appearance of diffuse airspace shadowing on plain chest x-ray (Figure 22.3) and the striking pattern on computed

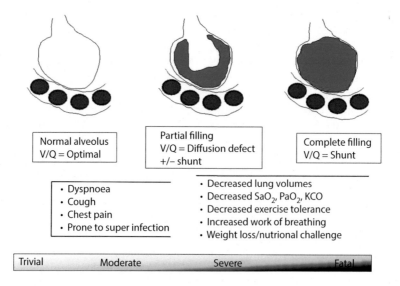

Figure 22.1 The gas exchange defect in PAP. (Abbreviations: KCO = carbon monoxide diffusion; SaO_2 = arterial oxygen saturation; V/Q = ventilation:perfusion ratio.)

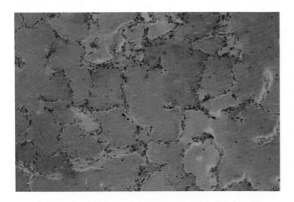

Figure 22.2 Photomicrograph of a lung biopsy specimen from typical PAP. (Note the essentially normal alveolar walls but the alveolar airspace is completely filled with protein stained pink in periodic acid-Schiff.)

tomography (CT) (Figure 22.4). The CT appearances are almost pathognomonic and include ground-glass shadowing from airspace filling, *crazy-paving* from accentuation of the interlobular septa and *geographic sparing* – that is the complete random pattern of involvement of different segments of the lung with no rational predilection for upper, lower, basal or anterior areas. This random distribution still has no plausible explanation but is

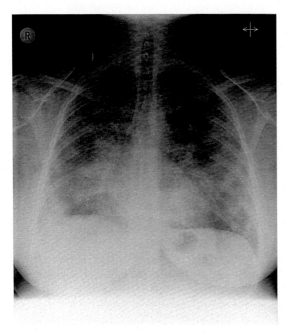

Figure 22.3 Plain chest radiograph from a 30-year-old woman with typical aPAP. There is diffuse airspace shadowing throughout both lungs.

an important diagnostic feature of PAP. The extent of the ground-glass opacification in terms of density and percentage of segments affected has an obvious correlation with the severity of the physiologic and therefore the clinical defect.

From this, it is easy to understand the leading clinical symptoms of dyspnoea and limitation of exercise capacity, and the range of severity usually correlates well with the CT-assessed extent of disease from mild to extremely severe with respiratory failure.

PAP VARIANTS

AUTOIMMUNE PAP

As discussed, PAP represents a syndrome with a common phenotype. The most common variant accounts for around 90% of all cases and is now known to be associated with very high serum concentration of an IgG antibody to circulating granulocyte–macrophage colony-stimulating factor (GM-CSF) (3). This anti-GM-CSF effectively 'neutralizes' and prevents GM-CSF expression. We now understand that GM-CSF is not required for normal haemopoiesis but is important in up-regulation of monocytes during inflammatory response and, more importantly perhaps, is vital for the normal migration, maturation and function of the alveolar macrophage. In the absence of normal GM-CSF tone, the alveolar macrophages can still become resident in the alveolar space and can ingest damaged surfactant but they are incapable of the normal processing and recycling of surfactant in concert with the type II pneumocytes that ensures perfect surface tension control and augmented host defence. So the alveolar space becomes full of damaged surfactant and enlarged macrophages packed with undigested surfactant globules. This explains the gas exchange defect and also the tendency to opportunistic infection with conventional and atypical pathogens. This variant of PAP is now often referred to as *auto-immune PAP* (aPAP) but it is not auto-immune in the classic sense of a destructive or pro-inflammatory antibody/antigen association. It is fascinatingly the only known example of disease caused by an antibody interacting with a regulatory cytokine. Even more fascinating is that the IgG anti-GM-CSF is present in normal subjects but is difficult to detect

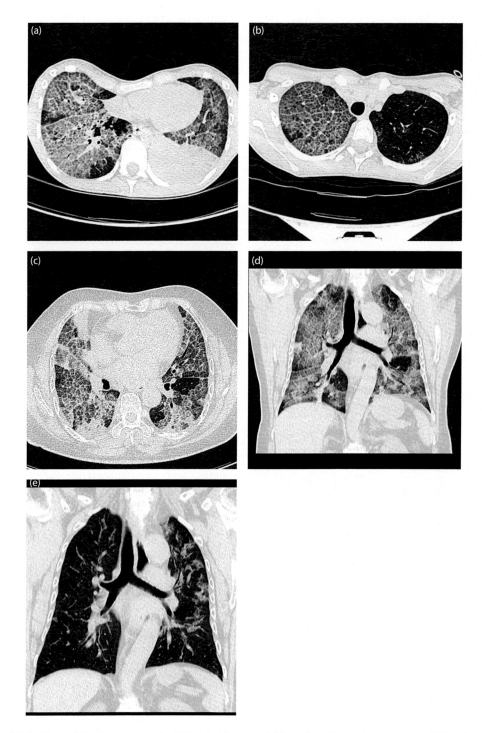

Figure 22.4 Chest CT appearances in PAP **(a)**. 12-year-old female with typical severe aPAP – note the extensive areas of opacification, accentuation of interlobular septa, classical 'crazy-paving' and small areas of 'geographic sparing'. Note also the unusually dense consolidation of the left lower lobe. **(b)** The same 12-year-old patient with slices further up the thorax with extensive disease on the right but remarkable sparing on the left. **(c)** 75-year-old female with typical severe aPAP and the usual CT features. **(d, e)** The same 75-year-old female with CT images before and after successful treatment by WLL and inhaled GM-CSF.

because it is bound to circulating GM-CSF where it appears to exert a modulating or cytokine down-regulating effect, perhaps having evolved to prevent over-expression of GM-CSF and unrestrained pro-inflammatory consequences.

The diagnosis of aPAP is based on the following:

- The typical clinical features of increasing breathlessness, exercise limitation, cough (which may be productive of lumpy white sputum) and non-specific chest pain
- Abnormal pulmonary function tests (reduced gas transfer, widened A-aDO2, reduced lung volumes and reduced resting and exertional arterial oxygen tension and saturation)
- Abnormal plain chest radiograph (diffuse airspace shadowing) and almost pathognomonic changes on the chest computed tomogram
- The presence of high concentrations of the anti-GM-CSF antibody in serum and elevation of other biomarkers like LDH, CEA and KL6

Treatment will be discussed in more detail later in this chapter but the gold standard option is massive WLL to literally wash the offending lipoprotein accumulation out of the alveolar space. The relatively recent understanding of the effect of the anti-GM-CSF antibody has opened up some additional treatment options.

CLINICAL CASES

Example 1: A 34-year-old male smoker with 14 pack-year exposure returned from a holiday in Spain with cough and increasing breathlessness. The family doctor suspected a community-acquired chest infection and prescribed oral antibiotics. There was no improvement after 10 days so a chest radiograph was ordered. This was abnormal with diffuse airspace shadowing but no other specific features. Routine blood tests and sputum cultures were unremarkable. He was referred to a pulmonary specialist at a local hospital who arranged chest CT, further blood tests and performed fibre-optic bronchoscopy with diagnostic bronchoalveolar lavage (BAL). The BAL fluid was remarkable in being milky and non-odorous. The CT was typical of PAP and this was suggested by the radiologist even though they had not seen a previous case. The

patient was set up for thoracoscopic lung biopsy to confirm the suspected diagnosis but a timely telephone and web-based discussion with an experienced PAP team including ILD specialist, chest radiologist and lung pathologist confirmed the diagnosis on the information already available and the biopsy procedure was cancelled. He was found to be positive for the anti-GM-CSF antibody. He was referred to a specialist PAP centre, underwent three separate bilateral whole lung lavage procedures, each with significant 'yield' of lipoproteinaceous material and improved from clinically limited with gas transfer of 46% predicted, A-aDO2 of 5.2 kPa and resting oxygen saturation in air of 87% (dropping to 70% during 6-minute walk test) with each repetition towards normal and then remained in long-term remission (and also on emphatic advice managed to stop smoking).

Example 2: A 42-year-old male with no significant past medical history apart from mild asthma and a 10 pack-year past smoking exposure suffered gradually worsening dyspnoea and non-productive cough. There was also some non-specific chest pain, possibly associated with the bouts of coughing. He was treated with oral antibiotics by his primary care doctor for presumed chest infection but there was no improvement and he was referred to his local hospital for investigation. The chest radiograph was abnormal and the CT confirmed widespread ground-glass opacification with areas of spared normal lung and a crazy-paving pattern in most segments. Bronchoscopy was performed and the BAL fluid was turbid and milky and stained intensively pink in PAS medium indicating highly concentrated lipoproteins. Lung function was severely abnormal with reduced lung volumes and gas transfer and 6-minute walk test was stopped after 2 minutes when SpO2 fell to 68%. He underwent selective bronchoscopic lavage of multiple segments in separate sessions under mild sedation but little progress was achieved so he underwent WLL at that hospital with limited improvement and using a relatively low lavage volume. He was then referred to a specialist PAP centre for further investigation and management. He underwent a series of massive WLL initially one lung per session but latterly both lungs and with an average of between 40 and 50 litres per lung to achieve a therapeutic endpoint. Each time he left hospital 'cured' with virtually normal pulmonary physiology but quickly relapsed each time and returned for further massive WLL within a month. He was confirmed positive for anti-GM-CSF and after approval by the Institutional Clinical Practice Committee was commenced on daily subcutaneous injections of GM-CSF (sargramastim) and carefully monitored for signs of improvement or toxicity but there were neither. So he was commenced on daily inhalation of GM-CSF using an ultra-efficient nebulizer (in order to maximize the benefit of the high-cost drug) and within weeks there was a dramatic improvement in general condition and gross reduction in requirements for WLL, initially down to every 6 weeks, then to 3 months, 6 months and finally to none at all. He continues on a small maintenance dose of two inhalations per week and remains well with no recent WLL.

HEREDITARY PAP

In some of the literature this has also been referred to as congenital PAP but *hereditary* or hPAP is becoming the preferred term because of the fairly wide range of gene defects (4) and timing of presentation that have been described. Better understanding of alveolar macrophage natural history and control suggest the possibility for radical treatment options, even 'cure' by *pulmonary macrophage transplantation* (5). In some cases there are clear inheritance patterns in a cohort of relatives while in others a more sporadic mutation may have occurred. The defect may be anywhere along the various surfactant control or alveolar macrophage control pathways culminating in the typical PAP phenotype. The easiest variants to understand are the mutations of *CSF2RA* or *CSF2RB* genes which encode GM-CSF receptor alpha or beta and subsequent macrophage failure typical of all forms of PAP. Some cases present in early infancy with a similar combination of physiology, imaging and histology to aPAP but with the added complication of afflicting small and immature children and babies with all that entails. In particular the WLL options in small children are much more complex when the child is too small for a typical double-lumen endobronchial tube used to safely separate left and right lungs during thoracic anaesthesia procedures.

Diagnosis of hPAP is based on the typical PAP phenotype features of all PAP together with the following:

- Absence of anti-GM-CSF antibody (or typical causes of secondary PAP)
- Family history of hPAP (or in some cases of unconfirmed pulmonary illness or syndromes)

- Specific genotype from gene sequence analysis
- Index patient + siblings and other family members

Treatment is WLL (including where necessary paediatric WLL variants) but this may have to be repeated many times depending on physiological and clinical condition of the patient. Lung transplant may be considered as a longer-term goal after a period of WLL supported health, maturation and growth (because of the generally poor results of lung transplantation in younger patients) but exciting prospects regarding pulmonary macrophage transplantation offer hope in the near future of a more selective and longer-term solution.

CLINICAL CASES

Example 1: A 2-year-old female child was referred to a specialist paediatric cardiothoracic unit for investigation of severe respiratory failure. The family had originated from Iraq and there had been several related children afflicted by severe respiratory failure and early death but no specific diagnosis had been made. The patient had experienced progressive failure to thrive and increasing lethargy and breathlessness for about 6 months and this may have been exacerbated by an upper respiratory tract infection resulting in critical deterioration and mechanical ventilation. Investigations included fibre-optic bronchoscopy and BAL and chest CT, both of which were typical of PAP. Gene sequence confirmed mutation of *CSF2RB* locus. She underwent multiple successful paediatric WLL operations in clusters of two or three per hospital admission at intervals of around 6 months and is thriving in all other respects but likely to continue to require a similar pattern of WLL procedures, which will possibly culminate in the need for a lung transplantation in her early teens.

Example 2: A 33-year-old woman was seen with short stature and deformity of arms and legs but normal intellectual development. Four sisters have a similar deformity and all have been previously investigated and found to have an inherited deletion at locus q22,33 of both X chromosomes (or *SHOX* gene) known to be associated with the deformity. Having been in perfect health otherwise she experienced gradual progressive deterioration in exercise tolerance until she started getting breathless at rest. Investigations included plain chest radiograph and CT which were both typical of PAP. Fibre-optic bronchoscopy and BAL also proved typical of PAP but the anti-GM-CSF antibody test was negative. She was referred to a specialist PAP centre and underwent two episodes of bilateral WLL with excellent result and sustained remission. Her other sisters are being followed up but none show any signs of pulmonary issues yet. It turns out that the *SHOX* gene overlaps a CSF receptor locus and this must explain the PAP phenotype. The timing of onset of PAP is not explained however, and neither is the fact that only one of the affected siblings has so far developed PAP. An interaction with an as-yet unidentified co-factor may be at play.

SECONDARY PAP

Again the phenotype is identical to other variants of PAP but the process is driven by an identifiable provoking disease, typically a haematological malignancy (6). Rarely, a patient may have sPAP without a positive underlying diagnosis. The importance of the underlying diagnosis is because, although the PAP may require typical treatment by WLL to control symptoms, the long-term prognosis is entirely determined by the diagnosis and management of the provoking disease.

Diagnosis of sPAP is based on the presence of typical PAP phenotype – plus the following:

- Absence of anti-GM-CSF antibody (on at least two tests)
- Nothing to suggest or prove hPAP
- Presence of a typical provoking disease including
- Haematological malignancy – leukaemia, lymphoma but most commonly myelodysplasia
- Other malignancy
- Severe infection, especially pulmonary
- Some cases of other ILD – where a degree of PAP complicates other patterns of disease such as NSIP or DIP
- Massive environmental exposure to pollutants such as silica dust

Regarding treatment, WLL can play a vital role in temporarily controlling symptoms of breathlessness and improving physiological function, but it is important to diagnose and control the underlying condition. There are many examples in the literature where fixing the provoking disease results in complete remission of the PAP.

CLINICAL CASES

Example 1: A 56-year-old woman with no significant past history presented with gradual progressively worsening dyspnoea and exercise limitation. She had severely reduced lung volumes and her gas transfer was less than 50% and A-aDO2 was 6 kPa with PaO2 in air around 6.5 kPa and SpO2 between 85% and 88% at rest. CT chest was typical of PAP, and BAL confirmed the typical milky appearance of PAP. She was subjected to video-assisted thoracoscopic surgery (VATS) lung biopsy to confirm the diagnosis, but this was complicated by delayed extubation after anaesthesia and wound infection. She also went on to suffer prolonged neuropathic chest pain at the wound site. She was referred to a specialist PAP centre and benefited from WLL treatments, but the boost in function and symptoms was always relatively brief (3 months) before repeat WLL was again required and she had frequent chest infections requiring oral antibiotics. The anti-GM-CSF antibody test was negative, but she did have atypical mycobacterium (*Mycobacterium kansasii*) in BAL cultures. Because of her recurrent PAP and significant infections she was further investigated and a bone marrow aspiration revealed a mild degree of myelodysplasia (MDS). A haematological multidisciplinary team meeting decided that the MDS was 'too mild to warrant treatment by bone marrow transplantation' and her PAP continued to worsen and the associated pulmonary infections also, despite frequent courses of systemic antibiotics and repetition of WLL. She subsequently died with worsening hypoxaemia and uncontrollable infection.

Example 2: A 22-year-old woman was seen with a history of frequent and recurrent infections including lower respiratory and vulvar warts. She developed a classical picture of PAP (chest radiograph, CT and milky appearance of BAL fluid) and required multiple WLL treatments at a PAP centre to control her symptoms. Because the anti-GM-CSF antibody was negative and because it was noted that she had absolute monocytopenia on multiple blood counts, it was decided to do a bone marrow aspiration that confirmed that she had autosomal dominant monocytopenia. She was referred back to the originating university hospital where she underwent successful matched unrelated donor stem cell transplant. The PAP completely resolved with no further treatment (7).

TREATMENT OF PAP

The established treatment for PAP is physical removal of the excess lipoprotein and foamy macrophages from the alveolar space by lavage. This can be accomplished by bronchial segmental lavage via a fibre-optic bronchoscope and this approach certainly has a role; for instance where general anaesthesia is contraindicated or not possible but in most cases rapid and effective improvement is better achieved by massive WLL. The first description of WLL was in 1963 (8), not long after the syndrome was first described. Variants of WLL have evolved over the years and Campo et al (9) recently published a survey of current practice. This confirms that a small number of centres are concentrating effort and delivering treatment that is both safe and effective.

WHOLE LUNG LAVAGE: GENERAL PRINCIPLES

The essence is simple; under general anaesthesia, a double-lumen endobronchial tube is placed to ensure safe and secure separation of left and right lungs. One lung is ventilated to ensure adequate oxygenation and the other is lavaged with a very large quantity of fluid to clear the lung of the accumulated lipoprotein and other debris. The initial returns are often strikingly turbid because of the concentration of the emulsion but gradually clear, and when visually clear, the therapeutic endpoint has been reached and all residual fluid is drained and the lung re-ventilated (Figure 22.5).

There are interesting variants in technique but most operators use plain 0.9% saline as the lavage fluid, often with a little sodium bicarbonate added (0.6 mmol of sodium bicarbonate per 1 litre of saline) to shift the pH to neutral. The saline must be instilled at body temperature to prevent hypothermia or scolding and should be sterile and, preferably micro-filtered to remove any particulate matter. Large total volumes may be required, perhaps as much as 30–40 litres per lung in normal-size adults with severe PAP. There are then two

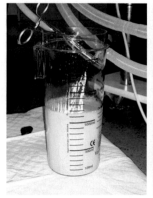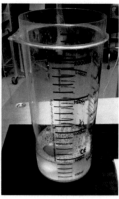

Figure 22.5 Typical fluid returns from WLL in severe PAP on the left at the start and on the right when the therapeutic endpoint has been reached and the returns are clear.

main variants of the WLL; simple tidal volumes of saline instilled and then immediately drained and degassing to convert the lung to saline ventilation.

SIMPLE TIDAL EXCHANGE WLL

The lavage lumen of the double-lumen tube (the treatment lung side) is connected to a funnel and a tidal volume of warm neutral saline of perhaps 500 mL to 1 litre is instilled and the lumen clamped shut. Many centres then use physiotherapy or some other variant of agitation to increase lavage efficiency. The saline is drained gravitationally by tipping the patient's head down and the process repeated until the returns are clear.

SALINE VENTILATION WLL

Both lungs are ventilated with 100% oxygen until there is no insoluble nitrogen left. The lavage lung lumen is clamped at end-expiration and the sterile saline delivery circuit attached. Saline is gradually let in from the closed circuit (Figure 22.6) as the residual oxygen is absorbed by ongoing perfusion until the lung is full to total lung capacity (TLC) with saline. A tidal volume of around 500 mL is let out into a measuring cylinder via the closed-loop circuit and replaced with 500 mL from the reservoir. The process is repeated, possibly with larger tidal volumes to recruit more lung until the returns are clear. Agitation of the lung is not required in this variant of WLL because it is inherently more efficient at reaching a high proportion of affected lung units.

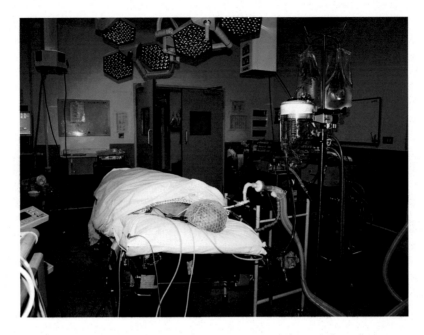

Figure 22.6 The scene in the operating room during WLL. Note the ventilator hoses are attached to the left lung lumen of the double-lumen tube and the lavage closed circuit is attached to the right lung lumen. There is a reservoir of saline for accurately instilling tidal volumes of saline into the right lung. The reservoir can be refilled from the large bags of saline by pump through a heat exchanger to ensure body temperature. Clamps control inlet and outlet into a collecting cylinder (not in view).

SINGLE VERSUS BILATERAL LUNG WLL

Some centres only ever perform WLL of one lung in a single session and this is perfectly reasonable. The procedure may take several hours and involve 30 to 50 litres of saline. The patient will need to be ventilated for a period of between 2 and 8 hours post-operatively until they are ready to resume spontaneous breathing and be extubated. However it is also routine in some centres to perform bilateral WLL in the same session. One lung is treated, both lungs are then ventilated to allow recovery of the treated lung before a trial of one lung ventilation of the just-treated lung is confirmed to be safe, then the second lung is treated. This more than doubles the treatment time and may require a little longer recovery, but the advantage is that the patient goes home with both lungs fixed and with relatively less disruption of their routine.

COMPLICATIONS OF WLL

Hazards and complications of WLL are probably equal for both main variants and the most important is hypoxia. The patient may already be severely compromised by severe disease, perhaps with SpO2 already less than 90% at rest in room air. They typically improve with anaesthesia and positive pressure ventilation because PAP is essentially a restrictive lung disease. The patient may well require a high FiO2 and relatively high airway pressure and positive end-expiratory pressure (PEEP) to recruit and ventilate adequately. The patient may tolerate one lung ventilation (OLV) very badly with a significant fall in oxygenation and potentially significant increase in arterial CO_2. In most cases the disturbance is tolerated with the most severe patients already habituated to chronic hypoxia so the massive therapeutic benefit of the WLL easily offsets the intra-operative gas exchange problem. But there are reports of successful temporary use of extracorporeal membrane oxygenation (ECMO) to support safe WLL in extreme hypoxia.

Other risks and issues include the standard risks of general anaesthesia such as anaphylaxis, etc. and more specific risks of WLL such as hypothermia (if the saline is not adequately warmed) and spillage of saline unintentionally into the ventilated lung (if the technique for lung separation is not secure). All of the risks are controllable with standard care for the anaesthesia and experience with a consistent WLL technique.

WLL should be confined to a small number of centres that thus have sufficient experience through numbers of treatments for the procedure to become 'routine' in their hands. Before embarking on a first WLL it would be wise to visit an active WLL centre to see how it is done.

RESPONSE TO TREATMENT AFTER WLL

Several publications confirm the durable and long-term benefit of WLL (10). A well-executed WLL in a patient with severe PAP will result in a dramatic improvement in symptoms, signs and objective measurements of gas exchange, respiratory function and exercise tolerance. Everything gets better and most importantly, the patient feels better. There may be a slight delay in maximal benefit however as not all of the lavage saline is recovered; some is stranded in the lung despite gravitational drainage and suction. It does no harm and is gradually absorbed and then maximum benefit is seen between 24 and 72 hours post-WLL.

In some cases the PAP never comes back but in most cases the accumulation of surfactant and macrophages recurs and eventually symptoms and objective deterioration prompt repeat treatment. The speed of decline is variable and somewhat unpredictable so the patients need to be monitored over time. Even before the recent understanding of the pathophysiology of PAP it was typical that the vast majority of patients eventually achieved satisfactory and sustained remission – but after a variable number of WLLs.

ALTERNATIVE TREATMENT OF PAP IN ADDITION TO WLL

There have been anecdotal reports of treatment of aPAP with immune-suppression (usually rituximab) to suppress the T lymphocytes producing the excess anti-GM-CSF and of plasma exchange to actually remove the antibody. However the alternative treatment with the greatest uptake and best promise is the use of exogenous GM-CSF. The first trials were using subcutaneous injected GM-CSF

with half of a small series showing significant improvement (11). No harm was done in the case of the non-responders but all were at risk of minor injection site irritation issues. It makes intuitive sense to deliver the drug to where the main action is and inhaling GM-CSF has been demonstrated to be safe, more effective and significantly cheaper than the injection route. There is yet a lack of powerful evidence from double-blinded prospective randomized trials of inhaled GM-CSF in aPAP, but the observational material from Japan, the United States and Europe is extremely encouraging (12–14).

One major issue with using inhaled GM-CSF in aPAP is that there is no licenced product anywhere in the world. Patients have been treated mostly with a branded version of GM-CSF produced for injection and licenced only for a limited range of bone marrow support in haematological malignancy and only in the United States. It is therefore being used off-licence, off-label and off-route. In fact it is impossible to obtain and prescribe in some jurisdictions. This situation should improve in the next few years.

CONCLUSION

The great progress in understanding the pathophysiology of aPAP, and to an extent for some of the variants of hPAP, has stimulated beneficial interest in macrophage signalling and control which should have direct benefit in PAP and potentially in several other serious pulmonary and non-pulmonary conditions. There is a real prospect in the near future (15,16) of taking pluri-potential cells and processing them *ex vivo* before re-introducing them, for example by bronchoscopic instillation back to the patient as a normal functional population of healthy pulmonary macrophages – effectively alveolar macrophage transplantation in selected cases of hPAP with otherwise untreatable disease. There may even be a role for cell-based manipulations in the more common aPAP variant but at present it would seem that conventional therapy with WLL, which is proven, safe and effective should be supported with trials of inhaled GM-CSF when WLL alone is not winning. Other treatments such as plasma exchange and immune suppression should be reserved for the rare circumstances where both WLL and inhaled GM-CSF have failed.

REFERENCES

1. Seymour JF, Presneill JJ. Pulmonary alveolar proteinosis: Progress in the first 44 years. *Am J Respir Crit Care Med.* 2002;166:215–35.

2. Trapnell BC, Whitsett JA, Nakata K. Pulmonary alveolar proteinosis. *N Engl J Med.* 2003;349:2527–39.

3. Kitamura T, Tanaka N, Watanabe J, Uchida K, Kanegasaki S, Yamada Y, Nakata K. Idiopathic pulmonary alveolar proteinosis as an autoimmune disease with neutralizing antibody against granulocyte-macrophage colony stimulating factor. *J Exp Med.* 1999;190:875–80.

4. Hildebrandt J, Yalcin E, Bresser HG, Cinel G, Gappa M, Haghighi A et al. Characterization of CSF2RA mutation related juvenile pulmonary alveolar proteinosis. *Orphanet J Rare Dis.* 2014;9:171.

5. Suzuki T, Arumugam P, Sakagami T, Lachmann N, Chalk C, Sallese A et al. Pulmonary macrophage transplantation therapy. *Nature.* 2014;514:450–4.

6. Chaulagain CP, Pilichowska M, Brinkerhoff L, Tabba M, Erban JK. Secondary pulmonary alveolar proteinosis in hematologic malignancies. *Hematol Oncol Stem Cell Ther.* 2014;7:127–35.

7. Bigley V, Haniffa M, Doulatov S, Wang XN, Dickinson R, McGovern N et al. The human syndrome of dendritic cell, monocyte, B and NK lymphoid deficiency. *J. Exp. Med.* 2011;208:227–34.

8. Ramirez RJ, Schult R, Dutton RE. Pulmonary alveolar proteinosis: A new technique and rationale for treatment. *Arch Intern Med.* 1963;112:419–31.

9. Campo I, Luisetti M, Griese M, Trapnell BC, Bonella F, Grutters J et al. Whole lung lavage therapy for pulmonary alveolar proteinosis: A global survey of current practices and procedures. *Orphanet J Rare Dis.* 2016;11:115.

10. Beccaria M, Luisetti M, Rodi G, Corsico A, Zoia MC, Colato S et al. Long-term durable benefit after whole lung lavage in pulmonary alveolar proteinosis. *Eur Respir J.* 2004;23:526–31.

11. Seymour JF, Dunn AR, Vincent JM, Presneill JJ, Pain MC. Efficacy of granulocyte-macrophage colony-stimulating factor in acquired alveolar proteinosis. *N Engl J Med.* 1996;335:1924–5.

12. Wylam ME, Ten R, Prakash UB, Nadrous HF, Clawson ML, Anderson PM. Aerosol granulocyte-macrophage colony-stimulating factor for pulmonary alveolar proteinosis. *Eur Respir J.* 2006;27:585–93.

13. Tazawa R, Trapnell BC, Inoue Y, Arai T, Takada T, Nasuhara Y et al. Inhaled granulocyte/macrophage-colony stimulating factor as therapy of pulmonary alveolar proteinosis. *Am J Respir Crit Care Med.* 2010;181:1345–54.

14. Tazawa R, Inoue Y, Arai T, Takada T, Kasahara Y, Hojo M et al. Duration of benefit in patients with autoimmune pulmonary alveolar proteinosis after inhaled granulocyte-macrophage colony-stimulating factor therapy. *Chest.* 2014;145:729–37.

15. Happle C, Lachmann N, Skuljec J, Wetzke M, Ackermann M, Brennig S et al. Pulmonary transplantation of macrophage progenitors as effective and long-lasting therapy for hereditary pulmonary alveolar proteinosis. *Sci Transl Med.* 2014;6(250):250ra113.

16. Kotton DN, Rossant J. Modeling pulmonary alveolar proteinosis with induced pluripotent stem cells. *Am J Respir Crit Care Med.* 2014;189:124–6.

23

Rare forms of interstitial lung disease

JAY H RYU

INTRODUCTION

There has been an increasing recognition that rare diseases represent a substantial global health burden. In the United States, rare or orphan disease is defined as a condition affecting less than 200,000 persons, which is approximately 63 per 100,000 persons (1,2). In Europe, a disorder is defined as rare when it affects less than 1 in 2,000 (approximately 50 per 100,000) persons. Because there are more than 6,000 rare diseases, it is estimated that 8% of the general population are affected by these rare disorders, and many of them remain undiagnosed (1,2).

There are many lung diseases that are rare. Indeed, nearly all interstitial lung diseases (ILDs) are rare using definitions cited above and pose challenges to appropriate diagnosis and management, even for experienced clinicians at large academic medical centres. This chapter covers several of these poorly recognized ILDs. Included in this chapter are amyloidosis, IgG4-related disease, follicular bronchiolitis, diffuse panbronchiolitis, diffuse aspiration bronchiolitis, Erdheim–Chester disease, pulmonary alveolar microlithiasis, diffuse pulmonary lymphatic diseases, Hermansky–Pudlak syndrome and other heritable disorders. Finally, neoplastic disorders that can mimic ILDs are also discussed.

AMYLOIDOSIS

Amyloidosis refers to a group of inherited or acquired conditions that result from extracellular deposition of insoluble fibrillar protein of β-pleated sheet structure that allows the characteristic binding of Congo red stain. Amyloid can form from a variety of precursor proteins. The three most common forms of amyloidosis are primary amyloidosis (immunoglobulin light chains, AL), transthyretin amyloidosis (ATTR), and amyloid A protein amyloidosis (AA) (3,4).

Clinical manifestations of amyloidosis are diverse and determined by the type of precursor protein, tissue distribution and extent of deposition. It can present in systemic or organ-limited (localized) forms. When amyloid is found in the

Table 23.1 Patterns of pulmonary amyloidosis

Tracheobronchial plaques/masses (focal
    or diffuse)
Parenchymal nodules (may contain calcification
    or cavitations)
Diffuse or localized interstitial infiltrates
    Reticular opacities and septal thickening
    Cystic lesions
Hilar/mediastinal lymphadenopathy
Pleural effusion
Pulmonary vascular disease
    Pulmonary hypertension
    Pulmonary vascular aneurysm

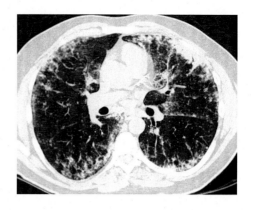

Figure 23.1 HRCT of diffuse interstitial pulmonary amyloidosis in a 56-year-old woman with systemic AL amyloidosis. Predominantly peripheral distribution of reticular and consolidative opacities is present.

lung, it may be part of a systemic process or limited to the lung (5–7).

Pulmonary involvement in amyloidosis usually results from primary (AL) amyloidosis (deposition of immunoglobulin light-chain fragments), which typically occurs in adults older than 50 years of age (5,6). Intra-thoracic manifestations of amyloidosis can be classified as tracheobronchial disease, parenchymal nodules (sometimes partially calcified or cavitated), localized or diffuse interstitial infiltrates, intra-thoracic lymphadenopathy, pleural disease and pulmonary vascular disease (Table 23.1). Tracheobronchial and interstitial infiltration with amyloid often causes symptoms including cough and dyspnoea, whereas nodular pulmonary amyloidosis generally does not.

Diffuse interstitial pulmonary amyloidosis manifests bilateral reticular or reticulonodular opacities on chest radiography. High-resolution CT (HRCT) of the chest demonstrates diffuse reticular opacities and inter-lobular septal thickening that may contain punctate calcifications (Figure 23.1) (8,9). These interstitial infiltrates may be associated with the presence of small nodules or patchy ground-glass/consolidation opacities as well as intra-thoracic lymphadenopathy. In recent years, it has been recognized that amyloidosis can also cause cystic lung lesions, which can at times be diffusely distributed in both lungs (10,11).

The diagnosis of pulmonary amyloidosis is confirmed by obtaining a biopsy that demonstrates the presence of amyloid deposits with positive staining by Congo red, which reveals the characteristic apple-green birefringence with polarized microscopy (3,12). The type of amyloid can be characterized by immunohistochemistry or mass spectroscopy. In systemic AL amyloidosis, a monoclonal immunoglobulin in the serum or monoclonal light chains in the urine are detectable in approximately 80% of cases (3,4).

Treatment of pulmonary amyloidosis is individualized based on the type of amyloid, pattern of involvement and clinical effects. Diffuse parenchymal pulmonary AL amyloidosis is treated with systemic chemotherapy aimed at the underlying amyloidosis along with autologous haematopoietic stem cell transplantation (13). The nodular form of pulmonary amyloidosis often does not need treatment. Tracheobronchial amyloidosis (usually AL amyloidosis), when symptomatic, can be treated with bronchoscopic resection or external beam radiation (14).

IMMUNOGLOBULIN G4-RELATED DISEASE

Immunoglobulin G4-related disease (IgG4-RD) is a recently described fibroinflammatory disorder of unknown cause and characterized by an infiltrate of IgG4-positive plasma cells and lymphocytes in a characteristic histopathologic pattern (15–18). Sometimes, a modest increase in eosinophils may be seen (17). Fibrosis, focally organized in a storiform pattern, is another characteristic finding of IgG4-RD (15,16). However, storiform fibrosis is not commonly seen in pulmonary lesions. Both pulmonary arteries and veins show an intimal inflammation and active fibrosis, resulting in obliterative phlebitis and arteritis (15,17). It should be noted, however, that IgG4-positive plasma cell infiltration can be seen in other conditions that can mimic IgG4–RD. These conditions include granulomatosis with polyangiitis (Wegener granulomatosis), eosinophilic granulomatosis and polyangiitis (Churg–Strauss syndrome), multicentric Castleman disease and some malignancies (16,19).

First described as a form of autoimmune pancreatitis, IgG4-RD has been recognized to frequently involve the salivary glands, kidneys, retroperitoneum and orbital adnexal structures, but virtually any organ can be affected. Elevated serum IgG4 level is demonstrated in about 60%–70% patients (17,20–22).

Pulmonary involvement has been reported in approximately 10%–15% of patients with IgG4-RD (15,17,21). Although initial reports of pulmonary involvement were described in those manifesting IgG4-related autoimmune pancreatitis, more recent reports indicate that IgG4-related lung disease may precede pancreatic involvement or be seen in the absence of pancreatic disease (23,24).

Pulmonary manifestations are heterogeneous and include parenchymal nodules or masses, patchy ground-glass or consolidative infiltrates and diffuse interstitial lung infiltrates (Table 23.2) (21,25). Airways may be involved as well with bronchial inflammation or tracheobronchial stenosis that causes patients to present with asthma-like symptoms (21,26). Other intra-thoracic findings are mediastinal lymphadenopathy (27), fibrosing mediastinitis (28) and pleural nodules or effusion (29). When IgG4-RD presents in the lung as ILD, widely varying HRCT patterns of interstitial lung infiltrates may be seen including reticular opacities, patchy ground-glass opacities, alveolar consolidation and thickening of the bronchovascular bundles and inter-lobular septa (21,23,30–35).

Earlier studies describing patients with IgG4-RD emphasized the association with elevated serum IgG4 level (>135 mg/dL), but this laboratory finding is not adequately sensitive or specific for diagnostic purposes (22,25,36–38). The serum IgG4 level has been reported to be elevated in 50%–95% of patients with active IgG4-RD (22,36,39,40). Conversely, only 10%–20% of patients with an

Table 23.2 Pulmonary manifestations of IgG4-RD

Lung Parenchyma
Focal opacities (nodules, masses)
Interstitial lung disease
Airway
Stenosis/endobronchial mass
Bronchospastic disease
Pulmonary Vasculature
Vasculitis
Pulmonary hypertension
Mediastinum
Lymphadenopathy
Fibrosing mediastinitis
Pleural
Thickening or mass
Effusion

elevated serum IgG4 level in clinical practice have IgG4-RD (25,41,42). Thus, an elevated serum IgG4 level is supportive of the diagnosis of IgG4-RD but not necessary nor diagnostically sufficient.

In general, the diagnosis of IgG4-RD requires judicious correlation of clinicoradiologic findings with histopathologic features, which typically include dense lymphoplasmacytic infiltrates, fibrosis with a storiform pattern and obliterative phlebitis combined with an increased number of IgG4+ plasma cells (21,37,38,43,44). None of the histopathologic features or laboratory findings, including a high serum IgG4 level, is specific for the diagnosis of IgG4-RD. Suggested cut-off values for quantitating IgG4+ plasma cells in the diagnosis of IgG4-RD vary depending on the organ, according to the current consensus statement on pathologic analysis (43). For the lung, >20 or >50 IgG4+ plasma cells per high power field in non-surgical biopsy and surgical biopsy specimens, respectively, with an IgG4+/IgG+ plasma cell ratio of >40% for both types of specimens have been proposed. The respective cut-off values for the pleura are >50 IgG4+ plasma cells per high power field and >40% IgG4+/IgG+ plasma cell ratio (43).

To identify the characteristic histopathologic features of IgG4-RD within the thorax, a surgical biopsy specimen is generally needed. However, bronchoscopic or transthoracic needle biopsy may sometimes yield features suggestive of IgG4-RD while allowing exclusion of competing diagnoses (21,38,43).

While histopathologic data are important in confirming the diagnosis of IgG4-RD lung involvement, lung or pleural biopsy may not be necessary in achieving this diagnosis if an extra-pulmonary organ has already been biopsied to confirm the presence of IgG4-RD. In the absence of another more likely explanation for the intra-thoracic lesion, the diagnosis of IgG4-RD can be assumed in most such cases. A subsequent clinical course that is atypical such as progressive lung disease despite treatment may warrant additional diagnostic evaluation including lung biopsy.

The goal for the treatment of IgG4-RD, in general, is the prevention of irreversible fibrosis and organ damage (16,37,45). Corticosteroids are generally considered the first-line therapy for IgG4-RD. Although the optimal dose of corticosteroid therapy in the treatment of IgG4-RD has not been rigorously determined, most authors recommend oral prednisone or equivalent at an initial dosage of 30–40 mg/day (16,37,46). This initial dose is maintained for 2–4 weeks with a favourable response typically seen by 2 weeks on treatment. Subsequently, the corticosteroid dose is gradually tapered over the following weeks to months, typically 3–6 months, while monitoring for possible recurrence or reactivation of disease.

As with extra-thoracic lesions, intra-thoracic manifestations of IgG4-RD respond well to corticosteroid therapy (16,21,23,24,27,30,33,37,45,47–50). However, it should be noted that there have been no randomized clinical trials conducted to investigate the efficacy of treatment for IgG4-RD. In addition, some patients with asymptomatic disease may not require pharmacologic therapy.

Although most patients respond well to initial therapy, the durability of response is variable, and relapses have been commonly observed (39). Thus, some authors have advocated the use of a low-dose maintenance therapy (e.g. prednisone 5 mg/day) for a longer period to reduce the risk of such relapse (16,51–54). In addition, various steroid-sparing immunosuppressive agents have been used in the treatment of IgG4-RD, but the evidence supporting their use is limited (16,37,39,45,55). These agents have included azathioprine, mycophenolate mofetil, methotrexate, cyclophosphamide, 6-mercaptopurine and tacrolimus (16,21,37,39,55–58). A relatively new concept in the treatment of IgG4-RD is B-cell depletion therapy. Several reports in recent years have described successful use of rituximab therapy, even in patients who failed to achieve a durable remission with steroid-sparing immunosuppressive agents (31,59–66).

Prompt recognition and effective treatment prevent irreversible organ damage from the fibrotic changes that can result from persistently active IgG4-RD (46,54,67). Deaths directly attributable to IgG4-RD are rare and have resulted from cardiac or aortic involvement (39,55,56,68,69).

BRONCHIOLITIS

The term 'bronchiolitis' refers to inflammation and/or fibrosis involving bronchioles, small airways that do not contain cartilage in their walls and have internal diameter ≤ 2 mm. There are multiple forms of bronchiolitis, and associated clinico-radiologic features are heterogeneous (70,71). For example, constrictive bronchiolitis manifests airflow obstruction physiologically along with mosaic pattern (due to air trapping) on HRCT, while others present with diffuse parenchymal opacities. The latter group includes respiratory bronchiolitis (discussed in Chapter 17), follicular bronchiolitis, diffuse panbronchiolitis and diffuse aspiration bronchiolitis.

FOLLICULAR BRONCHIOLITIS

Follicular bronchiolitis is a disorder characterized by the presence of hyperplastic lymphoid follicles with reactive germinal centres distributed along bronchiolar walls and associated with a mild degree of lymphocytic infiltration within the adjacent interstitium (72,73). Peribronchiolar nodules, 3–10 mm in diameter, formed by lymphoid follicles with reactive germinal centres are defining histopathological features in follicular bronchiolitis (70,74). Bronchiolar lumens may be compromised (75). An inflammatory infiltrate of T cells (CD3+) may be present in the immediate peribronchiolar interstitium, while the extensive parenchymal expansion that characterizes lymphoid interstitial pneumonia (LIP) is absent (76).

Follicular bronchiolitis likely results from repetitive antigen stimulation of bronchus-associated lymphoid tissue (BALT) with consequent polyclonal lymphoid expansion (73). It is usually associated with connective tissue diseases (72,77), such as Sjögren syndrome (78) and rheumatoid arthritis (74,79) as well as immunodeficiency syndromes (80,81). It may be idiopathic in some cases (72,74).

Typical presenting symptoms include dyspnoea and cough but pulmonary function findings are variable. Chest radiography may appear normal but generally demonstrates bilateral small nodular or reticulonodular infiltrates with intra-thoracic presentation. The cardinal features of follicular bronchiolitis on HRCT consist of centrilobular nodules measuring 1–12 mm in diameter that are variably associated with peribronchial nodules and patchy areas of ground-glass opacity (72,74,75). Nodules and ground-glass opacities are generally bilateral and diffuse in distribution (72,74,75). Treatment is usually directed at the underlying disease (e.g. connective tissue disease) and usually involves corticosteroids and other immunosuppressive agents. The prognostic implication of follicular bronchiolitis is uncertain, particularly when it is found in patients with underlying systemic diseases.

DIFFUSE PANBRONCHIOLITIS

Diffuse panbronchiolitis is an unusual form of bronchiolitis of unknown cause described mainly in Asia, particularly in Japanese adults, and is characterized by diffuse bronchiolar inflammation and chronic sinusitis (82,83). Few cases occurring in non-Asian patients have been described in the United States and Europe (84,85). Patients are typically middle aged and present with sub-acute onset of cough productive of purulent sputum, dyspnoea and evidence of airflow obstruction.

Histopathologic findings in diffuse panbronchiolitis are characteristic and consist of bronchiolocentric infiltration of lymphocytes, plasma cells and foamy macrophages at the level of the respiratory bronchioles (70,82,83). Accumulation of foam cells in the walls of the respiratory bronchioles, adjacent alveolar ducts and alveoli is the most distinctive feature of diffuse panbronchiolitis. However, similar histopathologic features can be seen in other inflammatory airway diseases such as bronchiectasis (86).

On chest radiography, diffuse panbronchiolitis is characterized by diffuse, small, ill-defined nodular opacities (up to 5 mm in diameter) that are most prominent over the lung bases and symmetrically distributed. In late stages, the radiographic features of cylindrical bronchiectasis and hyperinflation may become evident (82,83). Findings on HRCT depend on the stage of the disease and include centrilobular nodules, distal branching structures, thickened and ectatic bronchioles, bronchiectasis and peripheral air trapping (82,83).

The natural history of diffuse panbronchiolitis is characterized by progressive respiratory dysfunction with episodic bacterial superinfection, often with *Pseudomonas aeruginosa* in advanced stages (82,83). When untreated, nearly 50% of patients died within 5 years of diagnosis. Long-term (at least 6 months), low-dose erythromycin therapy, 400–600 mg per day, is the preferred treatment and improves symptoms, lung function, computed tomography scan abnormalities and survival. Other macrolides such as azithromycin and clarithromycin can be used for those who cannot tolerate erythromycin therapy. Macrolides have been demonstrated to possess immunomodulatory effects on inflammatory cells and suppress airway hypersecretion (82,83,87).

DIFFUSE ASPIRATION BRONCHIOLITIS

There is a diverse spectrum of airway and parenchymal pulmonary disorders related to aspiration (88–90). The two most commonly recognized forms of aspiration-related lung diseases are aspiration pneumonitis (acute lung injury following aspiration of gastric contents) and aspiration pneumonia (pneumonia developing after aspiration of oropharyngeal secretions) (88). Diffuse aspiration bronchiolitis (DAB) is a term used to define a clinical entity that is characterized by chronic inflammation of bronchioles caused by recurrent aspiration of foreign particles (89,91,92). Although earlier descriptions of this disorder comprised elderly and bed-ridden subjects, recent reports suggest that this disorder can be seen in adults of varying ages with gastro-oesophageal reflux disease (GERD) that may be clinically occult (92,93) Histologic findings of DAB are characterized by localization of chronic mural inflammation with foreign-body reaction in bronchioles (92).

Patients with DAB usually present with productive cough and exertional dyspnoea (92,93). Intermittent fevers and a history of 'pneumonias' are also common. Aspiration is occult in the majority of patients (92,93). Chest radiography demonstrates patchy or diffuse interstitial infiltrates suggestive of ILD. HRCT demonstrates findings characteristic of bronchiolitis with micronodules and tree-in-bud opacities.

Management of patients with DAB focuses on prevention of recurrent aspiration by addressing the underlying risk factors such as GERD and drug abuse. Corticosteroids and antimicrobial therapy are unlikely to be of benefit.

ERDHEIM–CHESTER DISEASE

Erdheim–Chester disease (ECD) is a rare non-Langerhans histiocytic disorder with multiorgan involvement characterized by tissue infiltration with foamy histiocytes along with interspersed inflammatory cells and multinucleated giant cells (Touton cells) (94–96). The aetiology of ECD remains unclear. It is not an infectious or inheritable disorder. Chronic uncontrolled inflammation appears to be a dominant process with evidence of intense systemic immune activation. Somatic mutations in the *BRAF* gene (*BRAF* V600E mutation) were recently identified in over one-half of patients with ECD (97,98).

The clinical presentation of ECD varies depending on the dominant sites of organ system involvement. Long bones are most commonly involved, and bone pain, particularly in the lower extremities, is the most common presenting symptom and related to bilateral, symmetric osteosclerotic diaphyseal and metaphyseal lesions (94,96,99,100). Approximately 50%–60% of ECD patients will have extra-osseous disease that includes the heart, lungs, central nervous system (CNS) and orbital structures.

Pulmonary involvement is seen in 25%–50% of patients with ECD and includes parenchymal infiltrates, mediastinal infiltration and pleural effusion/thickening (94,96,101,102). The most common pulmonary symptom is dyspnoea, the gender distribution for pulmonary involvement by ECD appears equal, and most cases arise in middle-aged patients. The most common parenchymal finding seen on chest CT is inter-lobular septal thickening (Figure 23.2), but other abnormalities including reticular opacities, centrilobular nodules, ground-glass opacities, cysts and visceral pleural thickening

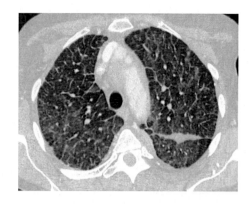

Figure 23.2 HRCT of Erdheim–Chester disease in a 62-year-old woman. A diffuse parenchymal infiltrative process consisting of inter-lobular septal thickening and patchy ground-glass opacities is seen. Also seen are focal thickening of the left major fissure and some reticular opacities.

can also be present (101–103). Pulmonary function testing typically shows a restrictive pattern with a decreased diffusing capacity.

The diagnosis of ECD is achieved by identifying the distinctive histopathologic findings of tissue infiltration by foamy histiocytes with non-Langerhans features (CD1a-negative and absence of Birbeck granules) in the context of appropriate clinical and imaging features. In the lung, the histiocytic infiltration and associated fibrosis exhibit a lymphangitic distribution (104). On immuno-histochemical staining, the foamy histiocytes are positive for CD68 but not CD1a, S100 and Langerin (CD207), which are all Langerhans cell markers. After ECD is diagnosed, the *BRAF* mutational status needs to be established, as these results have implications for therapy (94,96,105,106).

There are no randomized clinical trials in the treatment of ECD. ECD is currently not curable, but therapy can improve symptoms and outcomes (94,96). Therapy is recommended for most patients with ECD, although asymptomatic patients may not need to be treated. A variety of agents have been used in the treatment of ECD, but the treatment modality with the most favourable experience is interferon-α (96,107,108). Other treatments have included anti-cytokine therapies such as infliximab and anakinra, corticosteroids, imatinib and chemotherapeutic agents such as cladribine or combination cytotoxic agents (94,96). In ECD patients manifesting *BRAF* mutations, excellent response to vemurafenib, a *BRAF* kinase inhibitor, has recently been reported (105,106). Optimal treatment for pulmonary lesions in ECD has not been defined, but improvement with interferon-α and vemurafenib therapy (in patients with *BRAF* V600r mutation) has been reported (106,107).

The natural history of ECD is not well defined, but spontaneous regression appears to be uncommon. A five-year survival rate of 68% has been reported. CNS involvement is a major prognostic factor and an independent predictor of mortality.

PULMONARY ALVEOLAR MICROLITHIASIS

Pulmonary alveolar microlithiasis is a rare lung disease characterized by extensive intra-alveolar deposition of concentrically lamellated calcium phosphate spheres that results in a distinctive calcific micronodular infiltrate seen on chest radiography and CT (109–111). This disease was recently discovered to be a genetic disease caused by mutations of the *SLC34A2* gene, which encodes a type IIb sodium phosphate cotransporter (112,113). Mutations in the *SLC34A2* gene that impair normal co-transporter function (transporting the phosphorus ion from the alveolar space into the alveolar type II cells) cause formation of intra-alveolar calcium phosphate microliths (i.e. pulmonary alveolar microlithiasis). It is inherited in an autosomal recessive pattern.

Pulmonary alveolar microlithiasis is found world-wide but predominates in several countries including Turkey, Japan, China, India and Italy (109). The age at diagnosis spans a wide range with one-third being less than 20 years old (109–111). Many patients are asymptomatic at presentation and are diagnosed after abnormalities are detected on incidental chest imaging studies. Exertional dyspnoea and cough occur in later stages of the disease, usually in the third and fourth decades of life, and the disease course may eventually be complicated by respiratory failure and cor pulmonale (109,110). Expectoration of microliths is uncommon. Elevated serum concentrations of the surfactant proteins A and D have been reported in patients with pulmonary alveolar microlithiasis, but this is a non-specific finding.

Chest radiography reveals bilateral fine, sand-like calcified micronodules throughout both lungs ('sandstorm' appearance) that are more prominent in mid and lower lung zones (109,111,114). HRCT of the chest confirms micronodular calcifications but may also demonstrate ground-glass opacities and inter-lobular septal calcifications, which sometimes results in a 'crazy-paving' pattern (109,111,114). Coalescence of micronodules may give rise to consolidative opacities.

The diagnosis of pulmonary alveolar microlithiasis is usually achieved based on the characteristic appearance on chest CT. Lung biopsy, if needed, will demonstrate intra-alveolar microliths that may be associated with interstitial inflammation and fibrosis. Genetic testing demonstrating the presence of the *SLC34A2* gene mutation also confirms the diagnosis.

The clinical course of patients with pulmonary alveolar microlithiasis is variable, but many will show slow progression of disease over a course of 10–15 years that often results in death from respiratory failure and cor pulmonale, which typically occurs in the fifth decade of life (109–111). There is no known therapy, but lung transplantation, more commonly bilateral than unilateral, has been successfully employed in several cases (115–117). Use of bisphosphonate therapy has been described with improvement noted in some of these cases (118,119).

DIFFUSE PULMONARY LYMPHATIC DISEASES

There are several disorders related to proliferation of lymphatic tissue that can be seen in the thorax (120,121). For example, lymphangioma is a benign lesion that results from focal proliferation of lymphatics and can present as fluid-filled cystic masses that are typically located in the mediastinum (122). However, there are two notable lymphatic disorders that can involve the lung parenchyma diffusely and present as ILD: diffuse pulmonary lymphangiomatosis and pulmonary lymphangiectasis. Although these lymphatic disorders present mainly in childhood, both can be seen in adults (120,121,123–126). There is no sex predilection, and pulmonary disease can be seen with or without evidence of a generalized lymphatic disorder.

Clinical presentation of these two disorders is nonspecific and generally consists of chronic cough and exertional dyspnoea. Chyloptysis, wheezing, chest discomfort and fever can occur.

On chest radiography, both disorders present bilateral interstitial infiltrates, which are sometimes accompanied by pleural effusions (125,127–129). Chest HRCT demonstrates extensive inter-lobular septal thickening along with mediastinal soft-tissue thickening in both disorders. Ground-glass opacities are commonly present and reflect oedema or chylous congestion.

The diagnoses of diffuse pulmonary lymphangiomatosis and pulmonary lymphangiectasis typically require surgical lung biopsy (124). Diffuse pulmonary lymphangiomatosis is characterized by proliferation of anastomosing lymphatic vessels in the inter-lobular septa, bronchovascular bundles and sub-pleural space (124,125). Lymphangiectasis is characterized mainly by dilated lymphatic vessels (124). In adult cases of lymphangiectasis, mild-to-moderate fibrosis may be present around the dilated lymphatic vessels and cause some confusion in pathologic interpretation.

Management of diffuse lymphatic diseases in the lung can be difficult due to absence of established treatment of proven efficacy. The clinical course is characterized by slow progression for patients with both disorders (120,123–125). For diffuse pulmonary lymphangiomatosis, sirolimus (130–132), bevacizumab (133), propranolol (134), imatinib (135) and interferon-α (125,136) therapy have been reported to benefit some affected patients. Lung transplantation has been performed for few patients with diffuse pulmonary lymphangiomatosis (137).

HERMANSKY–PUDLAK SYNDROME AND OTHER HERITABLE DISORDERS

The Hermansky–Pudlak syndrome (HPS) refers to a group of autosomal recessive disorders characterized by a triad of oculocutaneous albinism, bleeding diathesis related to platelet aggregation dysfunction, and, in some cases, ILD (138,139). HPS occurs worldwide, and there are nine genetic subtypes. HPS, particularly types 1 and 3, is found in high frequency among Puerto Ricans, and types 1, 2 and 4 are associated with ILD (138,140).

The clinical manifestations of HPS are related the dysfunction of various lysosome-related organelles caused by defects in intracellular protein trafficking and accumulation of ceroid lipofuscin (138,141).

ILD occurring in patients with HPS manifests as progressive interstitial fibrosis that develops during the second decade and onward. The onset of respiratory symptoms, such as dry cough and exertional dyspnoea, typically appear in the fourth decade of life (139,142). Inspiratory crackles are heard on lung auscultation, and pulmonary function testing demonstrates abnormalities with a restrictive pattern (138–140).

In HPS patients with ILD, chest radiography demonstrates bilateral interstitial infiltrates with a reticulonodular pattern or perihilar fibrosis (140,143,144). HRCT demonstrates reticulation, traction bronchiectasis and subpleural cysts distributed throughout both lungs (143).

The diagnosis of HPS is established by clinical features and the absence of dense bodies in platelets demonstrated on electron microscopy (138,139). Genetic testing can be used to identify the HPS subtype.

There is no reliable treatment for pulmonary fibrosis, which is the most common cause of death in HPS patients (138,140). Corticosteroids and immunosuppressive agents have not demonstrated efficacy (138–140). Treatment with pirfenidone, an anti-fibrotic medication, did not appear to provide benefit in a 12-month study (145). Successful bilateral lung transplantation has been performed in a patient with HPS (146).

NEUROFIBROMATOSIS

Neurofibromatosis consists of three genetically distinct forms of autosomal dominant inherited conditions manifesting neurogenic tumours. Pulmonary manifestations have been reported mainly with neurofibromatosis type 1 (von Recklinghausen neurofibromatosis), which is the most common form of neurofibromatosis. Neurofibromatosis type 1 (NF1) affects approximately 1 in 3,500 individuals. NF1 results from mutations in the *NF1* gene, which is localized to chromosome 17q 11.2. Mutations in the

NF1 gene result in lack of expression of neurofibromin, the protein product of this gene. Neurofibromin is a tumour suppressor acting as a negative regulator of the Ras signalling pathway, which is involved in cell growth. Loss of neurofibromin activity results in overactive Ras signalling that can lead to tumour formation.

Thoracic manifestations of NF1 are more often skeletal (e.g. scoliosis, kyphosis, rib deformities) or mediastinal (e.g. paravertebral neurofibromas, lateral meningoceles) rather than parenchymal. The relationship of parenchymal lesions with NF1 has been controversial with conflicting results reported (147–149). Two types of parenchymal lesions have been associated with NF1; interstitial fibrosis and cysts (bullae). A proposed relationship between these parenchymal lesions and NF1 is confounded by smoking, which was not accounted for in some studies (149). It remains to be clarified whether NF1 is truly associated with parenchymal lung changes.

LIPID STORAGE DISORDERS

Lipid storage disorders refer to a group of inherited metabolic disorders in which deleterious amounts of lipids accumulate in cells and tissues. These disorders result from deficiency of one of the enzymes needed to metabolize lipids and are inherited in an autosomal recessive or X-linked recessive pattern.

The most common lipid storage disorder is Gaucher disease, which is caused by a deficiency of a lysosomal enzyme glucocerebrosidase (also called glucosylceramidase) that leads to accumulation of glucocerebroside and other glycolipids within the lysosomes of macrophages and reticuloendothelial cells. The clinical manifestations of this disease result from accumulation of lipid-laden cells (i.e. Gaucher cells) in various organs, but the clinical severity of the disease varies widely. Most patients manifest hepatosplenomegaly, haematologic abnormalities and bone involvement.

Pulmonary involvement has been reported with all three types of Gaucher disease and consists of ILD, pulmonary hypertension and restrictive lung disease related to hepatosplenomegaly and spinal deformities. ILD results from accumulation of Gaucher cells in the lung parenchyma, while pulmonary hypertension is a manifestation of Gaucher cells filling the pulmonary capillaries (139,150,151). On chest imaging, the ILD manifests reticular, reticulonodular or a miliary pattern. Enzyme replacement therapy is available for the treatment of Gaucher disease and can reverse and prevent many manifestations of the disease (139,150,151). Haematopoietic stem cell transplantation may be beneficial for some patients.

Niemann–Pick disease is a group of disorders characterized by accumulation of sphingomyelin, and it is inherited in an autosomal recessive pattern. These disorders are caused by mutations in the sphingomyelin phosphodiesterase-1 gene or genes that control cellular processing and transport of low-density cholesterol. Intracellular accumulation of sphingomyelin or unesterified cholesterol leads to disease manifestations that commonly include organomegaly and neurologic deficits with variable age of onset. ILD due to parenchymal accumulation of lipid-laden macrophages, alveolar proteinosis, recurrent respiratory infections and respiratory failure can occur in these patients (139,150–153). At present, there is no cure or enzyme replacement therapy for Niemann–Pick disease.

There are other lipid storage disorders in which the lung may become involved. These include Fabry disease, Farber disease, gangliosidoses, Krabbe disease, Wolman disease and metachromatic leukodystrophy (150,154,155). However, these disorders are rarer, and pulmonary involvement has been incompletely described or is overshadowed by extra-pulmonary manifestations.

MIMICS OF ILD

There are disease processes that are not ILD but can mimic various features associated with ILDs. These include congestive heart failure with interstitial edema, pulmonary vascular disease such as pulmonary veno-occlusive disease and chronic pulmonary infection. There are also several neoplastic disorders that can mimic ILD.

Lymphangitic carcinomatosis, most commonly associated with breast cancer, presents with progressive exertional dyspnoea, cough and diffuse interstitial lung infiltrates. Thickening (typically beaded rather than smooth) of the inter-lobular septa, fissures and bronchovascular bundles are seen on HRCT (156,157). The extent and distribution of these parenchymal findings may vary from unilateral to bilateral and diffuse. Associated findings on CT may include hilar and mediastinal lymphadenopathy and pleural effusion. The diagnosis of lymphangitic carcinomatosis is usually confirmed by bronchoscopic lung biopsy. Although generally indicative of poor prognosis, some patients with lymphangitic carcinomatosis may experience a response to chemotherapy and stability for a period of time (158).

Lymphoproliferative disorders can display a wide variety of clinico-radiologic patterns in various regions including in the thorax. Intra-thoracic lymphoma (both Hodgkin and non-Hodgkin), is more often a part of generalized disease rather than limited to primary pulmonary or mediastinal lymphoma. Although intra-thoracic lymphadenopathy is the most common imaging feature associated with intra-thoracic lymphoma, parenchymal involvement, including not only nodule(s)/mass(es) but also lymphangitic interstitial infiltrates, consolidative opacities and miliary pattern can be seen (159,160).

Lymphomatoid granulomatosis (LG) is a rare Epstein–Barr virus-associated, T-cell rich B-cell lymphoproliferative disorder that typically affects patients aged between 20 and 50 years (161,162). Nearly all patients will manifest lung involvement, although a variety of extrapulmonary organs can also be affected. While multiple nodular opacities (±cavitation) are the most common presentation on chest imaging, some patients with LG manifest reticulonodular or alveolar opacities (163).

Post-transplant lymphoproliferative disease (PTLD) is a serious and potentially fatal complication encountered after organ transplantation with the majority encountered during the first year following transplantation (164,165). PTLD represents a spectrum of lymphoid proliferation ranging from benign polyclonal hyperplasia to lymphoma. The majority of PTLD is of B-cell origin, and most of these are associated with EBV infection. The most common intra-thoracic presentation of PTLD is lung mass or nodules (159,160,166). Other manifestations in the thorax include lymphadenopathy, parenchymal consolidation, pleural or pericardial effusion and chest wall involvement (159,160,166). The diagnosis of PTLD requires histologic confirmation based on biopsy of the suspected lesion.

REFERENCES

1. Richter T, Nestler-Parr S, Babela R, Khan ZM, Tesoro T, Molsen E et al. Rare disease terminology and definitions – A systematic global review: Report of the ISPOR rare disease special interest group. *Value Health.* 2015;18(6):906–14.
2. Ryu JH, Richeldi L. Orphan lung diseases. *Semin Respir Crit Care Med.* 2016;37(3): 319–20.
3. Merlini G, Seldin DC, Gertz MA. Amyloidosis: Pathogenesis and new therapeutic options. *J Clin Oncol.* 2011;29(14):1924–33.
4. Gertz MA. Immunoglobulin light chain amyloidosis: 2014 update on diagnosis, prognosis, and treatment. *Am J Hematol.* 2014; 89(12):1132–40.
5. Lachmann HJ, Hawkins PN. Amyloidosis and the lung. *Chron Respir Dis.* 2006;3(4):203–14.
6. Gillmore JD, Hawkins PN. Amyloidosis and the respiratory tract. *Thorax.* 1999;54(5): 444–51.
7. Utz JP, Swensen SJ, Gertz MA. Pulmonary amyloidosis. The Mayo Clinic experience from 1980 to 1993. *Ann Intern Med.* 1996; 124(4):407–13.
8. Pickford HA, Swensen SJ, Utz JP. Thoracic cross-sectional imaging of amyloidosis. *AJR. Am J Roentgenol.* 1997;168(2):351–5.
9. Marchiori E, Franquet T, Gasparetto TD, Goncalves LP, Escuissato DL. Consolidation with diffuse or focal high attenuation: Computed tomography findings. *J Thorac Imaging.* 2008;23(4):298–304.
10. Baqir M, Kluka EM, Aubry M-C, Hartman TE, Yi ES, Bauer PR et al. Amyloid-associated cystic lung disease in primary Sjogren's syndrome. *Respir Med.* 2013;107(4):616–21.
11. Zamora AC, White DB, Sykes A-MG, Hoskote SS, Moua T, Yi ES et al. Amyloid-associated Cystic Lung Disease. *Chest.* 2016;149(5):1223–33.
12. Picken MM. Amyloidosis – Where are we now and where are we heading? *Arch Pathol Lab Med.* 2010;134(4):545–51.
13. Kastritis E, Dimopoulos MA. Recent advances in the management of AL Amyloidosis. *Br J Haematol.* 2016;172(2):170–86.

14. Neben-Wittich MA, Foote RL, Kalra S. External beam radiation therapy for tracheobronchial amyloidosis. *Chest.* 2007;132(1):262–7.

15. Yi ES, Sekiguchi H, Peikert T, Ryu JH, Colby TV. Pathologic manifestations of Immunoglobulin(Ig)G4-related lung disease. *Semin in Diagn Pathology.* 2012;29(4):219–25.

16. Khosroshahi A, Wallace ZS, Crowe JL, Akamizu T, Azumi A, Carruthers MN et al. International consensus guidance statement on the management and treatment of IgG4-related disease. *Arthritis Rheumatol.* 2015;67(7):1688–99.

17. Zen Y, Nakanuma Y. IgG4-related disease: A cross-sectional study of 114 cases. *Am J Surg Pathol.* 2010;34(12):1812–9.

18. Kamisawa T, Okamoto A. IgG4-related sclerosing disease. *World J Gastroenterol.* 2008;14(25):3948–55.

19. Chang SY, Keogh KA, Lewis JE, Ryu JH, Cornell LD, Garrity JA et al. IgG4-positive plasma cells in granulomatosis with polyangiitis (Wegener's): A clinicopathologic and immunohistochemical study on 43 granulomatosis with polyangiitis and 20 control cases. *Hum Pathol.* 2013;44(11): 2432–7.

20. Hamano H, Kawa S, Horiuchi A, Unno H, Furuya N, Akamatsu T et al. High serum IgG4 concentrations in patients with sclerosing pancreatitis.[see comment]. *N Engl J Med.* 2001;344(10):732–8.

21. Ryu JH, Sekiguchi H, Yi ES. Pulmonary manifestations of immunoglobulin G4-related sclerosing disease. *Eur Respir J.* 2012;39(1):180–6.

22. Sah RP, Chari ST. Serologic issues in IgG4-related systemic disease and autoimmune pancreatitis. *Curr Opin Rheumatol.* 2011;23(1):108–13.

23. Zen Y, Inoue D, Kitao A, Onodera M, Abo H, Miyayama S et al. IgG4-related lung and pleural disease: A clinicopathologic study of 21 cases. *Am J Surg Pathol.* 2009;33(12): 1886–93.

24. Shrestha B, Sekiguchi H, Colby TV, Graziano P, Aubry M-C, Smyrk TC et al. Distinctive pulmonary histopathology with increased IgG4-positive plasma cells in patients with autoimmune pancreatitis: Report of 6 and 12 cases with similar histopathology. *Am J Surg Pathol.* 2009;33(10):1450–62.

25. Ryu JH, Horie R, Sekiguchi H, Peikert T, Yi ES. Spectrum of disorders associated with elevated serum IgG4 levels encountered in clinical practice. *Int J Rheumatol.* 2012;2012:232960.

26. Sekiguchi H, Horie R, Aksamit TR, Yi ES, Ryu JH. Immunoglobulin G4-related disease mimicking asthma. *Can Respir J.* 2013;20(2):87–9.

27. Matsui S, Hebisawa A, Sakai F, Yamamoto H, Terasaki Y, Kurihara Y et al. Immunoglobulin G4-related lung disease: Clinicoradiological and pathological features. *Respirology.* 2013;18(3):480–7.

28. Peikert T, Shrestha B, Aubry MC, Colby TV, Ryu JH, Sekiguchi H et al. Histopathologic overlap between fibrosing mediastinitis and IgG4-related disease. *Int J Rheumatol.* 2012;2012:207056.

29. Ryu JH, Hu X, Yi ES. IgG4-related pleural disease. *Curr Pulmonol Rep.* 2015;4(1):22–7.

30. Duvic C, Desrame J, Leveque C, Nedelec G. Retroperitoneal fibrosis, sclerosing pancreatitis and bronchiolitis obliterans with organizing pneumonia. *Nephrol Dial Transplant.* 2004;19(9):2397–9.

31. Tsushima K, Tanabe T, Yamamoto H, Koizumi T, Kawa S, Hamano H et al. Pulmonary involvement of autoimmune pancreatitis. *Eur J Clin Invest.* 2009;39(8):714–22.

32. Fujinaga Y, Kadoya M, Kawa S, Hamano H, Ueda K, Momose M et al. Characteristic findings in images of extra-pancreatic lesions associated with autoimmune pancreatitis. *Eur J Radiol.* 2010;76(2):228–38.

33. Inoue D, Zen Y, Abo H, Gabata T, Demachi H, Kobayashi T et al. Immunoglobulin G4-related lung disease: CT findings with pathologic correlations. *Radiology.* 2009;251(1):260–70.

34. Yamashita K, Haga H, Kobashi Y, Miyagawa-Hayashino A, Yoshizawa A, Manabe T. Lung involvement in IgG4-related lymphoplasmacytic vasculitis and interstitial fibrosis: Report of 3 cases and review of the literature. *Am J Surg Pathol.* 2008;32(11):1620–6.

35. Matsui S, Taki H, Shinoda K, Suzuki K, Hayashi R, Tobe K et al. Respiratory involvement in IgG4-related Mikulicz's disease. *Mod Rheumatol.* 2012;22(1):31–9.

36. Carruthers MN, Khosroshahi A, Augustin T, Deshpande V, Stone JH. The diagnostic utility of serum IgG4 concentrations in IgG4-related disease. *Ann Rheum Dis.* 2015;74(1):14–8.

37. Kamisawa T, Zen Y, Pillai S, Stone JH. IgG4-related disease. *Lancet.* 2015;385(9976):1460–71.

38. Stone JH, Brito-Zeron P, Bosch X, Ramos-Casals M. Diagnostic approach to the complexity of IgG4-related disease. *Mayo Clin Proc.* 2015;90(7):927–39.

39. Wallace ZS, Deshpande V, Mattoo H, Mahajan VS, Kulikova M, Pillai S et al. IgG4-related disease: Clinical and laboratory features in one hundred twenty-five patients. *Arthritis Rheumatol.* 2015;67(9):2466–75.

40. Yu K-H, Chan T-M, Tsai P-H, Chen C-H, Chang PY. Diagnostic performance of serum IgG4 levels in patients with IgG4-related disease. *Medicine.* 2015;94(41):e1707.

41. Ebbo M, Grados A, Bernit E, Vely F, Boucraut J, Harle J-R et al. Pathologies associated with serum IgG4 elevation. *Int J Rheumatol.* 2012;2012:602809.

42. Ngwa TN, Law R, Murray D, Chari ST. Serum immunoglobulin g4 level is a poor predictor of immunoglobulin g4-related disease. *Pancreas.* 2014;43(5):704–7.

43. Deshpande V, Zen Y, Chan JK, Yi EE, Sato Y, Yoshino T et al. Consensus statement on the pathology of IgG4-related disease. *Mod Pathol.* 2012;25(9):1181–92.

44. Umehara H, Okazaki K, Masaki Y, Kawano M, Yamamoto M, Saeki T et al. Comprehensive diagnostic criteria for IgG4-related disease (IgG4-RD), 2011. *Mod Rheumatol.* 2012;22(1):21–30.

45. Stone JH, Zen Y, Deshpande V. IgG4-related disease. *N Engl J Med.* 2012;366(6):539–51.

46. Kamisawa T, Okazaki K, Kawa S, Ito T, Inui K, Irie H et al. Amendment of the Japanese consensus guidelines for autoimmune pancreatitis, 2013 III. Treatment and prognosis of autoimmune pancreatitis. *J Gastroenterol.* 2014;49(6):961–70.

47. Hamano H, Arakura N, Muraki T, Ozaki Y, Kiyosawa K, Kawa S. Prevalence and distribution of extrapancreatic lesions complicating autoimmune pancreatitis. *J Gastroenterol.* 2006;41(12):1197–205.

48. Cheuk W, Yuen HK, Chu SY, Chiu EK, Lam LK, Chan JK. Lymphadenopathy of IgG4-related sclerosing disease. *Am J Surg Pathol.* 2008;32(5):671–81.

49. Taniguchi T, Ko M, Seko S, Nishida O, Inoue F, Kobayashi H et al. Interstitial pneumonia associated with autoimmune pancreatitis. [comment]. *Gut.* 2004;53(5):770.

50. Campbell SN, Rubio E, Loschner AL. Clinical review of pulmonary manifestations of IgG4-related disease. *Ann Am Thorac Soc.* 2014;11(9):1466–75.

51. Ghazale A, Chari ST, Zhang L, Smyrk TC, Takahashi N, Levy MJ et al. Immunoglobulin G4-associated cholangitis: Clinical profile and response to therapy. *Gastroenterology.* 2008;134(3):706–15.

52. Raina A, Yadav D, Krasinskas AM, McGrath KM, Khalid A, Sanders M et al. Evaluation and management of autoimmune pancreatitis: Experience at a large US center. *Am J Gastroenterol.* 2009;104(9):2295–306.

53. Masaki Y, Shimizu H, Sato Nakamura T, Nakamura T, Nakajima A, Iwao Kawanami H et al. IgG4-related disease: Diagnostic methods and therapeutic strategies in Japan. *J Clin Exp Hematop.* 2014;54(2):95–101.

54. Khosroshahi A, Stone JH. Treatment approaches to IgG4-related systemic disease. *Curr Opin Rheumatol.* 2011;23(1):67–71.

55. Inoue D, Yoshida K, Yoneda N, Ozaki K, Matsubara T, Nagai K et al. IgG4-related disease: Dataset of 235 consecutive patients. *Medicine.* 2015;94(15):e680.

56. Fernandez-Codina A, Martinez-Valle F, Pinilla B, Lopez C, DeTorres I, Solans-Laque R et al. IgG4-related disease: Results from a multicenter Spanish registry. *Medicine.* 2015;94(32):e1275.

57. Sodikoff JB, Keilin SA, Cai Q, Bharmal SJ, Lewis MM, Raju GS et al. Mycophenolate mofetil for maintenance of remission in steroid-dependent autoimmune pancreatitis. *World J Gastroenterol.* 2012;18(18):2287–90.

58. Hart PA, Kamisawa T, Brugge WR, Chung JB, Culver EL, Czako L et al. Long-term outcomes of autoimmune pancreatitis: A multicentre, international analysis. *Gut*. 2013;62(12):1771–6.

59. Witzig TE, Inwards DJ, Habermann TM, Dogan A, Kurtin PJ, Gross JB, Jr. et al. Treatment of benign orbital pseudolymphomas with the monoclonal anti-CD20 antibody rituximab. *Mayo Clin Proc*. 2007;82(6):692–9.

60. Plaza JA, Garrity JA, Dogan A, Ananthamurthy A, Witzig TE, Salomao DR. Orbital inflammation with IgG4-positive plasma cells: Manifestation of IgG4 systemic disease. *Arch Ophthalmol*. 2011;129(4):421–8.

61. Khosroshahi A, Bloch DB, Deshpande V, Stone JH. Rituximab therapy leads to rapid decline of serum IgG4 levels and prompt clinical improvement in IgG4-related systemic disease. *Arthritis Rheum*. 2010;62(6):1755–62.

62. Topazian M, Witzig TE, Smyrk TC, Pulido JS, Levy MJ, Kamath PS et al. Rituximab therapy for refractory biliary strictures in immunoglobulin G4-associated cholangitis. *Clin Gastroenterol Hepatol*. 2008;6(3):364–6.

63. Carruthers MN, Topazian MD, Khosroshahi A, Witzig TE, Wallace ZS, Hart PA et al. Rituximab for IgG4-related disease: A prospective, open-label trial. *Ann Rheum Dis*. 2015;74(6):1171–7.

64. Della-Torre E, Feeney E, Deshpande V, Mattoo H, Mahajan V, Kulikova M et al. B-cell depletion attenuates serological biomarkers of fibrosis and myofibroblast activation in IgG4-related disease. *Ann Rheum Dis*. 2015;74(12):2236–43.

65. Khosroshahi A, Carruthers MN, Deshpande V, Unizony S, Bloch DB, Stone JH. Rituximab for the treatment of IgG4-related disease: Lessons from 10 consecutive patients. *Medicine*. 2012;91(1):57–66.

66. Murakami J, Matsui S, Ishizawa S, Arita K, Wada A, Miyazono T et al. Recurrence of IgG4-related disease following treatment with rituximab. *Mod Rheumatol*. 2013;23(6):1226–30.

67. Hirano K, Tada M, Isayama H, Yagioka H, Sasaki T, Kogure H et al. Long-term prognosis of autoimmune pancreatitis with and without corticosteroid treatment. *Gut*. 2007;56(12):1719–24.

68. Patel NR, Anzalone ML, Buja LM, Elghetany MT. Sudden cardiac death due to coronary artery involvement by IgG4-related disease: A rare, serious complication of a rare disease. *Arch Pathol Lab Med*. 2014;138(6):833–6.

69. Holmes BJ, Delev NG, Pasternack GR, Halushka MK. Novel cause of sudden cardiac death: IgG4-related disease. *Circulation*. 2012;125(23):2956–7.

70. Ryu JH, Myers JL, Swensen SJ. Bronchiolar disorders. *Am J Respir Crit Care Med*. 2003;168(11):1277–92.

71. Devakonda A, Raoof S, Sung A, Travis WD, Naidich D. Bronchiolar disorders: A clinical-radiological diagnostic algorithm. *Chest*. 2010;137(4):938–51.

72. Ryu JH. Classification and approach to bronchiolar diseases. *Curr Opin Pulm Med*. 2006;12(2):145–51.

73. Travis WD, Galvin JR. Non-neoplastic pulmonary lymphoid lesions. *Thorax*. 2001;56(12):964–71.

74. Aerni MR, Vassallo R, Myers JL, Lindell RM, Ryu JH. Follicular bronchiolitis in surgical lung biopsies: Clinical implications in 12 patients. *Respir Med*. 2008;102(2):307–12.

75. Howling SJ, Hansell DM, Wells AU, Nicholson AG, Flint JD, Muller NL. Follicular bronchiolitis: Thin-section CT and histologic findings. *Radiology*. 1999;212(3):637–42.

76. Guinee DG, Jr. Update on nonneoplastic pulmonary lymphoproliferative disorders and related entities. *Arch Pathol Lab Med*. 2010;134(5):691–701.

77. Fortoul TI, Cano-Valle F, Oliva E, Barrios R. Follicular bronchiolitis in association with connective tissue diseases. *Lung*. 1985;163(5):305–14.

78. Deheinzelin D, Capelozzi VL, Kairalla RA, Barbas Filho JV, Saldiva PH, de Carvalho CR. Interstitial lung disease in primary Sjogren's syndrome. Clinical-pathological evaluation and response to treatment. *Am J Respir Crit Care Med*. 1996;154(3 Pt 1):794–9.

79. Hayakawa H, Sato A, Imokawa S, Toyoshima M, Chida K, Iwata M. Bronchiolar disease in rheumatoid arthritis. *Am J Respir Crit Care Med*. 1996;154(5):1531–6.

80. Exley CM, Suvarna SK, Matthews S. Follicular bronchiolitis as a presentation of HIV. *Clin Radiol*. 2006;61(8):710–3.

81. Camarasa Escrig A, Amat Humaran B, Sapia S, Leon Ramirez JM. Follicular bronchiolitis associated with common variable immunodeficiency. *Arch Bronconeumol.* 2013;49(4):166–8.

82. Poletti V, Casoni G, Chilosi M, Zompatori M. Diffuse panbronchiolitis. *Eur Respir J.* 2006;28(4):862–71.

83. Kudoh S, Keicho N. Diffuse panbronchiolitis. *Clin Chest Med.* 2012;33(2):297–305.

84. Fitzgerald JE, King TE, Jr., Lynch DA, Tuder RM, Schwarz MI. Diffuse panbronchiolitis in the United States. *Am J Respir Crit Care Med.* 1996;154(2 Pt 1):497–503.

85. Poletti V, Chilosi M, Casoni G, Colby TV. Diffuse panbronchiolitis. *Sarcoidosis Vasc Diffuse Lung Dis.* 2004;21(2):94–104.

86. Iwata M, Colby TV, Kitaichi M. Diffuse panbronchiolitis: Diagnosis and distinction from various pulmonary diseases with centrilobular interstitial foam cell accumulations. *Hum Pathol.* 1994;25(4):357–63.

87. Spagnolo P, Fabbri LM, Bush A. Long-term macrolide treatment for chronic respiratory disease. *Eur Respir J.* 2013;42(1):239–51.

88. Marik PE. Pulmonary aspiration syndromes. *Curr Opin Pulm Med.* 2011;17(3):148–54.

89. Hu X, Lee JS, Pianosi PT, Ryu JH. Aspiration-related pulmonary syndromes. *Chest.* 2015;147(3):815–23.

90. Hu X, Yi ES, Ryu JH. Solitary lung masses due to occult aspiration. *Am J Med.* 2015;128(6):655–8.

91. Matsuse T, Teramoto S, Matsui H, Ouchi Y, Fukuchi Y. Widespread occurrence of diffuse aspiration bronchiolitis in patients with dysphagia, irrespective of age. *Chest.* 1998;114(1):350–1.

92. Barnes TW, Vassallo R, Tazelaar HD, Hartman TE, Ryu JH. Diffuse bronchiolar disease due to chronic occult aspiration. *Mayo Clinic Proc.* 2006;81(2):172–6.

93. Hu X, Yi ES, Ryu JH. Diffuse aspiration bronchiolitis: Analysis of 20 consecutive patients. *J Bras Pneumol.* 2015;41(2):161–6.

94. Munoz J, Janku F, Cohen PR, Kurzrock R. Erdheim-Chester disease: Characteristics and management. *Mayo Clin Proc.* 2014;89(7):985–96.

95. Haroche J, Arnaud L, Cohen-Aubart F, Hervier B, Charlotte F, Emile JF et al.

96. Diamond EL, Dagna L, Hyman DM, Cavalli G, Janku F, Estrada-Veras J et al. Consensus guidelines for the diagnosis and clinical management of Erdheim-Chester disease. *Blood.* 2014;124(4):483–92.

97. Haroche J, Charlotte F, Arnaud L, von Deimling A, Helias-Rodzewicz Z, Hervier B et al. High prevalence of BRAF V600E mutations in Erdheim-Chester disease but not in other non-Langerhans cell histiocytoses. *Blood.* 2012;120(13):2700–3.

98. Hervier B, Haroche J, Arnaud L, Charlotte F, Donadieu J, Neel A et al. Association of both Langerhans cell histiocytosis and Erdheim-Chester disease linked to the BRAFV600E mutation. *Blood.* 2014;124(7):1119–26.

99. Cavalli G, Guglielmi B, Berti A, Campochiaro C, Sabbadini MG, Dagna L. The multifaceted clinical presentations and manifestations of Erdheim-Chester disease: Comprehensive review of the literature and of 10 new cases. *Ann Rheum Dis.* 2013;72(10):1691–5.

100. Haroche J, Arnaud L, Amoura Z. Erdheim-Chester disease. *Curr Opin Rheumatol.* 2012;24(1):53–9.

101. Arnaud L, Pierre I, Beigelman-Aubry C, Capron F, Brun AL, Rigolet A et al. Pulmonary involvement in Erdheim-Chester disease: A single-center study of thirty-four patients and a review of the literature. *Arthritis Rheum.* 2010;62(11):3504–12.

102. Brun AL, Touitou-Gottenberg D, Haroche J, Toledano D, Cluzel P, Beigelman-Aubry C et al. Erdheim-Chester disease: CT findings of thoracic involvement. *Eur Radiol.* 2010;20(11):2579–87.

103. Wittenberg KH, Swensen SJ, Myers JL. Pulmonary involvement with Erdheim-Chester disease: Radiographic and CT findings. *AJR. Am J Roentgenol.* 2000;174(5):1327–31.

104. Nagarjun Rao R, Moran CA, Suster S. Histiocytic disorders of the lung. *Adv Anat Pathol.* 2010;17(1):12–22.

105. Hyman DM, Puzanov I, Subbiah V, Faris JE, Chau I, Blay J-Y et al. Vemurafenib in multiple nonmelanoma Cancers with BRAF V600 mutations. *N Engl J Med.* 2015;373(8):726–36.

106. Haroche J, Cohen-Aubart F, Emile J-F, Arnaud L, Maksud P, Charlotte F et al. Dramatic efficacy of vemurafenib in both multisystemic and refractory Erdheim-Chester disease and Langerhans cell histiocytosis harboring the BRAF V600E mutation. *Blood*. 2013;121(9):1495–500.

107. Hervier B, Arnaud L, Charlotte F, Wechsler B, Piette JC, Amoura Z et al. Treatment of Erdheim-Chester disease with long-term high-dose interferon. *Semin Arthritis Rheum*. 2012;41(6):907–13.

108. Braiteh F, Boxrud C, Esmaeli B, Kurzrock R. Successful treatment of Erdheim-Chester disease, a non-Langerhans-cell histiocytosis, with interferon-alpha. *Blood*. 2005;106(9):2992–4.

109. Castellana G, Castellana G, Gentile M, Castellana R, Resta O. Pulmonary alveolar microlithiasis: Review of the 1022 cases reported worldwide. *Eur Respir Rev*. 2015;24(138):607–20.

110. Ferreira Francisco FA, Pereira e Silva JL, Hochhegger B, Zanetti G, Marchiori E. Pulmonary alveolar microlithiasis. State-of-the-art review. *Respir Med*. 2013;107(1):1–9.

111. Tachibana T, Hagiwara K, Johkoh T. Pulmonary alveolar microlithiasis: Review and management. *Curr Opin Pulm Med*. 2009;15(5):486–90.

112. Huqun, Izumi S, Miyazawa H, Ishii K, Uchiyama B, Ishida T et al. Mutations in the SLC34A2 gene are associated with pulmonary alveolar microlithiasis. *Am J Respir Crit Care Med*. 2007;175(3):263–8.

113. Yin X, Wang H, Wu D, Zhao G, Shao J, Dai Y. SLC34A2 Gene mutation of pulmonary alveolar microlithiasis: Report of four cases and review of literatures. *Respir Med*. 2013;107(2):217–22.

114. Deniz O, Ors F, Tozkoparan E, Ozcan A, Gumus S, Bozlar U et al. High resolution computed tomographic features of pulmonary alveolar microlithiasis. *Eur J Radiol*. 2005;55(3):452–60.

115. Borrelli R, Fossi A, Volterrani L, Voltolini L. Right single-lung transplantation for pulmonary alveolar microlithiasis. *Eur J Cardiothorac Surg*. 2014;45(2):e40.

116. Shigemura N, Bermudez C, Hattler BG, Johnson B, Crespo M, Pilewski J et al. Lung transplantation for pulmonary alveolar microlithiasis. *J Thorac Cardiovasc Surg*. 2010;139(3):e50–2.

117. Stamatis G, Zerkowski HR, Doetsch N, Greschuchna D, Konietzko N, Reidemeister JC. Sequential bilateral lung transplantation for pulmonary alveolar microlithiasis. *Ann Thorac Surg*. 1993;56(4):972–5.

118. Cakir E, Gedik AH, Ozdemir A, Buyukpinarbasili N, Bilgin M, Ozgen IT. Response to disodium etidronate treatment in three siblings with pulmonary alveolar microlithiasis. *Respiration*. 2015;89(6):583–6.

119. Ozcelik U, Yalcin E, Ariyurek M, Ersoz DD, Cinel G, Gulhan B et al. Long-term results of disodium etidronate treatment in pulmonary alveolar microlithiasis. *Pediatr Pulmonol*. 2010;45(5):514–7.

120. Faul JL, Berry GJ, Colby TV, Ruoss SJ, Walter MB, Rosen GD et al. Thoracic lymphangiomas, lymphangiectasis, lymphangiomatosis, and lymphatic dysplasia syndrome. *Am J Respir Crit Care Med*. 2000;161(3):1037–46.

121. Radhakrishnan K, Rockson SG. The clinical spectrum of lymphatic disease. *Ann N Y Acad Sci*. 2008;1131:155–84.

122. Park JG, Aubry M-C, Godfrey JA, Midthun DE. Mediastinal lymphangioma: Mayo Clinic experience of 25 cases. *Mayo Clin Proc*. 2006;81(9):1197–203.

123. Luisi F, Torre O, Harari S. Thoracic involvement in generalised lymphatic anomaly (or lymphangiomatosis). *Eur Respir Rev*. 2016;25(140):170–7.

124. Boland JM, Tazelaar HD, Colby TV, Leslie KO, Hartman TE, Yi ES. Diffuse pulmonary lymphatic disease presenting as interstitial lung disease in adulthood: Report of 3 cases. *Am J Surg Pathol*. 2012;36(10):1548–54.

125. Tazelaar HD, Kerr D, Yousem SA, Saldana MJ, Langston C, Colby TV. Diffuse pulmonary lymphangiomatosis. *Hum Pathol*. 1993;24(12):1313–22.

126. Brown M, Pysher T, Coffin CM. Lymphangioma and congenital pulmonary lymphangiectasis: A histologic, immunohistochemical, and clinicopathologic comparison. *Mod Pathol*. 1999;12(6):569–75.

127. Raman SP, Pipavath SNJ, Raghu G, Schmidt RA, Godwin JD. Imaging of thoracic lymphatic diseases. *AJR. Am J Roentgenol*. 2009;193(6):1504–13.

128. Swensen SJ, Hartman TE, Mayo JR, Colby TV, Tazelaar HD, Muller NL. Diffuse pulmonary lymphangiomatosis: CT findings. *J Comput Assist Tomogr.* 1995;19(3): 348–52.

129. Yekeler E, Dursun M, Yildirim A, Tunaci M. Diffuse pulmonary lymphangiomatosis: Imaging findings. *Diagn Interv Radiol.* 2005;11(1):31–4.

130. Adams DM, Trenor CC, 3rd, Hammill AM, Vinks AA, Patel MN, Chaudry G et al. Efficacy and safety of sirolimus in the treatment of complicated vascular anomalies. *Pediatrics.* 2016;137(2):1–10.

131. Bassi A, Syed S. Multifocal infiltrative lymphangiomatosis in a child and successful treatment with sirolimus. *Mayo Clin Proc.* 2014;89(12):e129.

132. Hammill AM, Wentzel M, Gupta A, Nelson S, Lucky A, Elluru R et al. Sirolimus for the treatment of complicated vascular anomalies in children. *Pediatr Blood Cancer.* 2011;57(6):1018–24.

133. Aman J, Thunnissen E, Paul MA, van Nieuw Amerongen GP, Vonk-Noordegraaf A. Successful treatment of diffuse pulmonary lymphangiomatosis with bevacizumab. *Ann Intern Med.* 2012;156(11):839–40.

134. Ozeki M, Fukao T, Kondo N. Propranolol for intractable diffuse lymphangiomatosis. *N Engl J Med.* 2011;364(14):1380–2.

135. Libby LJ, Narula N, Fernandes H, Gruden JF, Wolf DJ, Libby DM. Imatinib treatment of lymphangiomatosis (Generalized Lymphatic Anomaly). *J Natl Compr Canc Netw.* 2016;14(4):383–6.

136. Laverdiere C, David M, Dubois J, Russo P, Hershon L, Lapierre JG. Improvement of disseminated lymphangiomatosis with recombinant interferon therapy. *Pediatr Pulmonol.* 2000;29(4):321–4.

137. Kinnier CV, Eu JPC, Davis RD, Howell DN, Sheets J, Palmer SM. Successful bilateral lung transplantation for lymphangiomatosis. *Am J Transplant.* 2008;8(9):1946–50.

138. Seward SL, Jr., Gahl WA. Hermansky-Pudlak syndrome: Health care throughout life. *Pediatrics.* 2013;132(1):153–60.

139. Devine MS, Garcia CK. Genetic interstitial lung disease. *Clin Chest Med.* 2012;33(1):95–110.

140. Pierson DM, Ionescu D, Qing G, Yonan AM, Parkinson K, Colby TC et al. Pulmonary fibrosis in Hermansky-Pudlak syndrome. A case report and review. *Respiration.* 2006;73(3):382–95.

141. Huizing M, Helip-Wooley A, Westbroek W, Gunay-Aygun M, Gahl WA. Disorders of lysosome-related organelle biogenesis: Clinical and molecular genetics. *Ann Rev Genomics Hum Genet.* 2008;9:359–86.

142. Brantly M, Avila NA, Shotelersuk V, Lucero C, Huizing M, Gahl WA. Pulmonary function and high-resolution CT findings in patients with an inherited form of pulmonary fibrosis, Hermansky-Pudlak syndrome, due to mutations in HPS-1. *Chest.* 2000;117(1):129–36.

143. Avila NA, Brantly M, Premkumar A, Huizing M, Dwyer A, Gahl WA. Hermansky-Pudlak syndrome: Radiography and CT of the chest compared with pulmonary function tests and genetic studies. *AJR. Am J Roentgenol.* 2002;179(4):887–92.

144. Bin Saeedan M, Faheem Mohammed S, Mohammed T-LH. Hermansky-Pudlak syndrome: High-resolution computed tomography findings and literature review. *Curr Probl Diagn Radiol.* 2015;44(4):383–5.

145. O'Brien K, Troendle J, Gochuico BR, Markello TC, Salas J, Cardona H et al. Pirfenidone for the treatment of Hermansky-Pudlak syndrome pulmonary fibrosis. *Mol Genet Metab.* 2011;103(2):128–34.

146. Lederer DJ, Kawut SM, Sonett JR, Vakiani E, Seward SL, Jr., White JG et al. Successful bilateral lung transplantation for pulmonary fibrosis associated with the Hermansky-Pudlak syndrome. *J Heart Lung Transplant.* 2005;24(10):1697–9.

147. Zamora AC, Collard HR, Wolters PJ, Webb WR, King TE. Neurofibromatosis-associated lung disease: A case series and literature review. *Eur Respir J.* 2007;29(1):210–4.

148. Ryu JH, Parambil JG, McGrann PS, Aughenbaugh GL. Lack of evidence for an association between neurofibromatosis and pulmonary fibrosis. *Chest.* 2005;128(4):2381–6.

149. Webb WR, Goodman PC. Fibrosing alveolitis in patients with neurofibromatosis. *Radiology.* 1977;122(2):289–93.

150. Santamaria F, Montella S, Mirra V, De Stefano S, Andria G, Parenti G. Respiratory manifestations in patients with inherited metabolic diseases. *Eur Respir Rev.* 2013;22(130):437–53.

151. Gulhan B, Ozcelik U, Gurakan F, Gucer S, Orhan D, Cinel G et al. Different features of lung involvement in Niemann-Pick disease and Gaucher disease. *Respir Med.* 2012;106(9):1278–85.

152. Sheth J, Joseph JJ, Shah K, Muranjan M, Mistri M, Sheth F. Pulmonary manifestations in Niemann-Pick type C disease with mutations in NPC2 gene: Case report and review of literature. *BMC Med Genet.* 2017;18(1):5.

153. Simoes RG, Maia H. *Niemann-Pick type B in adulthood.* BMJ Case Rep. 2015.

154. Krayenbuehl PA, Lidove O, Aubert J-D, Barbey F. Pulmonary involvement in Fabry disease: Overview and perspectives. *Eur J Intern Med.* 2013;24(8):707–13.

155. Pyeritz RE, Bernhardt BA, Casey M, Litt HI. Pulmonary manifestations of Fabry disease and positive response to enzyme replacement therapy. *Am J Med Genet Part A.* 2007;143(4):377–81.

156. Prakash P, Kalra MK, Sharma A, Shepard J-AO, Digumarthy SR. FDG PET/CT in assessment of pulmonary lymphangitic carcinomatosis. *AJR Am J Roentgenol.* 2010;194(1):231–6.

157. Acikgoz G, Kim SM, Houseni M, Cermik TF, Intenzo CM, Alavi A. Pulmonary lymphangitic carcinomatosis (PLC): Spectrum of FDG-PET findings. *Clin Nucl Med.* 2006;31(11):673–8.

158. Ikezoe J, Godwin JD, Hunt KJ, Marglin SI. Pulmonary lymphangitic carcinomatosis: Chronicity of radiographic findings in long-term survivors. *AJR Am J Roentgenol.* 1995;165(1):49–52.

159. Restrepo CS, Carrillo J, Rosado de Christenson M, Ojeda Leon P, Lucia Rivera A, Koss MN. Lymphoproliferative lung disorders: A radiologic-pathologic overview. Part II: Neoplastic disorders. *Semin Ultrasound CT MR.* 2013;34(6):535–49.

160. Hare SS, Souza CA, Bain G, Seely JM, Frcpc, Gomes MM et al. The radiological spectrum of pulmonary lymphoproliferative disease. *Br J Radiol.* 2012;85(1015): 848–64.

161. Roschewski M, Wilson WH. Lymphomatoid granulomatosis and other Epstein-Barr virus associated lymphoproliferative processes. *Curr Hematol Malig Rep.* 2012;7(3):208–15.

162. Katzenstein A-LA, Doxtader E, Narendra S. Lymphomatoid granulomatosis: Insights gained over 4 decades. *Am J Surg Pathol.* 2010;34(12):e35–48.

163. Dee PM, Arora NS, Innes DJ, Jr. The pulmonary manifestations of lymphomatoid granulomatosis. *Radiology.* 1982;143(3): 613–8.

164. Arcadu A, Moua T, Yi ES, Ryu JH. Lymphoid interstitial pneumonia and other benign lymphoid disorders. *Semin Respir Crit Care Med.* 2016;37(3):406–20.

165. Lyu DM, Zamora MR. Medical complications of lung transplantation. *Proc Am Thorac Soc.* 2009;6(1):101–7.

166. Borhani AA, Hosseinzadeh K, Almusa O, Furlan A, Nalesnik M. Imaging of post-transplantation lymphoproliferative disorder after solid organ transplantation. *Radiographics.* 2009;29(4):981–1000.

24

Childhood ILD

ANDREW BUSH

INTRODUCTION: WHY SHOULD ADULT PHYSICIANS CARE ABOUT INTERSTITIAL LUNG DISEASES IN CHILDREN?

These are a rare and disparate group of conditions; even specialist centres see less than 10 cases/year in total; and many are fatal in early life (1). So what is the relevance across the wider age spectrum? Mutations in the surfactant protein-(Sp)-C gene provide the most graphic illustration of the interactions between genetics, and developmental and environmental processes, and why we can no longer operate in developmental silos. The same gene mutation, in the same family, can present as a pulmonary alveolar proteinosis-like picture in newborns, and usual interstitial pneumonia (UIP, a condition unknown in children) in adults (2); furthermore, nearly 50% of SpC children present as slowly resolving respiratory syncytial virus (RSV) infection (3), and there are *in vitro* data showing that SpC mutation cells are especially vulnerable to the cytotoxic effects of RSV (4). Similarly, the same *Adenosine triphosphate binding cassette subfamily A member 3 (ABCA3)* mutation in the same family may have very differing clinical courses (5), and *ABCA3* mutations also confer vulnerability to the effects of RSV (6). Respiratory bronchiolitis associated ILD and isolated Langerhans cell histiocytosis are both diseases of adult smokers, as may be DIP (7); all three are seen in children passively exposed to tobacco smoke (8–10).

It is highly unlikely that these are the only diseases that cross developmental boundaries, and it is probable that many 'adult' ILDs have childhood manifestations of which paediatricians are currently unaware, with the converse also likely being true. Furthermore, progress in the treatment of interstitial lung disease in children (chILD) is desperately slow; paediatricians need to learn the lessons of adult randomized controlled trials. The scientific mechanisms of chILD are little studied: anything known in specific conditions is given in the relevant sections in this chapter. However, this too may be an area where paediatricians should learn from adult physicians. There are thus many areas where working in developmental silos has stunted progress. This chapter describes specific entities and an approach based on clinical presentations, rather than focusing on elaborate schemes of classification.

EPIDEMIOLOGY

chILD comprises a heterogeneous group of at least 200 different conditions, with a joint prevalence of less than 5/100,000 of the population (1). Classification has proved increasingly complex (Table 24.1). Conventionally, the 0–2 age group has

Table 24.1 Modified summary classification of chILD proposed by the current author

chILD 0–2	chILD 2–18	chILD all ages
Developmental disorders: ACD-CAD spectrum	*Non-infectious pneumonias: diffuse alveolar damage, organizing pneumonias*	**Other Sp mutations:** *Sp-C, ABCA3, TTF-1*
Abnormalities of alveolar growth: pulmonary hypoplastic syndromes	*Lymphoproliferative disorders*	**Disorders of the normal host, including hypersensitivity pneumonitis, aspiration syndromes,** *post-infectious disorders*
Sp-B mutations	*Others: granulomatous lung disease, haemosiderosis, LCH, alveolar microlithiasis*	**Disorders resulting from systemic diseases, including pulmonary capillaritis, collagen vascular disease,** *pulmonary alveolar proteinosis, storage disorder*
Specific conditions: NEHI, PIG		**Disorders of the immunocompromised host**
Rare genetic disorders, e.g. integrin mutations		**(Masquerades of chILD, especially cardiac mimics)**
		Rare genetic disorders
		Iatrogenic chILD; medications, radiation. A full list is beyond the scope of this chapter
		Chronic bronchiolitis spectrum: obliterative, constrictive, follicular, eosinophilic
		Unclassifiable

Notes: **Bold**, 0–2 US chILD classification; ***Bold Italic***, 0–18 Royal Brompton series; *Italic*, additional entities from the US 2–18 classification; Roman, entities from other sources such as case reports and case series. Note that there are overlaps between some of these conditions, and that the age ranges are not prescriptive; so for example, rare cases of NEHI have been described in older children.

Abbreviations: ABCA3 = Adenosine triphosphate binding cassette-3; ACD = alveolar-capillary dysplasia; CAD = capillary dysplasia; LCH = Langerhans cell histiocytosis; NEHI = neuroendocrine cell hyperplasia of infancy; PIG = pulmonary interstitial glycogenosis; Sp = surfactant protein; TTF-1 = thyroid transcription factor-1.

been split off from older children for several reasons: because many more biopsies are performed in this age group, developmental factors are likely to be more important than environmental, and the spectrum of disease thought likely to be very different. Thus, the initial manuscript from the US group identified eight different entities from studying 189 biopsies in the 0–2 age group (11). The subsequent Brompton study of more than 200 biopsies spanning the entire age range described additional entities, and highlighted that the histological patterns were by no means as discrete as was initially thought, with more than one histological pattern being found in the same biopsy (12). In the 0–2 age group, only 54/92 conditions (58%) were captured by the North American classification, and 23% of 118 biopsies in the 2–18 age range had conditions conventionally thought of as more common in infancy, again suggesting that developmental silos should be used cautiously. Further descriptions in the 2- to 18-year age group have recently been published by the US group (13), with less than 5% having disorders more prevalent in infancy and other countries have added their own classifications (14,15), leading to an increasingly confusing situation. I suggest that the best way forward is as follows:

- We need to acknowledge that increasingly chILD does not require a biopsy for diagnosis, so biopsy-based classifications will fail to capture the diversity of chILD.
- Many of these entities overlap histologically and overlap with normal developmental processes (below).
- Although there are conditions more common above and below the watershed age of 2 years, there is considerable overlap across the age range.
- Some chILD classifications have become too broad, including conditions such as bronchopulmonary dysplasia and obliterative bronchiolitis (11), which are respectively not a real diagnostic conundrum, and a primary airway disease.
- The complexity of chILD means that any classification system will be so unwieldy as to be unusable, and a more clinically practical approach is to delineate diagnostic pathways and approaches (16,17).
- Classing conditions together may obscure reasoning; so for example, thyroid transcription factor-1 (*TTF-1*, also known as *NKX2-1*)

mutations certainly affect surfactant protein gene expression, but also are important in non-surfactant developmental pathways (below).
- Novel entities are still being discovered (18) which may not fit into tidy classifications.

SPECIFIC chILD ENTITIES

A description of the more than 200 chILD entities is beyond the scope of this chapter; some of the most common considerations are described below.

INFANCY: DIFFUSE DEVELOPMENTAL DISORDERS

There is a spectrum of disorders comprising acinar dysplasia and alveolar-capillary dysplasia. Typically these present in a term baby who requires positive pressure ventilation soon after birth and progresses rapidly despite every attempted treatment into terminal respiratory failure. The histological pattern is of disrupted alveolar and capillary growth, with failure of normal apposition of capillaries and airspaces. Mutations in *FOXF1* and *STRA6* have been found in some patients (19,20). 'Alveolar-capillary dysplasia with misalignment of pulmonary veins' is in fact a misnomer; the 'misaligned' pulmonary veins have been shown by elegant morphometric studies to be dilated bronchial veins, with the anastomotic communications with the pulmonary venous system and distal pulmonary veins absent or obliterated (21).

INFANCY: DISORDERS OF ALVEOLAR GROWTH

Large, primitive alveoli are the hallmarks of these conditions. Causes include anything that interferes with foetal breathing movements, such as neuromuscular disease with antenatal origin, for example severe spinal muscular atrophy, abdominal masses, pleural effusion, oligohydramnios; reduced fetal pulmonary blood flow (pulmonary valve stenosis); chromosomal abnormalities such as trisomy 21 and mutations in the X-linked dominant Filamin-A (*FLNA-A*) (22); and postnatally, prematurity and its treatment, although it can be argued whether this is truly a chILD (23). Recent evidence suggesting alveolar growth may continue throughout the period of somatic growth (24–26), and a case report of improvement of an alveolar growth disorder with sildenafil (27) holds out some hope for improvement in these otherwise untreatable conditions.

INFANCY: SPECIFIC DISORDERS

These currently comprise neuroendocrine cell hyperplasia of infancy (NEHI) and pulmonary interstitial glycogenosis (PIG), although whether these are truly specific entities, or in fact whether NEHI and PIG cells merely represent persistence of the fetal airway and mesenchyme, respectively, is still not determined (below).

INFANCY: NEHI

In its purest form, NEHI condition presents as early onset of respiratory distress, usually with oxygen dependency (28). HRCT shows ground-glass shadowing in the lingula, right middle lobe and perihilar regions (Figure 24.1), allowing an experienced radiologist to make the diagnosis (29) (strictly, NEHI syndrome in the absence of biopsy

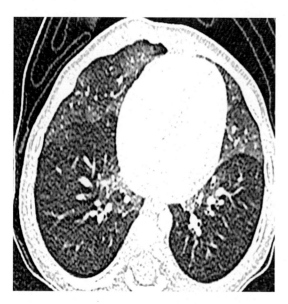

Figure 24.1 HRCT scan of an 8-month-old infant with persistent tachypnoea and oxygen requirement. There is ground-glass opacification in the right middle lobe and lingula, and also in the perihilar regions. The appearances are classical of neuroendocrine cell hyperplasia of infancy (NEHI).

confirmation [30]). If a biopsy is performed, the lung architecture looks normal on haematoxylin and eosin (H&E) staining, but on specific staining, increased bombesin positive cells are seen in the distal airways (31). Familial cases have been described (30). The clinical course is generally benign, but there may be prolonged oxygen dependency. No treatment is effective. If pulmonary function tests are performed they show hyperinflation and airflow obstruction (32), and a limited amount of follow-up data suggest that there is persistent fixed and variable airflow obstruction (33).

In real life, there are rather more uncertainties than this neat sketch would suggest. NEHI with atypical imaging is well described (34). Bombesin positive cells are not specific for NEHI, and are found in other disorders such as PIG, follicular bronchiolitis and surfactant protein disorders (35). Other histological features of these conditions preclude diagnostic confusion, but this finding raises the question as to whether these cells are of pathophysiological importance or merely persistence of a normal foetal phenomenon; how many bombesin positive cells are needed to make a diagnosis of NEHI has not really been determined. It seems likely that we will need more specific biomarkers for subgroups of what has been termed 'persistent tachypnoea of infancy (PTI)' (below) (34) if progress is to be made.

INFANCY: PIG

The hallmark of this condition is glycogen-containing cells in the pulmonary mesenchyme; as with NEHI cells, these are also a feature of normal antenatal lung development (36). There is no systemic abnormality of glycogen storage or underlying metabolic disorder. Treatment is expectant and the prognosis generally good, although fatalities have been recorded (37).

ACROSS THE AGE RANGE: SURFACTANT PROTEIN ABNORMALITIES

These are traditionally described as disorders of infancy, but most can present at any age including late adult life. The current (probably oversimplistic) view of Sp metabolism is shown in Figure 24.2. Furthermore, at least some of these genes may have functions additional to Sp homeostasis, so it would be more logical to include

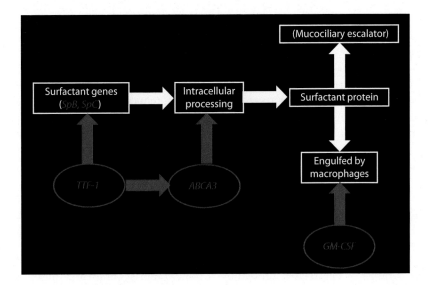

Figure 24.2 Surfactant synthesis and processing. (Abbreviations: ABCA3 = adenosine triphosphate binding cassette subfamily A member 3; GM-CSF = granulocyte–macrophage colony-stimulating factor; Sp = surfactant protein; TTF-1 = thyroid transcription factor 1.)

them in a broader category of genetic causes of chILD (below). Finally, given the complex post-transcriptional processing of Sps, it is likely that many more gene mutations impairing Sp homeostasis await discovery. The hallmark of these conditions is abnormal lamellar bodies on electron microscopy, and they can present with virtually any lung histology. In small series in which serial CT scans and biopsies have been reported, the appearances of both can change dramatically over time especially in *ABCA3* mutations (38) and Figure 24.3.

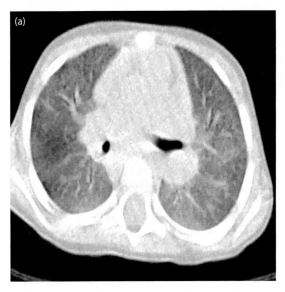

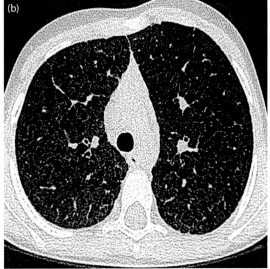

Figure 24.3 Progression of HRCT changes in a boy with two known disease-producing adenosine triphosphate binding cassette subfamily A member 3 (ABCA3) mutations in-*trans*. **(a)** There is diffuse non-specific ground-glass shadowing (child age 3 years). **(b)** Six years later, at age 9, the HRCT shows emphysema-like destruction most marked in the upper lobe. Such lung parenchyma as can be identified is relatively normal.

INFANCY: Sp-B MUTATIONS (AUTOSOMAL RECESSIVE, CHROMOSOME 22)

These present in the newborn period with relentlessly progressive respiratory failure, usually in a term baby, progressing to death or lung transplantation within months (39). Occasional milder forms with longer survival have been described (40).

ACROSS THE AGE RANGE: Sp-C MUTATIONS (AUTOSOMAL DOMINANT, CHROMOSOME 8)

Disease is due to gain of function mutations. Kindreds with a range of age-related presentations have been described (above). Sp-C chILD is part of the differential diagnosis of RSV bronchiolitis which fails to resolve. Although in the largest series, empirical treatment with systemic corticosteroids, hydroxychloroquine and azithromycin is associated with a good prognosis (3), fatalities are well described. Very prolonged survival with good lung function with just intermittent hydroxychloroquine therapy has been described (41). Interestingly, a Japanese kindred just presenting with UIP in adult life, although containing one child with asymptomatic radiological abnormalities has been described (42). Endoplasmic reticulum stress (BiP, IRE1α, cleaved Caspase-3) was reported to be increased *in vitro* by the mutant protein. Finding the reasons why the presentation of an inherited abnormality may be delayed may offer avenues for the discovery of new treatments.

ACROSS THE AGE RANGE: ABCA3 MUTATIONS (AUTOSOMAL RECESSIVE, CHROMOSOME 16)

This is a very large and complex gene, and mutations due to large deletions are easily missed (43). Babies with two severe (null) mutations in-*trans* present as SpB (above) and death or transplantation ensues in the first year of life (44). Those with mild mutations generally present later and have a better prognosis, with small series showing prolonged stability of spirometry. In terms of disease mechanism, wild-type and ABCA3 (R43L, R280C, L101P) mutation human A549 cells were studied. R280C and L101P, but not R43L ABCA3 was retained in the endoplasmic reticulum, and this was associated with endoplasmic reticulum stress (BiP/Grp78 upregulated, XBP1 splicing induced) and increased apoptosis (Annexin V/PI staining, reduced GSH, increased caspase 3 and 4) (45). This important study underscores that there may be different mechanisms of disease operative in different mutations in the same gene, analogous to the situation in cystic fibrosis.

ACROSS THE AGE RANGE: TTF-1 MUTATIONS (AUTOSOMAL DOMINANT, CHROMOSOME 14)

Presentation is at any age; the full-blown syndrome comprises brain and thyroid as well as lung disease, but only just over 50% have the full-blown triad, and, in the largest series, 24% solely had lung disease at presentation (46). Lung disease was diverse; typical Sp abnormalities (accumulation of foamy macrophages, pulmonary alveolar proteinosis [PAP], interstitial widening and pneumocyte hyperplasia, and abnormal lamellar bodies) were described, but also growth abnormalities and remodelling, as well as desquamative (DIP) and non-specific (NSIP) interstitial pneumonitis, the former perhaps reflecting the role of *TTF-1* in antenatal lung development (47).

An interesting family kindred demonstrated an interaction between *TTF-1* mutations and NEHI (48). The proband had classical NEHI, and five close relatives also had respiratory symptoms and failure to thrive in infancy. A *TTF-1* mutation was described in the proband and four of her relatives, but not found in any unaffected family member; no-one with the mutation had thyroid or brain disease. The exact cause of this intriguing relationship is unclear; the authors speculated that *TTF-1* mutations or one or more *TTF-1* target genes may underlie NEHI, and perhaps NEHI may be related to other genetic disorders. Clearly more work is needed, but this kindred underscores the need to think beyond apparently discrete chILD boxes.

ACROSS THE AGE RANGE: THE SPECTRUM OF PAP

PAP is not a diagnosis, merely a description of an abnormality with multiple underlying causes

Table 24.2 The spectrum of PAP

- Anti-GM-CSF auto-antibodies (adult type, but seen in children)
- Disorders of surfactant protein metabolism (adults and children); *SpB, SpC, ABCA3, TTF-1*
- GM-CSF receptor gene mutations (α- and β-chains) (49,50)
- Metabolic: lysinuric protein intolerance, Niemann–Pick disease
- Other genetic: MARS (51), GATA-2 (52)
- Associated with immune deficiency, including HIV
- Macrophage blockade (lymphoma; adult disease, not described in children)

(Table 24.2). It is one of the few diagnoses which can be diagnosed on HRCT alone (Figure 24.4). A precise diagnosis is essential, because treatment is not the same for all causes (below).

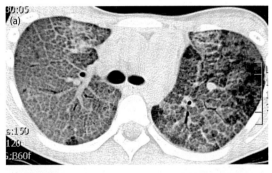

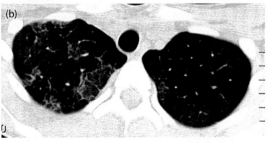

Figure 24.4 Pulmonary alveolar proteinosis in a 14-year-old boy who has circulating GM-CSF autoantibodies. **(a)** There is dense ground-glass opacification with outlining of the secondary pulmonary lobules giving the classical appearances of cobblestoning, **(b)** There is substantial clearing after sequential bilateral large volume lung lavages (Dr Cliff Morgan, Royal Brompton Hospital). Subsequent treatment with a good outcome was with nebulized GM-CSF.

ACROSS THE AGE RANGE: PULMONARY HAEMORRHAGIC SYNDROMES

These encompass conditions associated with pulmonary capillaritis, and cardiovascular and non-cardiovascular causes without capillaritis (Table 24.3). The diagnosis of acute pulmonary haemorrhage is likely if there is an acute rise in carbon monoxide transfer, and also on HRCT (Figure 24.5), confirmed by the finding of haemosiderin-laden macrophages on bronchoalveolar lavage. These likely persist for many days after an acute bleed (53). The old textbooks describe Heiner syndrome as being related to anti-IgD milk antibodies. These can no longer be measured, and I have never seen a case, or spoken to a paediatrician who has seen a case of pulmonary haemorrhage alleviated by a milk-free diet, so it is omitted from the table. The differential diagnosis of course includes any airway cause of haemoptysis. Pulmonary capillaritis is rare; in one series, more than 800 biopsies were analysed, of which 23 were from children with pulmonary haemorrhage; 8 were diagnosed with pulmonary capillaritis. Four had positive serology for ANA or ANCA, four had abnormal urinary sediment and six had a raised ESR; only two had none of these abnormalities (54). There are no clinical signs that can differentiate capillaritis from idiopathic pulmonary haemosiderosis (55), and so diagnosis of pulmonary capillaritis requires a lung biopsy. Many experts would consider treatment should be guided by clinical course rather than histopathology, but there is no evidence to support either view. A cluster of cases after an earthquake implicates a role for environmental factors in pulmonary haemorrhage (56).

ACROSS THE AGE RANGE: NON-SP GENETIC CAUSES OF chILD

There is an ever-increasing spectrum of rare genetic disorders which may either present with isolated chILD, or with chILD as part of the presenting disease (Table 24.4). Genetic causes should especially be suspected in early onset chILD associated with other organ disease, for example kidney and skin lesions as with integrin mutations (59,60), and central nervous system (CNS) disease (FLNA mutations [22]).

Table 24.3 Causes of pulmonary haemorrhage

Pulmonary capillaritis	• Idiopathic isolated • Idiopathic with renal disease • Goodpasture syndrome • Drug induced • Collagen vascular disease (including polyangiitis with granulomatosis, microscopic polynagiitis, SLE, anti-phospholipid syndrome, PAN) • HSP, IgA nephropathy • Behçet syndrome • Cryoglobulinemia
CVS causes without capillaritis	• Pulmonary venous hypertension • Pulmonary veno-occlusive disease • Pulmonary arteriovenous malformations • Pulmonary lymphangioleiomyomatosis • Pulmonary hypertension • Pulmonary capillary haemangiomatosis • Thrombosis with lung infarction
Non-CVS causes without capillaritis	• Idiopathic pulmonary haemosiderosis • Acute idiopathic pulmonary haemorrhage of infancy • Bone marrow transplantation • Immunodeficienccy • Coagulopathy (congenital or acquired) • Coeliac disease (57) • Child abuse
Non-CVS causes, capillaritis status unclear	• COPA mutations (58) • Down syndrome (57)

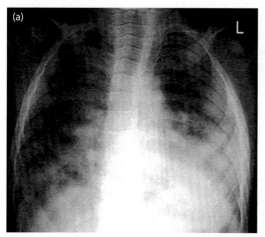
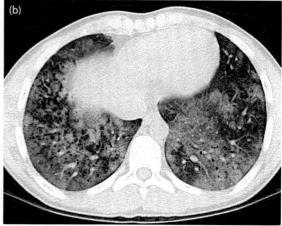

Figure 24.5 Acute pulmonary haemorrhage due to idiopathic pulmonary haemosiderosis which presented with iron deficiency anaemia. **(a)** Chest radiograph showing extensive confluent shadowing, particularly in the basal regions. **(b)** High-resolution CT scan showing widespread alveolar filling.

Table 24.4 Genetic disorders which may present as chILD; there are without doubt many more to be discovered

- Sp-B, Sp-C, ABCA-3, TTF-1 mutations
- GM-CSF receptor abnormalities (α- and β-chain)
- Storage disorders, e.g. Gaucher disease, Niemann–Pick disease
- Hermansky–Pudlak syndrome
- Lysinuric protein intolerance
- GM$_1$ agangliosidosis
- Fabry disease
- Neurofibromatosis
- FOXP3 mutations
- Pulmonary alveolar microlithiasis (mutations in the *SLC34A2* gene)
- STRA6 deficiency
- Telomerase gene mutations (*TERC, TERT*)
- Integrin mutations (59,60)
- *FLNA* mutations
- Ataxia telangiectasia (chILD as well as airway diseases, chronic infection and bronchiectasis secondary to immunodeficiency and aspiration)
- MARS (51)
- GATA-2 (52)
- COPA (autoimmune inflammatory arthritis and chILD) (58)
- STING (61)
- STAT3 (62)

Abbreviations: COPA = coatomer subunit alpha; FLNA = Filamin-A; GM-CSF = granulocyte–macrophage colony-stimulating factor; Sp = surfactant protein.

CHILDHOOD: ENVIRONMENTAL CAUSES OF chILD

EXTRINSIC ALLERGIC ALVEOLITIS

In the case of extrinsic allergic alveolitis (EAA) related to birds, typically avian IgG antibodies are implicated. Classically these are from a pet bird with a subacute presentation, but chronic presentations may occur from pigeon antigens inhaled from the parent's clothing (63) after they have emerged from the pigeon loft (the parent may present with acute disease as well). Feathers in the duvet have also been implicated (64). Treatment is allergen avoidance and corticosteroids (65).

KOREA: A NEW ENVIRONMENTAL chILD

A devastating ILD affecting both adults and children was reported from Korea; there were 138 cases between 2006 and 2011, with increasing annual incidence and a seasonal pattern (18). The mean age at presentation was 30.4 months, and presentation was with cough and dyspnoea, with rapid progression and no response to treatment. Air leaks were common, and 58% died. Histology showed combinations of centrilobular fibrosis, with bronchiolocentric destruction and foamy histiocytes, with sub-pleural sparing. Suspicion fell on a humidifier disinfectant, and when this was taken off the market there were no more new cases. This important outbreak reminds us to be wary of new environmental causes of chILD in the future.

HISTORY AND EXAMINATION

The presentation of chILD is very non-specific, and the condition should at least be remembered in children of any age with otherwise unexplained chronic or acute respiratory distress, hypoxaemia and failure to thrive. The US network has defined 'chILD syndrome' (18) to try to refine referrals for more detailed workup for chILD. This requires at least three of the following criteria in the absence of any other aetiology as the primary cause: (a) symptoms of impaired respiratory function; (b) hypoxaemia; (c) diffuse infiltrates on CXR or HRCT; (d) crackles on auscultation; and (e) abnormal lung function. It should be noted that although this is a good guide to the presence of chILD, it cannot replace clinical judgement, and over-reliance on the index may lead to diagnostic error. Additionally, chILD should be considered in the term baby with progressive respiratory distress; the baby with non-resolving bronchiolitis; unexplained iron deficiency anaemia, even in the absence of overt pulmonary haemorrhage; and children with a family history of unexpected respiratory deaths. Findings on history and examination are likely non-specific. A history of exposure to allergens, family history and any systemic features should be sought. A detailed medication history is essential; iatrogenic ILD is not uncommon (Figure 24.6). A full general and

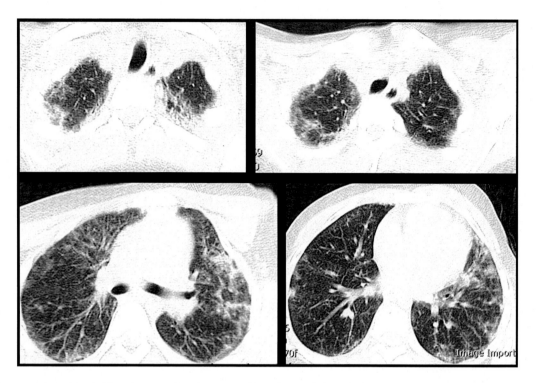

Figure 24.6 This child with neurodevelopmental handicap and a single kidney presented with cough. The HRCT shows patchy, quite dense consolidation, not in a distribution suggestive of aspiration, and with dilated airways within the consolidation in the upper lobes in particular. This is nitrofurantoin lung related to prophylactic treatment of the abnormal urinary tract with nitrofurantoin.

respiratory examination should be performed, and respiratory distress, hypoxaemia, digital clubbing, crackles and wheeze may all be found; however a clear chest to auscultation does not exclude chILD. Given the likely non-specific nature of the clinical findings, detailed further investigation is essential.

INVESTIGATIONS

Detailed protocols for the investigation and management of chILD have been published (16,17). The first essential step is to confirm the presence or otherwise of chILD, which usually requires HRCT (below). The pace and nature of further testing depend on the clinical urgency; in relatively well children, the results of blood tests can be awaited, whereas in a rapidly deteriorating neonate, an immediate lung biopsy may be the correct course of action. The severity of chILD is currently assessed by scoring symptoms, the degree of hypoxaemia

and the presence of pulmonary hypertension (66) (Table 24.5): this crude classification has stood the test of time. An echocardiogram is also essential to exclude vascular mimics of chILD (67). There is very little published on pulmonary function or exercise tests in children, but there is no reason to suppose these will be much different from adults, with restrictive spirometry, low lung volumes and reduced carbon monoxide transfer being expected. Serological tests which may be considered are listed in Table 24.6; again, the clinical situation will determine what tests are useful.

If serology is not diagnostic, then planning of further tests should aim to minimize the number of general anaesthetics to which the child is submitted. In general, FOB is reserved for children who are thought to have an opportunistic infection; most chILDs will not be definitively diagnosed by this procedure. Although FOB can demonstrate that there has been a pulmonary haemorrhage, it cannot distinguish primary from secondary causes, nor can it diagnose pulmonary capillaritis; and haemosiderin-laden macrophages

Table 24.5 Illness severity score used in chILD

Score	Symptoms	Hypoxaemia <90% sleep or exercise	Hypoxaemia <90% rest	Pulmonary hypertension
1	No	No	No	No
2	Yes	No	No	No
3	Yes	Yes	No	No
4	Yes	Yes	Yes	No
5	Yes	Yes	Yes	Yes

Source: Fan LL et al. Pediatr Pulmonol. 2004;38:369–78.

Table 24.6 Blood tests to be considered in the workup of chILD

Test	Disease	Comment
SpB, SpC, ABCA3, TTF-1 genes	Surfactant protein deficiency	Indicated in most children with ILD, unless there are extra-pulmonary features or another obvious diagnosis; especially in chILD presenting with neonatal respiratory distress
Angiotensin-converting enzyme	Sarcoidosis	Especially if extra-pulmonary features; isolated pulmonary sarcoidosis is rare (but described) in children
Anti-neutrophil cytoplasmic antibodies	Polyangiitis with granulomatosis, other vasculitides	Especially if upper airway disease, renal disease, pulmonary haemorrhage
Avian, M Faeni precipitins	Extrinsic allergic alveolitis	CT scan may be suggestive of this diagnosis
Viral and mycoplasma serology	Obliterative bronchiolitis	Not a true ILD, but may be confused on CT
Immune workup including HIV	Lymphoproliferative syndromes, including follicular bronchiolitis	Also perform if ILD in fact proves to be an opportunistic infection
Autoantibody studies; in this fast-moving field, consultation with a paediatric rheumatologist is advisable	Systemic lupus, rheumatoid diseases, scleroderma and other collagen vascular disease	Especially if extra-pulmonary features and renal disease
GM-CSF studies (serum autoantibody, receptor genetic studies)	Some of the variants of pulmonary alveolar proteinosis	Adult type with response to GM-CSF has been described in children

Note: Obviously, not all should be performed in all cases, and a selective approach taken according to the clinical circumstances.

are also seen in BAL from children with haemoglobinopathy but no obvious pulmonary haemorrhage (68). It is of course legitimate to perform a BAL at the time of lung biopsy under the same anaesthetic, at a site away from where the biopsy is to be performed.

RADIOLOGY

CXR is rarely diagnostic, and may indeed be essentially normal. HRCT should be performed without contrast, and minimizing the radiation

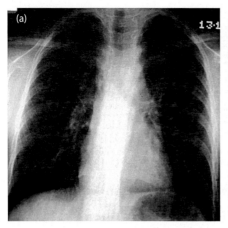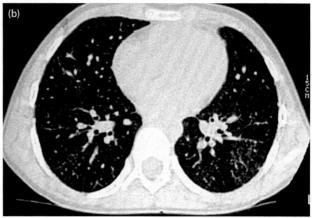

Figure 24.7 This 8-year-old boy had suffered from an undiagnosed respiratory illness with failure to thrive in infancy, which recovered spontaneously. He was well, but found to have digital clubbing and possible signs of pulmonary hypertension. **(a)** The chest radiograph is unremarkable. **(b)** The CT scan is non-diagnostic and shows a degree of basal ground-glass shadowing. A lung biopsy showed burnt out desquamative interstitial pneumonitis. No underlying cause was found.

dose. HRCT is used to confirm the presence of chILD (Figures 24.7 and 24.8); as a guide to severity of the disease, including the possible extent of fibrosis and traction bronchiectasis; occasionally to make a diagnosis of a specific condition (Langerhans cell histiocytosis, hypersensitivity pneumonitis) or group of conditions (PAP spectrum); and to guide the site of biopsy if one is planned. Unlike adult ILD, HRCT alone is not frequently diagnostic in chILD.

PATHOLOGY

An ongoing source of controversy is the indication and timing of lung biopsy in chILD. Clearly it is unnecessary if the diagnosis has been definitively made by less invasive means, such as a blood test or HRCT (above). If the child is gravely ill, and no diagnosis has been made, this author would proceed to lung biopsy rather than treat blindly, although not all would agree. In this circumstance, although findings such as granulomatous lung disease may strongly suggest specific diagnoses (e.g. sarcoidosis, hypersensitivity pneumonitis, chronic granulomatous disease), in many cases, although the pattern of abnormalities may be described (alveolar simplification, cholesterol clefts, for example), the underlying diagnosis may remain obscure. Conversely, an

unexpected finding, for example a lymphoproliferative disorder (Figure 24.9) may suggest a new line of investigation, in this case for a congenital or acquired immunodeficiency. A difficult issue is in PTI (above) (34). A recent manuscript defined this group as persistent tachypnoea, HCT with predominantly ground-glass opacities and only minor other abnormalities; and exclusion of specific entities such as Sp mutations. HRCT scans were described as typical (of NEHI) if they were parahilar and paramediastinal, and in right middle lobe and lingula; all other distributions and findings were regarded as atypical. A few had biopsies performed, and the atypical group showed NEHI, PIG or normal lung tissue. Both groups had a good outcome, with 50% asymptomatic at 2.6 years of age and no deaths. It was suggested that biopsy was not needed in this group unless there were red flags such as age of onset less than 4 weeks, very atypical HRCT findings, failure to thrive despite oxygen therapy, a positive family history, evidence of other organ involvement or relentless clinical deterioration.

Although the indications for biopsy are still a matter of debate, the technique is not. Transbronchial biopsy samples are too small for most diagnostic purposes, and the risk of the procedure is not trivial. Percutaneous CT-guided biopsy offers no advantage over a VATS procedure which should be performed to sample from more and less affected areas of the lung. The biopsy

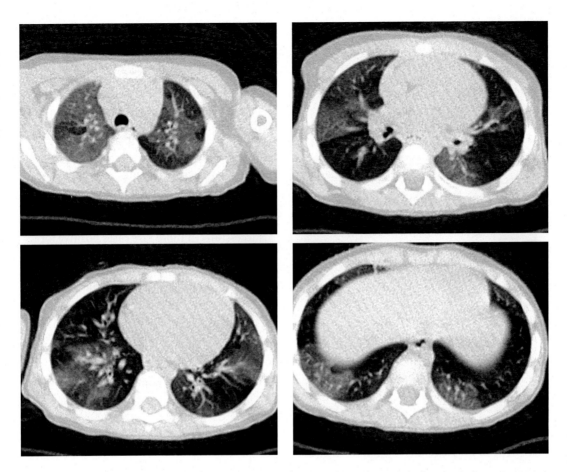

Figure 24.8 The CT scan shows alternating ground-glass shadowing and darker areas. It may sometimes be difficult to determine whether the black (air trapping?) or grey (ground-glass opacification?) areas are abnormal. In this case, the diagnosis is obliterative bronchiolitis secondary to adenovirus infection.

should be planned, and samples stored so as to maximize the information obtained (69).

GENERAL MANAGEMENT

There are no randomized controlled trials of treatment in chILD, so all recommendations, both general and specific, are not evidence based. Oxygen should be given to maintain normoxia. General respiratory care (full immunizations, avoidance of tobacco smoke and environmental pollution, exercise as far as possible) is mandated. Palivizumab should be considered in young children prescribed corticosteroids (70). Nutritional status must be optimized; a recent parent survey has shown that feeding disorders and reflux are common in chILD

patients. The families are needy, and as far as possible, full support including specialist nursing and psychological should be put in place (71).

Non-specific pharmacotherapy comprises systemic corticosteroids (oral daily or alternate day in mild cases, monthly pulsed methyl prednisolone sometimes combined with interval oral prednisolone), hydroxychloroquine and azithromycin, the last two for their immunological effects. The evidence for other non-specific therapies such as methotrexate and cyclosporine is more tenuous.

Lung transplantation is the only option for end-stage chILD. Results are comparable with other paediatric indications, but the risk of recurrence in the transplanted lung should always be considered in the non-genetic chILDs. For most, there are insufficient data to give an evidence-based estimate of risk.

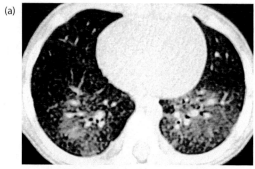

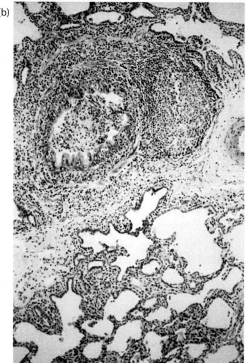

Figure 24.9 This infant presented with unexplained tachypnoea. **(a)** The CT scan shows bilateral ground-glass opacification with some nodularity. **(b)** The lung biopsy shows follicular bronchiolitis, with peribronchial inflammation and a lymphoid follicle. Immunological and rheumatological conditions were excluded, and no underlying cause could be found.

SPECIFIC ASPECTS OF MANAGEMENT

There are a few additional treatments for specific conditions, all non-evidence-based and discussed below; however, there are sufficient of these to

mandate a careful search for a specific diagnosis, rather than therapeutic nihilism or steroids for everyone. Disappointingly, anti-fibrotics such as Pirfenidone or Nintedanib (which have found a place in adult IPF) have never been trialed in children, despite EMEA and FDA strictures on the importance of trialing of medications in children.

PAP spectrum: Whole lung lavage can be performed in even very young children with considerable success (72). Inhaled or subcutaneous granulocyte–macrophage colony-stimulating factor (GM-CSF) has been used successfully in those rare cases positive for serum anti-GM-CSF autoantibodies (73).

Hypersensitivity pneumonitis: The key is identification of the allergen or chemical driving the disease, and prevention of exposure, in addition to steroid therapy (pulsed or oral, as above). Unfortunately, diagnosis may be significantly delayed and lung function may be severely impaired at presentation, and the outcome is not always favourable (Figure 24.10).

Sarcoidosis: (see Figure 24.11) The anti-TNF monoclonal infliximab, combined with methotrexate, may be effective (74), although evidence in childhood is anecdotal at best.

ChILD secondary to rheumatological conditions: These may respond to specific regimens, for example cyclophosphamide for granulomatosis with polyangiitis (formerly known as Wegener

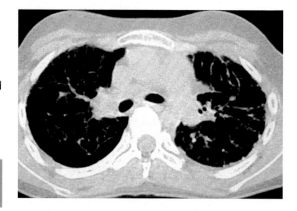

Figure 24.10 CT scan of a 16-year-old boy, showing a right pneumothorax, extensive lung destruction and fibrosis due to end-stage extrinsic allergic alveolitis.

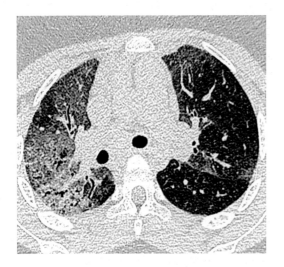

Figure 24.11 Bilateral ground-glass shadowing, more right-sided, in a 13-year-old Afro-Caribbean girl who presented with blurred vision due to anterior uveitis. She had severely restrictive spirometry. The underlying diagnosis was confirmed as sarcoidosis.

granulomatosis) (75); it would be wise to seek the advice of a paediatric rheumatologist in such cases.

Idiopathic pulmonary haemosiderosis: If bleeding is not controlled on the non-specific regime above, consider triple pulses of intravenous immunoglobulin, intravenous cyclophosphamide and methyl prednisolone. Plasmapheresis can be used if acute bleeding continues despite steroid pulses (76); again, there is not much evidence for this. These intensive regimes are especially important in pulmonary capillaritis, but should be used irrespective of the lung histology in those with ongoing bleeding despite standard treatment.

Pulmonary hypertension (PHT) and child: Possible mechanisms of PHT in chILD include reduction in the capillary bed due to developmental and acquired disorders, and hypoxaemia. It is speculative, but it may be in some cases that treatment of PHT with specific medications (Phosphodiesterase V inhibitors, endothelin antagonists and prostacyclin analogues) may be beneficial over and above the treatment of the underlying chILD. The advice of a PHT specialist should be sought before instituting such therapy.

PROGNOSIS AND LONG-TERM OUTLOOK

The prognosis of individual conditions has been discussed above. However, in general, prognostication for individual conditions is based on very small case series and should always be cautious. Surprisingly good responses to treatment are sometimes seen, but conversely, a rapid and unexpected spiral downhill may also be the clinical course.

CURRENT AND FUTURE AREAS OF RESEARCH

Individual chILD diseases are so rare that no country, let alone a single institution, will see enough cases to develop an evidence base for treatment, so international collaboration is essential, and this is increasingly happening across the world. Patient involvement is critical in this, and patient groups have already made significant discoveries about chILD. As should be clear from the above, we are profoundly ignorant about almost all aspects of chILD, and therefore the scope for future research is huge. I suggest the following priority areas:

1. We need to be alert for new entities, and especially think geographically – chILD in developed and low-/middle-income countries may be very different
2. Paediatric pulmonologists need to apply lessons from the huge adult ILD cohorts; so for example, MUC5B promotor (77) and ciliary genes (78) are implicated in adult ILD. We need to explore whether there is also a signature in chILD (79)
3. There are unlikely to be the same huge trials in chILD as in adult ILD; so paediatric pulmonologists must utilise adult data to do really focussed, probably *n*-of-1 trials in chILD.

ACKNOWLEDGEMENTS

AB is an NIHR Senior Investigator, and is funded through the Royal Brompton Hospital NIHR BRU and the chILD EU FP7 grant 'Orphans Unite: chILD better together – European Management Platform for Childhood Interstitial Lung Diseases'. My great thanks are due to Professors Hansell and Nicholson who have taught me so much about chILD, and even more so, Carlee Gilbert and other families who have children with chILD who have taught me so much more.

REFERENCES

1. Hime NJ, Zurynski Y, Fitzgerald D, Selvadurai H, Phu A, Deverell M et al. Childhood interstitial lung disease: A systematic review. *Pediatr Pulmonol.* 2015;50:1383–92.
2. Thomas AQ, Lane K, Phillips J 3rd, Prince M, Markin C, Speer M et al. Heterozygosity for a surfactant protein C gene mutation associated with usual interstitial pneumonitis and cellular nonspecific interstitial pneumonitis in one kindred. *Am J Respir Crit Care Med.* 2002;165:1322–8.
3. Thouvenin G, Abou Taam R, Flamein F, Guillot L, Le Bourgeois M, Reix P et al. Characteristics of disorders associated with genetic mutations of surfactant protein C. *Arch Dis Child.* 2010;95:449–54.
4. Glasser SW, Witt TL, Senft AP, Baatz JE, Folger D, Maxfield MD et al. Surfactant protein C-deficient mice are susceptible to respiratory syncytial virus infection. *Am J Physiol Lung Cell Mol Physiol.* 2009;297:L64–72.
5. Thavagnanam S, Cutz E, Manson D, Nogee LM, Dell SD. Variable clinical outcome of ABCA3 deficiency in two siblings. *Pediatr Pulmonol.* 2013;48:1035–8.
6. Kaltenborn E, Kern S, Frixel S, Fragnet L, Conzelmann KK, Zarbock R, Griese M. Respiratory syncytial virus potentiates ABCA3 mutation-induced loss of lung epithelial cell differentiation. *Hum Mol Genet.* 2012;21:2793–806.
7. Margaritopoulos GA, Vasarmidi E, Jacob J, Wells AU, Antoniou KM. Smoking and interstitial lung diseases. *Eur Respir Rev.* 2015;24:428–35.
8. Sismanlar T, Aslan AT, Turktas H, Memis L, Griese M. Respiratory bronchiolitis-associated interstitial lung disease in childhood: New sequela of smoking. *Pediatrics.* 2015;136:e1026–9.
9. Ischander M, Fan LL, Farahmand V, Langston C, Yazdani S. Desquamative interstitial pneumonia in a child related to cigarette smoke. *Pediatr Pulmonol.* 2014;49:E56–8.
10. Kale Y, Aslan A, Kose G. Pulmonary Langerhans cell histiocytosis in an infant: Can passive smoking accelerate the disease progress? *Pediatr Pulmonol.* 2007;42:565–7.
11. Deutsch GH, Young LR, Deterding RR, Fan LL, Dell SD, Bean JA et al.; Pathology Cooperative Group, ChILD Research Co-operative. Diffuse lung disease in young children: Application of a novel classification scheme. *Am J Respir Crit Care Med.* 2007;176:1120–8.
12. Rice A, Tran-Dang MA, Bush A, Nicholson AG. Diffuse lung disease in infancy and childhood: Expanding the chILD classification. *Histopathology.* 2013;63:743–55.
13. Fan LL, Dishop MK, Galambos C, Askin FB, White FV, Langston C et al. Children's Interstitial and Diffuse Lung Disease Research Network (chILDRN). Diffuse lung disease in biopsied children 2 to 18 years of age. Application of the chILD classification scheme. *Ann Am Thorac Soc.* 2015;12:1498–505.
14. Clement A; ERS Task Force. Task force on chronic interstitial lung disease in immunocompetent children. *Eur Respir J.* 2004;24:686–97.
15. Griese M, Haug M, Brasch F, Freihorst A, Lohse P, von Kries R et al. Incidence and classification of pediatric diffuse parenchymal lung diseases in Germany. *Orphanet J Rare Dis.* 2009;4:26.
16. Kurland G, Deterding RR, Hagood JS, Young LR, Brody AS, Castile RG et al. American Thoracic Society Committee on Childhood Interstitial Lung Disease (chILD) and the chILD Research Network. An official American Thoracic Society clinical practice guideline: Classification, evaluation, and management of childhood interstitial lung disease in infancy. *Am J Respir Crit Care Med.* 2013;188:376–94.
17. Bush A, Cunningham S, de Blic J, Barbato A, Clement A, Epaud R et al. ChILD-EU Collaboration. European protocols for the diagnosis and initial treatment of

interstitial lung diseass in children. *Thorax.* 2015;70:1078–84.

18. Kim KW, Ahn K, Yang HJ, Lee S, Park JD, Kim WK et al. Humidifier disinfectant-associated children's interstitial lung disease. *Am J Respir Crit Care Med.* 2014;189:48–56.

19. Dharmadhikari AV, Szafranski P, Kalinichenko VV, Stankiewicz P. Genomic and epigenetic complexity of the FOXF1 locus in 16q24.1: Implications for development and disease. *Curr Genomics.* 2015;16:107–16.

20. Pasutto F, Sticht H, Hammersen G, Gillessen-Kaesbach G, Fitzpatrick DR, Nürnberg G et al. Mutations in STRA6 cause a broad spectrum of malformations including anophthalmia, congenital heart defects, diaphragmatic hernia, alveolar capillary dysplasia, lung hypoplasia, and mental retardation. *Am J Hum Genet.* 2007;80:550–60.

21. Galambos C, Sims-Lucas S, Ali N, Gien J, Dishop MK, Abman SH. Intrapulmonary vascular shunt pathways in alveolar capillary dysplasia with misalignment of pulmonary veins. *Thorax.* 2015;70:84–5.

22. Masurel-Paulet A, Haan E, Thompson EM, Goizet C, Thauvin-Robinet C, Tai A et al. Lung disease associated with periventricular nodular heterotopia and an FLNA mutation. *Eur J Med Genet.* 2011;54:25–8.

23. Abel RM, Bush A, Chitty LS, Harcourt J, Nicholson AG. Congenital lung disease. In: Wilmott R, Boat T, Bush A, Chernick V, Deterding R, Ratjen F, eds. *Kendig and Chernick's Disorders of the Respiratory Tract in Children.* 8th ed. Philadelphia, PA: Elsevier Saunders; 2012:317–57.

24. Narayanan M, Owers-Bradley J, Beardsmore CS, Mada M, Ball I, Garipov R et al. Alveolarization continues during childhood and adolescence: New evidence from helium-3 magnetic resonance. *Am J Respir Crit Care Med.* 2012;185:186–91.

25. Narayanan M, Beardsmore CS, Owers-Bradley J, Dogaru CM, Mada M, Ball I et al. Catch-up alveolarization in ex-preterm children: Evidence from (3)He magnetic resonance. *Am J Respir Crit Care Med.* 2013;187:1104–9.

26. Hyde DM, Blozis SA, Avdalovic MV, Putney LF, Dettorre R, Quesenberry NJ et al. Alveoli increase in number but not size from birth to adulthood in rhesus monkeys. *Am J Physiol Lung Cell Mol Physiol.* 2007;293:L570–9.

27. Chaudhari M, Vogel M, Wright C, Smith J, Haworth SG. Sildenafil in neonatal pulmonary hypertension due to impaired alveolarisation and plexiform pulmonary arteriopathy. *Arch Dis Child Fetal Neonatal Ed.* 2005;90:F527–8.

28. Deterding RR, Pye C, Fan LL, Langston C. Persistent tachypnea of infancy is associated with neuroendocrine cell hyperplasia. *Pediatr Pulmonol.* 2005;40:157–65.

29. Brody AS, Crotty EJ. Neuroendocrine cell hyperplasia of infancy (NEHI). *Pediatr Radiol.* 2006;36:1328.

30. Popler J, Gower WA, Mogayzel PJ Jr., Nogee LM, Langston C, Wilson AC et al. Familial neuroendocrine cell hyperplasia of infancy. *Pediatr Pulmonol.* 2010;45:749–55.

31. Young LR, Brody AS, Inge TH, Acton JD, Bokulic RE, Langston C, Deutsch GH. Neuroendocrine cell distribution and frequency distinguish neuroendocrine cell hyperplasia of infancy from other pulmonary disorders. *Chest.* 2011;139:1060–71.

32. Kerby GS, Wagner BD, Popler J, Hay TC, Kopecky C, Wilcox SL et al. Abnormal infant pulmonary function in young children with neuroendocrine cell hyperplasia of infancy. *Pediatr Pulmonol.* 2013;48:1008–15.

33. Lukkarinen H, Pelkonen A, Lohi J, Malmström K, Malmberg LP, Kajosaari M et al. Neuroendocrine cell hyperplasia of infancy: A prospective follow-up of nine children. *Arch Dis Child.* 2013;98:141–4.

34. Rauch D, Wetzke M, Reu S, Wesselak W, Schams A, Hengst M et al. PTI (Persistent Tachypnea of Infancy) Study Group of the Kids Lung Register. Persistent tachypnea of infancy. Usual and aberrant. *Am J Respir Crit Care Med.* 2016;193:438–47.

35. Yancheva SG, Velani A, Rice A, Montero A, Hansell DM, Koo S et al. Bombesin staining in neuroendocrine cell hyperplasia of infancy (NEHI) and other childhood interstitial lung diseases (chILD). *Histopathology.* 2015;67:501–8.

36. Canakis AM, Cutz E, Manson D, O'Brodovich H. Pulmonary interstitial glycogenosis: A new variant of neonatal interstitial lung disease. *Am J Respir Crit Care Med.* 2002;165:1557–65.

37. King BA, Boyd JT, Kingma PS. Pulmonary maturational arrest and death in a patient with pulmonary interstitial glycogenosis. *Pediatr Pulmonol.* 2011;46:1142–5.

38. Doan ML, Guillerman RP, Dishop MK, Nogee LM, Langston C, Mallory GB et al. Clinical, radiological and pathological features of ABCA3 mutations in children. Clinical, radiological and pathological features of ABCA3 mutations in children. *Thorax.* 2008;63:366–73.

39. Hamvas A, Nogee LM, deMello DE, Cole FS. Pathophysiology and treatment of surfactant protein-B deficiency. *Biol Neonate.* 1995;67:18S–31S.

40. Dunbar AE 3rd, Wert SE, Ikegami M, Whitsett JA, Hamvas A, White FV et al. Prolonged survival in hereditary surfactant protein B (SP-B) deficiency associated with a novel splicing mutation. *Pediatr Res.* 2000;48:275–82.

41. Avital A, Hevroni A, Godfrey S, Cohen S, Maayan C, Nusair S et al. Natural history of five children with surfactant protein C mutations and interstitial lung disease. *Pediatr Pulmonol.* 2014;49:1097–105.

42. Ono S, Tanaka T, Ishida M, Kinoshita A, Fukuoka J, Takaki M et al. Surfactant protein C G100S mutation causes familial pulmonary fibrosis in Japanese kindred. *Eur Respir J.* 2011;38:861–9.

43. Henderson LB, Melton K, Wert S, Couriel J, Bush A, Ashworth M, Nogee LM. Large ABCA3 and SFTPC deletions resulting in lung disease. *Ann Am Thorac Soc.* 2013;10:602–7.

44. Wambach JA, Casey AM, Fishman MP, Wegner DJ, Wert SE, Cole FS et al. Genotype-phenotype correlations for infants and children with ABCA3 deficiency. *Am J Respir Crit Care Med.* 2014;189:1538–43.

45. Weichert N, Kaltenborn E, Hector A, Woischnik M, Schams A, Holzinger A et al. Some ABCA3 mutations elevate ER stress and initiate apoptosis of lung epithelial cells. *Respir Res.* 2011;12:4.

46. Hamvas A, Deterding RR, Wert SE, White FV, Dishop MK, Alfano DN et al. Heterogeneous pulmonary phenotypes associated with mutations in the thyroid transcription factor gene NKX2-1. *Chest.* 2013;144:794–804.

47. Zscheppang K, Giese U, Hoenzke S, Wiegel D, Dammann CE. ErbB4 is an upstream regulator of TTF-1fetal mouse lung type II cell development in vitro. *Biochim Biophys Acta.* 2013;1833:2690–702.

48. Young LR, Deutsch GH, Bokulic RE, Brody AS, Nogee LM. A mutation in TTF1/NKX2.1 is associated with familial neuroendocrine cell hyperplasia of infancy. *Chest.* 2013;144:1199–206.

49. Hildebrandt J, Yalcin E, Bresser HG, Cinel G, Gappa M, Haghighi A et al. Characterization of CSF2RA mutation related juvenile pulmonary alveolar proteinosis. *Orphanet J Rare Dis.* 2014;9:171.

50. Suzuki T, Maranda B, Sakagami T, Catellier P, Couture CY, Carey BC et al. Hereditary pulmonary alveolar proteinosis caused by recessive CSF2RB mutations. *Eur Respir J.* 2011;37:201–4.

51. Hadchouel A, Wieland T, Griese M, Baruffini E, Lorenz-Depiereux B, Enaud L et al. Biallelic mutations of methionyl-tRNA synthetase cause a specific type of pulmonary alveolar proteinosis prevalent on Réunion Island. *Am J Hum Genet.* 2015;96:826–31.

52. Griese M, Zarbock R, Costabel U, Hildebrandt J, Theegarten D, Albert M et al. GATA2 deficiency in children and adults with severe pulmonary alveolar proteinosis and hematologic disorders. *BMC Pulm Med.* 2015;15:87–1.

53. Epstein CE, Elidemir O, Colasurdo GN, Fan LL. Time course of hemosiderin production by alveolar macrophages in a murine model. *Chest.* 2001;120:2013–20.

54. Fullmer JJ, Langston C, Dishop MK, Fan LL. Pulmonary capillaritis in children: A review of eight cases with comparison to other alveolar hemorrhage syndromes. *J Pediatr.* 2005;146:376–81.

55. Wang H, Sun L, Tan W. Clinical features of children with pulmonary microscopic polyangiitis: Report of 9 cases. *PLoS One.* 2015;10:e0124352.

56. Ebisawa K, Yamada N, Kobayashi M, Katahira M, Konno H, Okada S. Cluster of diffuse alveolar hemorrhage cases after the 2011 Tohoku Region Pacific Coast Earthquake. *Respir Investig*. 2013;51:2–8.

57. Taytard J, Nathan N, de Blic J, Fayon M, Epaud R, Deschildre A et al.; French RespiRare® group. New insights into pediatric idiopathic pulmonary hemosiderosis: The French RespiRare(®) cohort. *Orphanet J Rare Dis*. 2013;8:161.

58. Watkin LB, Jessen B, Wiszniewski W, Vece TJ, Jan M, Sha Y et al. COPA mutations impair ER-Golgi transport and cause hereditary autoimmune-mediated lung disease and arthritis. *Nat Genet*. 2015;47:654–60.

59. Nicolaou N, Margadant C, Kevelam SH, Lilien MR, Oosterveld MJ, Kreft M et al. Gain of glycosylation in integrin α3 causes lung disease and nephrotic syndrome. *J Clin Invest*. 2012;122:4375–87.

60. Has C, Spartà G, Kiritsi D, Weibel L, Moeller A, Vega-Warner V et al. Integrin α3 mutations with kidney, lung, and skin disease. *N Engl J Med*. 2012;366:1508–14.

61. Liu Y, Jesus AA, Marrero B, Yang D, Ramsey SE, Montealegre Sanchez GA et al. Activated STING in a vascular and pulmonary syndrome. *N Engl J Med*. 2014;371:507–18.

62. Flanagan SE, Haapaniemi E, Russell MA, Caswell R, Lango Allen H, De Franco E et al. Activating germline mutations in STAT3 cause early-onset multi-organ autoimmune disease. *Nat Genet*. 2014;46:812–4.

63. Rosal-Sanchez M, Alvarez J, Torres MJ, Mayorga C, Pérez J, Blanca M. Pigeon Fancier's Lung after low exposure. *Allergy*. 2002;57:649.

64. Griese M, Haug M, Hartl D, Teusch V, Glöckner-Pagel J, Brasch F; National EAA Study Group. Hypersensitivity pneumonitis: Lessons for diagnosis and treatment of a rare entity in children. *Orphanet J Rare Dis*. 2013;8:121.

65. Buchvald F, Petersen BL, Damgaard K, Deterding R, Langston C, Fan LL et al. Frequency, treatment, and functional outcome in children with hypersensitivity pneumonitis. *Pediatr Pulmonol*. 2011;46:1098–107.

66. Fan LL, Deterding RR, Langston C. Pediatric interstitial lung disease revisited. *Pediatr Pulmonol*. 2004;38:369–78.

67. Sondheimer HM, Lung MC, Brugman SM, Ikle DN, Fan LL, White CW. Pulmonary vascular disorders masquerading as interstitial lung disease. *Pediatr Pulmonol*. 1995;20:284–288.

68. Priftis KN, Anthracopoulos MB, Tsakanika C, Tapaki G, Ladis V, Bush A, Nicolaidou P. Quantification of siderophages in bronchoalveolar fluid in transfusional and primary pulmonary hemosiderosis. *Pediatr Pulmonol*. 2006;41:972–977.

69. Langston C, Patterson K, Dishop MK; chILD Pathology Co-operative Group, Askin F, Baker P, Chou P et al. A protocol for the handling of tissue obtained by operative lung biopsy: Recommendations of the chILD pathology co-operative group. *Pediatr Dev Pathol*. 2006;9:173–80.

70. Drummond D, Thumerelle C, Reix P, Fayon M, Epaud R, Clement A et al. Effectiveness of palivizumab in children with childhood interstitial lung disease: The French experience. *Pediatr Pulmonol*. 2015. doi:10.1002/ppul.23354. [Epub ahead of print].

71. Gilbert C, Bush A, Cunningham S. Childhood interstitial lung disease: Family experiences. *Pediatr Pulmonol*. 2015;50:1301–3.

72. Reiter K, Schoen C, Griese M, Nicolai T. Whole-lung lavage in infants and children with pulmonary alveolar proteinosis. *Paediatr Anaesth*. 2010;20:1118–23.

73. Robinson TE, Trapnell BC, Goris ML, Quittell LM, Cornfield DN. Quantitative analysis of longitudinal response to aerosolized granulocyte-macrophage colony-stimulating factor in two adolescents with autoimmune pulmonary alveolar proteinosis. *Chest*. 2009;135:842–8.

74. Saleh S, Ghodsian S, Yakimova V, Henderson J, Sharma OP. Effectiveness of infliximab in treating selected patients with sarcoidosis. *Respir Med*. 2006;100:2053–9.

75. Cabral DA, Uribe AG, Benseler S, O'Neil KM, Hashkes PJ, Higgins G et al. ARChiVe (A Registry for Childhood Vasculitis: E-entry) Investigators Network. Classification, presentation, and initial treatment of Wegener's

granulomatosis in childhood. *Arthritis Rheum.* 2009;60:3413–24.

76. Kupfer O, Ridall LA, Hoffman LM, Dishop MK, Soep JB, Wagener JS, Fan LL. Pulmonary capillaritis in monozygotic twin boys. *Pediatrics.* 2013;132:e1445–8.

77. Seibold MA, Wise AL, Speer MC, Steele MP, Brown KK, Loyd JE et al. A common MUC5B promoter polymorphism and pulmonary fibrosis. *N Engl J Med.* 2011;364:1503–12.

78. Yang IV, Coldren CD, Leach SM, Seibold MA, Murphy E, Lin J et al. Expression of cilium-associated genes defines novel molecular subtypes of idiopathic pulmonary fibrosis. *Thorax.* 2013;68:1114–21.

79. Liptzin DR, Watson AM, Murphy E, Kroehl ME, Dishop MK, Galambos C et al. MUC5B expression and location in surfactant protein C mutations in children. *Pediatr Pulmonol.* 2015;50:1270–6.

25

Understanding the role of co-morbidities in interstitial lung diseases

ADRIAN SHIFREN, TONYA RUSSELL, ADAM L ANDERSON
AND STEVEN D NATHAN

INTRODUCTION

Patients with interstitial lung diseases have a higher prevalence of both pulmonary and extra-pulmonary co-morbidities compared to age- and gender-matched controls. These include respiratory failure, pulmonary hypertension (PH), coronary artery disease (CAD), gastro-oesophageal reflux disease (GERD), pneumothorax, lung cancer and obstructive sleep apnoea. Patients will frequently have multiple co-morbidities. While a unifying basis for the increased prevalence of co-morbidities in patients with interstitial lung disease (ILD) remains unknown, potential causes include up-regulation of disease mediators in the lung, telomere shortening as noted in patients with idiopathic pulmonary fibrosis (IPF), which may increase the risk for age-related diseases and cigarette smoking, which is common

to a number of the known co-morbidities (1–3). While most of the literature pertaining to complications emanates from investigations of IPF, these maladies may occur in many other forms of ILD. An awareness of the propensity, impact and management of these complications is important in the holistic care of patients with various forms of ILD.

ACUTE EXACERBATIONS

Acute exacerbation of fibrotic lung disease has a significant impact on morbidity and mortality. In one series, acute exacerbations were the most frequent cause of respiratory decompensation in IPF patients, accounting for 55.2% of respiratory decompensation events (4). The 1- and 3-year incidences of acute exacerbations in IPF have been reported as 14.2% and 20.7%, respectively.

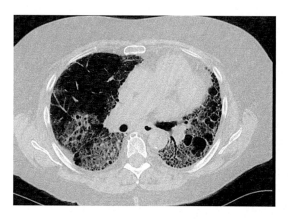

Figure 25.1 Acute exacerbation. Bilateral ground-glass opacities on the background of UIP in an IPF patient with an acute exacerbation. (Image courtesy of Andrew Bierhals, Mallinckrodt Institute of Radiology, Washington University School of Medicine.)

Acute exacerbation in the setting of IPF has been defined as the onset of worsening dyspnoea over the course of <30 days, ground-glass opacities on chest high-resolution computed tomography (HRCT) on the background of a usual interstitial pneumonia (UIP) pattern (Figure 25.1), exclusion of respiratory infection and exclusion of other causes of respiratory decompensation such as heart failure or pulmonary embolism (5). Definitive exclusion of these other conditions is often difficult, and, therefore, the bar is set high to confirm the diagnosis of a true acute exacerbation. For example, it is difficult to obtain adequate sampling to rule out respiratory infection, as patients can be severely hypoxaemic during acute exacerbations. In this setting, the condition has previously been referred to as 'suspected acute exacerbation'. Patients with known triggers for respiratory decompensation can have similar outcomes as patients with idiopathic acute exacerbation. A growing appreciation for these factors has resulted in a recent revision to the definition of acute exacerbations of IPF with modifications and broadening of the defining criteria. Specifically, the temporal requirements now allow for acute exacerbations that may initially manifest outside the 30-day window. In addition, exclusion of other conditions includes only overt pulmonary edema, which is easy to recognize and should be imminently reversible with diuresis. Therefore, acute exacerbations may now have an identifiable precipitating factor or could still be idiopathic (6).

Classically, the histopathology of acute exacerbations has demonstrated diffuse alveolar damage (DAD) on a background of UIP, although diffuse alveolar haemorrhage has been reported in a very small number of patients (5,7,8). Therefore, the more recent definition of acute exacerbation has been modified to focus more on the acute worsening of respiratory status in a pattern suggestive of lung injury with DAD, rather than the idiopathic nature of the episodes (9).

Although the current definition of acute exacerbation is specific to IPF, acute exacerbations can occur in other fibrotic lung diseases, such as collagen vascular disease related interstitial lung disease (CVD-ILD), chronic hypersensitivity pneumonitis (HP) and unclassifiable ILD. Prognosis of an acute exacerbation is overall poor with in-hospital survival in one patient cohort of 37% and a 1-year survival of only 14%. A second cohort of patients with a higher number of non-IPF patients demonstrated a slightly better outcome with a 90-day survival of 60%. In both study populations, IPF patients who experienced an acute exacerbation had significantly worse outcomes than non-IPF patients with acute exacerbations (7,10).

Acute exacerbations can occur after surgical lung biopsy (SLB) or lung resection. The incidence is 4%–5% after lung biopsy with a nearly uniform mortal outcome for those who develop an exacerbation. In the setting of SLB or resection, acute exacerbations appear to occur almost solely in patients with IPF (8,11,12). For this reason, SLB should be reserved for patients in whom the diagnosis remains unclear after a thorough review of clinical and radiographic data. Lower forced vital capacity (FVC), reduced single breath diffusing capacity for carbon monoxide (DLCO), and longer exposure time to 100% oxygen intra-operatively appear to be risk factors for the development of acute exacerbation after surgery (12).

Workup for acute exacerbation should include evaluation for left ventricular dysfunction, pulmonary embolism, pneumothorax and infection, along with respiratory sampling if feasible. Treatment options are limited. Patients often receive broad-spectrum antibiotics for potential infection, as well as high-dose corticosteroids tapered over a few weeks, although the data to support corticosteroid use are limited. Interestingly, a recent study from Japan demonstrated that the use of sulfamethoxazole/trimethoprim (odds ratio [OR] 0.28) and macrolides (OR 0.37) were associated with significantly improved prognosis (13). In addition, the dosage of sulfamethoxazole/trimethoprim correlated significantly with a survival effect, and both agents have well-described anti-inflammatory properties. The use of plasmapheresis and rituximab has also been reported to show promising results (14).

PULMONARY INFECTIONS

The lower respiratory tract is a very common site for serious infection in ILD patients, and pneumonia is associated with an increase in both morbidity and mortality (15,16). Acute pulmonary infections rank second only to acute exacerbations as a cause of respiratory decompensation in IPF patients. In one study, acute infections accounted for almost a third of all episodes of respiratory decompensation in this patient group (4). Host risk factors for infection in ILD patients include abnormal macrophage, neutrophil and lymphocyte function, immune senescence and abnormal mucociliary clearance of pathogens from the lower respiratory tract (17–22). In addition, immunosuppression, particularly that used in the treatment of ILD secondary to auto-immune diseases, predisposes patients to a wide variety of bacterial, viral and fungal infections. In an older study of IPF patients with acute infections, opportunistic organisms accounted for 57.1% of all documented infections. The infections usually developed in IPF patients treated with corticosteroids, regardless of co-administration of additional immunosuppressive agents (4). This practice has fortunately fallen out of favour since the publication of the PANTHER-IPF study in 2012 (23). However, this phenomenon was also noted in a large multicentre study of rheumatoid arthritis patients who demonstrated no increase in hospitalization for pneumonia when treated with disease-modifying anti-rheumatic drugs, but a significantly increased risk of hospitalization for pneumonia when taking oral corticosteroids was observed, and this risk increased in a corticosteroid dose-dependent manner (24).

Patients with fibrotic ILDs are also susceptible to more indolent (but no less severe), chronic pulmonary infections. Risk factors include structural remodelling of the pulmonary parenchyma, bronchiectasis, co-existing chronic obstructive pulmonary disease (COPD), pneumothorax, previous thoracic surgery and long-term immunosuppression therapy (22,25,26). Both corticosteroids and TNF-α-inhibiting agents, used extensively in rheumatoid arthritis and sarcoidosis, confer an increased risk of chronic pulmonary fungal and mycobacterial infections (27,28), and the diagnosis of infection in these patients may be difficult to distinguish from disease progression. Chest imaging can be challenging to interpret as interstitial disease frequently obscures the typical findings associated with these pulmonary infections (22,28).

HYPOXAEMIC RESPIRATORY FAILURE

As ILD progresses, worsened hypoxaemia and respiratory insufficiency are expected complications, usually related to ventilation-perfusion (V/Q) mismatch, shunt pathophysiology and, not infrequently, concomitant PH. In ILD patients, hypoxaemia is much more common than hypercapnoea (29,30). No clinical trials have assessed the impact of long-term oxygen therapy in ILD; however, data are extrapolated from the COPD literature. Societal guidelines (31) support oxygen supplementation for a $PaO_2 \leq 55$ mm Hg or $SpO_2 \leq 88\%$. Additional indications include $PaO_2 \leq 59$ mm Hg or $SpO_2 \leq 89\%$ in the setting of physiologic evidence of hypoxaemia (cor pulmonale, polycythaemia). Objective measurements of oxygenation are imperative during rest, exercise and sleep to ensure an optimal oxygen prescription. In the setting of isolated nocturnal desaturation, screening and appropriate therapy for obstructive sleep apnoea (OSA) is warranted in addition to oxygen supplementation. Despite generic guidelines for in-flight oxygen recommendations (32), air travel is discouraged if oxygen requirements are greater than 4 L/min (33).

As pharmacotherapy may or may not alter the disease process, goals of care discussions are necessary. Non-invasive and invasive ventilation have been retrospectively studied in these settings (34–36); however, data suggest poor outcomes with a mortality rate that may be as high as 100% despite these interventions (35). For insults that are felt to be rapidly reversible clinically (e.g. cardiogenic pulmonary edema), or for palliative purposes, a short course of non-invasive ventilation is reasonable. Unless lung transplantation is an option, mechanical ventilation should be offered judiciously and discouraged in most cases (37).

Although not directly correlated, dyspnoea related to deconditioning, irrespective of oxygenation, is common. A regimented rehabilitation program has been shown to improve exercise capacity, health-related quality of life (38–41) and oxygen consumption without significantly altering oxygenation (42). However, sustained benefits may not be evident after graduation from the program (39). The positive impact of pulmonary rehabilitation has been validated in a Cochrane meta-analysis in patients with ILD, specifically for patients with IPF (43), therefore providing support for its routine implementation.

Once hypoxaemia develops, discussions regarding lung transplantation become necessary. Hopefully, with the implementation of newly available pharmacotherapy including pirfenidone and nintedanib, the rate of lung function decline will decrease, allowing delay of transplant for patients who meet eligibility criteria. However, the availability of anti-fibrotic therapy does not obviate, nor should it delay, the early referral of appropriate candidates for transplant evaluation (37).

PULMONARY HYPERTENSION

Fibrotic interstitial lung disease can be associated with the development of PH, right ventricular dysfunction and eventually right-sided heart failure. Clinical, radiographic and laboratory findings suggesting the presence of underlying PH in ILD patients are summarized in Table 25.1 and illustrated in Figure 25.2.

PH is defined as a mean pulmonary artery (PA) pressure >25 mm Hg at rest as measured on right heart catheterization (RHC) (44). PH is further divided into five distinct groups by the Pulmonary Hypertension World Health Organization (WHO) clinical classification system (Dana Point 2008):

group 1 – pulmonary arterial hypertension, group 2 – PH in left heart disease (pulmonary capillary wedge pressure [PCWP] >15 mm Hg), group 3 – PH due to chronic lung disease or hypoxia, group 4 – PH due to chronic thromboembolic disease, and group 5 – PH of unclear mechanisms (44,45). Both groups 2 and 3 PH can occur in ILD. The presence of PH has a significant association with worse outcomes.

The prevalence of PH in IPF can be highly variable depending upon the population evaluated. In a retrospective analysis of over 6,000 patients with IPF who were listed for lung transplantation, 44.2% had PH. As a group, these patients had severe restrictive lung disease with a mean FVC of 47% predicted. Of those with PH, the mean PA pressure was 33.8 mm Hg (46). Although IPF patients with more mild to moderate disease tend to have less PH, the prevalence in these patients can be surprisingly high. Specifically, among patients enrolled in the ARTEMIS-IPF trial, 14% had WHO group 3 PH, while 5% percent had WHO group 2 PH. The WHO group 3 patients had a mean PA pressure of 33.4 mm Hg, similar to the severe patients listed for lung transplant in the prior study, despite having mild-moderate restriction (mean FVC of approximately 68%) (47). ARTEMIS-IPF was a large, randomized controlled study evaluating the effect of ambrisentan on progression-free survival in patients IPF. There were over 500 patients enrolled, all of whom underwent RHC.

PH can also occur in non-IPF forms of fibrotic ILD. Among a cohort of CVD-ILD patients, 8.1% had a mean PA pressure >25 mm Hg and 21.6% had a mean PA pressure >20 mm Hg (48). When Doppler echocardiography was used to evaluate for PH with a cut-off of an estimated PA systolic pressure >50 mm Hg, the prevalence of PH in a group of chronic HP patients was 19%, while in a group of chronic HP patients who underwent RHC, 44% had WHO group 3 PH (49,50).

As demonstrated by the previously discussed studies, it is not clear that the severity of PH directly correlates to the severity of the ILD. Nathan and colleagues demonstrated that there was a greater prevalence of PH in their IPF patient population in those patients with an FVC >70% of predicted as compared to those patients with an FVC <40% of predicted. However, when controlled for patients with group 2 PH, the prevalence was similar between the two groups. There was no significant correlation

Table 25.1 Factors suggesting pulmonary hypertension in ILD

History	Physical exam	PFTs	6MWT	CT scan	Laboratory markers	Echocardiogram
SOB out of proportion to the extent of ILD	Increased P2 component of the second heart sound	DLCO <30% predicted	Distance <200 m	PA: aorta diameter >1	Elevated BNP or pro-NT BNP levels	Elevated RVSP
Presyncope or syncope	Evidence of right heart failure including hepatomegaly, ascites, pitting lower extremity edema, poor peripheral perfusion	FVC%: DLCO% >1.5	SpO2 <85% on room air	Right-sided chamber enlargement		Dilated RA, RV, or both
			Pulse rate recovery <13 beats/min following 6MWT	Reflux of IV contrast into the IVC		RV dysfunction

Source: Modified from Peacock AJ, Naeije R, Rubin LJ, eds. *Pulmonary Circulation: Diseases and Their Treatment*. 4th ed. Boca Raton, FL: CRC Press/Taylor & Francis Group; 2016, and King CS, Nathan SD. *Lancet Respir Med*. 2017;5(1):72–84.

Notes: BNP = brain natriuretic peptide; DLCO = single breath diffusing capacity of the lung for carbon monoxide; DLCO% = single breath diffusing capacity of the lung for carbon monoxide percent predicted; FVC% = forced vital capacity percent predicted; IVC = inferior vena cava; PA = pulmonary artery; PFTs = pulmonary function tests; pro-NT BNP = pro-n terminal brain natriuretic peptide; RA = right atrium; RV = right ventricle; RVSP = right ventricular systolic pressure; 6MWT = 6-minute walk test; SOB = shortness of breath.

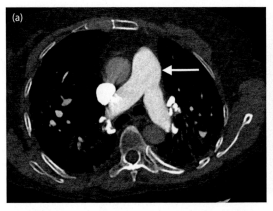
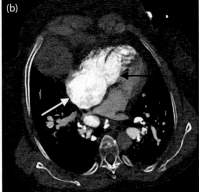

Figure 25.2 Pulmonary hypertension. **(a)** Enlargement of the pulmonary trunk (arrow) and main pulmonary arteries suggests the presence of pulmonary hypertension in a patient with interstitial lung disease. **(b)** Enlargement of the right ventricle (*black arrow*) and right atrium (*white arrow*) provide additional evidence in support of the diagnosis of pulmonary hypertension in a patient with interstitial lung disease. (Images courtesy of Andrew Bierhals, Mallinckrodt Institute of Radiology, Washington University School of Medicine.)

between FVC, DLCO or FVC/DLCO and mean PA pressure (51). However, a DLCO <40% of predicted and supplemental oxygen requirements indicate an increased risk of PH being present (52). Other clues to the presence of PH include an elevated BNP or pro-NT BNP, an enlarged pulmonary artery segment on chest HRCT and suggestive echocardiographic findings (see Table 25.1).

Overall, the prognosis of patients with ILD and PH is worse than ILD patients without PH. Mean PA pressure is associated with an increased risk of mortality among IPF patients (46,52). For patients with CVD-ILD, increasing mean PA pressure is also associated with decreased survival with a mean PA pressure that is only >20 mm Hg portending worse outcomes (48). PH as defined by echocardiography parameters is also associated with worse survival in chronic HP patients, however it should be stressed that RHC is always required for a definitive diagnosis (48).

The pathophysiology of the development of PH in fibrotic ILD is likely a multifactorial process. While hypoxic vasoconstriction and regression of vasculature within fibrotic areas play a role in the development of PH, there are clearly other factors involved including an imbalance between angiogenesis and angiostasis. Factors such as transforming growth factor beta (TGF-β), vascular endothelial growth factor (VEGF), platelet-derived growth factor (PDGF), angiotensin II (AT) and endothelin-1(ET) are all likely involved. Mediators that can lead to fibroblast activation and increased extracellular matrix deposition after epithelial cell injury can also lead to endothelial cell activation, which can further lead to an imbalance in angiogenic and angiostasis factors as well as shifting the balance towards vasoconstriction rather than vasodilation (53).

There are no clear-cut data at this time for the treatment of PH in IPF, and many of the clinical trials using PH therapies in IPF patients have not been specifically directed towards patients with PH. Clinical trials with bosentan (endothelin receptor antagonist) or sildenafil (phosphodiesterase inhibitor) have shown no benefit, although there may be some improvement in exercise tolerance in IPF patients with right ventricular dysfunction with sildenafil (54,55). In the case of ambrisentan, the trial was terminated early due to lack of efficacy (47). Macitentan, another endothelin receptor antagonist, also showed no benefit on mortality or disease progression (56). The RISE-IIP study of riociguat targeted patients with PH due to any of the idiopathic interstitial pneumonias (unpublished data). This study was stopped early for apparent increased mortality and adverse events in the treatment arm. The 2015 updated American Thoracic Society recommendations give a conditional recommendation against the use of all of these medications in IPF (57). Whether or not there is a specific phenotype of patients with PH due to ILD who might benefit from therapy remains to be determined. There does appear to be a very small subgroup of patients with hemodynamic profiles similar to those patients with WHO group 1 PAH. However, if there is any consideration to treating these patients, it should be done under the guidance of an expert centre with adequate experience in treating patients with ILD with or without PH.

CORONARY ARTERY DISEASE

ILD, and specifically IPF, is associated with multiple cardiovascular co-morbidities, including CAD, congestive heart failure (CHF), arrhythmias, systemic hypertension and cerebrovascular accidents (58,59). Coronary ischaemia and CHF should be considered in the differential diagnoses for any IPF patient with worsening dyspnoea or declining functional status.

The prevalence of CAD in IPF patients varies widely depending on the study and ranges from 3.2% to 68% (Figure 25.3) (60). In a cohort of 73 patients with IPF who underwent left heart catheterization for lung transplant assessment, 28.8% had severe CAD (61). In fact, pulmonary fibrosis

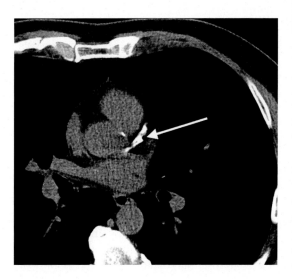

Figure 25.3 Coronary artery disease. Coronary artery calcification (*arrow*) is a marker of diseased coronary arteries in a patient with IPF. (Image courtesy of Andrew Bierhals, Mallinckrodt Institute of Radiology, Washington University School of Medicine.)

appears to be an independent risk factor for the development of CAD with an associated OR of 2.64 (62). One study comparing the prevalence of CAD in lung transplant candidates with IPF and those with COPD found that patients with IPF were more likely to have CAD than those with COPD despite a lower prevalence of heavy smoking in the IPF group (31% versus 98%) (63).

Despite an increased prevalence of CAD in IPF patients, mild to moderate CAD does not result in significant perioperative complications or adversely affect either short- or long-term survival in IPF patients undergoing lung transplantation (64). However, IPF patients with severe CAD demonstrate an increased risk of death compared to IPF patients with no or non-severe CAD with an unadjusted hazard ratio of 3.3 (61). Aggressive treatment of CAD in this population seems appropriate, particularly considering the concomitant pulmonary function impairment.

HRCT scans provide a tool that can screen for CAD in IPF patients. The presence of moderate-to-severe coronary artery calcifications on HRCT had a sensitivity of 81% and specificity of 85% for the diagnosis of CAD with an associated OR of 25.2 (65).

GASTRO-OESOPHAGEAL REFLUX DISEASE

GERD is a frequently encountered co-morbidity in patients with chronic pulmonary diseases. Prevalence estimates have ranged from 57% in COPD (66) to over 50% in cystic fibrosis (67) and up to 90% in IPF (68,69). GERD is a hallmark of systemic sclerosis and is seen in up to 90% of patients (Figure 25.4) (70). Reflux in IPF may be silent in nearly a third of patients and may only be identified using invasive diagnostic testing such as manometry and esophageal pH probe monitoring (71,72). Chronic aspiration alone can result in a range of pulmonary disease evidenced by an associated decrease in DLCO (73) and the presence of GERD-associated pulmonary fibrosis (74). Although a recent meta-analysis found no significant causal relationship between reflux and IPF (75), some experts consider GERD and chronic micro-aspiration to play a role in disease genesis, progression and mortality (76–79). Additionally, reflux may trigger acute exacerbations, as elevated levels of pepsin

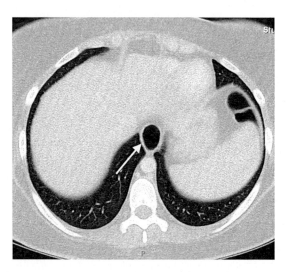

Figure 25.4 GERD. The presence of a patulous esophagus (*arrow*) in a patient with scleroderma may be a marker for oesophageal dysfunction and GERD. (Image courtesy of Andrew Bierhals, Mallinckrodt Institute of Radiology, Washington University School of Medicine.)

have been identified in bronchoalveolar lavage fluid sampled at the time of acute exacerbations (80).

Several studies have assessed the impact of GERD therapy on progression of IPF, although none have been specifically designed for this purpose. A two-centre retrospective analysis of 204 patients identified a positive relationship between GERD treatment, including pharmacotherapy ($p < 0.01$) and fundoplication ($p = 0.04$), and improved survival (81).

In a much larger cohort, patients from placebo arms in three randomized trials (82–84) were analyzed with regards to GERD treatment, and it was found that treatment with a histamine-2 blocker or a proton pump inhibitor led to a slower decline in FVC over 30 weeks (-0.06 liters versus -0.12 liters, p-value $= 0.05$), decreased frequency of acute exacerbations (no events versus nine events, p-value < 0.01), but no difference in mortality (p-value $= 0.40$) (85). A similar study design using placebo group data from the pirfenidone studies CAPACITY 004, 006 and ASCEND demonstrated opposite results (86,87). This cohort analysis showed no difference in disease progression, and actually showed an increase in both overall ($p = 0.0174$) and pulmonary infections ($p = 0.0214$) in patients with advanced IPF on GERD therapy (88). Because these initial trials

were not designed to assess the impact of GERD therapy, cautious interpretation of these observations is warranted.

Pharmacotherapy alone may be insufficient to control symptoms, and silent reflux with aspiration may still occur in over half of treated patients (89). Therefore, behavioural modifications may be equally as critical. Pharmacotherapy may limit gastric acidity and reflux of acidic contents, but acid-suppressing drugs may increase non-acid reflux events (90) and the risk of pneumonia (91). Usual supportive care for reflux including weight loss, limiting oral intake 3 hours prior to bedtime, head of the bed elevation and avoidance of reflux-precipitating foods are imperative (92). Some argue for early surgical intervention (93), although no official guidelines exist. Regardless, fundoplication may be a reasonable option in patients with refractory disease and continued decline in lung function despite appropriate therapies.

The 2011 American Thoracic Society (ATS) guidelines (37) provided a weak recommendation for asymptomatic GERD to be medically treated in most patients with IPF. After evaluating several publications in the interim, the 2015 ATS guidelines (57) suggest a conditional recommendation for regular anti-acid treatments in patients with IPF, regardless of symptoms, given the high rate of asymptomatic disease. However, this recommendation was given prior to the publication of the pooled pirfenidone studies.

Although a distinct pathophysiologic entity, esophageal disease is nearly universal in systemic sclerosis and common in anti-synthetase syndrome, where it has been associated with higher mortality (70,94–97). In addition to usual care as above, pro-kinetic agents may be beneficial in systemic sclerosis (and possibly anti-synthetase syndrome), as oesophageal hypomotility may play a role in GERD pathogenesis.

In summary, GERD is highly prevalent in ILD and especially in IPF and some forms of CVD-ILD. Given the high mortality in fibrotic lung disease, any therapy that might delay progression of fibrosis may have a profound impact on disease progression, and dedicated prospective studies to assess the impact of GERD therapy are needed. Aggressive screening including esophageal manometry and 24-hour pH probe is necessary to accurately diagnose patients given the low sensitivity of patient-reported symptoms (93,94).

Similarly, GERD should be aggressively managed if lung transplantation is anticipated, as GERD increases the risk of chronic lung allograft dysfunction (98).

PNEUMOTHORAX

Pneumothoraces are frequently described in cystic lung diseases such as lymphangiomyelomatosis, pulmonary Langerhans cell histiocytosis (PLCH) and Birt–Hogg–Dubé syndrome. They occur less commonly in fibrotic lung disease such as IPF, chronic HP and non-specific interstitial pneumonitis (NSIP). However, given the underlying lung disease and smaller reserve of lung function in all ILD patients, a pneumothorax can be devastating and cause significant worsening of dyspnoea and respiratory failure. Clinical suspicion for a pneumothorax must remain high for any patient presenting with chest discomfort, worsened dyspnoea or a decline in lung function.

Although the incidence of pneumothorax in IPF has been estimated at 7% in cross-sectional studies (99,100), a retrospective analysis of 56 patients in Japan showed an incidence closer to 30%. Patients with pneumothorax in this study also had poorer outcomes with death occurring a mean of 9 months following an initial pneumothorax (101). Interestingly, the incidence of pneumothorax in pleuroparenchymal fibroelastosis (PPFE) with UIP histology was as high as 66% in one study and was felt to contribute to mortality in roughly half of patients (102). Though frequently discouraged for oxygenation issues, air travel had no obvious impact on the incidence of pneumothorax in a mixed population of IPF and sarcoidosis patients (103).

Management of pneumothoraces on a background of ILD mirrors that of other conditions (104–106). Given the underlying fibrosis and architectural distortion of lung tissue, the risk of bronchopleural fistulae is increased. Prolonged tube thoracostomy may ensue when the non-compliant lung fails to expand with the fistula less inclined to heal due to the lack of chest wall apposition. If the aetiology for the ILD is unknown and the patient proceeds to video-assisted thoracoscopic surgery (VATS), a simultaneous SLB may provide invaluable histopathologic information.

MALIGNANCY

The first reported link between pulmonary fibrosis and lung cancer was published in 1939 (107). Since then, patients with several subtypes of fibrotic lung disease have been described as being at increased risk for lung cancer compared to the general population.

Large studies have clearly demonstrated that patients with IPF are at increased risk of developing lung cancer. The reported incidence of lung cancer in IPF patients varies widely (4.4%–48%) (108–110). However, when compared to the general population, the incidence of lung cancer in patients with IPF is 1.51 times higher (95% CI 1.20–1.90) (108). In the same study, no increased risk for other cancer types was demonstrable. IPF patients who develop lung cancer are more frequently male (M:F ratio 7:1), smokers (91.3% versus 71.6%) and more likely to have combined pulmonary fibrosis and emphysema (52% versus 32%) (110,111). These data most likely reflect the overlapping risk factors for developing lung cancer with the presence of both emphysema and IPF in subjects who smoke (112,113). Interestingly, the prevalence of familial IPF appears similar in IPF patients with and without lung cancer, although the numbers studied have been small (114).

Most lung cancers in IPF are described as well-defined nodular lesions. More than 80% of tumours are located within the lung periphery and more than 50% within the lower lobes (115–117). However, biopsy-confirmed tumours resembling pleural thickening, ground-glass opacities and airspace consolidation have been described (118). Squamous cell carcinomas are the most common histologic subtype, with adenocarcinomas being the next most common (108–110,114).

The development of lung cancer in IPF patients has a profoundly negative impact on survival. Lung cancer significantly increases the risk of death (HR = 7; 95% CI 3.81–12.90) compared to patients with IPF alone (114). This mortality is attributable not only to cancer progression (13%) but also to complications arising during the diagnosis and treatment of the cancer (18%) (119). Surgical resection of lung cancers in IPF patients is associated with higher post-operative mortality, higher risk of acute lung injury and longer hospital stays than non-IPF controls (119). Surgery results in significantly higher post-operative morbidity (33.3% versus 2%) and mortality (18.2% versus 1.3%) in IPF patients compared to non-IPF controls (120). The increased mortality persists regardless of the extent of surgery, with both pneumonectomy (33% versus 5.1%) and lobectomy (12% versus 2.6%) resulting in higher mortality in IPF patients (121). Systemic chemotherapy appears to also carry significant treatment risks, primarily that of IPF exacerbation. In one study, the incidence of acute respiratory deterioration following chemotherapy was 28% compared to 16% after surgical resection (122). In general, chemotherapy appears to trigger IPF exacerbations in 13%–30% of IPF patients, with a resultant mortality ranging from 9% to 16% (122–125). As a result of diagnosis and treatment-related morbidity and mortality, there is currently no consensus on the treatment of IPF-related lung cancer. Treatment strategies should be individualized based on patient goals of care, baseline physiology and expertise of the treating centre.

The association between inflammatory myopathies and cancer is well recognized (126). Epidemiologic evidence from large population studies clearly supports the association between inflammatory myopathy and malignancy (127–129). This association appears to be stronger for patients with dermatomyositis (DM) than polymyositis (PM). The incidence of cancer for patients with DM appears to be increased between three- and sixfold compared with the general population (127,129,130), but the relationship between cancer and inflammatory myopathies is less clear-cut than in IPF (131). Cancer may be diagnosed prior to, simultaneously with, or following the diagnosis of an inflammatory myopathy (129), and in several patients, the temporal relationship between myopathy and cancer suggests the existence of a paraneoplastic disorder.

Adenocarcinomas of the lung, ovaries, cervix, stomach, pancreas, colon, rectum and bladder, along with non-Hodgkin lymphoma account for the majority of inflammatory myopathy-associated malignancies in dermatomyositis. Patients with polymyositis are at increased risk for lung and bladder adenocarcinomas as well as non-Hodgkin lymphoma (132–134).

Patients with newly diagnosed inflammatory myopathy should be evaluated for underlying malignancy. Interestingly, autoantibody types tend to predict the risk of malignancy. TIF-1γ (anti-p155/140) and NXP-2 (anti-p140) have both been associated with increased cancer risk (135), while anti-synthetase antibodies (e.g. anti Jo-1) appear to predict a lower risk of cancer (but an increased risk of ILD). Studies indicate that the risk of cancer is highest at the time of diagnosis and during the first year thereafter, but risk then appears to decline annually over 5 years (129,133).

OBSTRUCTIVE SLEEP APNOEA

Sleep architecture in patients with ILD is abnormal. They experience decreased sleep efficiency, increased stage 1 and 2 sleep, and decreased slow wave sleep (SWS) and rapid eye movement (REM) sleep. Sleep disruption may come from symptoms related to the ILD such as nocturnal coughing. There is a markedly increased risk of OSA in IPF with a reported prevalence as high as 85%–88% (136,137). However, it appears that sleep apnoea in IPF patients is significantly under recognized by both primary care physicians and pulmonary specialists (137). Untreated OSA can lead to poor sleep quality, which can decrease quality of life in patients with IPF (138). IPF and scleroderma are also more likely to be associated with other conditions that can affect sleep quality or disrupt sleep such as restless leg syndrome or periodic limb movements.

OSA among middle-aged adults, as defined by an apnoea-hypopnoea index (AHI) of greater than 5, is present in about 24% of men and 9% of women (139). Although the prevalence of OSA in ILD is consistently higher than within the general population, the prevalence varies between studies. In a study of 50 patients with either IPF, scleroderma ILD, or sarcoidosis the prevalence of OSA was noted to be 82%, 56% and 67%, respectively. In all three groups, the severity of OSA based on the AHI was mild overall, but severity became moderate during REM sleep (140).

A study of 27 newly diagnosed IPF patients undergoing polysomnography demonstrated that 22% had moderate OSA with an AHI greater than 20 (141). A second study using a larger group of newly diagnosed IPF patients demonstrated a higher prevalence of OSA with 65% of patients having at least moderate OSA as defined by an AHI >15. An additional 20% of the patients had mild

OSA, with the remaining 15% having a normal AHI (142). In a group of lung transplant recipients, the prevalence of OSA was 52% for those with a pre-transplant diagnosis of IPF (143).

The presence of OSA does not clearly correlate with the severity of impairment of lung function in IPF patients (138,140,141). The study by Mermgikis et al., in which 65% of newly diagnosed IPF patients were found to have OSA, demonstrated a survival benefit at 24 months in the group noted to have good compliance with continuous positive airway pressure (CPAP). All patients who were CPAP compliant were alive at 24 months; whereas 17% of the patients who were intolerant of CPAP had died by 24 months. There was no difference in baseline lung function between those who were and those who were not compliant with CPAP therapy (142).

Serious consideration should be given to performing polysomnography in patients with fibrotic lung disease given the increased prevalence of OSA in this population (137). Polysomnography allows for the diagnosis of OSA as well as other forms of sleep-disordered breathing including periodic limb movements, which may disrupt sleep. Treatment of OSA may positively impact quality of life by lessening sleep disruption. In addition, a number of studies suggest a potential survival benefit with OSA treatment for patients with IPF.

THERAPEUTIC DRUG PULMONARY TOXICITY

Many of the medications utilized for the treatment of ILD have been associated with pulmonary toxicity. It is often difficult to prove causality between worsening ILD and adverse effects of specific therapeutic agents because ILD patients are prone to disease exacerbations, lung infections and treatment failure. In addition, patients may be on more than one therapeutic agent, and significant drug-drug interactions may occur.

Pulmonary toxicity remains an important consideration in the differential diagnosis of patients treated for ILD who present with progressive respiratory symptoms or worsening infiltrates. Prognosis varies depending on the type and severity of pulmonary toxicity; however, in the face of already compromised lung function, drug-induced pulmonary disease may result in significant patient morbidity and mortality.

The spectrum and management of drug-related toxicity is very broad and beyond the scope of this current chapter. The more common pulmonary toxicities are presented in Table 25.2. The references in Table 25.2 provide an excellent resource

Table 25.2 Pulmonary toxicities of drugs used to treat ILD

	GLD	DAD	Pneumonitis	Fibrosis	Infection risk	OP	OB	EP	DAH
Cyclophosphamide		X	x	x	x	x			x
Methotrexate	X (HP)	x		?	Small	x			
Leflunomide			x	?	x				
TNF-α inhibitors	x				Mycobacteria	x			
Mycophenolate			x	?	x				
Azathioprine		x	x	x	x	x		x	
Rituximab			x		x	x			x
Gold			x			x	x		
Sulfasalazine	x			x	x	x	x	x	
Penicillamine				x	x		?		x

Source: Data from Camus P, Rosenow III E. In: Camus P, Rosenow III E, eds. *Drug-induced and Iatrogenic Respiratory Disease*. Boca Raton, FL: CRC Press; 2010:3–11; Rossi SE et al. *Radiographics* 2000;20(5):1245–59; Camus PH et al. *Eur Respir J Suppl*. 2001;32:93s–100s; Camus P et al. *Clin Chest Med*. 2004;25(3):479–519; Pneumotox. www.pneumotox.com. Accessed 5 July 2016.

Notes: ? = reported but relation between drug and effect uncertain; DAD = diffuse alveolar damage; EP = eosinophilic pneumonia; GLD = granulomatous lung disease; HP = hypersensitivity pneumonitis; OB = obliterative bronchiolitis; OP = organizing pneumonia.

for further investigation with respect to toxicities, treatment and response.

PALLIATIVE CARE

Palliative care is specialized medical care centred on the prevention and relief of symptoms in advanced illness. For patients with ILD who are not lung transplant candidates, their illness often evolves to end-stage disease without effective options for curative treatment. Palliative care is an important part of the treatment process for these patients.

In 2008, the American Thoracic Society released a statement regarding palliative care in chronic lung disease. The statement advocates for the 'individualized integrated model' of palliative care in which patients receive palliative care at all stages of ILD, starting from the moment of diagnosis and including the period during which therapeutic treatments are implemented. The intensity of palliative care is titrated to the needs of both the patient and the patient's family over the course of the illness (144).

Compared to metastatic cancers, palliative care in the setting of chronic lung diseases is significantly under-utilized. A Swedish study comparing end-of-life care for oxygen-dependent ILD patients with lung cancer patients found that deaths among ILD patients were more likely to be considered unexpected and to occur in a non-palliative care setting. In addition, ILD patients were less likely to experience relief or partial relief of their breathlessness as compared to the lung cancer patients (145). A retrospective review of 277 deceased IPF patients with an initial visit to the University of Pittsburgh Dorothy P. and Richard P. Simmons Center for Interstitial Lung Disease between 2000 and 2012 revealed that more than half the patients died in hospital. Only around 15% of patients received a formal palliative care consult, and the consults occurred within 1 month of death in almost two-thirds of the patients (146). A third study from the University of Washington compared palliative care in the intensive care unit (ICU) setting between patients with chronic lung disease (COPD or ILD) and patients with metastatic cancer. In contrast to the cancer patients, patients with chronic lung disease were less likely to have a pain assessment, a do not resuscitate order or a discussion of prognosis (147).

A comprehensive palliative care program should provide attention to the physical, psychological and spiritual needs of the patient as well as the psychological and spiritual needs of the family. Over half of patients with ILD report uncontrolled symptoms such as dyspnoea and cough. The same patients also report a sense of social isolation due to increasing difficulty leaving the home and a loss of a sense of purposefulness as spouses and caregivers assume more of the patient's daily care (148). The pulmonary physician can help guide a thoughtful discussion of prognosis and goals of care (144). It is important to remember that the patient and their family members may not process or accept information at the same rate (149).

Outcomes for IPF patients requiring mechanical ventilation for acute respiratory failure are extremely poor, and less data are available for other fibrotic lung diseases. Most intubated patients with IPF died while receiving mechanical ventilation in the ICU with only a small minority of patients being extubated and leaving the ICU. Of those that left the ICU and were eventually discharged from hospital, a substantial percentage died shortly thereafter (150–152). It is imperative, therefore, that patients are made aware of this fact and that they plan for end-of-life care and clearly indicate their preferences regarding intubation, mechanical ventilation and cardiopulmonary resuscitation. This allows the patient to discuss goals of care with their loved ones, surrogates and physicians, and patients can clearly delineate their plans for the period surrounding their death.

Palliative medical therapies for symptoms of end-stage fibrotic lung disease include opioids and anxiolytics for dyspnoea, anti-depressants for depression and stool softeners for constipation (144). In a study of ILD patients who died from exacerbations of their disease, IV morphine in opioid naïve patients was effective in alleviating dyspnoea in 77% of the patients without significantly depressing the respiratory rate (153). If withdrawal from a ventilator is to be performed, pre-treatment with opioids and benzodiazepines should be given to prevent air hunger. In addition, IV fluids should be stopped and consideration given to the use of anti-cholinergics to help prevent the build-up of airway secretions leading to gurgling noises, which can be distressing to the patient's family (144).

TIPS FOR THE PRACTITIONER

1. There are a wide variety of fibrotic lung diseases.
2. These diseases vary widely in their onset, natural history and prognosis.
3. Treatments of variable efficacy are available for fibrotic lung diseases, but in general, these are chronic diseases characterized by progressive lung function decline despite therapy.
4. Functional capacity and quality of life have both been shown to be significantly impaired in patients with lung fibrosis.
5. While patients may die because of their lung fibrosis, several patients will die with it.
6. This is particularly the case with older patients, such as those with IPF, who may have considerable co-morbidities.
7. Co-morbidities may include respiratory failure, pulmonary hypertension, coronary artery disease, GERD, pneumothorax, lung cancer, pulmonary infections and obstructive sleep apnoea.
8. Screening for, diagnosing and managing these co-morbidities may not only have an impact on patient well-being but also survival.
9. Because of the progressive nature of fibrotic lung diseases, palliative care is an important part of holistic management of fibrotic lung disease.

REFERENCES

1. Kreuter M, Ehlers-Tenenbaum S, Palmowski K, Bruhwyler J, Oltmanns U, Muley T et al. Impact of comorbidities on mortality in patients with idiopathic pulmonary fibrosis. *PLoS One.* 2016;11(3):e0151425.
2. Navaratnam V, Fogarty AW, McKeever T, Thompson N, Jenkins G, Johnson SR et al. Presence of a prothrombotic state in people with idiopathic pulmonary fibrosis: A population-based case-control study. *Thorax.* 2014;69(3):207–15.
3. Tsoutsou PG, Gourgoulianis KI, Petinaki E, Germenis A, Tsoutsou AG, Mpaka M et al. Cytokine levels in the sera of patients with idiopathic pulmonary fibrosis. *Respir Med.* 2006;100(5):938–45.
4. Song JW, Hong SB, Lim CM, Koh Y, Kim DS. Acute exacerbation of idiopathic pulmonary fibrosis: Incidence, risk factors and outcome. *Eur Respir J.* 2011;37(2):356–63.
5. Collard HR, Moore BB, Flaherty KR, Brown KK, Kaner RJ, King TE Jr et al. Idiopathic Pulmonary Fibrosis Clinical Research Network Investigators. Acute exacerbations of idiopathic pulmonary fibrosis. *Am J Respir Crit Care Med.* 2007;176(7):636–43.
6. Collard HR, Ryerson CJ, Corte TJ, Jenkins G, Kondoh Y, Lederer DJ et al. Acute exacerbation of idiopathic pulmonary fibrosis. An International Working Group Report. *Am J Respir Crit Care Med.* 2016;194(3):265–75.
7. Huie TJ, Olson AL, Cosgrove GP, Janssen WJ, Lara AR, Lynch DA et al. A detailed evaluation of acute respiratory decline in patients with fibrotic lung disease: Aetiology and outcomes. *Respirology.* 2010;15(6):909–17.
8. Sakamoto S, Homma S, Mun M, Fujii T, Kurosaki A, Yoshimura K. Acute exacerbation of idiopathic interstitial pneumonia following lung surgery in 3 of 68 consecutive patients: A retrospective study. *Intern Med.* 2011;50:77–85.
9. Ryerson CJ, Cottin V, Brown KK, Collard HR. Acute exacerbation of idiopathic pulmonary fibrosis: Shifting the paradigm. *Eur Respir J.* 2015;46:512–20.
10. Tachikawa R, Tomii K, Ueda H, Nagata K, Nanjo S, Sakurai A et al. Clinical features and outcome of acute exacerbation of interstitial pneumonia: Collagen vascular diseases-related versus idiopathic. *Respiration.* 2012;83(1):20–7.
11. Kreider ME, Hansen-Flaschen J, Ahmad NN, Rossman MD, Kaiser LR, Kucharczuk JC et al. Complications of video-assisted thoracoscopic lung biopsy in patients with interstitial lung disease. *Ann Thorac Surg.* 2007;83(3):1140–4.
12. Bando M, Ohno S, Hosono T, Yanase K, Sato Y, Sohara Y et al. Risk of acute exacerbation after video-assisted thoracoscopic lung biopsy for interstitial lung disease. *J Bronchology Interv Pulmonol.* 2009;16(4):229–35.
13. Oda K, Yatera K, Fujino Y, Ishimoto H, Nakao H, Hanaka T et al. Efficacy of concurrent treatments in idiopathic pulmonary

fibrosis patients with a rapid progression of respiratory failure: An analysis of a national administrative database in Japan. *BMC Pulm Med.* 2016;16(1):91.

14. Donahoe M, Valentine VG, Chien N, Gibson KF, Raval JS, Saul M, et al. Autoantibody-targeted treatments for acute exacerbations of idiopathic pulmonary fibrosis. *PLoS One.* 2015;10(6):e0127771.

15. Kelly C, Hamilton J. What kills patients with rheumatoid arthritis? *Rheumatology (Oxford).* 2007;46(2):183–4.

16. Coyne P, Hamilton J, Heycock C, Saravanan V, Coulson E, Kelly CA. Acute lower respiratory tract infections in patients with rheumatoid arthritis. *J Rheumatol.* 2007;34(9):1832–6.

17. Kaplan MJ. Role of neutrophils in systemic autoimmune diseases. *Arthritis Res Ther.* 2013;15(5):219.

18. Mathieu A, Cauli A, Pala R, Satta L, Nurchis P, Loi GL et al. Tracheo-bronchial mucociliary clearance in patients with primary and secondary Sjögren's syndrome. *Scand J Rheumatol.* 1995;24(5):300–4.

19. Evans CM, Fingerlin TE, Schwarz MI, Lynch D, Kurche J, Warg L et al. Idiopathic pulmonary fibrosis: A genetic disease that involves mucociliary dysfunction of the peripheral airways. *Physiol Rev.* 2016;96(4):1567–91.

20. Ren P, Rosas IO, Macdonald SD, Wu HP, Billings EM, Gochuico BR. Impairment of alveolar macrophage transcription in idiopathic pulmonary fibrosis. *Am J Respir Crit Care Med.* 2007;175(11):1151–7.

21. Fingerlin TE, Murphy E, Zhang W, Peljto AL, Brown KK, Steele MP et al. Genome-wide association study identifies multiple susceptibility loci for pulmonary fibrosis. *Nat Genet.* 2013;45(6):613–20.

22. Margaritopoulos GA, Antoniou KM, Wells AU. Comorbidities in interstitial lung diseases. *Eur Respir Rev.* 2017;26(143):pii:160027.

23. Idiopathic Pulmonary Fibrosis Clinical Research Network, Raghu G, Anstrom KJ, King TE Jr, Lasky JA, Martinez FJ. Prednisone, azathioprine, and N-acetylcysteine for pulmonary fibrosis. *N Engl J Med.* 2012;366(21): 1968–77.

24. Wolfe F, Caplan L, Michaud K. Treatment for rheumatoid arthritis and the risk of hospitalization for pneumonia: Associations with prednisone, disease-modifying antirheumatic drugs, and anti-tumor necrosis factor therapy. *Arthritis Rheum.* 2006;54(2):628–34.

25. Denning DW, Riniotis K, Dobrashian R, Sambatakou H. Chronic cavitary and fibrosing pulmonary and pleural aspergillosis: Case series, proposed nomenclature change, and review. *Clin Infect Dis.* 2003;37(Suppl 3):S265–80.

26. Camuset J, Nunes H, Dombret MC, Bergeron A, Henno P, Philippe B et al. Treatment of chronic pulmonary aspergillosis by voriconazole in nonimmunocompromised patients. *Chest.* 2007;131(5):1435–41.

27. Smith NL, Denning DW. Underlying conditions in chronic pulmonary aspergillosis including simple aspergilloma. *Eur Respir J.* 2011;37(4):865–72.

28. Park SW, Song JW, Shim TS, Park MS, Lee HL, Uh ST et al. Mycobacterial pulmonary infections in patients with idiopathic pulmonary fibrosis. *J Korean Med Sci.* 2012;27(8):896–900.

29. Javaheri S, Sicilian L. Lung function, breathing pattern, and gas exchange in interstitial lung disease. *Thorax.* 1992;47(2):93–7.

30. Young IH, Bye PT. Gas exchange in disease: Asthma, chronic obstructive pulmonary disease, cystic fibrosis, and interstitial lung disease. *Compr Physiol.* 2011;1(2):663–97.

31. Qaseem A, Wilt TJ, Weinberger SE, Hanania NA, Criner G, van der Molen T et al. American College of Physicians, American College of Chest Physicians, American Thoracic Society, European Respiratory Society. Diagnosis and management of stable chronic obstructive pulmonary disease: A clinical practice guideline update from the American College of Physicians, American College of Chest Physicians, American Thoracic Society, and European Respiratory Society. *Ann Intern Med.* 2011;155(3):179–91.

32. Ahmedzai S, Balfour-Lynn IM, Bewick T, Buchdahl R, Coker RK, Cummin AR et al. British Thoracic Society Standards of Care

Committee. Managing passengers with stable respiratory disease planning air travel: British Thoracic Society recommendations. *Thorax.* 2011;66 (Suppl 1):i1–i30.

33. Nicholson TT, Sznajder JI. Fitness to fly in patients with lung disease. *Ann Am Thorac Soc.* 2014;11(10):1614–22.

34. Aliberti S, Messinesi G, Gamberini S, Maggiolini S, Visca D, Galavotti V et al. Non-invasive mechanical ventilation in patients with diffuse interstitial lung diseases. *BMC Pulm Med.* 2014;14:194.

35. Vianello A, Arcaro G, Battistella L, Pipitone E, Vio S, Concas A et al. Noninvasive ventilation in the event of acute respiratory failure in patients with idiopathic pulmonary fibrosis. *J Crit Care.* 2014;29(4):562–7.

36. Mollica C, Paone G, Conti V, Ceccarelli D, Schmid G, Mattia P et al. Mechanical ventilation in patients with end-stage idiopathic pulmonary fibrosis. *Respiration.* 2010;79(3):209–15.

37. Raghu G, Collard HR, Egan JJ, Martinez FJ, Behr J, Brown KK et al. ATS/ERS/JRS/ALAT Committee on Idiopathic Pulmonary Fibrosis. An official ATS/ERS/JRS/ALAT statement: Idiopathic pulmonary fibrosis: Evidence-based guidelines for diagnosis and management. *Am J Respir Crit Care Med.* 2011;183(6):788–824.

38. Nishiyama O, Kondoh Y, Kimura T, Kato K, Kataoka K, Ogawa T et al. Effects of pulmonary rehabilitation in patients with idiopathic pulmonary fibrosis. *Respirology.* 2008;13(3):394–9.

39. Holland AE, Hill CJ, Conron M, Munro P, McDonald CF. Short term improvement in exercise capacity and symptoms following exercise training in interstitial lung disease. *Thorax.* 2008;63(6):549–54.

40. Ferreira A, Garvey C, Connors GL, Hilling L, Rigler J, Farrell S et al. Pulmonary rehabilitation in interstitial lung disease: Benefits and predictors of response. *Chest.* 2009;135(2):442–7.

41. Huppmann P, Sczepanski B, Boensch M, Winterkamp S, Schönheit-Kenn U, Neurohr C et al. Effects of inpatient pulmonary rehabilitation in patients with interstitial lung disease. *Eur Respir J.* 2013;42(2):444–53.

42. Jackson RM, Gómez-Marín OW, Ramos CF, Sol CM, Cohen MI, Gaunaurd IA et al. Exercise limitation in IPF patients: A randomized trial of pulmonary rehabilitation. *Lung.* 2014;192(3):367–76.

43. Dowman L, Hill CJ, Holland AE. Pulmonary rehabilitation for interstitial lung disease. *Cochrane Database Syst Rev.* 2014;10:CD006322.

44. Hoeper MM, Bogaard HJ, Condliffe R, Frantz R, Khanna D, Kurzyna M et al. Definitions and diagnosis of pulmonary hypertension. *J Am Coll Cardiol.* 2013;62(25 Suppl):D42–50.

45. Simonneau G, Gatzoulis MA, Adatia I, Celermajer D, Denton C, Ghofrani A et al. Updated clinical classification of pulmonary hypertension. *J Am Coll Cardiol.* 2013;62(25 Suppl):D34–41.

46. Hayes D Jr, Black SM, Tobias JD, Kirkby S, Mansour HM, Whitson BA. Influence of pulmonary hypertension on patients with idiopathic pulmonary fibrosis awaiting lung transplantation. *Ann Thorac Surg.* 2016;101(1):246–52.

47. Raghu G, Nathan SD, Behr J, Brown KK, Egan JJ, Kawut SM et al. Pulmonary hypertension in idiopathic pulmonary fibrosis with mild-to-moderate restriction. *Eur Respir J.* 2015;46(5):1370–7.

48. Takahashi K, Taniguchi H, Ando M, Sakamoto K, Kondoh Y, Watanabe N et al. Mean pulmonary arterial pressure as a prognostic indicator in connective tissue disease associated with interstitial lung disease: A retrospective cohort study. *BMC Pulm Med.* 2016;16(1):55.

49. Koschel DS, Cardoso C, Wiedemann B, Höffken G, Halank M. Pulmonary hypertension in chronic hypersensitivity pneumonitis. *Lung.* 2012;190(3):295–302.

50. Oliveira RK, Pereira CA, Ramos RP, Ferreira EV, Messina CM, Kuranishi LT et al. A haemodynamic study of pulmonary hypertension in chronic hypersensitivity pneumonitis. *Eur Respir J.* 2014;44(2):415–24.

51. Nathan SD, Shlobin OA, Ahmad S, Urbanek S, Barnett SD. Pulmonary hypertension and pulmonary function testing in idiopathic pulmonary fibrosis. *Chest.* 2007;131(3):657–63.

52. Lettieri CJ, Nathan SD, Barnett SD, Ahmad S, Shorr AF. Prevalence and outcomes of pulmonary arterial hypertension in advanced idiopathic pulmonary fibrosis. *Chest*. 2006;129(3):746–52.

53. Farkas L, Gauldie J, Voelkel NF, Kolb M. Pulmonary hypertension and idiopathic pulmonary fibrosis: A tale of angiogenesis, apoptosis, and growth factors. *Am J Respir Cell Mol Biol*. 2011;45(1):1–15.

54. Corte TJ, Keir GJ, Dimopoulos K, Howard L, Corris PA, Parfitt L et al. BPHIT Study Group. Bosentan in pulmonary hypertension associated with fibrotic idiopathic interstitial pneumonia. *Am J Respir Crit Care Med*. 2014;190(2):208–17.

55. Idiopathic Pulmonary Fibrosis Clinical Research Network; Zisman DA, Schwarz M, Anstrom KJ, Collard HR, Flaherty KR, Hunninghake GW. A controlled trial of sildenafil in advanced idiopathic pulmonary fibrosis. *N Engl J Med*. 2010;363(7):620–8.

56. Raghu G, Million-Rousseau R, Morganti A, Perchenet L, Behr J; MUSIC Study Group. Macitentan for the treatment of idiopathic pulmonary fibrosis: The randomised controlled MUSIC trial. *Eur Respir J*. 2013;42(6):1622–32.

57. Raghu G, Rochwerg B, Zhang Y, Garcia CA, Azuma A, Behr J et al. American Thoracic Society, European Respiratory Society, Japanese Respiratory Society, Latin American Thoracic Association. An Official ATS/ERS/JRS/ALAT Clinical Practice Guideline: Treatment of Idiopathic Pulmonary Fibrosis. An Update of the 2011 Clinical Practice Guideline. *Am J Respir Crit Care Med*. 2015;192(2):e3–19.

58. Ponnuswamy A, Manikandan R, Sabetpour A, Keeping IM, Finnerty JP. Association between ischaemic heart disease and interstitial lung disease: A case-control study. *Respir Med*. 2009;103(4):503–7.

59. Kizer JR, Zisman DA, Blumenthal NP, Kotloff RM, Kimmel SE, Strieter RM et al. Association between pulmonary fibrosis and coronary artery disease. *Arch Intern Med*. 2004;164(5):551–6.

60. Raghu G, Amatto VC, Behr J, Stowasser S. Comorbidities in idiopathic pulmonary fibrosis patients: A systematic literature review. *Eur Respir J*. 2015;46(4):1113–30.

61. Nathan SD, Basavaraj A, Reichner C, Shlobin OA, Ahmad S, Kiernan J et al. Prevalence and impact of coronary artery disease in idiopathic pulmonary fibrosis. *Respir Med*. 2010;104(7):1035–41.

62. Kim WY, Mok Y, Kim GW, Baek SJ, Yun YD, Jee SH, Kim DS. Association between idiopathic pulmonary fibrosis and coronary artery disease: A case-control study and cohort analysis. *Sarcoidosis Vasc Diffuse Lung Dis*. 2015;31(4):289–96.

63. Izbicki G, Ben-Dor I, Shitrit D, Bendayan D, Aldrich TK, Kornowski R et al. The prevalence of coronary artery disease in end-stage pulmonary disease: Is pulmonary fibrosis a risk factor? *Respir Med*. 2009;103(9):1346–9.

64. Choong CK, Meyers BF, Guthrie TJ, Trulock EP, Patterson GA, Moazami N. Does the presence of preoperative mild or moderate coronary artery disease affect the outcomes of lung transplantation? *Ann Thorac Surg*. 2006;82(3):1038–42.

65. Nathan SD, Weir N, Shlobin OA, Urban BA, Curry CA, Basavaraj A et al. The value of computed tomography scanning for the detection of coronary artery disease in patients with idiopathic pulmonary fibrosis. *Respirology*. 2011;16(3):481–6.

66. Kempainen RR, Savik K, Whelan TP, Dunitz JM, Herrington CS, Billings JL. High prevalence of proximal and distal gastroesophageal reflux disease in advanced COPD. *Chest*. 2007;131(6):1666–71.

67. Robinson NB, DiMango E. Prevalence of gastroesophageal reflux in cystic fibrosis and implications for lung disease. *Ann Am Thorac Soc*. 2014;11(6):964–8.

68. Tobin R, Pope C, Pelligrini C, Emond M, Sillery J, Raghu G. Increased prevalence of gastroesophageal reflux in patients with idiopathic pulmonary fibrosis. *Am J Respir Crit Care Med*. 1998;158(6):1804–8.

69. Pashinsky YY, Jaffin BW, Litle VR. Gastroesophageal reflux disease and idiopathic pulmonary fibrosis. *Mt Sinai J Med*. 2009;76(1):24–9.

70. Forbes A, Marie I. Gastrointestinal complications: The most frequent internal complications of systemic sclerosis. *Rheumatology (Oxford)*. 2009;48(Suppl 3):iii36–9.

71. Sweet MP, Patti MG, Leard LE, Golden JA, Hays SR, Hoopes C et al. Gastroesophageal reflux in patients with idiopathic pulmonary fibrosis referred for lung transplantation. *J Thorac Cardiovasc Surg.* 2007;133(4):1078–84.

72. Patti MG, Tedesco P, Golden J, Hays S, Hoopes C, Meneghetti A et al. Idiopathic pulmonary fibrosis: How often is it really idiopathic? *J Gastrointest Surg.* 2005;9(8):1053–6.

73. Schachter LM, Dixon J, Pierce RJ, O'Brien P. Severe gastroesophageal reflux is associated with reduced carbon monoxide diffusing capacity. *Chest.* 2003;123(6):1932–8.

74. Cardasis JJ, MacMahon H, Husain AN. The spectrum of lung disease due to chronic occult aspiration. *Ann Am Thorac Soc.* 2014;11(6):865–73.

75. Hershcovici T, Jha LK, Johnson T, Gerson L, Stave C, Malo J et al. Systematic review: The relationship between interstitial lung diseases and gastro-oesophageal reflux disease. *Aliment Pharmacol Ther.* 2011;34(11–12):1295–305.

76. Lee JS, Collard HR, Raghu G, Sweet MP, Hays SR, Campos GM et al. Does chronic microaspiration cause idiopathic pulmonary fibrosis? *Am J Med.* 2010;123(4):304–11.

77. Raghu G. The role of gastroesophageal reflux in idiopathic pulmonary fibrosis. *Am J Med.* 2003;115(Suppl 3A):60S–4S.

78. Ing AJ. Interstitial lung disease and gastroesophageal reflux. *Am J Med.* 2001;111(Suppl 8A):41S–4S.

79. Salvioli B, Belmonte G, Stanghellini V, Baldi E, Fasano L, Pacilli AM. Gastro-oesophageal reflux and interstitial lung disease. *Dig Liver Dis.* 2006;38(12):879–84.

80. Lee JS, Song JW, Wolters PJ, Elicker BM, King TE, Jr, Kim DS et al. Bronchoalveolar lavage pepsin in acute exacerbation of idiopathic pulmonary fibrosis. *Eur Respir J.* 2012;39(2):352–8.

81. Lee JS, Ryu JH, Elicker BM, Lydell CP, Jones KD, Wolters PJ et al. Gastroesophageal reflux therapy is associated with longer survival in patients with idiopathic pulmonary fibrosis. *Am J Respir Crit Care Med.* 2011;184(12):1390–4.

82. Noth I, Anstrom KJ, Calvert SB, de Andrade J, Flaherty KR, Glazer C et al. Idiopathic Pulmonary Fibrosis Clinical Research Network (IPFnet). A placebo-controlled randomized trial of warfarin in idiopathic pulmonary fibrosis. *Am J Respir Crit Care Med.* 2012;186(1):88–95.

83. Raghu G, Anstrom KJ, King TEJ, Lasky JA, Martinez FJ. Prednisone, azathioprine, and N-acetylcysteine for pulmonary fibrosis. *N Engl J Med.* 2012;366(21):1968–77.

84. Idiopathic Pulmonary Fibrosis Clinical Research Network; Zisman DA, Schwarz M, Anstrom KJ, Collard HR, Flaherty KR, Hunninghake GW. A controlled trial of sildenafil in advanced idiopathic pulmonary fibrosis. *N Engl J Med.* 2010;363(7):620–8.

85. Lee JS, Collard HR, Anstrom KJ, Martinez FJ, Noth I, Roberts RS et al.; IPFnet Investigators. Anti-acid treatment and disease progression in idiopathic pulmonary fibrosis: An analysis of data from three randomised controlled trials. *Lancet Respir Med.* 2013;1(5):369–76.

86. King TE, Jr, Bradford WZ, Castro-Bernardini S, Fagan EA, Glaspole I, Glassberg MK et al. A phase 3 trial of pirfenidone in patients with idiopathic pulmonary fibrosis. *N Engl J Med.* 2014;370(22):2083–92.

87. Noble PW, Albera C, Bradford WZ, Costabel U, Glassberg MK, Kardatzke D et al. CAPACITY Study Group. Pirfenidone in patients with idiopathic pulmonary fibrosis (CAPACITY): Two randomised trials. *Lancet.* 2011;377(9779):1760–9.

88. Kreuter M, Wuyts W, Renzoni E, Koschel D, Maher TM, Kolb M et al. Antacid therapy and disease outcomes in idiopathic pulmonary fibrosis: A pooled analysis. *Lancet Respir Med.* 2016;4(5):381–9.

89. Raghu G, Freudenberger TD, Yang S, Curtis JR, Spada C, Hayes J. High prevalence of abnormal acid gastro-oesophageal reflux in idiopathic pulmonary fibrosis. *Eur Respir J.* 2006;27(1):136–42.

90. Orr WC, Craddock A, Goodrich S. Acidic and non-acidic reflux during sleep under conditions of powerful acid suppression. *Chest.* 2007;131(2):460–5.

91. Laheij R, Sturkenboom M, Hassing R, Dieleman J, Stricker B, Jansen J. Risk of community-acquired pneumonia and use of gastric acid-suppressive drugs. *JAMA*. 2004;292(16):1955–60.

92. Katz PO, Gerson LB, Vela MF. Guidelines for the diagnosis and management of gastroesophageal reflux disease. *Am J Gastroenterol*. 2013;108(3):308–28.

93. Allaix ME, Fisichella PM, Noth I, Herbella FA, Borraez Segura B, Patti MG. Idiopathic pulmonary fibrosis and gastroesophageal reflux. Implications for treatment. *J Gastrointest Surg*. 2014;18(1):100–4.

94. Marie I, Hatron PY, Cherin P, Hachulla E, Diot E, Vittecoq O et al. Functional outcome and prognostic factors in anti-Jo1 patients with antisynthetase syndrome. *Arthritis Res Ther*. 2013;15(5):R149.

95. Marie I, Josse S, Decaux O, Diot E, Landron C, Roblot P et al. Clinical manifestations and outcome of anti-PL7 positive patients with antisynthetase syndrome. *Eur J Intern Med*. 2013;24(5):474–9.

96. Solomon J, Swigris JJ, Brown KK. Myositis-related interstitial lung disease and anti-synthetase syndrome. *J Bras Pneumol*. 2011;37(1):100–9.

97. Soares R, Forsythe A, Hogarth K, Sweiss N, Noth I, Patti MG. Interstitial lung disease and gastroesophageal reflux disease: Key role of esophageal function tests in the diagnosis and treatment. *Arg Gastroenterol*. 2011;48(2):91–7.

98. Meyer KC, Raghu G, Verleden GM, Corris PA, Aurora P, Wilson KC et al. ISHLT/ATS/ERS BOS Task Force Committee, ISHLT/ATS/ERS BOS Task Force Committee. An international ISHLT/ATS/ERS clinical practice guideline: Diagnosis and management of bronchiolitis obliterans syndrome. *Eur Respir J*. 2014;44(6):1479–503.

99. McLoud T, Carrington C, Gaensler E. Diffuse infiltrative lung disease: A new scheme for description. *Radiology*. 1983;149(2):353–63.

100. Franquet T, Gimenez A, Torrubia S, Sabate J, Rodriguez-Arias J. Spontaneous pneumothorax and pneumomediastinum in IPF. *Eur Radiol*. 2000;10(1):108–13.

101. Iwasawa T, Ogura T, Takahashi H, Asakura A, Gotoh T, Yazawa T et al. Pneumothorax and idiopathic pulmonary fibrosis. *Jpn J Radiol*. 2010;28(9):672–9.

102. Oda T, Ogura T, Kitamura H, Hagiwara E, Baba T, Enomoto Y et al. Distinct characteristics of pleuroparenchymal fibroelastosis with usual interstitial pneumonia compared with idiopathic pulmonary fibrosis. *Chest*. 2014;146(5):1248–55.

103. Taveira-DaSilva AM, Burstein D, Hathaway OM, Fontana JR, Gochuico BR, Avila NA et al. Pneumothorax after air travel in lymphangioleiomyomatosis, idiopathic pulmonary fibrosis, and sarcoidosis. *Chest*. 2009;136(3):665–70.

104. Baumann M, Strange C, Heffner J, Light R, Kirby T, Klein J et al. AACP Pneumothorax Consensus Group. Management of spontaneous pneumothorax: An American College of Chest Physicians Delphi consensus statement. *Chest*. 2001;119(2):590–602.

105. Bintcliffe OJ, Hallifax RJ, Edey A, Feller-Kopman D, Lee YC, Marquette CH et al. Spontaneous pneumothorax: Time to rethink management? *Lancet Respir Med*. 2015;3(7):578–88.

106. MacDuff A, Arnold A, Harvey J; BTS Pleural Disease Guideline Group. Management of spontaneous pneumothorax: British Thoracic Society Pleural Disease Guideline 2010. *Thorax*. 2010;65(Suppl 2):ii18–31.

107. Friedrich G. Periphere Lungenkrebse auf dem Bodem pleuranaher Narben. *Virchows Arch Path Anat*. 1939;304:230–46.

108. Le Jeune I, Gribbin J, West J, Smith C, Cullinan P, Hubbard R. The incidence of cancer in patients with idiopathic pulmonary fibrosis and sarcoidosis in the UK. *Respir Med*. 2007;101(12):2534–40.

109. Matsushita H, Tanaka S, Saiki Y, Hara M, Nakata K, Tanimura S et al. Lung cancer associated with usual interstitial pneumonia. *Pathol Int*. 1995;45(12):925–32.

110. Turner-Warwick M, Lebowitz M, Burrows B, Johnson A. Cryptogenic fibrosing alveolitis and lung cancer. *Thorax*. 1980;35(7):496–9.

111. Aubry MC, Myers JL, Douglas WW, Tazelaar HD, Washington Stephens TL, Hartman TE et al. Primary pulmonary carcinoma in patients with idiopathic pulmonary fibrosis. *Mayo Clin Proc.* 2002;77(8):763–70.

112. Antoniou KM, Walsh SL, Hansell DM, Rubens MR, Marten K, Tennant R et al. Smoking-related emphysema is associated with idiopathic pulmonary fibrosis and rheumatoid lung. *Respirology.* 2013;18(8):1191–6.

113. Vancheri C. Common pathways in idiopathic pulmonary fibrosis and cancer. *Eur Respir Rev.* 2013;22(129):265–72.

114. Tomassetti S, Gurioli C, Ryu JH, Decker PA, Ravaglia C, Tantalocco P et al. The impact of lung cancer on survival of idiopathic pulmonary fibrosis. *Chest.* 2015;147(1):157–64.

115. Sakai S, Ono M, Nishio T, Kawarada Y, Nagashima A, Toyoshima S. Lung cancer associated with diffuse pulmonary fibrosis: CT-pathologic correlation. *J Thorac Imaging.* 2003;18(2):67–71.

116. Kishi K, Homma S, Kurosaki A, Motoi N, Yoshimura K. High-resolution computed tomography findings of lung cancer associated with idiopathic pulmonary fibrosis. *J Comput Assist Tomogr.* 2006;30(1):95–9.

117. Lee T, Park JY, Lee HY, Cho YJ, Yoon HI, Lee JH et al. Lung cancer in patients with idiopathic pulmonary fibrosis: Clinical characteristics and impact on survival. *Respir Med.* 2014;108(10):1549–55.

118. Lee HJ, Im JG, Ahn JM, Yeon KM. Lung cancer in patients with idiopathic pulmonary fibrosis: CT findings. *J Comput Assist Tomogr.* 1996;20(6):979–82.

119. Antoniou KM, Tomassetti S, Tsitoura E, Vancheri C. Idiopathic pulmonary fibrosis and lung cancer: A clinical and pathogenesis update. *Curr Opin Pulm Med.* 2015;21(6):626–33.

120. Kushibe K, Kawaguchi T, Takahama M, Kimura M, Tojo T, Taniguchi S. Operative indications for lung cancer with idiopathic pulmonary fibrosis. *Thorac Cardiovasc Surg.* 2007;55(8):505–8.

121. Kumar P, Goldstraw P, Yamada K, Nicholson AG, Wells AU, Hansell DM et al. Pulmonary fibrosis and lung cancer: Risk and benefit analysis of pulmonary resection. *J Thorac Cardiovasc Surg.* 2003;125(6):1321–7.

122. Isobe K, Hata Y, Sakamoto S, Takai Y, Shibuya K, Homma S. Clinical characteristics of acute respiratory deterioration in pulmonary fibrosis associated with lung cancer following anti-cancer therapy. *Respirology.* 2010;15(1):88–92.

123. Watanabe N, Taniguchi H, Kondoh Y, Kimura T, Kataoka K, Nishiyama O et al. Efficacy of chemotherapy for advanced non-small cell lung cancer with idiopathic pulmonary fibrosis. *Respiration.* 2013;85(4):326–31.

124. Watanabe N, Taniguchi H, Kondoh Y, Kimura T, Kataoka K, Nishiyama O et al. Chemotherapy for extensive-stage small-cell lung cancer with idiopathic pulmonary fibrosis. *Int J Clin Oncol.* 2014;19(2):260–5.

125. Kenmotsu H, Naito T, Kimura M, Ono A, Shukuya T, Nakamura Y et al. The risk of cytotoxic chemotherapy-related exacerbation of interstitial lung disease with lung cancer. *J Thorac Oncol.* 2011;6(7):1242–6.

126. Stertz O. Polymyositis. *Berl Klin Wochenschr.* 1916;53:489.

127. Buchbinder R, Forbes A, Hall S, Dennett X, Giles G. Incidence of malignant disease in biopsy-proven inflammatory myopathy. A population-based cohort study. *Ann Intern Med.* 2001;134(12):1087–95.

128. Yang Z, Lin F, Qin B, Liang Y, Zhong R. Polymyositis/dermatomyositis and malignancy risk: A meta-analysis study. *J Rheumatol.* 2015;42(2):282–91.

129. Chen YJ, Wu CY, Huang YL, Wang CB, Shen JL, Chang YT. Cancer risks of dermatomyositis and polymyositis: A nationwide cohort study in Taiwan. *Arthritis Res Ther.* 2010;12(2):R70.

130. Chow WH, Gridley G, Mellemkjaer L, McLaughlin JK, Olsen JH, Fraumeni JF Jr. Cancer risk following polymyositis and dermatomyositis: A nationwide cohort study in Denmark. *Cancer Causes Control.* 1995;6(1):9–13.

131. Levine SM. Cancer and myositis: New insights into an old association. *Curr Opin Rheumatol.* 2006;18(6):620–4.

132. Hill CL, Zhang Y, Sigurgeirsson B, Pukkala E, Mellemkjaer L, Airio A et al. Frequency of specific cancer types in dermatomyositis and polymyositis: A population-based study. *Lancet.* 2001;357(9250):96–100.

133. Sigurgeirsson B, Lindelöf B, Edhag O, Allander E. Risk of cancer in patients with dermatomyositis or polymyositis. A population-based study. *N Engl J Med.* 1992;326(6):363–7.

134. Stockton D, Doherty VR, Brewster DH. Risk of cancer in patients with dermatomyositis or polymyositis, and follow-up implications: A Scottish population-based cohort study. *Br J Cancer.* 2001;85(1):41–5.

135. Fiorentino DF, Chung LS, Christopher-Stine L, Zaba L, Li S, Mammen AL et al. Most patients with cancer-associated dermatomyositis have antibodies to nuclear matrix protein NXP-2 or transcription intermediary factor 1γ. *Arthritis Rheum.* 2013;65(11):2954–62.

136. Troy LK, Corte TJ. Sleep disordered breathing in interstitial lung disease: A review. *World J Clin Cases.* 2014;2(12):828–34.

137. Lancaster LH, Mason WR, Parnell JA, Rice TW, Loyd JE, Milstone AP et al. Obstructive sleep apnea is common in idiopathic pulmonary fibrosis. *Chest.* 2009;136(3):772–8.

138. Milioli G, Bosi M, Poletti V, Tomassetti S, Grassi A, Riccardi S et al. Sleep and respiratory sleep disorders in idiopathic pulmonary fibrosis. *Sleep Med Rev.* 2016;26:57–63.

139. Young T, Palta M, Dempsey J, Skatrud J, Weber S, Badr S. The occurrence of sleep-disordered breathing among middle-aged adults. *N Engl J Med.* 1993;328(17):1230–5.

140. Pihtili A, Bingol Z, Kiyan E, Cuhadaroglu C, Issever H, Gulbaran Z. Obstructive sleep apnea is common in patients with interstitial lung disease. *Sleep Breath.* 2013;17(4):1281–8.

141. Reid T, Vennelle M, McKinley M, MacFarlane PA, Hirani N, Simpson AJ et al. Sleep-disordered breathing and idiopathic pulmonary fibrosis—Is there an association? *Sleep Breath.* 2015;19(2):719–21.

142. Mermigkis C, Bouloukaki I, Antoniou K, Papadogiannis G, Giannarakis I, Varouchakis G et al. Obstructive sleep apnea should be treated in patients with idiopathic pulmonary fibrosis. *Sleep Breath.* 2015;19(1):385–91.

143. Sommerwerck U, Kleibrink BE, Kruse F, Scherer MJ, Wang Y, Kamler M et al. Predictors of obstructive sleep apnea in lung transplant recipients. *Sleep Med.* 2016;21:121–5.

144. Lanken PN, Terry PB, Delisser HM, Fahy BF, Hansen-Flaschen J, Heffner JE et al.; ATS End-of-Life Care Task Force. An official American Thoracic Society clinical policy statement: Palliative care for patients with respiratory diseases and critical illnesses. *Am J Respir Crit Care Med.* 2008;177(8):912–27.

145. Lindell KO, Liang Z, Hoffman LA, Rosenzweig MQ, Saul MI, Pilewski JM et al. Palliative care and location of death in decedents with idiopathic pulmonary fibrosis. *Chest.* 2015;147(2):423–9.

146. Brown CE, Engelberg RA, Nielsen EL, Curtis JR. Palliative care for patients dying in the intensive care unit with chronic lung disease compared with metastatic cancer. *Ann Am Thorac Soc.* 2016;13(5):684–9.

147. Bajwah S, Higginson IJ, Ross JR, Wells AU, Birring SS, Riley J et al. The palliative care needs for fibrotic interstitial lung disease: A qualitative study of patients, informal caregivers and health professionals. *Palliat Med.* 2013;27(9):869–76.

148. Overgaard D, Kaldan G, Marsaa K, Nielsen TL, Shaker SB, Egerod I. The lived experience with idiopathic pulmonary fibrosis: A qualitative study. *Eur Respir J.* 2016;47(5):1472–80.

149. Ahmadi Z, Wysham NG, Lundström S, Janson C, Currow DC, Ekström M. End-of-life care in oxygen-dependent ILD compared with lung cancer: A national population-based study. *Thorax.* 2016;71(6):510–6.

150. Fumeaux T, Rothmeier C, Jolliet P. Outcome of mechanical ventilation for acute respiratory failure in patients with pulmonary fibrosis. *Intensive Care Med.* 2001;27(12):1868–74.

151. Blivet S, Philit F, Sab JM, Langevin B, Paret M, Guérin C et al. Outcome of patients with idiopathic pulmonary fibrosis admitted to the ICU for respiratory failure. *Chest.* 2001;120(1):209–12.

152. Al-Hameed FM, Sharma S. Outcome of patients admitted to the intensive care unit for acute exacerbation of idiopathic pulmonary fibrosis. *Can Respir J.* 2004;11(2):117–22.

153. Takeyasu M, Miyamoto A, Kato D, Takahashi Y, Ogawa K, Murase K et al. Continuous intravenous morphine infusion for severe dyspnea in terminally ill interstitial pneumonia patients. *Intern Med.* 2016;55(7):725–9.

HENRY YUNG AND JASVIR S PARMAR

GENERAL INTRODUCTION

Lung transplantation is the treatment of choice for end-stage lung disease in individuals who have failed maximal therapy. In carefully selected patients it offers both prognostic benefit and an improvement in quality of life. However, it is not a risk-free enterprise and has significant associated short- and long-term morbidity and mortality; for these reasons it is reserved for patients who have exploited all other tolerable treatment options. Chronic obstructive pulmonary disease (COPD), pulmonary fibrosis, cystic fibrosis (CF) and pulmonary hypertension (PH) account for 95% of lung transplants performed. In this chapter we focus in on the challenges and opportunities for patients with interstitial lung disease (ILD).

BACKGROUND

The first lung transplant was performed in 1963 in Mississippi for a patient who was a prisoner with lung cancer. The surgery was successful with the patient returning to the intensive care unit; although he was successfully extubated, he unfortunately failed to leave the intensive care unit and died of sepsis on day 19 post-transplant. While this was not the success that was hoped for, it was the first demonstration that the principle of human lung transplantation was achievable. Subsequently, over the next 30 years lung transplants were only sporadically performed with mostly poor results, most often related to airway complications. These poor results led to a period of surgical refinement in the laboratory with two divergent approaches emerging as potential options. At Stanford, the group of Shumway pioneered heart-lung transplantation and performed their first transplant in 1981 followed by two additional transplants in the same year. Two years later in 1983 a group in Toronto performed an isolated single lung transplant in a patient with pulmonary fibrosis who survived for 10 years. Synchronous with these developments in surgery, the first formulations of cyclosporine became available, and this immunomodulatory drug undoubtedly added to the improvement in survival. These pioneering approaches heralded the start of the modern era of lung transplantation, and

since 1981 (a year in which three lung transplants were performed) there has been an exponential rise in the number of patients transplanted to over 4,000 worldwide in 2015.

As lung transplantation has matured as a treatment, survival rates have improved significantly since the broad adoption of the procedure over 30 years ago. This has been driven by improvements at each step of the patient pathway to successful transplantation. The key components to this success include better candidate selection, surgical innovation, improved intensive care management and enhancements in post-transplant care. Among the many other factors that help to improve outcomes, there is an appreciable centre effect with odds ratios for survival improving in centres preforming more than 40 transplants per year.

However, despite this improved survival, the prognosis for lung transplant recipients remains less than that for other solid organ transplant recipients. Multiple factors are considered to contribute to this; key among them is the persistent exposure of the allograft to the environment, which predisposes to infectious complications and possibly to bronchiolitis obliterans syndrome (1). There are few effective therapies for chronic rejection, and it remains a key contributor to long-term mortality.

Sadly, there is an enormous unmet need that arises from a significant shortfall in the number of donor organs available in comparison to the number of potential candidates. This has necessitated the careful selection of recipients to try and maximize the benefits from a scarce resource. Even with careful selection there is still a high risk of waiting list mortality, which is highest for patients with IPF. In this chapter we examine the process of referral, listing and transplantation, and we outline and discuss some the salient challenges that candidates face.

CRITERIA FOR REFERRAL

Lung transplantation is now an established therapy for idiopathic pulmonary fibrosis (IPF) and other forms of ILD that have reached end stage. Accumulated experience over the last three decades has led to the distillation of practice across centres (predominantly in Europe and North America) performing lung transplantation and the development of international guidelines on referral practice. The latest iteration of the International Society for Heart and Lung Transplantation (ISHLT) Guidelines for the Referral and Selection of Lung Transplant Candidates describes current consensus (2). The intention of these referral guidelines is to identify the subset of individuals who have the worst prognosis without a transplant and, therefore, likely derive the greatest survival benefit from a transplant.

Potential candidates should have a disease that is severe enough to make the risk profile of a transplant acceptable. In general this means that they should have an estimated median survival of less than 2 years and be in functional NYHA status class III or IV. In addition, potential candidates should also demonstrate ability to understand issues surrounding transplant, make informed decisions and demonstrate good compliance with medical therapy.

Early referral is to be encouraged, especially for patients with IPF, in view of high waiting list mortality and overall poor prognosis for this group. A narrow window of opportunity often exists between initial symptoms and decline. The unpredictability of acute exacerbations also makes the timing of referral difficult. In recognition of this, in the new consensus guidelines it is suggested that clinicians should consider an automatic referral for anyone with a new diagnosis of IPF or fibrosing non-specific interstitial pneumonia (NSIP). This should allow prompt review of these individuals by the transplant team and allow them time to explore underlying issues and complete the pre-transplant assessment process.

The opportunity to offer treatment with the newer licensed drugs for IPF (pirfenidone and nintedanib) has increased the complexity of the pathway of patients with IPF and has made the understanding of the timing of lung transplantation as an intervention more challenging. However, given the proven benefits (as shown by the CAPACITY, ASCEND and INPULSIS clinical trials) in some patients, it remains desirable (where patients meet the criteria) to offer these therapies prior to or concurrent with a referral for lung transplantation. Reassuringly, the theoretical concerns over the deleterious effects of both pirfenidone and nintedanib on transplant recipients have not so far translated into any short-term increase in mortality. However, there remains an open question as to any impact that pre-transplant treatment with these anti-fibrotic agents may have on long-term survival, which will only be answerable with time.

As the scope and range of medical therapies evolve, the opportunity to treat previously life-shortening conditions has necessitated a constant re-examination of the relative and absolute contraindications for listing for lung transplantation. Examples of these have been the relaxation of the age limits on transplantation, the ability to treat and control human immunodeficiency virus (HIV) and hepatitis B and C infections (2,3). With each of these developments there is a necessity to ensure that overall outcomes are preserved and that organ utilization remains optimal.

DISEASE PROGRESSION

While the diagnosis of IPF carries a relatively poor prognosis, the natural history of the disease course differs among patients with IPF. Some individuals have a slow and prolonged gradual deterioration, whereas others can experience rapid worsening in symptoms and early mortality. Additionally, acute exacerbations can happen at anytime, even in a relatively stable patient with relatively preserved lung function. In one recent study the 1- and 2-year incidence of acute exacerbations was 8.5% and 9.6%, respectively (4), which adds further uncertainty to prognostication and timing of referral for transplantation.

Selman et al. (5) examined patients with IPF in an attempt to identify factors that differentiated patients with high risk of disease progression from those with lower risk. They defined two cohorts as either 'slow' or 'rapid' progressors and then examined their characteristics. Those with the progressive IPF phenotype were characterized by symptom onset <6 months before first presentation and were more likely to be of male gender and smokers. These investigators also identified overexpression of genes associated with fibrosis and higher levels of active MMP-9 in bronchoalveolar lavage (BAL) fluid in the 'rapid' progressors.

While a low FVC measurement on lung function tests at the time of transplant pre-assessment are an indicator of waiting list mortality, it is increasingly recognized that the accelerated phase of the disease accounts for a significant proportion of the waiting list mortality (6).

PROGNOSTIC MARKERS FOR IPF AND TRANSPLANT ASSESSMENT

A number of studies have attempted to address the factors that could predict disease progression in IPF. Serological tests that may act as surrogate markers include surfactant protein D (SP-D), KL-6, LDH and erythrocyte sedimentation rate (ESR) (7). Limited data suggest that KL-6 may predict response to treatment in the rapidly progressive IPF group (8). Prasse et al. suggested that elevated levels of CCL18 predict change in forced vital capacity (FVC) and total lung capacity (TLC) at 6 months (9). Interestingly, SP-D levels decrease following bilateral lung transplant (BLT) but remain elevated after single lung transplant (SLT), perhaps indicating that in some individuals this biomarker may be useful (10). Hypoalbuminaemia at the time of transplantation has also been shown to be an independent risk factor for mortality in an analysis of United Network for Organ Sharing (UNOS) data (11). However, despite these promising studies no single biomarker has yet been universally adopted for lung transplantation assessment.

Patients with systemic manifestations of connective tissue disease are often considered to be poor transplant candidates. Interestingly, in a single centre study, Lee et al. (12) found that transplant-free survival is longer for IPF patients with circulating autoantibodies. Collard et al. (13) identified change in dyspnoea score, TLC/FVC, DLCO, partial pressure of arterial oxygen and A-a oxygen gradient as prognostic factors in IPF. Severe impairment in FVC and DLCO have also been implicated in some studies, although serial lung function is probably more informative (14). Flaherty et al. (15) identified decrease in FVC >10% over a 6-month period as a risk factor for mortality in a multivariate analysis (hazard ratio 2.47, 95% CI 1.29–4.73). Richeldi et al. (16) suggested the use of relative rather than absolute change in FVC over 12 months to allow inclusion of more individuals with meaningful decline while still predicting survival. Ryerson et al. (17) found that long-term oxygen therapy, TLC and DLCO predict time to death or transplantation.

Right ventricular dilatation and dysfunction are also associated with higher mortality in patients with IPF, this association is most marked when there is high pulmonary vascular resistance on right heart catheterization (18). Secondary PH is commonly found in IPF, and other studies have correlated this with worse physiological findings and survival.

Cardiopulmonary exercise testing can also offer some insight into the prognosis of patients listed for lung transplantation. Kawut et al. (19) found worse waiting list survival for 6-minute walk distance less than 350 m, reduced peak VO2/kg; and desaturation less than 95% on unloaded exercise. Lama et al. (20) noted that desaturation less than 88% on 6-minute walk test is associated with higher mortality in both IPF and NSIP. This was particularly pronounced in patients who desaturated early into the test. Desaturation areas and lowest saturation on a 15-stair climbing test are also linked with increased death rates (21).

Histopathology specimens from surgical lung biopsies may also provide insight into survival. The extent of fibroblastic foci has been shown to predict survival in some studies (22,23). However, the findings have been refuted in another study (24) that did not find any association with survival. While the data are conflicting, it is likely that fibroblastic foci correspond with IPF progression, and extent of fibroblastic foci may provide some additional insight into prognosis. Mogulkoc et al. (25) suggested one based on lung function (DLCO) and high-resolution computed tomography (HRCT) fibrosis score, which reflects the degree of reticular opacities and honeycombing in each lobe. The study found good survival prediction with optimal cut-off of DLCO 39% predicted and fibrosis score 2.25. However, this study excluded patients over the age of 65 years, which now represent a significant proportion of referrals. Ley et al. (26) proposed a staging system for prognostic modelling and validated this with data from three large cohorts. The gender age physiology (GAP) model used gender, age and two physiology variables (FVC and DLCO), and the three stages had 1-year mortality of 6%, 16% and 39%, respectively. Another similar model (27) based on HRCT fibrosis scoring, gender, age and FVC (CT-GAP) also has comparable prediction ability.

King et al. (28) used a composite clinical-radiologic-physiologic (CRP) model to predict survival in IPF, which was based on variables found to be significant on a previous study. The parameters include dyspnoea, clubbing, inspiratory crackles, radiographic abnormalities, pulmonary function and exercise testing. Du Bois et al. (29) formulated an alternative mortality risk score using age, history of respiratory hospitalization, predicted FVC and 24-week change in predicted FVC. While none of these models have been universally adopted at present, it seems likely that the best prognostic model would need to use multiple variables to optimize predictive potential.

PROGNOSTIC MARKERS FOR NON-IPF ILDs

Overall the prognosis of patients with a NSIP pattern of pulmonary fibrosis is generally better than with a UIP pattern, and patients with NSIP are more likely to respond to treatment (30). Nonetheless, there is a subgroup of NSIP patients who have a progressive phenotype and should be considered for transplantation. Flaherty et al. (31) found significant differences in survival between those with histological diagnoses of UIP versus NSIP. Those patients with idiopathic NSIP and fibrosing pattern on lung biopsy have poorer outcomes than those with a cellular pattern. Deteriorating lung function at 12 months is a mortality predictor for both UIP and NSIP diagnoses (32). The majority of connective tissue disease (CTD)–associated ILD is associated with a NSIP pattern on imaging and histology. In systemic sclerosis, both NSIP and UIP patterns have similar survival outcomes at 5 years, and the DLCO and FVC trends are the main survival predictors (33). Indeed, HRCT appearances may not be helpful in predicting survival in patients with scleroderma (34). The differences from the IPF group may be related to decreased profusion of fibroblastic foci on histology (35).

An analysis of patients with sarcoidosis (36) at a single centre found that mortality from respiratory failure is associated with fibrosis on imaging and a FVC value less than 1.5 L. In a retrospective review of United Network for Organ Sharing (UNOS) data, 27.4% with sarcoidosis died on the waiting list, and predictive variables for mortality included African American race, supplemental oxygen requirements and mean pulmonary artery pressure (37).

For patients with hypersensitivity pneumonitis, evidence of fibrosis on CT scan, abnormal lung function and presence of crackles on examination were predictive of poor survival (38,39). In pulmonary Langerhans cell histiocytosis, increasing age and low FEV1/FVC ratio were identified as risk factors for poorer survival (40).

CRITERIA FOR LISTING AND CONTRAINDICATIONS

TRANSPLANT ASSESSMENT

Each individual lung transplant centre has its own approach to managing transplant assessments. However, a few guiding principles unify this individualized approach. The ambition of the process is to try and evaluate each patient's illness with particular attention to the trajectory of decline and the likely net benefit from lung transplantation. This is contextualized with the individual's co-morbidities and personal psychosocial situation to attempt to ensure that the therapy is targeted to the most appropriate candidates.

In general, this assessment will involve an elective admission lasting up to 5 days. During this period a comprehensive assessment of the individual's illness is made by various professionals including a transplant physician and surgeon, an anaesthetist, transplant nurses, physiotherapist, psychiatrist, social worker, dietitians, transplant recipient coordinator and the palliative care specialists. These assessments are supported by up-to-date investigations, which usually include a comprehensive respiratory, cardiac, liver and renal function evaluation. Detailed evaluation of the sensitization status of the patient is characterized by determining the presence of pre-formed anti-human leukocyte antigen (HLA) antibodies. An extensive virological screen is also undertaken, examining for the infection status in relation to cytomegalovirus (CMV), hepatitis B/C/E and HIV. Very careful consideration is given to the impact of any co-morbidities that may have a significant impact on the short- and long-term survival post-transplant.

The assessment culminates in a multidisciplinary discussion that involves all health professionals who have been involved in the evaluation of the patient's illness. The outcome may take one of three forms depending on the circumstances.

There may be agreement to put the candidate on the active waiting list, in which case they will be offered listing. Alternatively, some patients may be felt to be suitable candidates, but the timing is not correct or they need to meet certain criteria (i.e. losing or gaining weight or further investigations may be required). These patients will be kept under review and the outstanding issues re-examined regularly. Unfortunately, some patients may not be perceived as suitable candidates and, therefore, listing is not offered. This can be a very demoralizing situation for patients, who often are at the end of a long line of medical interventions and have invested a lot of hope in the prospect of transplantation. This is a delicate situation and one that needs to be handled in a very careful and sensitive manner. Central to this is communicating with the referring team and, where appropriate, involving the palliative care team.

GENERAL LISTING CRITERIA

The general listing criteria for ILD including both IPF and NSIP are displayed in Table 26.1. These reflect poor prognostic indicators described earlier.

In previous guidelines (3), the following criteria are recommended for sarcoidosis: hypoxaemia at rest, pulmonary hypertension and finding of elevated right atrial pressure >15 mm Hg. Similarly, hypoxaemia at rest and low VO2 maximum <50% with impaired lung function are indicators for lymphangioleiomyomatosis and Langerhans cell histiocytosis. It is important to take into context the rate of the decline and impact on quality of life in the decision-making process.

ABSOLUTE AND RELATIVE CONTRAINDICATIONS

Any condition that contributes to perioperative risk or significantly limits life expectancy may be considered a contraindication. Relative contraindications are concerns that are not necessarily strong enough reasons to preclude transplant but that may limit the survival outcome for a recipient. While one relative contraindication may not be a concern, a combination of these may make the risk profile for the individual unattractive and result in a patient not being offered transplantation (see Table 26.2 for a list of contraindications). A prime

Table 26.1 Referral and listing criteria for transplant in interstitial lung disease

Interstitial lung disease	
Referral criteria	• Histopathologic or radiographic evidence of usual interstitial pneumonitis (UIP) or fibrosing non-specific interstitial pneumonitis (NSIP), regardless of lung function. • Abnormal lung function: forced vital capacity (FVC) <80% predicted or diffusion capacity of the lung for carbon monoxide (DLCO) <40% predicted • Any dyspnoea or functional limitation • Any dyspnoea or functional limitation attributable to lung disease. • Any oxygen requirement, even if only during exertion. • For inflammatory interstitial lung disease (ILD), failure to improve dyspnoea, oxygen requirement, and/or lung function after a clinically indicated trial of medical therapy.
Listing criteria	• Decline in FVC >10% during 6 months of follow-up (note: a 5% decline is associated with a poorer prognosis and may warrant listing). • Decline in DLCO >15% during 6 months of follow-up. • Desaturation to o 88% or distance <250 m on 6-minute-walk test or >50 m decline in 6-minute-walk distance over a 6-month period. • Pulmonary hypertension on right heart catheterization or 2-dimensional echocardiography. • Hospitalization because of respiratory decline, pneumothorax or acute exacerbation.

Source: Reprinted from *J Heart Lung Transplant*, 34(1), Weill D et al., A consensus document for the selection of lung transplant candidates: 2014—an update from the Pulmonary Transplantation Council of the International Society for Heart and Lung Transplantation, 1–15, Copyright 2015, with permission from Elsevier.

Table 26.2 List of absolute and relative contraindications for lung transplantation

Absolute Contraindications

- Recent history of malignancy. A 2-year disease-free interval combined with a low predicted risk of recurrence after lung transplantation may be reasonable, for instance, in non-melanoma localized skin cancer that has been treated appropriately. However, a 5-year disease-free interval is prudent in most cases, particularly for patients with a history of hematologic malignancy, sarcoma, melanoma, or cancers of the breast, bladder or kidney. Unfortunately, for a portion of patients with a history of cancer, the risk of recurrence may remain too high to proceed with lung transplantation even after a 5-year disease-free interval.
- Untreatable significant dysfunction of another major organ system (e.g. heart, liver, kidney or brain) unless combined organ transplantation can be performed.
- Uncorrected atherosclerotic disease with suspected or confirmed end-organ ischaemia or dysfunction and/or coronary artery disease not amenable to revascularization.
- Acute medical instability, including, but not limited to, acute sepsis, myocardial infarction and liver failure.
- Uncorrectable bleeding diathesis.
- Chronic infection with highly virulent and/or resistant microbes that are poorly controlled pre-transplant.
- Evidence of active Mycobacterium tuberculosis infection.
- Significant chest wall or spinal deformity expected to cause severe restriction after transplantation.
- Class II or III obesity (body mass index [BMI] >35.0 kg/m^2).
- Current non-adherence to medical therapy or a history of repeated or prolonged episodes of non-adherence to medical therapy that are perceived to increase the risk of non-adherence after transplantation.
- Psychiatric or psychologic conditions associated with the inability to cooperate with the medical/allied health care team and/or adhere with complex medical therapy.
- Absence of an adequate or reliable social support system.
- Severely limited functional status with poor rehabilitation potential.
- Substance abuse or dependence (e.g. alcohol, tobacco, marijuana or other illicit substances). In many cases, convincing evidence of risk reduction behaviours, such as meaningful and/or long-term participation in therapy for substance abuse and/or dependence, should be required before offering lung transplantation. Serial blood and urine testing can be used to verify abstinence from substances that are of concern.

Relative Contraindications

- Age >65 years in association with low physiologic reserve and/or other relative contraindications. Although there cannot be endorsement of an upper age limit as an absolute contraindication, adults >75 years old are unlikely to be candidates for lung transplantation in most cases. Although age by itself should not be considered a contraindication to transplant, increasing age generally is associated with comorbid conditions that are either absolute or relative contraindications.
- Class I obesity (BMI 30.0–34.9 kg/m^2), particularly truncal (central) obesity.
- Progressive or severe malnutrition.
- Severe, symptomatic osteoporosis.
- Extensive prior chest surgery with lung resection.
- Mechanical ventilation and/or extracorporeal life support (ECLS). However, carefully selected candidates without other acute or chronic organ dysfunction may be successfully transplanted.

(Continued)

Table 26.2 (*Continued*) List of absolute and relative contraindications for lung transplantation

- Colonization or infection with highly resistant or highly virulent bacteria, fungi and certain strains of mycobacteria (e.g. chronic extrapulmonary infection expected to worsen after transplantation).
- For patients infected with hepatitis B and/or C, a lung transplant can be considered in patients without significant clinical, radiologic, or biochemical signs of cirrhosis or portal hypertension and who are stable on appropriate therapy. Lung transplantation in candidates with hepatitis B and/or C should be performed in centres with experienced hepatology units.
- For patients infected with human immunodeficiency virus (HIV), a lung transplant can be considered in patients with controlled disease with undetectable HIV-RNA, and compliant on combined anti-retroviral therapy. The most suitable candidates should have no current acquired immunodeficiency syndrome-defining illness. Lung transplantation in HIV-positive candidates should be performed in centres with expertise in the care of HIV-positive patients.
- Infection with Burkholderia cenocepacia, Burkholderia gladioli and multi-drug–resistant Mycobacterium abscessus if the infection is sufficiently treated preoperatively and there is a reasonable expectation for adequate control post-operatively. For patients with these infections to be considered suitable transplant candidates, the patients should be evaluated by centres with significant experience managing these infections in the transplant setting, and patients should be aware of the increased risk of transplant because of these infections.
- Atherosclerotic disease burden sufficient to put the candidate at risk for end-organ disease after lung transplantation. With regard to coronary artery disease, some patients will be candidates for percutaneous coronary intervention or coronary artery bypass graft (CABG) preoperatively or, in some instances, combined lung transplant and CABG. The preoperative evaluation, type of coronary stent used (bare metal vs drug eluting), and degree of coronary artery disease deemed acceptable vary among transplant centres.
- Other medical conditions that have not resulted in end-stage organ damage, such as diabetes mellitus, systemic hypertension, epilepsy, central venous obstruction, peptic ulcer disease, or gastroesophageal reflux, should be optimally treated before transplantation.

Source: Reprinted from Reprinted from *J Heart Lung Transplant*, 34(1), Weill D et al., A consensus document for the selection of lung transplant candidates: 2014—an update from the Pulmonary Transplantation Council of the International Society for Heart and Lung Transplantation, 1–15, Copyright 2015, with permission from Elsevier.

example of a relative contraindication is obesity, which has been associated with an increased rate of surgical complications and primary graft dysfunction. A recent retrospective analysis of BLT for IPF revealed that those with BMI >30 had a significantly higher 90-day mortality compared to those with BMI between 18.5 and 30 (41). In the most recent consensus guidelines the threshold has been raised from a BMI of greater than 30 to Class I obesity (BMI 30–34.9) as a relative contraindication (2).

Cardiothoracic surgery with video-assisted thoracoscopic (VATS) biopsies is commonly performed to establish a diagnosis for ILD. Pleurodesis, lung resection or pleurectomy may also be indicated for recurrent pneumothoraces. Previous thoracic surgery is not an absolute contraindication but may prolong native lung explantation and necessitate cardiopulmonary bypass with its associated complications. Prior pleurodesis is also associated with increased bleeding risk, primary graft dysfunction and renal impairment. This may be an issue for older or frail candidates who may struggle with a longer procedure.

Historically HIV was considered an absolute contraindication to lung transplantation. The concern with HIV-positive individuals is the risk of infectious complications in the setting of additional immunosuppression and the potential for drug-drug interactions. However, the improvement in prognosis with modern anti-retroviral drugs has led to a re-examination of this approach. Kern et al. (42) reported a series of three HIV-seropositive recipients including two with IPF. Although both developed acute rejection, they remained alive at 4- and 2-year follow-up. This has led to reconsideration of offering lung transplantation in selected cases, and candidates with good HIV control and CD4 >400 with no AIDS-defining illness may be assessed (43).

MANAGEMENT OF CO-MORBIDITIES

Prior to a recipient being placed on the transplant waiting list, any underlying co-morbidities should be aggressively managed. Overweight individuals should be encouraged to join a weight loss program. Risk factors such as systemic hypertension or diabetes mellitus should be controlled with medical treatment. Coronary artery disease may be treated with percutaneous intervention if lesions are amenable to angioplasty and/or stent placement. Osteoporotic individuals should receive supplementation and anti-resorptive therapies to lower fracture risk.

PRE-TRANSPLANT OPTIMIZATION

Dyspnoea and limitations in exercise capacity are universal features in many forms of ILD. Pulmonary rehabilitation consists of physical training, breathing exercises, nutritional counselling, educational and psychological support. It has been shown to improve 6-minute walk distances and health-related quality-of-life measures (SF-36) in ILD and also other advanced lung conditions (44). In 24 ILD lung transplant candidates, physical activity was higher in rehabilitation versus non-rehabilitation days (45). Vainshelboim et al. (46) conducted a randomized study that examined the longer-term outcomes of a 12-week exercise training program in IPF transplant candidates. At 11-month follow-up, 6-minute walk distance deteriorated in the control group but was preserved in the treatment group. Benefits were also seen in 30-second chair stand test and St. George's Respiratory Questionnaire impact. If there was any difference in survival remains unknown, because the study was underpowered to examine this. Nonetheless, there may be a significant advantage to better recovery post-transplant in individuals who are more physically robust.

In addition to physical rehabilitation, oxygen assessment is essential for resting hypoxaemia or exertional desaturation. Early treatment of hypoxaemia is favourable, as the development of secondary PH will add significant risk to the patients' profile. Routine review of waiting list status provides an opportunity to re-evaluate the recipient's candidacy. HLA antibody screen should be performed routinely at least every 3 months or earlier in the presence of potential sensitizing events (e.g. blood transfusion). In the event of an acute exacerbation or deterioration, candidates may need to be temporarily suspended or removed from the waiting list.

Assessment for transplant candidacy should be viewed as a continuous, ongoing process and not just a single event that occurs at the listing stage. Any major change in clinical state should prompt a re-evaluation of transplant candidacy. Pulmonary rehabilitation should be recommended for ILD candidates to improve exercise tolerance and functional status prior to transplant.

DISEASE-SPECIFIC CONSIDERATIONS

ESTABLISHING THE ILD SUBTYPE

Differentiation of the ILD subtype prior to transplantation is important for several reasons. Understanding the natural progression of the disease would help to guide the timing for referral and listing. Some CTD-associated ILD are associated with extrapulmonary features that could influence candidacy for transplant. In addition, an accurate diagnosis enables effective management of the underlying disease prior to transplant. The diagnosis should ideally be confirmed via an ILD multidisciplinary (clinician-radiologist-pathologist) meeting.

IDIOPATHIC PULMONARY FIBROSIS

IPF is the most commonly encountered form of idiopathic interstitial pneumonia with an incidence rate of 4.6 per 100,000 in the United Kingdom (47). The finding of a definite usual interstitial pneumonia (UIP) pattern of fibrosis on HRCT scan is usually diagnostic, while surgical lung biopsy may be required in uncertain cases. IPF is the second most frequent indication for lung transplantation, and the unadjusted survival rates for IPF at 1, 3, 5 and 10 years are 76.5%, 60.6%, 47.7% and 25.1%, respectively. These are significantly lower than for other lung transplant indications (www.ishlt.org/registries). This is supported by the observation that the median survival for IPF of 4.7 years is lower than that for other diagnoses such as CF (8.5 years), α-1-anti-tripsin deficiency emphysema (6.5 years) and COPD (5.5 years). However, in the context that the median survival of untreated IPF is about 2.4 years (48), lung transplantation still offers a survival benefit for recipients. Waiting list mortality for IPF is high compared to other lung conditions, ranging from 14% to 67% (49). Both BLT and SLT are viable options for the IPF population. In 2013, the proportions were BLT (60.2%) and SLT (39.8%), representing a reversal of practice over the last decade. The choice between the two procedures for uncomplicated IPF remains controversial. For those with secondary PH, many would opt for BLT in the view that this would reduce primary graft dysfunction. However, evidence has not shown a clear-cut advantage in the early post-operative phase.

SARCOIDOSIS

Sarcoidosis is a multisystem disease characterized by non-caseating granulomatous inflammation. The incidence varies across the world; in the United Kingdom it is approximately 5 per 100,000 person-years (47). There is a predilection for the lungs with 95% of cases having some form of pulmonary involvement (50). In one large case series of biopsy-confirmed sarcoidosis approximately half also had some degree of extrapulmonary involvement. Respiratory failure is a potential cause of mortality in sarcoidosis, and transplantation is indicated in advanced disease not responding to medical treatment.

PH is frequently associated with stage 4 sarcoidosis and may be secondary to extensive lung disease or sarcoid vasculopathy. It can manifest with right ventricular failure and occur in 28% of individuals with sarcoidosis (51) and up to 74% in those awaiting lung transplantation (52). There is higher mortality in those with PH (53); one study of individuals with sarcoidosis awaiting lung transplant found that right atrial pressure $\geq$15 mm Hg was a profoundly adverse prognostic indicator (RR 5.2, 95% CI 1.6–16.7) (54).

Patients with multisystem sarcoidosis may have cardiac, hepatic and neurological disease, and the involvement of more than one organ requires careful assessment of the extent of the disease prior to transplantation. Myocardial fibrosis can lead to left ventricular dysfunction, which may itself contribute to PH. Other cardiac abnormalities include conduction defects, arrhythmias, heart failure and sudden death (55). In these cases, cardiac magnetic resonance imaging may offer additional information on the extent and nature of cardiac disease. Impaired left ventricular systolic function is a strong contraindication for lung transplant, but

heart-lung transplantation may be warranted in highly selected cases.

Neurosarcoidosis can involve any part of the nervous system and has a whole spectrum of disease that can have severe consequences. While isolated cranial nerve involvement may not be an issue, patients with central nervous system lesions and seizures have a poor prognosis and are unlikely to be transplant candidates (56). Hepatic involvement can lead to portal hypertension and cirrhosis, and combined lung-liver transplant may be considered in some cases. Severe cutaneous sarcoid may also predispose to infection post-transplantation (57).

Cavitary lesions are frequent occurrences in advanced cystic sarcoidosis and may predispose to aspergilloma formation (58) (see Figure 26.1).

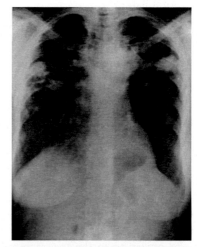

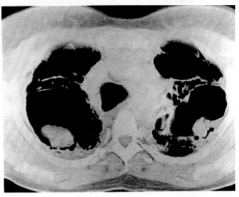

Figure 26.1 Chest radiograph and cross-sectional CT chest imaging of sarcoidosis individual with mycetomas. (Reprinted from *Chest*. 121(1), Hadjiliadis D et al., Outcome of lung transplantation in patients with mycetomas, 128–34, Copyright 2002, with permission from Elsevier.)

In a small case series looking at the outcome of six sarcoid recipients with mycetomas, survival was markedly reduced in comparison to controls with three patients dying within 30 days despite extensive anti-fungal treatment in some cases (59). These authors recommended aggressive anti-fungal prophylaxis and consideration of BLT to eliminate the risk of contamination from the native lung.

Intra-operatively, surgery is often complicated by fibrosis, pleural thickening and adhesions. PH increases the risk of haemodynamic instability and may obligate cardiopulmonary bypass. In the presence of mycetomas, there is a theoretical risk of seeding on explantation, and pleural disease may prolong surgery and ischaemic times. Some transplant centres adopt the practice of irrigating the pleural cavity with anti-fungal agents in high-risk cases (60).

Over the last 20 years there is an increasing shift away from BLT (2.9%) compared with SLT (1.9% total). This may reflect the increased incidence of bronchiectasis, mycetomas and PH in sarcoidosis. Unadjusted 1, 3, 5 and 10-year survival for transplant recipients are 75.9%, 62.3%, 55% and 34.7%. The median survival is 6.1 years (www.ishlt.org/registries). Poor prognostic factors for post-operative mortality included mechanical ventilation time in ICU, African American race, heart-lung transplant and pre-transplant physiology (61). There does not appear to be any difference in long-term survival or bronchiolitis obliterans syndrome (BOS) rates between sarcoid and IPF (62).

Disease recurrence post-transplant in sarcoidosis is a recognized potential issue in patients (63–65). The diagnosis may first come to light on the basis of granulomatous inflammation found on routine transbronchial biopsies, although it could also manifest with clinical changes or radiological evidence of pulmonary infiltrates or changes in the BAL fluid (increased CD4:CD8 ratio and lymphocyte count) (66). Granuloma recurrence has also been described on fluorescence in situ hybridization (FISH) analysis of cells recovered from biopsies (67). Given the rarity of this condition, there is no consensus on treatment regimes. Most patients are treated with augmentation of their immunosuppression.

SYSTEMIC SCLEROSIS

Systemic sclerosis (SSc) is a CTD that is characterized by excessive collagen deposition, vasculopathy and fibrosis. Annual incidence is estimated at 19.3 per million adults per year (68). It is a multi-organ disease that may involve the renal, cutaneous and gastrointestinal systems (69). ILD and PH are the major causes of mortality in this group of patients. SSc may be associated with a NSIP pattern on HRCT (70), and significant pulmonary involvement occurs in up to 25% of individuals (71). SSc-related ILD has a median survival of 2–5 years from time of diagnosis (72).

PH is more prevalent in SSc versus other forms of CTD. A meta-analysis of European studies (73) found 9% of SSc patients had pre-capillary PH, and this is associated with higher mortality independent of the presence of ILD (74). Waiting list mortality is also higher in CTD-related PH compared to other causes of PH (75).

Oesophageal dysmotility is a major concern in patients with SSc and is related to impaired peristalsis of the oesophageal body and/or laxity of the lower oesophageal sphincter. Gasper et al. (76) found 83% of SSc individuals have reflux, and 78% have impaired oesophageal motility. Fundoplication can worsen dysphagia in these individuals, and oesophagectomy is not without its complications. One group proposed Roux-en-Y gastric bypass as an alternative option, although this remains experimental (77). Significant dysmotility or aperistalsis is a relative contraindication for lung transplantation.

Studies in this group of patients have produced conflicting data, which likely reflect the heterogeneity of the patient group but also different approaches by transplant teams. Khan et al. (72) performed a systematic review of post-transplant survival rates of SSc recipients. Seven studies were identified with reported 1-year survival ranging from 59% to 93.4%, and 3-year survival ranged from 45.9% to 73%. However, Bernstein et al. analyzed UNOS registry data and found elevated 1-year mortality for SSc individuals compared to non-SSc related ILD (hazard ratio 1.48, 95% CI 1.01–2.17). These authors noted that survival was equivalent to those with non-SSc related PH. Saggar et al. (78) found no difference in survival between their SSc and IPF recipients, but there was significantly higher acute rejection rate for the SSc group at 1 year. There was also reduced freedom from BOS, but this result was not significant in this limited sample size; it was acknowledged in this paper that significant gastro-oesophageal reflux disease (GORD) may have contributed to higher rejection rates (see section on GORD), although objective measurements of oesophageal function were lacking. The highest survival rates are reported by transplant centres that adopt careful selection criteria (see Table 26.3, for example). Careful patient screening is essential, and all potential candidates should undergo investigations to assess oesophageal dysmotility and extrapulmonary involvement. It is likely that patients may be best served by centralizing expertise in a few centres that specialize in patients with SSc.

RHEUMATOID ARTHRITIS

Up to 8% of rheumatoid arthritis (RA) patients will develop ILD in their lifespan. Risk factors for ILD include advanced age at time of diagnosis, male gender, smoking and joint disease severity, and in this selected group the mortality is high with a median survival of 2.6 years (79). RA-related ILD is usually histologically indistinguishable from other fibrotic processes with UIP histopathology such as IPF (80). Prognosis is generally somewhat better in RA-related ILD with slower disease progression compared to IPF.

Yazdani et al. (81) found that there was no survival difference between RA-ILD, SSc- ILD and IPF up to 5 years post-transplant. In this study of 10 with RA-ILD, the- year survival for RA-ILD recipients was 67%. The authors also noticed substantial improvements in health-related quality-of-life (HRQOL) outcomes post-transplant (SF-36 and St. George's Respiratory Questionnaire). There are isolated reports of pulmonary capillaritis and diffuse alveolar haemorrhage post-transplant, which may represent a form of acute vascular rejection (82). In view of limited evidence, it is difficult to make recommendations for transplantation. Important considerations include anaesthetic complications as well as poor mobility and rehabilitation potential in those with extensive joint involvement. Also, there is a risk of atlanto-axial subluxation leading to spinal cord compression and quadriplegia at the time of anaesthesia induction and tracheal intubation when transplantation is performed, And cricoarytenoid arthritis may lead to soft tissue oedema and airway problems post-extubation (83). Finally, pre-existing disease-modifying therapies

may predispose to infectious complications following transplantation, and all potential candidates should have a formal assessment including an expert opinion from an anaesthesiology consultant prior to transplant listing.

SYSTEMIC LUPUS ERYTHEMATOSUS

Systemic lupus erythematosus (SLE) is a multisystem auto-immune disorder that often has a remitting and relapsing course. Pulmonary manifestations take the form of interstitial fibrosis and vasculitis. At post-mortem lung examination, disease-specific change in the lung parenchyma is detected in 18% of SLE individuals (84). Only anecdotal evidence exists for lung transplantation in this subgroup of CTD patients. Levy et al. (85) reported successful heart-lung transplant in a young female with SLE and progressive PH. She required treatment for BOS after 18 months but remained functionally stable at 4-year follow-up. A case series at Papworth Hospital (86) reported early mortality in two out of three SLE patients, both of which had positive anti-cardiolipin antibodies. The presence of these antibodies may predispose to coagulopathy and thrombosis.

INFLAMMATORY MYOPATHIES

Dermatomyositis and polymyositis are both associated with ILD and are often accompanied by antibodies against tRNA-synthetase (e.g. anti-Jo 1). Candidates should be carefully screened for malignancy given the higher incidence of adenocarcinomas with inflammatory myopathies. Patients should also be screened for respiratory muscle and diaphragmatic involvement. There are only anecdotal reports regarding lung transplantation (87,88). One reported successful bridging to transplant with extracorporeal membrane oxygenation (ECMO) support in a polymyositis sufferer. Despite post-operative infections, reperfusion injury and pulmonary artery stenosis, he was eventually discharged and remained well at 3-year follow-up. Lung transplantation has also been performed for anti-synthetase syndrome (89). Disease recurrence is reported in one case of polymyositis resulting in mortality 9 months following transplant (90). Given the limited data, it is advisable to assess each case on an individual basis.

Table 26.3 Sample selection criteria for systemic sclerosis associated ILD undergoing transplant assessment

University of California, Los Angeles Lung Transplant program algorithm in consideration of bilateral lung transplantation (LT) for individuals with underlying systemic sclerosis (SSc)

General

Adherence to established guidelines for referral and active listing for LT of patients with underlying usual interstitial pneumonia/non-specific interstitial pneumonia and/or pulmonary arterial hypertension[a] (78)

Age ≤60 yrs for bilateral LT

SSc diagnosis for ≥5 yrs defined from the date of first non-Raynaud's phenomenon (limited or diffuse scleroderma)

Baseline 6-min walk distance ≥100 m (with oxygen supplementation)

No chronic (≥6 months) scheduled narcotic requirement or dependence

Oral corticosteroid dose ≤10 mg prednisone (or equivalent) at time of LT

Extrapulmonary Disease

Gastrointestinal[b]

Absence of symptomatic oesophageal stricture, active upper GI ulceration, oesophageal aperistalsis, achalasia or abnormal gastric emptying (<25% clearance at 90 min post-ingestion) despite aggressive medical therapy[c]

Mild to moderate GER or oesophageal/gastric dysmotility is acceptable if controlled by aggressive medical therapy[+] based on patient self-report

Absence of chronic gastrointestinal bleeding with or without associated anaemia

Skin/musculoskeletal

Chest skin induration score of ≤2 (by modified Rodnan skin score of 0–3)

Absence of rapidly progressive diffuse skin thickening, and/or active digital ulceration with concern for digital necrosis

Absence of uncontrolled active myositis or progressive myopathy/neuropathy

Renal

Preserved and stable (≥3 months) renal function with creatinine clearance >50 mL · min^{-1}

A minimum time interval of 5 yrs between renal crisis and active listing for LT

Cardiac[d]

Normal right and left ventricular systolic function without prior clinical leftsided congestive heart failure (without associated pulmonary vascular disease)

Absence of obstructive coronary artery disease requiring concurrent artery bypass grafting during LT

Acceptable right ventricular function in the setting of known pulmonary vascular disease, without overt clinical signs of right sided congestive heart failure[e] or consideration of heart-lung transplantation

Source: Reproduced from Saggar R et al. Systemic sclerosis and bilateral lung transplantation: A single centre experience. *Eur Respir J.* 2010;36(4):893–900, Copyright 2010, with permission from European Respiratory Society.

Note: GI: gastrointestinal; GER: gastro-oesophageal reflux.

[a] The relatively poorer prognosis of SSc pulmonary arterial hypertension (PAH) compared to idiopathic PAH might warrant earlier referral and active listing for LT.

[b] We recommend the following tests to performed for all potential SSc LT recipients: barium oesophagram, nuclear medicine quantitative gastric emptying study, oesophageal manometry and upper endoscopy; and the following tests considered; dual pH probe study and/or impedance testing.

[c] Combination of high-dose proton-pump inhibitor and/or H$_2$ blocker, high-dose pro-motility agent and antireflux measure, including lifestyle modification counselling.

[d] Consider cardiac magnetic resonance imaging.

[e] Absence of clinical congestive heart failure, and preservation of liver function testing (including synthetic function).

HYPERSENSITIVITY PNEUMONITIS

Extrinsic allergic alveolitis (EAA) or what is now termed hypersensitivity pneumonitis (HP) is an inflammatory condition caused by repeated exposure to inhaled antigens. Common antigens include microbial organisms, chemicals and fungal spores. Its estimated incidence is 0.9 per 100,000 person years in the United Kingdom (91). The underlying immune mechanism is a type III hypersensitivity reaction, although the presence of granulomata and antibody responses suggest involvement of type IV hypersensitivity (92). Chronic progressive EAA leads to pulmonary fibrosis that can be indistinguishable from other end-stage fibrotic ILD.

Kern et al. (93) reported a case series of 31 EAA individuals who underwent lung transplantation. Survival was superior in the EAA group compared to IPF. Survival at 1, 3 and 5 years was reported as 96%, 89% and 89%, respectively, and the survival advantage persisted following adjustment for age and transplant procedure type. Acute rejection rates were lower in the first year, and a non-significant increase in freedom from BOS as compared to the IPF group was observed. The authors also reported disease recurrence in 2 out of 31 patients (6%) post-transplant, while a third patient had poorly formed granulomata on transbronchial biopsy. Despite augmented immunosuppression in two recipients, these patients developed allograft dysfunction, which emphasizes the need for antigen avoidance if the antigen is known (36.7% of patients with HP had known antigen sensitization in one study [39]), which may make prevention difficult.

OCCUPATIONAL-RELATED ILD

Occupational lung disease (OLD) consists of a heterogenous group of disorders that may manifest with ILD or airway abnormalities. Mao et al. (94) reported five transplants for silicosis, two of whom died within the first year, and the rest are alive at medium-term follow-up. Redondo et al. (95) reported a series of six lung transplants for end-stage silicosis. All recipients were alive at mean follow-up of 32 months, and this was associated with improved lung physiology and HRQOL outcomes. Singer et al. (96) performed an analysis on UNOS data comparing silicosis with other occupational lung diseases. These authors found increased mortality for the non-silicotic OLD group in the first

year post-transplant (hazard ratio 3.1, 95% CI 1.5–6.6). Survival at 1 and 3 years for the silicosis group was 86% and 76%, respectively. Coal workers' pneumoconiosis (CWP) remains a major problem in developing countries. It can present with progressive massive fibrosis and respiratory failure. Hayes et al. (97) presented a case series of eight patients with CWP who underwent transplant. Six individuals remained alive at mean follow-up of 1,013 days. Due to higher incidence of lung cancer in this group, all recipients received a positron emission tomography-computed tomography (PET-CT) scan. Analysis of UNOS data (98) revealed worse survival in the CWP group ($n = 30$) when compared with IPF and silicosis. The difference persisted following adjustments for multiple variables including age and functional status. Median survival in this study was 2.75 years for CWP as opposed to 4.6 years for ILD. It is difficult to draw any firm conclusions, as the data are based on a small patient subset.

PULMONARY LANGERHANS CELL HISTIOCYTOSIS

Pulmonary Langerhans cell histiocytosis (PLCH) is a rare ILD associated with smoking exposure, and some individuals develop pulmonary fibrosis and honeycombing even after smoking cessation. PH was universally found on right heart catheterization (mean PAP 59 mm Hg) in a group of 21 patients awaiting lung transplant with advanced disease due to PLCH (99). However, the presence or severity of PH may not correlate with lung function, and survival for patients with PLCH is better than that for patients with IPF.

Dauriat et al. (100) conducted a retrospective multicentre analysis of 39 patients who underwent transplantation. The survival rates at 1, 2, 5 and 10 years were 76.9%, 63.6%, 57.2% and 53.7%, respectively. Disease reoccurred in 20.5% of cases in this study, and multiple cases have reported this phenomenon (101,102). In two cases of recurrent disease (103), both subjects had continued to smoke despite counselling to quit.

LYMPHANGIOLEIOMYOMATOSIS

Lymphangioleiomyomatosis (LAM) is a rare form of ILD affecting women of reproductive age, and it is linked to the tuberous sclerosis gene complex. Disease progression is variable and may respond to sirolimus therapy, while others may progress to respiratory failure. Important extrapulmonary manifestations include chyloperitoneum, renal angiomyolipomas and meningiomas.

Pechet et al. (104) reported a single centre experience of 12 LAM patients who underwent lung transplantation. There were multiple perioperative complications but all survived to discharge. Boehler et al. (105) conducted a questionnaire survey of 34 LAM transplant recipients. The 1- and 2-year survival rates were 69% and 58%, respectively. Disease recurrence occurred in one individual who died from invasive aspergillosis. Benden et al. (106) reported a series of 61 LAM transplants in a multicentre study, with 1- and 3-year survival of 79% and 73%, respectively. Pleural adhesions and haemorrhage are cited as major intra-operative complications. Post-operatively, native lung pneumothorax and chylothorax occur more frequently than other conditions. Disease recurrence occurred in one recipient in the first and second case series; and four recipients in the latter. Other cases of recurrence have been documented in the literature (107–109). In this study the authors speculated that this was due to migration of benign LAM cells to the lung allograft (110).

DESQUAMATIVE INTERSTITIAL PNEUMONIA

Desquamative interstitial pneumonia (DIP) is a rare condition marked by accumulation of pigment-laden macrophages in the alveoli. It is more frequently encountered in smokers than non-smokers. There are scattered case reports of disease recurrence post-transplant, identified by the presence of intra-alveolar macrophages on transbronchial biopsy (111) or thoracoscopic lung biopsy (112). One improved with high-dose corticosteroids, whereas the other succumbed to infection despite treatment. There are very limited data on outcomes in these patients.

CO-MORBIDITIES IN ILD

GASTRO-OESOPHAGEAL REFLUX DISEASE

Gastro-oesophageal reflux disease (GORD) commonly occurs in IPF and may play a role in its pathogenesis. Early studies in the 1960s using dogs exposed to intra-bronchial hydrochloric acid revealed evidence of hyaline membrane formation and acute pneumonitis in lung biopsies (113). Following these observations multiple studies have suggested a significant association between IPF and acid reflux. Unfortunately there is poor correlation of reflux and symptoms with patients often not reporting typical symptoms of regurgitation or heartburn (114,115).

Both pre- and post-transplant GORD is extremely common in IPF patients. Sweet et al. (116) found that the majority of IPF patients referred for lung transplant have abnormalities on 24-hour pH monitoring with 67% and 30% displaying abnormal distal and proximal acid exposure, respectively. Linden et al. performed surgical fundoplication on 19 IPF individuals placed on the transplant waiting list (117), and although there were anaesthetic concerns over surgery in such a high-risk group, there were no substantial post-operative complications, and fundoplication stabilized supplemental oxygen requirements compared to controls. However, only limited inferences can be made due to the small sample size. This demonstrated that fundoplication could be safely performed in the pre-transplant phase.

A number of issues are likely to exacerbate the tendency to have significant GOR post-transplant. These include changes in diaphragmatic position, injury to the vagus nerve, and immunosuppressive drug side effects. GORD has increasingly become recognized as a risk factor for BOS (118). Laparoscopic fundoplication has been shown to improve long-term outlook in lung transplant recipients with significant reflux. Surgical fundoplication has been associated with improved FEV1 in early BOS and also may influence survival (5-year survival was 71% in fundoplication group versus 48% in overall series) (119). Cantu et al. (120) also showed enhanced freedom from BOS in the early fundoplication group compared to conservative management without anti-reflux surgery.

Thus, it is considered good practice to screen for GORD symptoms in pre-transplant assessment, and candidates with significant reflux symptoms or a history of GORD should be referred for 24-hour pH monitoring to determine its severity.

CARDIOVASCULAR DISEASE

Significant coronary artery disease (CAD) (defined as >50% stenosis of ≥1 coronary arteries) is common in patients with IPF, with one series suggesting a prevalence as high as 30% (121). Severe CAD in the context of poor ventricular function is viewed as an absolute contraindication to lung transplantation, and heart-lung transplant may need to be considered. However, revascularization techniques have evolved, and candidates may be considered if the disease is amenable to stent placement in the absence of left ventricular dysfunction (2,3). Left ventricular impairment may contribute to reduction in exercise tolerance and functional capacity, a phenomenon that is often under-appreciated in studies. Subtle decrease in LV diameters and capacities has been observed on echocardiography on waiting list ILD candidates (122). Sherman et al. (123) looked at the efficacy of interventional techniques in lung transplant recipients with CAD and a preserved left ventricular ejection fraction; concomitant coronary artery bypass graft was performed at the time of surgery, or alternatively, percutaneous coronary

intervention (PCI) was undertaken prior to transplant (see Figure 26.2 for algorithm). Survival outcomes were comparable to recipients without CAD for at least 5 years post-transplant. This suggests that similar algorithms could be adapted for selected candidates on the transplant waiting list.

In addition, cardiac involvement can coexist in some forms of ILD (e.g. sarcoidosis), and pre-transplant workup should include coronary angiograms to assess atherosclerotic burden in high-risk groups.

CORTICOSTEROID USE

Corticosteroids are commonly used to treat a variety of ILDs and present two issues for transplant. First, high-dose steroids pre-transplant are thought to predispose to anastomotic airway complications, although multivariate analyses of airway complication events have not reflected steroid use as a major factor (124,125). Another study detected no differences in hospitalization, intensive care stay and post-operative lung function in the steroid-treated group (126). Many transplant

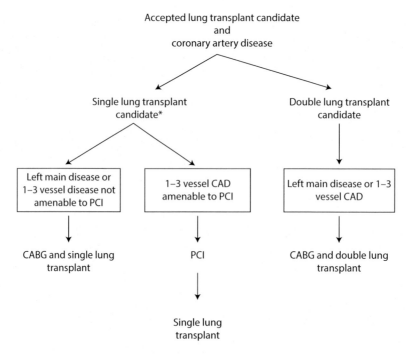

Figure 26.2 Sample coronary artery intervention algorithm for potential lung transplant recipients with coronary artery disease and preserved LV function. (Abbreviations: PCI = percutaneous coronary intervention, CABG = coronary artery bypass graft, CAD = coronary artery disease.) (Reprinted from *Ann Thorac Surg.*, 92(1), Sherman W et al., Lung transplantation and coronary artery disease, 303–8, Copyright 2011, with permission from Elsevier.)

centres insist on an upper steroid threshold prior to listing. Previous guidelines suggest attempting to wean to ≤20 mg prednisolone/day (127). Venuta et al. (128) presented a case where cyclosporine was used as a steroid-sparing agent in IPF, allowing reduction to an acceptable dose.

Second, long-term corticosteroid use may lead to osteoporosis. Risk factors for the ILD group include advanced age, physical inactivity, low muscle mass from deconditioning and smoking history. Lung transplantation often accelerates loss in bone mineral density 6–12 months post-transplant despite vitamin D and calcium supplementation, and osteoporotic fractures were detected in 5 out of 28 transplant patients in one study (129). Early screening using dual-energy x-ray absorptiometry (DEXA) scans, and institution of anti-resorptive therapy is recommended. Pamidronate and hormone replacement therapy prevent bone loss and increase bone mineral density in lung transplant recipients (130).

MALIGNANCY

Le Jeune et al. (131) analysed frequency of malignancies in two ILD subgroups; comparing with age-, gender- and smoking-adjusted controls. They found a higher incidence of lung cancer in IPF (rate ratio 4.96, 95% CI 3.00–8.18). In sarcoidosis, lymphomas were more frequently encountered (rate ratio 7.04, 95% CI 1.54–32.1); as well as skin cancers (rate ratio 1.86, 95% CI 1.11–3.11). Cross-sectional imaging should be carefully scrutinized in pre-assessment, and there should be a low threshold to investigate any suspicious lesions. Mediastinal and hilar nodes are frequently enlarged in ILD patients and may require further imaging modalities such as PET-CT imaging. Enlarged nodes (>10 mm short axis diameter) are also found in sarcoidosis (84%), IPF (67%), CTD (70%), EAA (53%) and cryptogenic organizing pneumonia (36%) (132). If there is any uncertainty, biopsies should be performed to exclude malignancy as this will have implications on eligibility.

PULMONARY HYPERTENSION

Secondary PH is frequently associated with ILD. In one study the frequency was as high as 32%in IPF patients, and this was associated with lower DLCO, need for supplemental oxygen, reduced 6-minute walk distance and exertional desaturation (133).

Mortality risk is higher when PH is present in patients with IPF (odds ratio 2.6, 95% CI 2.3–3.1), and PH is likewise associated with poorer outcomes when present in other ILD, e.g. sarcoidosis. The presence of PH may also influence transplant procedure choice. BLT is traditionally favoured over SLT when ILD is complicated by secondary PH. Pre-transplant PH may predispose to primary graft dysfunction (PGD), and previous studies have suggested that an increase in mean pulmonary artery pressure correlates with the risk of PGD in IPF recipients (134). Bando et al. (135) looked at the effect of SLT on 48 recipients with PH, and although mean pulmonary artery pressure and pulmonary vascular resistance improved post-transplant, it remained higher than the control group. They also discovered increased incidence of haemodynamic instability, pulmonary oedema and prolonged stay in the intensive care unit. However, this study combined patients with primary pulmonary arterial hypertension with those with secondary PH due to other parenchymal diseases. Studies that focused on secondary PH as an individual group observed no clear advantage in survival or complication rates for the BLT group (136,137). Fitton et al. noted slightly higher risk of reperfusion injury, but survival outcomes were preserved in the SLT group (138).

NT-pro BNP and echocardiography are helpful in the diagnosis of PH. However, echocardiographic estimation of pulmonary artery pressures is not always accurate in end-stage lung disease (139). Treatment of secondary PH includes management of the underlying ILD, diuretics for fluid overload and oxygen therapy. For those with CTD-associated ILD, referral to a centre that specializes in treatment of PH is recommended for vasodilator therapy. There are no established guidelines on vasodilator treatment for other ILD groups. There have been anecdotal reports of successful bridging to transplant with sildenafil (140) and treprostinil (141) when used to improve pulmonary haemodynamics pre-transplant, the former with PLCH and the latter with IPF.

ADVANCED AGE

Increasing recipient age is associated with worse long-term survival, which is probably related to frailty and other co-morbid conditions. Allograft survival half-life was 3.5 years for recipients over age 65 years as opposed to 6.7 years for recipients aged

35–49 years (142). In a UK study, the average age at presentation of IPF was 71 years, whereas average age for other ILD conditions such as sarcoidosis was 47 years (47). This makes the issue particularly relevant for IPF due to its usual presentation later in life. Previously published guidelines for the selection of lung transplant candidates suggested the following age limits: HLT 55 years, BLT 60 years and SLT 65 years (127). However, subsequent updates have relaxed this requirement and changed the age over 65 category to a relative contraindication (2,3). Older recipients must be carefully assessed for comorbidities, and the decision to list should be based on 'physiological age' rather than chronological age. Candidates over 75 years of age are unlikely to be suitable candidates for lung transplantation.

ALLOCATION OF ORGANS

INTRODUCTION

Allocation systems attempt to provide a framework for the optimal matching between a potential donor and recipient. A number of different systems are currently in existence across the world. In the United States, high waiting list mortality for patients with IPF was the major driving factor for the adoption of the Lung Allocation Score (LAS) as a means of optimizing lung allocation. Previously, prioritization was based on waiting times, which disadvantaged IPF patients due to rapid disease progression and leads to a high waiting list mortality. The LAS was developed in an attempt to circumvent this problem. Each potential recipient receives a waiting list urgency score, based on a cumulative score of their predicted pre- and post-transplant survival (143). The model is weighted towards waiting list mortality risk rather than post-transplant survival. The result has been substantial increase in the number of lung transplants performed for IPF, for one, combined with the desired reduction in waiting list deaths. This has come at the cost of increased perioperative mortality, length of hospital stay and decreased survival. Currently, such a lung allocation system does not exist in the United Kingdom. Each transplant centre allocates the organ according to greatest clinical need. Some centres keep a list of the sickest patients, who are given priority consideration. With the rapidly progressive nature

of IPF, it is vital that these individuals are escalated promptly in the event of deterioration.

SELECTION OF DONORS

Functional characteristics of the donor determine the likely viability of the transplanted organ. Investigations include chest radiograph, PaO_2/FiO_2 ratio, smoking history, evidence of aspiration or sepsis, history of trauma, bronchoscopy findings and positive microbiology results. Once the organ is removed, it is externally inspected and palpated for underlying nodules. The decision on whether to use the organ is based on all the clinical findings. The logistics of the procurement process also play an important role due to the influence on anticipated donor lung ischaemic times.

Recipients are matched primarily in terms of ABO blood type and lung size, and these two variables are also the major determinants of a candidate's time spent on the waiting list. Those with blood type AB generally have the shortest waiting times, as they can receive organs from any donor. Average waiting time is currently approximately 1 year for lung transplantation. Newer methods are currently being developed to expand the pool of available organs (see section on *ex vivo* lung perfusion). Risk factors associated with the donor, quality of the graft and recipient preferences may also need to be taken into account by the patient and the team. When patients are listed they are given a series of donor options to consider that include donor age, smoker or non-smoker and previous history of cerebral malignancy. These are discussed at the time of listing, and an agreement is reached on what is acceptable for the recipient.

BILATERAL VERSUS SINGLE LUNG TRANSPLANT IN IPF

Both types of transplant procedures are viable options for patients with IPF. Cumulative evidence from a number of studies has provided conflicting observations. Some studies suggest that there is no survival difference between the BLT versus SLT procedures (144), while others suggest better long-term survival in BLT versus SLT recipients (145–147). Thabut et al. (148) analyzed UNOS data and suggested that short-term mortality may be higher in the first year post-BLT, although this early mortality is offset by better long-term survival. There are, however, multiple confounders in this argument, not least of which is the propensity to offer BLT to younger and fitter individuals. Additionally the opportunity of a transplant is the major issue, and this may be significantly higher for a SLT versus BLT procedure. In support of this, Force et al. (149) performed a similar retrospective analysis of UNOS data for IPF. Although the crude data appeared to show a survival advantage of BLT over SLT, the difference was no longer significant following adjustment for 25 covariates including recipient age. Additionally, BLT recipients have higher rates of PGD, need for cardiopulmonary bypass, prolonged time on mechanical ventilation and length of hospitalization (144). Furthermore, there are also reports of increased airway dehiscence and need for dialysis in the BLT group (146). In the longer term, BLT may be less prone to the effects of BOS compared to SLT, and one study found reduced rate of FEV1 decline among BLT recipients (150). BLT also eliminates the occurrence of native lung complications such as pneumothoraces, infection or recurrent ILD.

However, as highlighted earlier, there is a significant lack of donor organ availability, leading to long waiting times and persistent high waiting list mortality. Thus, one must consider whether a set of lungs from one lung donor should be implanted separately into two recipients versus offering slight survival benefit to one recipient by performing a BLT. These considerations are supported by a study that found that when IPF patients were listed only for BLT, they had significantly higher waiting times and increased mortality risk while on the transplant list. While this has improved by the implementation of the LAS in the United States, a debate continues about the most ethical and efficacious way to allocate organs. The argument for or against SLT versus BLT as the right procedure for patients with IPF or non-IPF forms of ILD remains unresolved, and opinions are counterbalanced by advantages and disadvantages for each procedure (see Table 26.4).

Current practice is weighted towards a preference for BLT, especially in younger individuals with fewer co-morbidities that may have a significant impact on long-term survival. SLT tends to be reserved for higher-risk individuals or older candidates. The presence of PH may also sway the opinion for BLT, though practice differs widely among transplant institutions when secondary PH complicates fibrotic ILD.

GENERAL OUTCOMES

The ISHLT registry is an international repository of information on outcomes for lung transplant recipients, and these data are collected and collated from over 250 hospitals performing lung transplants. The registry has been running for over 25 years and has a wealth of patient data that allow macro-examination of outcomes in lung transplantation. While there is a wealth of data in the registry, there is also a very broad range of practice among contributing centres, and this may be reflected in limitations and accuracy of the available information.

For example, insights into the impact of age can be gleaned from the large number of recipients enrolled, and these data indicate that crude survival is worse in older age groups, especially in recipients who are over 65 years of age. Positive donor CMV status and recipient colonization with multiresistant organisms may also predict poorer outcomes (142).

Table 26.4 Advantages and disadvantages of BLT compared to SLT

Advantages of BLT	Disadvantages of BLT
Better long-term survival	Increased time on the waiting list which may translate to higher mortality rates
Reduced BOS related mortality	More complicated procedure
Better functional outcome	Increased ischaemic times
Less native lung complications (pneumothorax, opportunistic infections)	Increased use of cardiopulmonary bypass (risk of coagulopathy, neurological sequelae and prolonged wean from mechanical ventilation)
	Increased rates of primary graft dysfunction, airway complications and short term mortality
	Only benefits one recipient

Examining the registry for factors that favour long-term over (>10 years) medium-term (1–5 years) outcomes reveals positive signals for BLT, recipient age less than 35, higher levels of HLA-matching and less frequent hospitalization for rejection episodes (151). These data provide interesting pointers for discussion and allow programs to have some guidance about how to assess risk for groups of patients.

Historically, lung transplant outcomes were always reported in terms of survival at fixed time points. However, the assessment of the intervention on the recipient's quality of life is increasingly favoured. It is recognized that lung transplantation may also confer enhancement in physiological measurements with significant improvements in FEV1, FVC and 6-minute walk distance (152). Studies that have used HRQOL tools have been limited because there is no universally adopted scoring system for lung transplantation. However, one cross-sectional study revealed that lung transplant recipients have significantly higher scores (St. George's Respiratory Questionnaire/SGRQ) compared with a control group with obstructive pulmonary disease (153). The majority of the lung recipients in this study were satisfied with their outcome with 92% saying they would undergo a repeat operation. Kugler et al. (154) found that HRQOL outcomes post-transplant are comparable to the healthy population with the exception of social functioning. Reduction in HRQOL scores was associated with infection, late acute rejection and BOS. Singer et al. (155) similarly compared functional scores using SGRQ, 36-item short form health survey (SF-36) and other tools. They found improvement in all quality-of-life measures following lung transplantation, although the benefit is not as high in the ILD group compared to other transplant indications. These studies are limited by their design and selection bias, and while they provide some insight, these investigations are by no means comprehensive.

CHALLENGES

The rapidly progressive nature of IPF produces a narrow window between first presentation and eventual decline. Early referral and assessment are thus essential for all potential candidates; this is reflected in the most recent guidelines LINK (see section on referral). Post-transplant complications affect the long-term success of ILD recipients, especially BOSLINK (see section 'Complications and follow-up').

Re-transplantation is increasingly indicated for PGD, airway complications or BOS. In the case of SLT, the failed allograft is often removed due to infection risk and potential for sustained alloimmune stimulation. BLT is a common alternative option. To be eligible for re-transplantation, recipients must not have contraindications but must have preserved post-transplant rehabilitation potential. However, survival outcomes are poorer when compared with primary transplantation. Survival at 1, 3, 5 and 10 years is 65%, 46.5%, 37.2% and 18.5%, respectively, for all recipients, and median survival is 2.5 years compared with 5.7 years for primary transplantation (www.ishlt.org/registries).

The current climate of donor organ insufficiency limits the number of life-prolonging procedures carried out each year, which makes decisions regarding re-transplantation a difficult issue for transplant centres that offer re-transplantation.

COMPLICATIONS AND FOLLOW-UP

CHALLENGES

Transplant candidates with ILD can have many idiosyncratic, disease-associated problems that can present serious challenges to successful transplantation. First, certain forms of ILD such as CTD can be associated with extrapulmonary features and vasculitic processes that can present barriers to transplant (see section 'Disease-specific considerations'). Patients with ILD are also prone to having co-morbidities such as PH, which can influence the decision process as to type of transplant. Many patients with IPF can have rapidly declining lung function, which may provide a narrow window between first presentation and precipitous decline. Early referral and assessment are thus essential for all potential candidates, and this is reflected in the most recent guidelines (see section 'Criteria for referral').

POST-TRANSPLANT COMPLICATIONS

Post-transplant complications are often classified according to the time when they occur after

Table 26.5 Post-transplant complications categorized into different time stages

Immediate Complications (<24hrs)
- Primary graft dysfunction
- Hyperacute rejection
- Pneumothorax and persistent air leak
- Haemorrhage
- Phrenic nerve dysfunction

Acute Complications (<3mths)
- Acute rejection
- Infection (bacterial, viral and fungal)
- Airway dehiscence
- Wound or sternal dehiscence
- Thromboembolic disease
- Vascular anastomotic complications
- Neurological complications e.g. PRES
- Gastrointestinal complications

Chronic Complications (>3mths)
- Bronchiolitis obliterans syndrome
- Post-transplant lymphoproliferative disease (PTLD) and other malignancies
- Late airway complications (airway stenosis, fistula, bronchomalacia)
- Hernia
- Drug interactions and side effects
- Transbronchial biopsy associated complications

Source: Adapted from Vigneswaran WT. Lung transplantation. In: *Lung Biology in Health and Disease.* London, UK: Informa Healthcare. 2010, xix, 448 p., 8 p. of plates. Chapter 25. Copyright 2010, Taylor & Francis Group; Informa Healthcare. With permission.

transplant. Immediate complications are considered to occur within 24 hours of the procedure, acute complications within the first 3 months, and chronic complications beyond 3 months (see Table 26.5). This section gives an overview of frequently encountered complications following transplantation. Early identification and management of these complications are essential to optimize post-transplant outcomes.

IMMEDIATE COMPLICATIONS

PRIMARY GRAFT DYSFUNCTION

Primary graft dysfunction (PGD) is a form of reperfusion injury following lung transplantation and represents a complex phenomenon that has multiple potential contributory factors. The reperfusion of the lungs with recipient blood can cause a sequence of host and donor interactions which can result in damage to the alveolar endothelium and trigger a pro-inflammatory cascade. Clinically, this is characterized by severe hypoxaemia (by definition within the first 72 hours), pulmonary oedema and diffuse radiographic infiltrates (156) (see Figures 26.3 and 26.4). The ISHLT working group proposed a grading system for PGD based on chest radiograph appearance and PaO₂/FiO₂ ratio (see Table 26.6). Blood gas analysis is based on 24-hour time points up to 72 hours (T0 to T72), which in combination with the chest radiograph allows the PGD severity to be graded from 0 to 3. The main differential diagnostic considerations in this situation are hyperacute rejection, infection and cardiogenic pulmonary oedema.

The incidence of PGD for restrictive lung diseases has been estimated to range between 10% and 40%. Risk factors for PGD can be subdivided into donor, recipient and surgical factors (157,158) (see Table 26.7). Donor risk factors include patient demographics, smoking history, older donors and the mechanism of death. Recipient risk factors

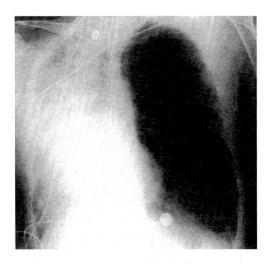

Figures 26.3 Portable chest radiograph depicting primary graft dysfunction post right SLT, showing typical diffuse infiltrates in the allograft. (Reprinted from *Chest.*, 114(1), Christie JD et al., Primary graft failure following lung transplantation, 51–60, Copyright 1998, with permission from Elsevier.)

that have been identified include the presence of PH, obesity and recipient age. In contrast, there is no firm evidence for secondary PH as a risk factor for PGD in IPF. Other considerations that are perceived as likely to have an impact on risk of PGD include pleural adhesions, intra-operative bleeding, donor-recipient size mismatch and use of cardiopulmonary bypass.

The importance of PGD cannot be understated as it significantly increases the risk of in-hospital mortality, prolonged need for mechanical ventilation and length of stay in the intensive care unit (159). Prekker et al. (160) found that the early 12-hour trend in the PaO2/FiO2 ratio may help to predict 90-day mortality. Christie et al. (161) found impaired functional recovery and reduced 6-minute walk test distance up to 1 year following discharge in recipients with PGD (previously referred to as primary graft failure) versus recipients who did not develop PGD. Additionally, PGD may increase risk of developing BOS, and this risk is apparent even after adjustment for other

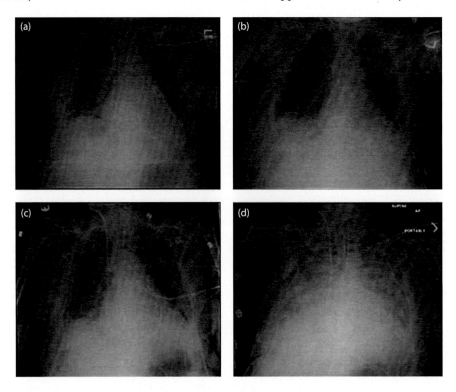

Figure 26.4 Radiographic progression of infiltrates seen on serial chest radiographs for an individual who developed primary graft dysfunction. Radiographs were taken on consecutive days from immediate post-operative date **(a-d)**. (Reprinted from Vigneswaran WT. Lung transplantation. In: *Lung Biology in Health and Disease*. London, UK: Informa Healthcare. 2010, xix, 448 p., 8 p. of plates. Chapter 26. Copyright 2010, Taylor & Francis Group; Informa Healthcare. With permission.)

Table 26.6 Recommended severity grading criteria for primary graft dysfunction

Grade	PaO$_2$/FiO$_2$	Radiographic infiltrates consistent with pulmonary oedema
0	>300	Absent
1	>300	Present
2	200–300	Present
3	<200	Present

Source: Reprinted from *J Heart Lung Transplant*, 24(10), Christie JD et al., Report of the ISHLT Working Group on Primary Lung Graft Dysfunction part II: Definition. A consensus statement of the International Society for Heart and Lung Transplantation, 1454–9, Copyright 2005, with permission from Elsevier.

Table 26.7 Potential risk factors for primary graft dysfunction organized into donor, recipient and surgical variables

	Risk factors for PGD
Donor variables	Female gender
	African American ethnicity
	Age >45yr or <21yr
	Possibly smoking history >20 pck yr
	Prolonged mechanical ventilation
	Aspiration pneumonia/Trauma
	Multiple blood transfusions
	Haemodynamic instability
Recipient variables	Primary pulmonary hypertension (secondary pulmonary hypertension unclear)
Surgical variables	Ischaemic time >7–8hrs
	Preservation solution (temperature, volume and flush technique)
	Storage temperature
	Vascular anastomotic obstruction

significant risk factors including acute rejection, lymphocytic bronchitis and viral infections (162).

The management of PGD consists of managing any identifiable cause and providing supportive measures. The major pathology is increased capillary permeability with resultant pronounced alveolar oedema that can cause profound hypoxaemia. One essential component of management is careful fluid restriction with the use of high-dose diuretics and renal replacement therapy if required. There are limited data on ventilation strategies, but a lung-protective approach is recommended that is similar to management of acute respiratory distress syndrome (ARDS). Other theoretical approaches include using inhaled nitric oxide, intravenous prostaglandin (PGE2) or nebulized surfactant (163). Early institution of ECMO is a potential option and can reduce the risk of potential of barotrauma from aggressive ventilatory support.

HYPERACUTE REJECTION

Hyperacute rejection is caused by pre-formed donor-specific antibodies in the recipient that bind to donor antigens and cause massive endothelial injury when the implanted lung is reperfused. This injury appears to occur via predominantly complement-mediated pathways. Fortunately, this complication is significantly less frequent with the improved screening of recipients for pre-formed anti-HLA antibodies pre-transplant. Hyperacute rejection is associated with significant mortality and should be distinguished from PGD. The manifestation is similar to PGD with sudden-onset pulmonary oedema and haemodynamic instability. There is histopathological evidence of alveolar damage and IgG deposition in the alveolar septa (164). Anecdotal cases have been treated with plasmapheresis, antithymocyte globulin and cyclophosphamide (165).

PLEURAL COMPLICATIONS

Pneumothorax is the most common pleural complication and may be caused by issues in the donor lung, disruption of a bronchial anastomosis, a native lung complication or pleural space chest drain dysfunction. Pneumothoraces may be relatively transient; however, if there is a major airway or parenchymal problem, resolution may be delayed. Other potential pleural problems include parapneumonic effusion, haemothorax and chylothorax. The majority of these resolve with conservative measures or chest tube insertion. Empyema can be associated with sepsis and increased mortality post-transplant (166). Thoracoscopic or surgical intervention may be required for recurrent pneumothorax or the presence of complex pleural disease (167).

NERVE INJURY

Phrenic nerve injury may be encountered after any form of cardiothoracic surgery. Suggested mechanisms include direct injury during dissection, indirect stretching during pericardial manipulation or hypothermic nerve injury. Ferdinand et al. (168) found evidence of phrenic nerve dysfunction in 42.8% of heart-lung recipients and 9.3% of lung transplant recipients using nerve conduction studies. Phrenic nerve dysfunction can lead to significantly increased time on mechanical ventilation and length of stay in intensive care. Non-invasive ventilation may help the weaning process from mechanical ventilation as diaphragmatic function recovers (169). Finally, the left vocal cord is supplied by the recurrent laryngeal nerve, which loops under the left main bronchus; if this is transected, the patient may end up with a hoarse voice due to vocal fold paresis/paralysis and be at increased risk of aspiration.

ACUTE COMPLICATIONS

BACTERIAL INFECTIONS

Bacterial infections account for the majority of post-transplant infections. Nosocomial infections and multidrug-resistant pathogens can invade the host in the hospital setting, and opportunistic organisms can colonize the allograft. This infection risk is increased by heavy immunosuppression, lack of cough reflex from denervation, and impaired mucociliary clearance (170). Recurrent infection also increases the risk of BOS via alloimmune stimulation. Frequently identified organisms causing allograft and/or native lung infections include *Klebsiella pneumoniae*, *Pseudomonas aeruginosa*, *Escherichia coli* and *Staphylococcus aureus* (171). Other potential culprits include *Legionella*, *Nocardia* and *Listeria monocytogenes*.

In the presence of positive donor cultures, a prolonged course of appropriate antibiotics is usually mandatory. Emphasis should be placed on strict hand hygiene and early removal of invasive devices (e.g. intravenous lines, endotracheal tube and urinary catheters) as soon as possible post-transplant. A low threshold for commencing empirical antimicrobial treatment may be warranted with a switch to subsequent targeted therapy according to culture results. Pneumococcal vaccination should be recommended for all recipients to help protect against *Streptococcus pneumoniae*.

VIRAL INFECTIONS

CMV infection can either be due to reactivation of latent infection or be acquired *de novo* from a seropositive donor (or, rarely, other routes of transmission). CMV viraemia may lead to multiple end-organ involvement, including CMV pneumonia, gastrointestinal disease, hepatitis and retinitis (172). Morbidity from CMV infection has declined due to introduction of prophylactic anti-virals plus early detection with quantitative viral polymerase chain reaction assays. Oral valganciclovir has revolutionized the ability to provide long-term prophylaxis, especially in CMV mismatched individuals. Treatment of severe infection includes intravenous ganciclovir or foscarnet in drug-resistant cases, and response can be monitored with serial CMV serum titres. CMV pneumonia treated successfully with ganciclovir appears not to be associated with BOS or affect survival (173).

Epstein–Barr virus (EBV), which causes infectious mononucleosis, can be acquired or reactivate and drive post-transplant lymphoproliferative disease (PTLD). Other respiratory viruses, which can be seasonally quite prevalent in the community in both immunosuppressed and immunocompetent individuals also represent a significant risk to transplant recipients. Influenza, parainfluenza, respiratory syncytial virus (RSV) and adenovirus can all cause community-acquired respiratory virus infections, and vaccination to protect from influenza A is recommended for all lung transplant recipients. Oral ribavirin therapy may be a safer alternative than inhaled, nebulized ribavirin for the treatment of RSV infection (174). Recent guidelines have also advocated transplantation in hepatitis B and C and in HIV-positive patients (2), but these individuals should be referred to centres experienced in managing these conditions.

FUNGAL INFECTIONS

Aspergillus and *Candida* spp. are frequent fungal colonizers in the immunosuppressed population. In a retrospective study of 251 recipients, *Aspergillus* was found to be present in 28% of pulmonary fibrosis cases (175). Pathology ranges from simple colonization to tracheobronchial mucosal lesions and invasive aspergillosis. The presence of *Aspergillus* is associated with reduced 5-year survival, and mortality of invasive aspergillosis is very high (78%). Diagnosis is usually detected and confirmed on specimens retrieved from airways (e.g. via direct aspiration or BAL) or histopathologic tissue samples for invasive disease. The presence of ulceration and pseudomembrane formation at bronchoscopy should trigger suspicion for the presence of tracheobronchial aspergillosis. Prophylaxis and treatment with anti-fungal agents such as imidazoles are key in preventing complications, and treatment with amphotericin may be required for invasive disease.

Candida is another common commensal that colonizes the skin and mucosa. In a large retrospective analysis, 8.3% of lung and heart-lung transplant recipients had evidence of *Candida* infection (176). Tracheobronchitis is the most common form of infection, but bloodstream and invasive infections may occur, and *Candida* infection has been associated with higher 1-year mortality. Other potential fungal pathogens include *Cryptococcus neoformans* which can lead to meningitis, and histoplasmosis can occur in endemic regions (and endogenous reactivation is possible). Most transplant centres deploy prophylactic co-trimoxazole,

which has brought down the incidence of *Pneumocystis jiroveci* pneumonia.

ACUTE REJECTION

Acute cellular rejection is a common post-transplant event and usually occurs within the first 3–6 months. It may present with worsening respiratory symptoms or a drop in lung function, but in some cases it is only detected on routine surveillance transbronchial biopsies, and recipients may be asymptomatic. Histologically, acute cellular rejection is divided into grade A (perivascular inflammatory infiltrates) and grade B (lymphocytic bronchiolitis) categories. Each category is then ranked (e.g. A1 to A3 for acute cellular rejection) depending on the severity of lymphocyte influx and inflammation, and it is important to exclude other etiologies such as infection before confirming the diagnosis. Early treatment is considered to be essential, as both perivascular infiltrates and lymphocytic bronchiolitis are risk factors for the subsequent development of BOS (177). First-line treatment is with high-dose corticosteroids. Antibody treatments (e.g. alemtuzumab, anti-thymoglobulin or addition of sirolimus) may be considered in refractory cases.

AIRWAY COMPLICATIONS

Anastomotic dehiscence is a complication that affects the early post-transplant phase. The incidence has declined due to improved surgical techniques, reduced ischaemic times and improved perioperative management. Moreno et al. (178) identified 12.6% of their patients with airway complications with a mortality of 1%. Significant risk factors included BLT, intubation more than 72 hours, and airway colonization with pathogenic bacteria or fungi. Antibiotic and anti-fungal prophylaxis may play a preventive role as well as reduce the extent of fungal membranes in anastomotic tissues at subsequent bronchoscopies (179). Dehiscence is detected on bronchoscopy or on CT scan. In the case of failure with surgical repair, transplant pneumonectomy may be necessary. Airway stenosis usually presents at a much later stage post-transplant. Conventional management includes balloon dilatation, endobronchial stent placement or surgical intervention in severe cases.

PULMONARY VASCULAR ANASTOMOTIC STENOSES

Stenoses of vascular anastomoses are unusual complications but can severely affect graft function and viability. Clark et al. (180) reported a case series of vascular complications in 109 patients (4 females and 1 male). They proposed possible donor-recipient bronchus size mismatch and difficult intra-operative access when constructing the anastomoses to explain the gender disparity. The characteristic appearance on chest radiograph is infiltrates in a lobar distribution. Confirmatory investigative techniques include isotope perfusion scanning, HRCT imaging, transoesophageal echocardiography, and pulmonary angiography. Some cases can be managed conservatively, whereas others require angioplasty, stent insertion or re-operation.

NEUROLOGICAL COMPLICATIONS

Neurological symptoms post-transplant include headaches and neuromuscular complications. A retrospective analysis of lung transplant recipients found that complications often relate to immunosuppressant toxicity or opportunistic infections (181). In younger recipients, high immunosuppressive drug levels can predispose to posterior reversible encephalopathy syndrome (PRES). This manifests with symptoms of headaches and seizures early post-transplant. In these cases, temporary suspension or change of the calcineurin inhibitor usually leads to symptom resolution.

THROMBOEMBOLIC EVENTS

Lung transplant recipients are prone to thromboembolic events and should receive appropriate prophylaxis. Due to disruption of the bronchial circulation and a lack of collateral circulation, the threat of infarcts should pulmonary embolism occur is substantially higher. There should be a low threshold for performing investigations with V/Q scan or CT pulmonary angiogram if pulmonary embolism is suspected. Patients should be treated with standard anti-coagulation, although urokinase infusion with selective pulmonary artery catheter placement has also been performed (182). In this cohort of 116 lung or heart-lung recipients,

12.1% developed thromboembolic events and 6% had pulmonary embolism.

GASTROENTEROLOGICAL COMPLICATIONS

Gastrointestinal complications are very common post-transplant. In a retrospective analysis of 208 recipients, 16% of IPF recipients developed some form of gastrointestinal complications. Frequently encountered problems include biliary complications, diarrhoea, peptic ulceration, small bowel obstruction, gastroparesis, reflux, cholecystitis and choledocholithiasis (183). Diarrhoea and colitis are common issues which may be related to the use of antibiotics or immunosuppression. Transplant-specific issues such as CMV colitis need to be borne in mind as well as colitis caused by *Clostridium difficile*.

Gastroparesis may arise from intra-operative vagal nerve damage, medications, metabolic issues or infections. Untreated, it can predispose to GORD and aspiration. The diagnosis can be confirmed with gastric emptying scintigraphy studies. Prokinetic agents may be tried if refractory to other interventions, and jejunal feeding tubes may be instituted as a last resort (184). Transcutaneous electrical nerve stimulation (TENS) has been trialed in the treatment of gastroparesis in lung transplant recipients (185). Some patients who are symptomatic may require Botox injections to alleviate acute gastric distension.

CHRONIC COMPLICATIONS

BRONCHIOLITIS OBLITERANS SYNDROME

BOS is the most profound contributor to long-term mortality post-transplant. It is characterized by progressive small airways disease and persistent airflow obstruction. Histologically, inflammation and fibroblast proliferation are present and lead to an obliteration of bronchioles. BOS is usually a diagnosis of exclusion that is made in the presence of deteriorating lung function that cannot be attributed to concomitant infection, acute rejection or airway complications. Freedom from BOS for patients with IPF is 91.1%, 68.2%, 51.1% and 23.7%

at 1, 3, 5 and 10 years, respectively, post-transplant (www.ishlt.org/registries). Currently, therapies for BOS have limited success, and limited progress in finding effective therapies has been made over the last decade.

Acute cellular rejection episodes and lymphocytic bronchiolitis are both associated with the development of BOS (186). CMV pneumonitis, human leucocyte antigen (HLA) mismatches and late-onset acute rejection were also identified as risk factors in a multivariate analysis (187). CMV prophylaxis has been associated with a reduction in infectious complications and incidence of BOS (188), and has become the standard treatment in many transplant centres. PGD (162) and bacterial infections such as *Pseudomonas aeruginosa* (189) may also play important roles. GORD is a known risk factor (118), and surgical fundoplication is indicated for significant reflux disease.

Current prevention of BOS relies on minimizing risk factors and optimizing immunosuppression regimens. Tacrolimus may be slightly better than cyclosporine when looking at freedom from acute rejection at 6 months and 1 year (190) and freedom from BOS stage 0p (191). However, differences in BOS rates were not significant, and none of these studies were blinded. Earlier studies suggested superiority of mycophenolate mofetil over azathioprine as an anti-metabolite (given in addition to a calcineurin inhibitor), although no differences in BOS rates were observed in a multicentre randomized trial (192). Azithromycin may have an immunomodulatory effect and slow progression of BOS (193), and more recent data show that it may arrest BOS progression and improve lung function in some recipients. Other therapies that have been used to treat BOS include antithymocyte globulin, total lymphoid irradiation and extracorporeal photophoresis. Re-transplantation may be the last resort option for some refractory cases.

DRUG INTERACTION AND TOXICITY

Immunosuppression regimes vary across different transplant centres. Standard triple therapy includes a calcineurin inhibitor (tacrolimus or cyclosporine), antimetabolite (azathioprine or mycophenolate) and low-dose corticosteroids. All of these treatment regimens are associated with

side effects and potential drug-drug interactions (see Tables 26.8 and 26.9). Most immunosuppressants predispose to systemic hypertension, hyperlipidaemia, renal dysfunction and diabetes mellitus, all of which increase cardiovascular risk. These issues necessitate regular appraisal of the medication regime for any patient in order to limit toxicities.

Renal impairment is commonly related to calcineurin inhibitor toxicity, and this risk may be exacerbated by systemic hypertension, diabetes and other nephrotoxic drugs. Worsening renal function should prompt a thorough medication review, particularly to ensure that calcineurin inhibitor levels are not excessive and that systemic hypertension is properly controlled. If proteinuria is absent, mTOR inhibitors (e.g. sirolimus or everolimus) may be considered. Referral to transplant nephrology may be advisable if renal impairment continues to worsen.

MALIGNANCY

PTLD and skin cancer are the most common malignancies encountered post-transplant. The incidence of PTLD has been estimated to range from 6.4% to 20% of lung transplant recipients (194). It is driven by immunosuppression and EBV infection, and primary EBV infection may be more influential than EBV re-activation (195). Histological classification helps prognostication and management strategies. The allograft is commonly involved, but PTLD may involve extrapulmonary organs, which portends a worse prognosis. Good cores of involved tissue are required for histological analysis of the architecture and lymphocyte clonality, which are needed to establish the diagnosis. The first line of therapy is to reduce the level of immunosuppression (the cell cycle inhibitor in particular), and approximately 20% of patients will respond favourably to this. If relaxing the intensity of immunosuppression fails to induce remission, additional measures must be taken. If the tumour is CD20-positive, rituximab as a single agent may be an option (194). However, if this is not the case, standard chemotherapy for lymphoma may be required.

Dermatological malignancies occur frequently in transplant recipients. Squamous cell carcinoma is the most common skin cancer, and it is strongly linked to cumulative immunosuppression over time and extent of sun exposure. Transplant

Table 26.8 Common side effects of immunosuppressive medications

Drug	Mechanism of action	Side effects	Interactions
Tacrolimus (FK-506)	Binds with FK-binding protein 12 and inhibits calcineurin and T cell activation	• Hypertension • Hypercholesterolaemia • Diabetes mellitus • Renal toxicity • Neurotoxicity (headaches, seizures and PRES)	Cytochrome P450 metabolism (needs drug monitoring)
Cyclosporine	Binds to cyclophilin and inhibits calcineurin and T cell activation	• Hypertension • Hypercholesterolaemia • Gingival hyperplasia • Hirsutism • Renal toxicity (acute reversible, chronic nephrotoxicity • Neurotoxicity (tremor, headaches, seizures, PRES)	Cytochrome P450 metabolism (needs drug monitoring)
Sirolimus (rapamycin)	Binds with FK-binding protein 12 and blocks activation of mTOR, inhibits cell cycle progression of T cells	• Hypertension • Hyperlipidaemia • Delayed wound healing • Haematological (anaemia, thrombocytopaenia) • Pulmonary toxicity (pneumonitis) • Peripheral oedema	Cytochrome P-450 3A4 (CYP3A4) and p-glycoprotein (P-gp) metabolism (needs drug monitoring)
Mycophenolate Mofetil	Inhibits *de novo* guanine nucleotide synthesis and T/B cell proliferation	• Gastrointestinal (vomiting, diarrhoea, oral ulceration) • Haematological (anaemia, leucopaenia) • Increased cytomegalovirus infection risk	Levels decreased by magnesium, aluminium hydroxide antacids, cholestyramine, cyclosporin Levels increased by aciclovir and probenecid
Azathioprine	Inhibits *de novo* purine nucleotide synthesis and T/B cell proliferation	• Haematological (anaemia, leucopaenia, thrombocytopaenia - check TPMT genotype) • Gastrointestinal (vomiting, diarrhoea, abnormal liver function) • Pancreatitis	Levels increased fivefold by allopurinol Reduces warfarin levels
Corticosteroids	Reduce transcription of proinflammatory cytokines IL1, IL 2, IFN-γ, TNF-α	• Hypertension • Diabetes mellitus • Osteoporosis • Hyperlipidaemia • Gastritis/peptic ulcer disease • Weight gain • Avascular necrosis • Skin atrophy • Muscle wasting • Cataracts and glaucoma	Cytochrome P450 metabolism

(Continued)

Table 26.8 (*Continued*) Common side effects of immunosuppressive medications

Drug	Potential complications
Corticosteroids	Glucose intolerance
	Diabetes mellitus
	Infection
	Systemic hypertension
	Increased risk of cardiovascular disease
	Dyslipidaemia
	Excessive weight gain obesity/change in physical appearance
	Growth retardation in children
	Osteoporosis
	Avascular necrosis
	Myopathy
	Glaucoma/cataracts
	Skin atrophy
	Psychological change/sleep disturbance
Cyclosporin A	Nephrotoxicity
	Systemic hypertension
	Hyperkalaemia, hypomagnesaemia
	Seizure, headache, tremor
	Hepatotoxicity
	Gastrointestinal (nausea, vomiting, diarrhoea, rarely pancreatitis)
	Hirsutism, pruritus, gingival hypertrophy
	Haemolytic uremic syndrome (rare)
Tacrolimus	Nephrotoxicity
	Systemic hypertension
	Hyperkalaemia, hypomagnesemia
	Hyperglycemia, diabetes mellitus
	Prolonged QT interval
	Nausea, vomiting, diarrhoea, constipation
	Tremor, headache, insomnia
Mycophenolate	Systemic hypertension
	Hematologic (myelosuppression, leukopenia, neutropenia)
	Gastrointestinal haemorrhage
	Peripheral oedema
	Neurologic (confusion, tremor, headache)
	Gastrointestinal (nausea, vomiting diarrhoea, constipation)
	Cough
Azathioprine	Hematologic (leukopenia, thrombocytopenia, megaloblastic anaemia)
	Pancreatitis (2%–12%)
	Hepatotoxicity (3%–13%)
	Gastrointestinal (gastritis, nausea, vomiting)
	Malignancy
Sirolimus	Pulmonary toxicity
	Delayed healing
	Systematic hypertension
	Hematologic (pancytopenia, thrombocytopenia, anaemia)

(*Continued*)

Table 26.8 (*Continued*) Common side effects of immunosuppressive medications

Drug	Potential complications
	Hyperlipidemia/hypercholesterolemia
	Hepatotoxicity
	Neurologic (asthenia, headache)
	Arthralgia
	Peripheral oedema

Source: Reprinted from Vigneswaran WT. Lung transplantation. In: *Lung Biology in Health and Disease*. London, UK: Informa Healthcare. 2010, xix, 448 p., 8 p. of plates. Chapter 37. Copyright 2010, Taylor & Francis Group; Informa Healthcare. With permission.

Table 26.9 Various drugs that can interfere with metabolism of immunosuppressive medications via cytochrome p450 pathway

Drugs that inhibit cytochrome P450 (increase levels of cyclosporine/tacrolimus)	Drugs that induce cytochrome P450 (decrease levels of cyclosporine/tacrolimus)
Calcium channel blockers	Anti-convulsants
Diltiazem	Carbamazepine
Nicardipine	Phenobarbital
Nifedipine	Phenytoin
Verapamil	Antibiotics
Anti-arrhythmics	Nafcillin
Amiodarone	Rifabutin
Macrolide antibiotics	Rifampin
Clarithromycin	Octreotide
Erythromycin	Ticlopidine
Antifungals	Orlistat
Fluconazole	St John's wart
Itraconazole	
Ketoconazole	
Pro-kinetic agents	
Cisapride	
Metoclopramide	
H2 antagonists	
Cimetidine	
Proton pump inhibitors	
Lansoprazole	
Rabeprazole	
Antigout drugs	
Allopurinol	
Colchicine	
Bromocriptine	
Danazole	
Methylprednisolone	
Grapefruit juice	

Source: Reprinted from Vigneswaran WT. Lung transplantation. In: *Lung Biology in Health and Disease*. London, UK: Informa Healthcare. 2010, xix, 448 p., 8 p. of plates. Chapter 29. Copyright 2010, Taylor & Francis Group; Informa Healthcare. With permission.

recipients are all warned about importance of sun protection and should undergo regular skin examination. Retinoid chemoprophylaxis (e.g. oral acitretin) has been tried in other transplant groups. Skin cancers are managed with surgery, cryotherapy, photodynamic therapy and reduced immunosuppression (196). Recurrence rate is high, and secondary skin cancer develops within 3.5 years in half of the cases.

NATIVE LUNG COMPLICATIONS

In SLT recipients, the native lung is prone to any complications that may affect the original disease process. Examples include bacterial pneumonia, secondary pneumothorax and lung malignancy as mentioned above. Lung cancer incidence is reported at 3.4%–4% in the pulmonary fibrosis group (197). Lowering the level of immunosuppression, if needed to deal with native lung complications, must be balanced with the risks of chronic rejection.

Acute exacerbation has been reported in a case of fibrotic NSIP despite maintenance immunosuppression (198). Significant native lung complications are associated with worsening survival, and native lung pneumonectomy may be feasible in selected cases (199). Disease recurrence has also been reported in the allograft for a variety of conditions (e.g. sarcoidosis).

FOLLOW-UP

Lung transplant recipients are routinely monitored for potential complications and require lifelong follow-up. Post-transplant care should be delivered by specialized transplant centres experienced in dealing with post-transplant issues. Drug levels (e.g. calcineurin) inhibitors should be carefully monitored due to the narrow therapeutic window, and high levels can cause significant toxicity. Recipients should also have regular serological tests to look for myelosuppression and renal impairment. Opportunistic infections and malignancies should be detected at an early stage and managed accordingly. On acute presentation to a peripheral hospital, standard investigations should be performed and there should be close liaison with the transplant team.

FUTURE DEVELOPMENTS

EXTRACORPOREAL MEMBRANE OXYGENATION

The outcome of acute exacerbations in IPF and other types of ILD is extremely poor, and there is general reluctance at initiating mechanical ventilation when acute respiratory failure occurs. Gaudry et al. (200) confirmed poor outcomes in a group of 27 IPF or fibrotic NSIP individuals who required mechanical ventilator support, and only 30% of these patients were successfully weaned from mechanical ventilation. Survival rates for those who did not undergo transplant were very poor (4% at 6 months). Mechanical ventilation is also associated with complications such as barotrauma and ventilator-acquired pneumonia.

Extracorporeal life support (ECLS) has evolved and is now increasingly used to support critically ill individuals. It can be used as a bridge to lung transplantation for patients who have progressed to respiratory failure pre-transplant, to provide haemodynamic support intra-operatively when transplantation is performed or as rescue therapy for severe PGD.

In a retrospective analysis of 108 lung transplant recipients, Bittner et al. (201) found that 25% required veno-arterial ECMO at any stage, and survival was reduced in this group. The 90-day, 1-year and 5-year survival were 44%, 33% and 21%, respectively, in the ECMO group. Hayes et al. (202) examined pooled UNOS data for recipients who required pre-transplant ECMO support and found that post-transplant survival was lower in the ECMO group, especially for recipients with an IPF diagnosis and those who underwent re-transplantation, which were labelled as poor prognostic factors. Several cases on ECMO bridging to transplant have been reported for ILD. One patient with IPF received a lung transplant following 3 days on ECMO support (203), and another with stage 4 pulmonary sarcoidosis was successfully transplanted following 35 days on ECMO (204).

In the most recent consensus for the selection of lung transplant candidates, ECLS is recognized formally for bridging in acute decompensation (2), and it is recommended for younger individuals without

Table 26.10 Mechanical bridge to lung transplantation selection criteria

	Selection criteria
ECLS recommended	• Young age • Absence of multiple-organ dysfunction • Good potential for rehabilitation
ECLS not recommended	• Septic shock • Multi-organ dysfunction • Severe arterial occlusive disease • Heparin-induced thrombocytopenia • Prior prolonged mechanical ventilation • Advanced age • Obesity

Source: Reprinted from *J Heart Lung Transplant*, 34(1), Weill D et al., A consensus document for the selection of lung transplant candidates: 2014—an update from the Pulmonary Transplantation Council of the International Society for Heart and Lung Transplantation, 1–15, Copyright 2015, with permission from Elsevier.

other end-organ dysfunction (see Table 26.10). There should be prior involvement and assessment by the transplant team. ECLS is associated with various risks including vascular complications, haematomas, infections and haemorrhage. There are also ethical issues regarding unfair resource allocation and inadequate donor organ availability. However, ECLS is an advancing field and can hopefully improve post-transplant outcomes for lung conditions that progress to respiratory failure before lung transplantation can be performed.

LIVING DONOR LOBAR LUNG TRANSPLANTATION

Living donor lobar lung transplantation (LDLLT) is another evolving technique. It is designed for rapidly deteriorating individuals who cannot wait for a cadaveric organ or who may deteriorate before one becomes available. Usually, two lower lobes are transplanted from separate living donors to the recipient in a planned simultaneous procedure. There are isolated case reports for LDLLT in dermatomyositis and scleroderma-associated pneumonitis (205–207). Date et al. (208) reported LDLLT in nine individuals with IPF or fibrotic NSIP. There was one early death due to acute rejection, but early results were otherwise favourable. Reservations over this procedure remain high, as there may be significant issues (including risk of perioperative death) faced by the donors and the recipients.

EX VIVO LUNG PERFUSION

In a world with immense donor organ shortage, there is a desperate need for techniques that can expand organ availability. *Ex vivo* lung perfusion (EVLP) allows functional assessment of borderline organs in a controlled fashion. It consists of a closed-circuit system that provides artificial ventilation via endotracheal tube, and the pulmonary vasculature can be perfused with blood or an acellular perfusate via cannulas and a centrifugal pump (see Figure 26.5). The lungs are perfused with an albumin-based extracellular solution (143), and this system allows for continuous assessment of haemodynamic and ventilatory parameters. The technique can potentially resuscitate oedematous lungs and improve functional quality, thereby increasing the number of organs available for transplantation. Additionally, the opportunities to attempt to repair the organ with novel anti-inflammatory approaches (such as gene transfection) offer new approaches to organ resuscitation.

CONCLUSION

Transplantation for patients with ILD is a rapidly expanding field that holds exciting promises for the future. However, numerous challenges must be overcome to deliver this therapy in a timely manner to extremely sick individuals. Increasing the

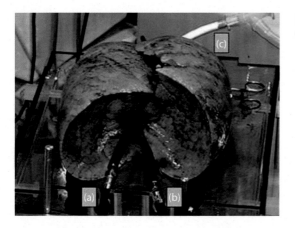

Figure 26.5 The lungs are explanted and mounted in a Plexiglas box for *ex vivo* lung perfusion. The illustration depicts the inflow and outflow cannulas for blood perfusion (a+b); and endotracheal tube used to ventilate the lungs (c). (Reprinted from Vigneswaran WT. *Lung transplantation. In: Lung Biology in Health and Disease.* London, UK: Informa Healthcare. 2010, xix, 448 p., 8 p. of plates. Chapter 18. Copyright 2010, Taylor & Francis Group; Informa Healthcare. With permission.)

availability of donor organs to prevent death from respiratory failure is a key unmet need, and this requires a coordinated approach from a number of agencies to raise the profile of organ donation. A number of different models existing for achieving increased organ donation, and one of the common themes across these models is improving the level of engagement and discussion in society of the merits of organ donation. Most importantly, increased knowledge of the benefits of organ transplantation will allow potential donors and their families to have an *a priori* understanding of what is involved in donation and the benefits it can bring to patients with progressive disease who have failed medical therapies.

Although the improvement in survival for lung transplant recipients has been gratifying, a number of challenges remain to ensure that more patients survive longer with a better quality of life. Key among these is reducing the toxicities that every patient is exposed to from the immunosuppression. While ILD patients are among the most challenging patients to transplant, good outcomes are achievable with careful candidate selection.

REFERENCES

1. Witt CA, Meyers, BF. Hachem, RR. Pulmonary infections following lung transplantation. *Thorac Surg Clin.* 2012;22(3):403–12.
2. Weill D et al. A consensus document for the selection of lung transplant candidates: 2014—An update from the Pulmonary Transplantation Council of the International Society for Heart and Lung Transplantation. *J Heart Lung Transplant.* 2015;34(1):1–15.
3. Orens JB et al. International guidelines for the selection of lung transplant candidates: 2006 update—A consensus report from the Pulmonary Scientific Council of the International Society for Heart and Lung Transplantation. *J Heart Lung Transplant.* 2006;25(7):745–55.
4. Kim DS, Park JH, Park BK, Lee JS, Nicholson AG, Colby T. Acute exacerbation of idiopathic pulmonary fibrosis: Frequency and clinical features. *Eur Respir J.* 2006;27(1):143–50.
5. Selman M et al. Accelerated variant of idiopathic pulmonary fibrosis: Clinical behavior and gene expression pattern. *PLoS One.* 2007;2(5):e482.
6. Reed A et al. Outcomes of patients with interstitial lung disease referred for lung transplant assessment. *Intern Med J.* 2006;36(7):423–30.
7. Takahashi H et al. Monitoring markers of disease activity for interstitial lung diseases with serum surfactant proteins A and D. *Respirology.* 2006;11(Suppl):S51–4.
8. Yokoyama A et al. Circulating KL-6 predicts the outcome of rapidly progressive idiopathic pulmonary fibrosis. *Am J Respir Crit Care Med.* 1998;158(5 Pt 1):1680–4.
9. Prasse A et al. Serum CC-chemokine ligand 18 concentration predicts outcome in idiopathic pulmonary fibrosis. *Am J Respir Crit Care Med.* 2009;179(8):717–23.
10. Sims MW et al. Effect of single vs bilateral lung transplantation on plasma surfactant protein D levels in idiopathic pulmonary fibrosis. *Chest.* 2011;140(2):489–96.

11. Zisman DA et al. Serum albumin concentration and waiting list mortality in idiopathic interstitial pneumonia. *Chest.* 2009;135(4):929–35.

12. Lee JS et al. Prevalence and clinical significance of circulating autoantibodies in idiopathic pulmonary fibrosis. *Respir Med.* 2013;107(2):249–55.

13. Collard HR et al. Changes in clinical and physiologic variables predict survival in idiopathic pulmonary fibrosis. *Am J Respir Crit Care Med.* 2003;168(5):538–42.

14. Alhamad EH, Lynch JP 3rd, Martinez FJ. Pulmonary function tests in interstitial lung disease: What role do they have? *Clin Chest Med.* 2001;22(4):715–50, ix.

15. Flaherty KR et al. Prognostic implications of physiologic and radiographic changes in idiopathic interstitial pneumonia. *Am J Respir Crit Care Med.* 2003;168(5): 543–8.

16. Richeldi L et al. Relative versus absolute change in forced vital capacity in idiopathic pulmonary fibrosis. *Thorax.* 2012;67(5):407–11.

17. Ryerson CJ et al. Cough predicts prognosis in idiopathic pulmonary fibrosis. *Respirology.* 2011;16(6):969–75.

18. Rivera-Lebron BN et al. Echocardiographic and hemodynamic predictors of mortality in idiopathic pulmonary fibrosis. *Chest.* 2013;144(2):564–70.

19. Kawut SM et al. Exercise testing determines survival in patients with diffuse parenchymal lung disease evaluated for lung transplantation. *Respir Med.* 2005;99(11):1431–9.

20. Lama VN et al. Prognostic value of desaturation during a 6-minute walk test in idiopathic interstitial pneumonia. *Am J Respir Crit Care Med.* 2003;168(9):1084–90.

21. Shitrit D et al. The 15-step oximetry test: A reliable tool to identify candidates for lung transplantation among patients with idiopathic pulmonary fibrosis. *J Heart Lung Transplant.* 2009;28(4):328–33.

22. King TE Jr. et al. Idiopathic pulmonary fibrosis: Relationship between histopathologic features and mortality. *Am J Respir Crit Care Med.* 2001;164(6): 1025–32.

23. Nicholson AG et al. The relationship between individual histologic features and disease progression in idiopathic pulmonary fibrosis. *Am J Respir Crit Care Med.* 2002;166(2):173–7.

24. Hanak V et al. Profusion of fibroblast foci in patients with idiopathic pulmonary fibrosis does not predict outcome. *Respir Med.* 2008;102(6):852–6.

25. Mogulkoc N et al. Pulmonary function in idiopathic pulmonary fibrosis and referral for lung transplantation. *Am J Respir Crit Care Med.* 2001;164(1):103–8.

26. Ley B et al. A multidimensional index and staging system for idiopathic pulmonary fibrosis. *Ann Intern Med.* 2012;156(10):684–91.

27. Ley B et al. Idiopathic pulmonary fibrosis: CT and risk of death. *Radiology.* 2014;273(2):570–9.

28. King TE Jr. et al. Predicting survival in idiopathic pulmonary fibrosis: Scoring system and survival model. *Am J Respir Crit Care Med.* 2001;164(7):1171–81.

29. du Bois RM et al. Ascertainment of individual risk of mortality for patients with idiopathic pulmonary fibrosis. *Am J Respir Crit Care Med.* 2011;184(4):459–66.

30. Daniil ZD et al. A histologic pattern of nonspecific interstitial pneumonia is associated with a better prognosis than usual interstitial pneumonia in patients with cryptogenic fibrosing alveolitis. *Am J Respir Crit Care Med.* 1999;160(3):899–905.

31. Flaherty KR et al. Radiological versus histological diagnosis in UIP and NSIP: Survival implications. *Thorax.* 2003;58(2): 143–8.

32. Latsi PI et al. Fibrotic idiopathic interstitial pneumonia: The prognostic value of longitudinal functional trends. *Am J Respir Crit Care Med.* 2003;168(5):531–7.

33. Bouros D et al. Histopathologic subsets of fibrosing alveolitis in patients with systemic sclerosis and their relationship to outcome. *Am J Respir Crit Care Med.* 2002;165(12):1581–6.

34. Wells AU et al. The predictive value of appearances on thin-section computed tomography in fibrosing alveolitis. *Am Rev Respir Dis.* 1993;148(4 Pt 1):1076–82.

35. Flaherty KR et al. Fibroblastic foci in usual interstitial pneumonia: Idiopathic versus collagen vascular disease. *Am J Respir Crit Care Med.* 2003;167(10):1410–5.

36. Baughman RP et al. Predicting respiratory failure in sarcoidosis patients. *Sarcoidosis Vasc Diffuse Lung Dis.* 1997;14(2):154–8.

37. Shorr AF, Davies DB, Nathan SD. Predicting mortality in patients with sarcoidosis awaiting lung transplantation. *Chest.* 2003;124(3):922–8.

38. Hanak V et al. High-resolution CT findings of parenchymal fibrosis correlate with prognosis in hypersensitivity pneumonitis. *Chest.* 2008;134(1):133–8.

39. Mooney JJ et al. Radiographic fibrosis score predicts survival in hypersensitivity pneumonitis. *Chest.* 2013;144(2):586–92.

40. Delobbe A et al. Determinants of survival in pulmonary Langerhans' cell granulomatosis (histiocytosis X). Groupe d'Etude en Pathologie Interstitielle de la Societe de Pathologie Thoracique du Nord. *Eur Respir J.* 1996;9(10):2002–6.

41. Gries CJ et al. Obese patients with idiopathic pulmonary fibrosis have a higher 90-day mortality risk with bilateral lung transplantation. *J Heart Lung Transplant.* 2015;34(2):241–6.

42. Kern RM et al. The feasibility of lung transplantation in HIV-seropositive patients. *Ann Am Thorac Soc.* 2014;11(6):882–9.

43. George MP. Time to reconsider transplant criteria for candidacy? Lung transplantation feasibility in HIV-infected patients. *Ann Am Thorac Soc.* 2014;11(6):962–3.

44. Florian J et al. Impact of pulmonary rehabilitation on quality of life and functional capacity in patients on waiting lists for lung transplantation. *J Bras Pneumol.* 2013;39(3):349–56.

45. Wickerson L et al. Physical activity profile of lung transplant candidates with interstitial lung disease. *J Cardiopulm Rehabil Prev.* 2013;33(2):106–12.

46. Vainshelboim B et al. Long-term effects of a 12-week exercise training program on clinical outcomes in idiopathic pulmonary fibrosis. *Lung.* 2015;193(3):345–54.

47. Gribbin J et al. Incidence and mortality of idiopathic pulmonary fibrosis and sarcoidosis in the UK. *Thorax.* 2006;61(11):980–5.

48. Rudd RM et al. British Thoracic Society Study on cryptogenic fibrosing alveolitis: Response to treatment and survival. *Thorax.* 2007;62(1):62–6.

49. Kistler KD et al. Lung transplantation in idiopathic pulmonary fibrosis: A systematic review of the literature. *BMC Pulm Med.* 2014;14:139.

50. Baughman RP et al. Clinical characteristics of patients in a case control study of sarcoidosis. *Am J Respir Crit Care Med.* 2001;164(10 Pt 1):1885–9.

51. Sulica R et al. Distinctive clinical, radiographic, and functional characteristics of patients with sarcoidosis-related pulmonary hypertension. *Chest.* 2005;128(3):1483–9.

52. Shorr AF et al. Pulmonary hypertension in advanced sarcoidosis: Epidemiology and clinical characteristics. *Eur Respir J.* 2005;25(5):783–8.

53. Baughman RP et al. Survival in sarcoidosis-associated pulmonary hypertension: The importance of hemodynamic evaluation. *Chest.* 2010;138(5):1078–85.

54. Arcasoy SM et al. Characteristics and outcomes of patients with sarcoidosis listed for lung transplantation. *Chest.* 2001;120(3):873–80.

55. Silverman KJ, Hutchins GM, Bulkley BH. Cardiac sarcoid: A clinicopathologic study of 84 unselected patients with systemic sarcoidosis. *Circulation.* 1978;58(6):1204–11.

56. Oksanen V. Neurosarcoidosis. *Sarcoidosis.* 1994;11(1):76–9.

57. Judson MA. Lung transplantation for pulmonary sarcoidosis. *Eur Respir J.* 1998;11(3):738–44.

58. Wollschlager C, Khan F. Aspergillomas complicating sarcoidosis. A prospective study in 100 patients. *Chest.* 1984;86(4):585–8.

59. Hadjiliadis D et al. Outcome of lung transplantation in patients with mycetomas. *Chest.* 2002;121(1):128–34.

60. Shlobin OA, Nathan SD. Management of end-stage sarcoidosis: Pulmonary hypertension and lung transplantation. *Eur Respir J.* 2012;39(6):1520–33.

61. Shorr AF et al. Sarcoidosis, race, and short-term outcomes following lung transplantation. *Chest*. 2004;125(3):990–6.

62. Wille KM et al. Bronchiolitis obliterans syndrome and survival following lung transplantation for patients with sarcoidosis. *Sarcoidosis Vasc Diffuse Lung Dis*. 2008;25(2):117–24.

63. Martinez FJ et al. Recurrence of sarcoidosis following bilateral allogeneic lung transplantation. *Chest*. 1994;106(5):1597–9.

64. Kiatboonsri C et al. The detection of recurrent sarcoidosis by FDG-PET in a lung transplant recipient. *West J Med*. 1998;168(2):130–2.

65. Collins J et al. Frequency and CT findings of recurrent disease after lung transplantation. *Radiology*. 2001;219(2):503–9.

66. Slebos DJ et al. Bronchoalveolar lavage in a patient with recurrence of sarcoidosis after lung transplantation. *J Heart Lung Transplant*. 2004;23(8):1010–3.

67. Milman N et al. Recurrent sarcoid granulomas in a transplanted lung derive from recipient immune cells. *Eur Respir J*. 2005;26(3):549–52.

68. Mayes MD et al. Prevalence, incidence, survival, and disease characteristics of systemic sclerosis in a large US population. *Arthritis Rheum*. 2003;48(8):2246–55.

69. Simeon CP et al. Survival prognostic factors and markers of morbidity in Spanish patients with systemic sclerosis. *Ann Rheum Dis*. 1997;56(12):723–8.

70. Solomon JJ et al. Scleroderma lung disease. *Eur Respir Rev*. 2013;22(127):6–19.

71. McNearney TA et al. Pulmonary involvement in systemic sclerosis: Associations with genetic, serologic, sociodemographic, and behavioral factors. *Arthritis Rheum*. 2007;57(2):318–26.

72. Khan IY et al. Survival after lung transplantation in systemic sclerosis. A systematic review. *Respir Med*. 2013;107(12):2081–7.

73. Avouac J et al. Prevalence of pulmonary hypertension in systemic sclerosis in European Caucasians and metaanalysis of 5 studies. *J Rheumatol*. 2010;37(11):2290–8.

74. Trad S et al. Pulmonary arterial hypertension is a major mortality factor in diffuse systemic sclerosis, independent of interstitial lung disease. *Arthritis Rheum*. 2006;54(1):184–91.

75. de Perrot M et al. Outcome of patients with pulmonary arterial hypertension referred for lung transplantation: A 14-year single-center experience. *J Thorac Cardiovasc Surg*. 2012;143(4):910–8.

76. Gasper WJ et al. Lung transplantation in patients with connective tissue disorders and esophageal dysmotility. *Dis Esophagus*. 2008;21(7):650–5.

77. Kent MS et al. Comparison of surgical approaches to recalcitrant gastroesophageal reflux disease in the patient with scleroderma. *Ann Thorac Surg*. 2007;84(5):1710–5; discussion 1715–6.

78. Saggar R et al. Systemic sclerosis and bilateral lung transplantation: A single centre experience. *Eur Respir J*. 2010;36(4):893–900.

79. Bongartz T et al. Incidence and mortality of interstitial lung disease in rheumatoid arthritis: A population-based study. *Arthritis Rheum*. 2010;62(6):1583–91.

80. Lamblin C et al. Interstitial lung diseases in collagen vascular diseases. *Eur Respir J Suppl*. 2001;32:69s–80s.

81. Yazdani A et al. Survival and quality of life in rheumatoid arthritis-associated interstitial lung disease after lung transplantation. *J Heart Lung Transplant*. 2014;33(5):514–20.

82. Badesch DB et al. Pulmonary capillaritis: A possible histologic form of acute pulmonary allograft rejection. *J Heart Lung Transplant*. 1998;17(4):415–22.

83. Samanta R, Shoukrey K, Griffiths R. Rheumatoid arthritis and anaesthesia. *Anaesthesia*. 2011;66(12):1146–59.

84. Haupt HM, Moore GW, Hutchins GM. The lung in systemic lupus erythematosus. Analysis of the pathologic changes in 120 patients. *Am J Med*. 1981;71(5):791–8.

85. Levy RD et al. Prolonged survival after heart-lung transplantation in systemic lupus erythematosus. *Chest*. 1993;104(6):1903–5.

86. Yeatman M et al. Lung transplantation in patients with systemic diseases: An eleven-year experience at Papworth Hospital. *J Heart Lung Transplant*. 1996;15(2):144–9.

87. Kim J et al. Successful lung transplantation in a patient with dermatomyositis and acute form of interstitial pneumonitis. *Clin Exp Rheumatol*. 2009;27(1):168–9.

88. Broome M et al. Prolonged extracorporeal membrane oxygenation and circulatory support as bridge to lung transplant. *Ann Thorac Surg.* 2008;86(4):1357–60.

89. Sem M, Lund MB, Molberg O. Long-term outcome of lung transplantation in a patient with the anti-synthetase syndrome. *Scand J Rheumatol.* 2011;40(4):327–8.

90. Arboleda R et al. Recurrent polymyositis-associated lung disease after lung transplantation. *Interact Cardiovasc Thorac Surg.* 2015;20(4):560–2.

91. Solaymani-Dodaran M et al. Extrinsic allergic alveolitis: Incidence and mortality in the general population. *QJM.* 2007;100(4):233–7.

92. Ismail T, McSharry C, Boyd G. Extrinsic allergic alveolitis. *Respirology.* 2006;11(3):262–8.

93. Kern RM et al. Lung transplantation for hypersensitivity pneumonitis. *Chest.* 2015;147(6):1558–65.

94. Mao WJ et al. Lung transplantation for end-stage silicosis. *J Occup Environ Med.* 2011;53(8):845–9.

95. Redondo MT, Vaz M, Damas C. End-stage silicosis and lung transplantation: A way forward. *Rev Port Pneumol.* 2014;20(6):341.

96. Singer J.P et al. Survival following lung transplantation for silicosis and other occupational lung diseases. *Occup Med (Lond).* 2012;62(2):134–7.

97. Hayes D Jr. et al. Lung transplantation in patients with coal workers' pneumoconiosis. *Clin Transplant.* 2012;26(4):629–34.

98. Enfield KB et al. Survival after lung transplant for coal workers' pneumoconiosis. *J Heart Lung Transplant.* 2012;31(12):1315–8.

99. Fartoukh M et al. Severe pulmonary hypertension in histiocytosis X. *Am J Respir Crit Care Med.* 2000;161(1):216–23.

100. Dauriat G et al. Lung transplantation for pulmonary Langerhans' cell histiocytosis: A multicenter analysis. *Transplantation.* 2006;81(5):746–50.

101. Habib SB et al. Recurrence of recipient Langerhans' cell histiocytosis following bilateral lung transplantation. *Thorax.* 1998;53(4):323–5.

102. Gabbay E et al. Recurrence of Langerhans' cell granulomatosis following lung transplantation. *Thorax.* 1998;53(4):326–7.

103. Etienne B et al. Relapsing pulmonary Langerhans cell histiocytosis after lung transplantation. *Am J Respir Crit Care Med.* 1998;157(1):288–91.

104. Pechet TT et al. Lung transplantation for lymphangioleiomyomatosis. *J Heart Lung Transplant.* 2001;20(2):174.

105. Boehler A et al. Lung transplantation for lymphangioleiomyomatosis. *N Engl J Med.* 1996;335(17):1275–80.

106. Benden C et al. Lung transplantation for lymphangioleiomyomatosis: The European experience. *J Heart Lung Transplant.* 2009;28(1):1–7.

107. Bittmann I et al. Recurrence of lymphangioleiomyomatosis after single lung transplantation: New insights into pathogenesis. *Hum Pathol.* 2003;34(1):95–8.

108. Nine JS et al. Lymphangioleiomyomatosis: Recurrence after lung transplantation. *J Heart Lung Transplant.* 1994;13(4):714–9.

109. O'Brien JD et al. Lymphangiomyomatosis recurrence in the allograft after single-lung transplantation. *Am J Respir Crit Care Med.* 1995;151(6):2033–6.

110. Karbowniczek M et al. Recurrent lymphangiomyomatosis after transplantation: Genetic analyses reveal a metastatic mechanism. *Am J Respir Crit Care Med.* 2003;167(7):976–82.

111. Verleden GM. Recurrence of desquamative interstitial pneumonia after lung transplantation. *Am J Respir Crit Care Med.* 1998;157(4 Pt 1):1349–50.

112. King MB, Jessurun J, Hertz MI. Recurrence of desquamative interstitial pneumonia after lung transplantation. *Am J Respir Crit Care Med.* 1997;156(6):2003–5.

113. Greenfield LJ et al. Pulmonary effects of experimental graded aspiration of hydrochloric acid. *Ann Surg.* 1969;170(1):74–86.

114. Raghu G et al. High prevalence of abnormal acid gastro-oesophageal reflux in idiopathic pulmonary fibrosis. *Eur Respir J.* 2006;27(1):136–42.

115. Tobin RW et al. Increased prevalence of gastroesophageal reflux in patients with idiopathic pulmonary fibrosis. *Am J Respir Crit Care Med.* 1998;158(6):1804–8.

116. Sweet MP et al. Gastroesophageal reflux in patients with idiopathic pulmonary fibrosis referred for lung transplantation. *J Thorac Cardiovasc Surg.* 2007;133(4):1078–84.

117. Linden PA et al. Laparoscopic fundoplication in patients with end-stage lung disease awaiting transplantation. *J Thorac Cardiovasc Surg.* 2006;131(2):438–46.

118. Hadjiliadis D et al. Gastroesophageal reflux disease in lung transplant recipients. *Clin Transplant.* 2003;17(4):363–8.

119. Davis RD Jr. et al. Improved lung allograft function after fundoplication in patients with gastroesophageal reflux disease undergoing lung transplantation. *J Thorac Cardiovasc Surg.* 2003;125(3):533–42.

120. Cantu E 3rd et al. J. Maxwell Chamberlain Memorial Paper. Early fundoplication prevents chronic allograft dysfunction in patients with gastroesophageal reflux disease. *Ann Thorac Surg.* 2004;78(4):1142–51; discussion 1142-51.

121. Izbicki G et al. The prevalence of coronary artery disease in end-stage pulmonary disease: Is pulmonary fibrosis a risk factor? *Respir Med.* 2009;103(9):1346–9.

122. Jastrzebski D et al. Left ventricular dysfunction in patients with interstitial lung diseases referred for lung transplantation. *J Physiol Pharmacol.* 2007;58 (Suppl 5)(Pt 1):299–305.

123. Sherman W et al. Lung transplantation and coronary artery disease. *Ann Thorac Surg.* 2011;92(1):303–8.

124. Wilson IC et al. Healing of the bronchus in pulmonary transplantation. *Eur J Cardiothorac Surg.* 1996;10(7):521–6; discussion 526-7.

125. Van De Wauwer C et al. Risk factors for airway complications within the first year after lung transplantation. *Eur J Cardiothorac Surg.* 2007;31(4):703–10.

126. Park SJ et al. Pre-transplant corticosteroid use and outcome in lung transplantation. *J Heart Lung Transplant.* 2001;20(3):304–9.

127. Maurer JR et al. International guidelines for the selection of lung transplant candidates. The International Society for Heart and Lung Transplantation, the American Thoracic Society, the American Society of Transplant Physicians, the European Respiratory Society. *J Heart Lung Transplant.* 1998;17(7):703–9.

128. Venuta F et al. Efficacy of cyclosporine to reduce steroids in patients with idiopathic pulmonary fibrosis before lung transplantation. *J Heart Lung Transplant.* 1993;12(6 Pt 1):909–14.

129. Spira A et al. Osteoporosis and lung transplantation: A prospective study. *Chest.* 2000;117(2):476–81.

130. Trombetti A et al. Bone mineral density in lung-transplant recipients before and after graft: Prevention of lumbar spine post-transplantation-accelerated bone loss by pamidronate. *J Heart Lung Transplant.* 2000;19(8):736–43.

131. Le Jeune I et al. The incidence of cancer in patients with idiopathic pulmonary fibrosis and sarcoidosis in the UK. *Respir Med.* 2007;101(12):2534–40.

132. Niimi H et al. CT of chronic infiltrative lung disease: Prevalence of mediastinal lymphadenopathy. *J Comput Assist Tomogr.* 1996;20(2):305–8.

133. Lettieri CJ et al. Prevalence and outcomes of pulmonary arterial hypertension in advanced idiopathic pulmonary fibrosis. *Chest.* 2006;129(3):746–52.

134. Fang A et al. Elevated pulmonary artery pressure is a risk factor for primary graft dysfunction following lung transplantation for idiopathic pulmonary fibrosis. *Chest.* 2011;139(4):782–7.

135. Bando K et al. Impact of pulmonary hypertension on outcome after single-lung transplantation. *Ann Thorac Surg.* 1994;58(5):1336–42.

136. Huerd SS et al. Secondary pulmonary hypertension does not adversely affect outcome after single lung transplantation. *J Thorac Cardiovasc Surg.* 2000;119(3):458–65.

137. Conte JV et al. Lung transplantation for primary and secondary pulmonary hypertension. *Ann Thorac Surg.* 2001;72(5):1673–9; discussion 1679–80.

138. Fitton TP et al. Impact of secondary pulmonary hypertension on lung transplant outcome. *J Heart Lung Transplant.* 2005;24(9):1254–9.

139. Arcasoy SM et al. Echocardiographic assessment of pulmonary hypertension in patients with advanced lung disease. *Am J Respir Crit Care Med.* 2003;167(5):735–40.

140. Yoshida T et al. Severe pulmonary hypertension in adult pulmonary Langerhans cell histiocytosis: The effect of sildenafil as a bridge to lung transplantation. *Intern Med.* 2014;53(17):1985–90.

141. Saggar R et al. Treprostinil to reverse pulmonary hypertension associated with idiopathic pulmonary fibrosis as a bridge to single-lung transplantation. *J Heart Lung Transplant.* 2009;28(9):964–7.

142. Christie JD et al. The Registry of the International Society for Heart and Lung Transplantation: Twenty-eighth Adult Lung and Heart-Lung Transplant Report—2011. *J Heart Lung Transplant.* 2011;30(10):1104–22.

143. Vigneswaran WT. Lung transplantation. In: Vigneswaran WT, Garrity ER, eds. *Lung Biology in Health and Disease.* London, UK: Informa Healthcare; 2010:xix, 448 p., 8 p. of plates.

144. De Oliveira NC et al. Lung transplant for interstitial lung disease: Outcomes for single versus bilateral lung transplantation. *Interact Cardiovasc Thorac Surg.* 2012;14(3):263–7.

145. Mason DP et al. Lung transplantation for idiopathic pulmonary fibrosis. *Ann Thorac Surg.* 2007;84(4):1121–8.

146. Gulack BC et al. What is the optimal transplant for older patients with idiopathic pulmonary fibrosis? *Ann Thorac Surg.* 2015;100(5):1826–33.

147. Schaffer JM et al. Single- vs double-lung transplantation in patients with chronic obstructive pulmonary disease and idiopathic pulmonary fibrosis since the implementation of lung allocation based on medical need. *JAMA.* 2015;313(9):936–48.

148. Thabut G et al. Survival after bilateral versus single-lung transplantation for idiopathic pulmonary fibrosis. *Ann Intern Med.* 2009;151(11):767–74.

149. Force SD et al. Bilateral lung transplantation offers better long-term survival, compared with single-lung transplantation, for younger patients with idiopathic pulmonary fibrosis. *Ann Thorac Surg.* 2011;91(1):244–9.

150. Lama VN et al. Course of FEV(1) after onset of bronchiolitis obliterans syndrome in lung transplant recipients. *Am J Respir Crit Care Med.* 2007;175(11):1192–8.

151. Weiss ES et al. Factors indicative of long-term survival after lung transplantation: A review of 836 10-year survivors. *J Heart Lung Transplant.* 2010;29(3):240–6.

152. Jastrzebski DT et al. A functional assessment of patients two years after lung transplantation in Poland. *Kardiochir Torakochirurgia Pol.* 2014;11(2):162–8.

153. Smeritschnig B et al. Quality of life after lung transplantation: A cross-sectional study. *J Heart Lung Transplant.* 2005;24(4):474–80.

154. Kugler C et al. Health-related quality of life in two hundred-eighty lung transplant recipients. *J Heart Lung Transplant.* 2005;24(12):2262–8.

155. Singer LG et al. Effects of recipient age and diagnosis on health-related quality-of-life benefit of lung transplantation. *Am J Respir Crit Care Med.* 2015;192(8):965–73.

156. Christie JD et al. Report of the ISHLT Working Group on Primary Lung Graft Dysfunction part II: Definition. A consensus statement of the International Society for Heart and Lung Transplantation. *J Heart Lung Transplant.* 2005;24(10):1454–9.

157. de Perrot M et al. Report of the ISHLT Working Group on Primary Lung Graft Dysfunction part III: Donor-related risk factors and markers. *J Heart Lung Transplant.* 2005;24(10):1460–7.

158. Barr ML et al. Report of the ISHLT Working Group on Primary Lung Graft Dysfunction part IV: Recipient-related risk factors and markers. *J Heart Lung Transplant.* 2005;24(10):1468–82.

159. King RC et al. Reperfusion injury significantly impacts clinical outcome after pulmonary transplantation. *Ann Thorac Surg.* 2000;69(6):1681–5.

160. Prekker ME et al. Early trends in PaO(2)/fraction of inspired oxygen ratio predict outcome in lung transplant recipients with severe primary graft dysfunction. *Chest.* 2007;132(3):991–7.

161. Christie JD et al. Impact of primary graft failure on outcomes following lung transplantation. *Chest.* 2005;127(1):161–5.

162. Daud SA et al. Impact of immediate primary lung allograft dysfunction on bronchiolitis obliterans syndrome. *Am J Respir Crit Care Med.* 2007;175(5):507–13.

163. Shargall Y et al. Report of the ISHLT Working Group on Primary Lung Graft Dysfunction part VI: Treatment. *J Heart Lung Transplant.* 2005;24(10):1489–500.

164. Frost AE, Jammal CT, Cagle PT. Hyperacute rejection following lung transplantation. *Chest.* 1996;110(2):559–62.

165. Bittner HB et al. Hyperacute rejection in single lung transplantation—Case report of successful management by means of plasmapheresis and antithymocyte globulin treatment. *Transplantation.* 2001;71(5): 649–51.

166. Herridge MS et al. Pleural complications in lung transplant recipients. *J Thorac Cardiovasc Surg.* 1995;110(1):22–6.

167. Sugimoto S et al. Thoracoscopic operation with local and epidural anesthesia in the treatment of pneumothorax after lung transplantation. *J Thorac Cardiovasc Surg.* 2005;130(4):1219–20.

168. Ferdinande P et al. Phrenic nerve dysfunction after heart-lung and lung transplantation. *J Heart Lung Transplant.* 2004;23(1):105–9.

169. Berk Y et al. Non-invasive ventilation in phrenic nerve dysfunction after lung transplantation: An attractive option. *J Heart Lung Transplant.* 2006;25(12):1483–5.

170. Patel R, Paya CV. Infections in solid-organ transplant recipients. *Clin Microbiol Rev.* 1997;10(1):86–124.

171. Deusch E et al. Early bacterial infections in lung transplant recipients. *Chest.* 1993;104(5):1412–6.

172. Ljungman P, Griffiths P, Paya C. Definitions of cytomegalovirus infection and disease in transplant recipients. *Clin Infect Dis.* 2002;34(8):1094–7.

173. Tamm M et al. Treated cytomegalovirus pneumonia is not associated with bronchiolitis obliterans syndrome. *Am J Respir Crit Care Med.* 2004;170(10):1120–3.

174. Pelaez A et al. Efficacy of oral ribavirin in lung transplant patients with respiratory syncytial virus lower respiratory tract infection. *J Heart Lung Transplant.* 2009;28(1):67–71.

175. Sole A et al. Aspergillus infections in lung transplant recipients: Risk factors and outcome. *Clin Microbiol Infect.* 2005;11(5):359–65.

176. Schaenman JM et al. Trends in invasive disease due to *Candida* species following heart and lung transplantation. *Transpl Infect Dis.* 2009;11(2):112–21.

177. Husain AN et al. Analysis of risk factors for the development of bronchiolitis obliterans syndrome. *Am J Respir Crit Care Med.* 1999;159(3):829–33.

178. Moreno P et al. Incidence, management and clinical outcomes of patients with airway complications following lung transplantation. *Eur J Cardiothorac Surg.* 2008;34(6):1198–205.

179. Weder W et al. Airway complications after lung transplantation: Risk factors, prevention and outcome. *Eur J Cardiothorac Surg.* 2009;35(2):293–8; discussion 298.

180. Clark SC et al. Vascular complications of lung transplantation. *Ann Thorac Surg.* 1996;61(4):1079–82.

181. Zivkovic SA et al. Neurologic complications following lung transplantation. *J Neurol Sci.* 2009;280(1-2):90–3.

182. Kroshus TJ et al. Deep venous thrombosis and pulmonary embolism after lung transplantation. *J Thorac Cardiovasc Surg.* 1995;110(2):540–4.

183. Paul S et al. Gastrointestinal complications after lung transplantation. *J Heart Lung Transplant.* 2009;28(5):475–9.

184. Berkowitz N et al. Gastroparesis after lung transplantation. Potential role in postoperative respiratory complications. *Chest.* 1995;108(6):1602–7.

185. Weinkauf JG, Yiannopoulos A, Faul JL. Transcutaneous electrical nerve stimulation for severe gastroparesis after lung transplantation. *J Heart Lung Transplant.* 2005;24(9):1444.

186. Reichenspurner H et al. Stanford experience with obliterative bronchiolitis after lung and heart-lung transplantation. *Ann Thorac Surg.* 1996;62(5):1467–72; discussion 1472-3.

187. Kroshus TJ et al. Risk factors for the development of bronchiolitis obliterans syndrome after lung transplantation. *J Thorac Cardiovasc Surg.* 1997;114(2):195–202.

188. Chmiel C et al. Ganciclovir/valganciclovir prophylaxis decreases cytomegalovirus-related events and bronchiolitis obliterans syndrome after lung transplantation. *Clin Infect Dis.* 2008;46(6):831–9.

189. Botha P et al. *Pseudomonas aeruginosa* colonization of the allograft after lung transplantation and the risk of bronchiolitis obliterans syndrome. *Transplantation.* 2008;85(5):771–4.

190. Treede H et al. Tacrolimus versus cyclosporine after lung transplantation: A prospective, open, randomized two-center trial comparing two different immunosuppressive protocols. *J Heart Lung Transplant.* 2001;20(5):511–7.

191. Hachem RR et al. A randomized controlled trial of tacrolimus versus cyclosporine after lung transplantation. *J Heart Lung Transplant.* 2007;26(10):1012–8.

192. McNeil K et al. Comparison of mycophenolate mofetil and azathioprine for prevention of bronchiolitis obliterans syndrome in de novo lung transplant recipients. *Transplantation.* 2006;81(7):998–1003.

193. Shitrit D et al. Long-term azithromycin use for treatment of bronchiolitis obliterans syndrome in lung transplant recipients. *J Heart Lung Transplant.* 2005;24(9):1440–3.

194. Reams BD et al. Posttransplant lymphoproliferative disorder: Incidence, presentation, and response to treatment in lung transplant recipients. *Chest.* 2003;124(4):1242–9.

195. Levine SM et al. A low incidence of posttransplant lymphoproliferative disorder in 109 lung transplant recipients. *Chest.* 1999;116(5):1273–7.

196. Zafar SY, Howell DN, Gockerman JP. Malignancy after solid organ transplantation: An overview. *Oncologist.* 2008;13(7):769–78.

197. Kotloff RM, Ahya VN. Medical complications of lung transplantation. *Eur Respir J.* 2004;23(2):334–42.

198. Yang D et al. Acute exacerbation of pulmonary fibrosis following single lung transplantation. *Can Respir J.* 2012;19(1):e3–4.

199. King CS et al. Native lung complications in single-lung transplant recipients and the role of pneumonectomy. *J Heart Lung Transplant.* 2009;28(8):851–6.

200. Gaudry S et al. Invasive mechanical ventilation in patients with fibrosing interstitial pneumonia. *J Thorac Cardiovasc Surg.* 2014;147(1):47–53.

201. Bittner HB et al. Outcome of extracorporeal membrane oxygenation as a bridge to lung transplantation and graft recovery. *Ann Thorac Surg.* 2012;94(3):942–9; author reply 949–50.

202. Hayes D Jr. et al. Extracorporeal membrane oxygenation and retransplantation in lung transplantation: An analysis of the UNOS registry. *Lung.* 2014;192(4):571–6.

203. Mangi AA et al. Bridge to lung transplantation using short-term ambulatory extracorporeal membrane oxygenation. *J Thorac Cardiovasc Surg.* 2010;140(3):713–5.

204. Bozso S et al. Canada's longest experience with extracorporeal membrane oxygenation as a bridge to lung transplantation: A case report. *Transplant Proc.* 2015;47(1):186–9.

205. Shoji T et al. Living-donor lobar lung transplantation for interstitial pneumonia associated with dermatomyositis. *Transpl Int.* 2010;23(5):e10–1.

206. Shoji T et al. Living-donor lobar lung transplantation for rapidly progressive interstitial pneumonia associated with clinically amyopathic dermatomyositis: Report of a case. *Gen Thorac Cardiovasc Surg.* 2013;61(1):32–4.

207. Laratta C et al. A case report of living-donor lobar lung transplantation for scleroderma-associated usual interstitial pneumonia: Eight years and counting. *Transplant Proc.* 2015;47(1):190–3.

208. Date H et al. A new treatment strategy for advanced idiopathic interstitial pneumonia: Living-donor lobar lung transplantation. *Chest.* 2005;128(3):1364–70.

209. Christie JD et al. Primary graft failure following lung transplantation. *Chest.* 1998;114(1):51–60.

27

Diagnosis and management of critical illness in patients with interstitial lung disease

TENG MOUA

INTRODUCTION

Issues of critical care involving the interstitial lung diseases (ILDs) are dominated by the progression of hypoxaemia and acute-on-chronic respiratory failure. Medical intensivists must often manage rapidly declining respiratory function caused by both the underlying interstitial process as well as superimposed complications, which are often related to co-morbidities. A commonly recognized phenomenon is acute exacerbation (AE), which is defined by the appearance of new diffuse pulmonary infiltrates superimposed on radiologic changes of underlying lung fibrosis accompanied by acute dyspnoea and worsening hypoxaemia that are not attributable to a secondary cause. An AE event is associated with high morbidity and mortality, particularly if mechanical ventilation is required. Co-morbidities such as pulmonary hypertension (PH) with related congestive heart failure (CHF), cardiac ischaemia, community-acquired infection, and deep-vein thrombosis/pulmonary embolism (DVT/PE) may also cause or contribute to clinical worsening, leading to intensive care unit (ICU) admission. This chapter highlights the incidence and presentation of AE and other known co-morbidities associated with ILD that may contribute to critical illness.

This is followed by a review of current management strategies including the delineation of secondary causes of respiratory failure and a discussion of the evidence and rationale for supportive treatments such as antibiotics, high-dose intravenous (IV) steroids, and mechanical ventilation. Finally, a review of both in-hospital and long-term survival will be discussed along with end-of-life and palliative care perspectives.

AETIOLOGIES OF CRITICAL ILLNESS ASSOCIATED WITH INTERSTITIAL LUNG DISEASE

ACUTE EXACERBATION

First described by Kondo and colleagues in 1993 (1), AE was formally recognized as a complication of idiopathic pulmonary fibrosis (IPF) by international consensus in 2007 (2). It was defined as abrupt worsening of dyspnoea and hypoxaemia over a time period of less than 30 days not explained by secondary causes such as infection, congestive heart failure (CHF) or pulmonary embolism (PE). New and superimposed diffuse bilateral infiltrates as seen on chest computed tomography (CT) or chest x-ray (CXR) are important to the definition. Despite consensus diagnostic criteria, difficulty in meeting all components in clinical practice is common, particularly as a standardized approach to excluding secondary causes is not well established. Acuity of presentation, which is often accompanied by severe hypoxaemia, may preclude elective bronchoscopy or endotracheal suction as a means to effectively rule out infection. Recent efforts have been made to describe 'suspected acute exacerbation', where careful history and assessment of clinical symptoms along with blood and sputum cultures may be sufficient to rule out infectious causes (3). A recent revision of the international guideline highlights the presence of parenchymal findings not related to volume overload or heart failure, moving away from the need to distinguish other specific triggers. In essence, the term 'idiopathic' now applies primarily to being unable to find a trigger for an AE event, with known aetiologies such as infection or drug toxicity now falling under the umbrella of AE diagnosis (4).

Though prior and current criteria were constructed for identification of AE in IPF, AE has also been described in connective-tissue disease associated ILD (CTD-ILD) (5) and hypersensitivity pneumonitis (HP) (6,7). The incidence of AE events in patients with IPF varies among reported case series and is affected by selected definitions of an AE event and the duration of assessment. The largest series to date noted a 14.2% incidence at 1 year and 20.7% at 3 years (8). This was comparable to other series suggesting an incidence of 7% to 8.7% (9,10) at 1 year and up to 23.9% and 28% at 3 years (10,11). The reported AE incidence in the placebo arm of a randomized clinical trial of nintedanib in IPF was 8% at 1 year (12). A recent review of acute respiratory worsening among ILD patients found that 29% of patients presented with acute respiratory failure as a first presentation of fibrotic lung disease (13). Parambil and colleagues reported that three of seven (43%) fatal AE cases undergoing autopsy presented as previously undiagnosed ILD (14). Other described triggers have included viral infection (15), aspiration (16), air pollution (17), bronchoscopy (18,19) and surgical lung biopsy (19,20).

The underlying pathophysiology of AE remains unknown, whereas autopsy and biopsy studies note diffuse alveolar damage (DAD) superimposed on underlying fibrotic patterns (14) (Figure 27.1). Associated histopathologic findings have included usual interstitial pneumonia (UIP) (14), non-specific interstitial pneumonia (NSIP) (21) and features of concomitant or superimposed organizing pneumonia (OP) (14) (Figure 27.2). Theoretical frameworks include the rapid progression of already present and underlying fibrosis, a unique or alternate phenomenon of progression separate from inherent fibrosis, or a non-specific lung injury in response to an unspecified trigger outside of the fibrotic process (4). In one large series, association of a bronchoalveolar lavage (BAL) lymphocyte-predominant differential cell count was noted in those with suspected AE as compared to neutrophil predominance in patients in whom infection was identified (8). Because the benefit of the historical use of high-dose steroids in the acute setting for suppression of possible overwhelming inflammation has proven equivocal, whether lymphocytes or lymphocyte-derived cytokines drive processes that are responsible for acute infiltrates and worsening hypoxaemia that characterize AE

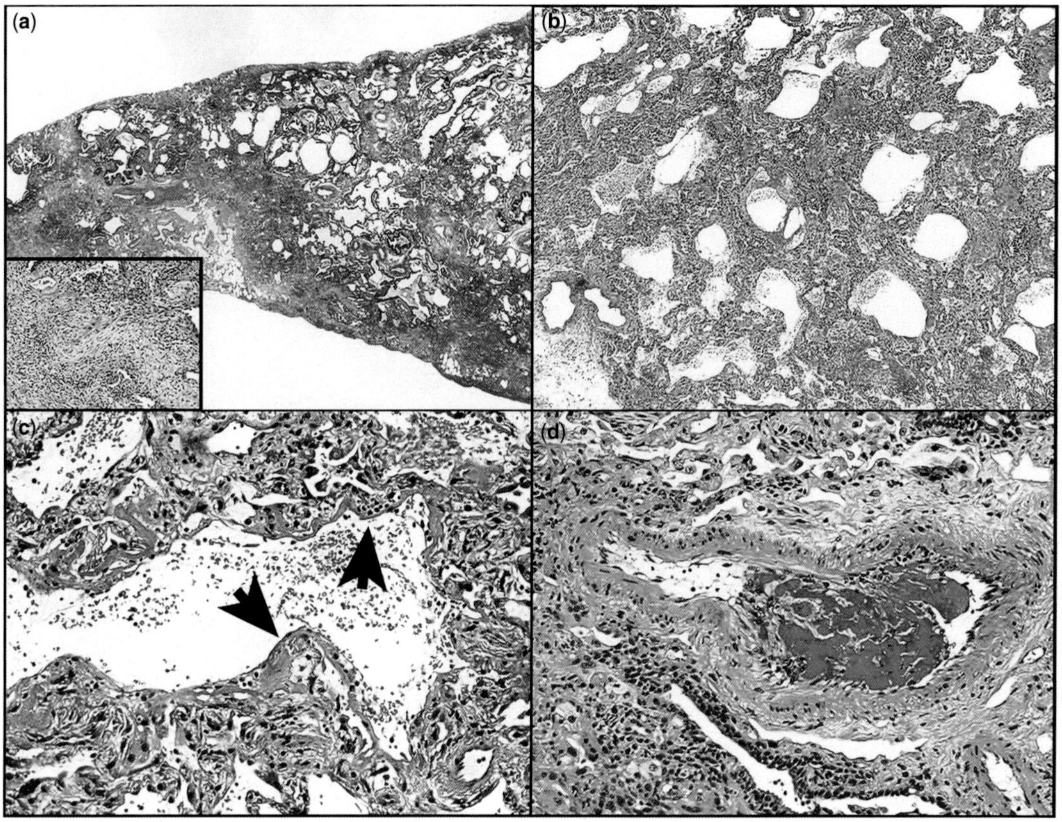

Figure 27.1 DAD superimposed on UIP. **(a)** A low-power view from a section of the lower lobe lung reveals interstitial peripheral/subpleural collagen fibrosis with honeycomb changes and fibroblast foci (inset). Focally, architectural preserved lung parenchyma is present (upper right hand). These morphologic features are consistent with UIP. **(b)** Sections from the lower and upper lobe also show interstitial thickening, which predominantly is due to fibroblast proliferation, type II pneumocyte hyperplasia and chronic inflammation. **(c)** Hyaline membranes are identified (c, arrows). These features are supportive of acute and organizing DAD. **(d)** Fibrin thrombi, as often seen in acute lung injury, are present. Haematoxylin & eosin, magnification × 12.5 (a), × 100 (a inset), × 40 (b), × 200 (c, d). (Courtesy of Dr Anja C Roden, Mayo Clinic Rochester.)

remain unknown (13,22). Nonetheless, underlying inflammation or cytokine-induced injury as a cause of AE is suggested by the recovery of some patients when managed with haemoperfusion (23,24).

Previously described risk factors associated with in-hospital mortality include mechanical ventilation (13,25,26), AE associated with a diagnosis of IPF (13,27), increased age, lower forced vital capacity (FVC) and diffusing capacity for carbon monoxide (DLCO) on presentation and treatment with immunosuppressive agents (8). In-hospital mortality associated with AE ranges from 20% to 100% (2,4), which is an ongoing concern for research studies using endpoints of FVC decline where

disease progression may be punctuated and confounded by rapid clinical deterioration and death due to an AE event. Efforts to define AE or acute respiratory worsening with hospitalization as clinical endpoints in treatment trials are ongoing (28).

INFECTION

While the 2007 AE criteria support the exclusion of infection in the diagnosis of AE, lack of a routine or specific approach to defining an infection as a culprit may underestimate its true incidence. In particular, timing of bronchoscopy or endotracheal aspiration, which specific microbiologic tests are performed (array of bacterial and viral studies)

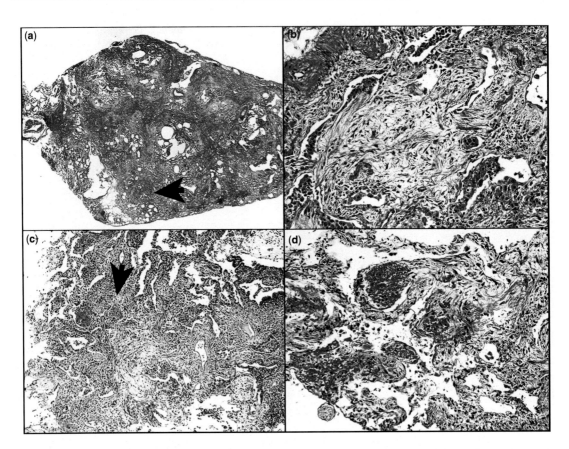

Figure 27.2 Organizing fibrinous pneumonia superimposed on UIP in a patient with rheumatoid arthritis presenting in acute exacerbation. **(a)** The lower lobe lung shows peripheral/subpleural collagen fibrosis with honeycomb changes, scattered lymphoid follicles (arrow) and fibroblast foci **(b)** in the vicinity to architectural preserved lung parenchyma (upper left hand). These morphologic features are consistent with UIP. **(c)**, **(d)**. In the upper lobe lung, in the areas of non-fibrotic lung parenchyma, intraalveolar fibrin (arrow) and plugs of proliferating fibroblasts are suggestive of organizing fibrinous pneumonia. Haematoxylin & eosin, magnification × 12.5 (a), × 200 (b, d), × 100 (c). (Courtesy of Dr Anja C Roden, Mayo Clinic Rochester.)

and early use of empiric broad-spectrum antibiotics may confound the ability to detect infection. Additionally, the use of recent immunosuppression (especially in the absence of prophylaxis) may lead to more infectious complications, though the exact incidence or prevalence of this scenario is unknown. In one large series reviewing bronchoscopic findings indicative of infection in patients with acute respiratory worsening and ILD, the prevalence of immunosuppression was not associated with a greater risk of infection (29). In contrast, Song et al. noted that 57.1% of diagnosed infections in their series were associated with the presence of opportunistic pathogens and recent immunosuppression with or without steroid-sparing agents (8). Other large series reviewing broadly

defined respiratory decline in patients with IPF or ILD note the prevalence of an infectious cause ranges from 11% to 31.3% (8,13,27). Finally, an autopsy series of 52 consecutive patients with IPF dying from suspected AE found bronchopneumonia in 28.8% (30), which suggests that empiric treatment of infection as a potential underlying cause of acute respiratory failure is not unreasonable (Figure 27.3).

PULMONARY HYPERTENSION

Pulmonary hypertension (PH) has been extensively reported in association with IPF (31–34). Its prevalence ranges from 32% (35) to 86.4% (36) by the time of lung transplantation evaluation, contributing significantly to morbidity and mortality. In one series of patients undergoing right heart catheterization (RHC), the prevalence of PH was as high as 46.1% (37). Diagnosis may often be obtained by screening transthoracic echo (TTE) using pulmonary artery systolic pressure (PASP) or right ventricular systolic pressure (RVSP) as surrogates for disease not assessed or confirmed by RHC. Echocardiographic measures have been shown to be predictive of poorer survival in IPF (38). Using TTE criteria of PASP > 36 mm Hg, PH was found in 55% of evaluated IPF patients (39). A recent study of 52 patients with IPF noted impaired RV function compared to controls even when PH was not fully diagnosed, suggesting the value of TTE findings in the assessment of early disease (40). The presence of PH has been assumed to be associated with more advanced clinical disease, though correlation with degree or severity of fibrosis on CT was not identified in one study (41). Rather, the severity of abnormal RVSP values appears to correlate inversely with DLCO (38,39).

Several pathologic mechanisms that cause PH have been previously proposed including intrinsic fibrosis leading to decreased vascular cross-sectional area for arterial vessels (42,43), vascular remodeling that is perhaps driven by the same fibrotic and microthrombotic process (44) and reflexive arterial vasoconstriction due to hypoxaemia. Because cor pulmonale may develop over

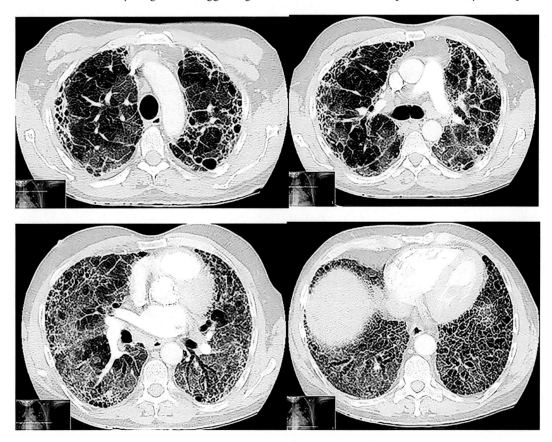

Figure 27.3 A 57-year-old male presented with Raynaud's, elevated ANA and UIP CT pattern initially concerning for undifferentiated ILD. Given poor response to 16 months of prednisone and mycophenolate, the patient was transitioned to nintedanib for 6 months, returning at follow-up with worsening dyspnoea and decline in lung function. A trial of high-dose prednisone was reinitiated and by week 3, the patient presented with severe hypoxemia and the CT findings of diffuse ground glass infiltrates. Sputum PCR was positive for pneumocystis pneumonia leading to a 4-week hospitalization with directed antibiotics and supportive treatments (steroids and high flow nasal cannula oxygen). The patient was assessed for transplantation but died on hospital day 29 from progressive respiratory failure.

time, both left- and right-sided heart disease may contribute to acute clinical decline that warrants assessment of cardiac function at the time of critical care admission. Indeed, in the setting of an acutely hypoxaemic patient with progressive dyspnoea and absence of pulmonary infiltrates, PH should be on the differential and assessed. Baseline PH has been described as increasing risk of AE by 2.2 times and is associated with poorer survival (43) and prognosis (45,46). Specific management strategies for PH in IPF are limited and often not pursued acutely other than to treat hypoxaemia, as there is concern for worsening shunt with the use of vasodilators in World Health Organization (WHO) Class III PH patients as a whole. While it is hoped that directed treatment of PH may extend life in patients with ILD, published treatment trials in IPF have not shown efficacy (47,48). A sparse amount of literature exists in terms of directed treatment of PH associated with other forms of ILD (49,50), and considering the heterogeneity of ILD types and presentations, further study is needed.

CORONARY ARTERY DISEASE/ CONGESTIVE HEART FAILURE

Risk of acute coronary syndrome (ACS) in IPF was previously described as greater than that of non-IPF controls and increased after IPF diagnosis as compared to the pre-diagnosis period (51). Despite the described association of coronary artery disease (CAD) with lung fibrosis, the incidence or frequency of ACS associated with ICU level care is unknown. Prior studies suggest increased prevalence of CAD in IPF ranging from 40% (52) to 65.8% (53), and Kizer et al. found an odds ratio (OR) of 2.18 for the prevalence of CAD in fibrotic lung disease when compared with non-fibrotic lung diseases (54). Kizer and colleagues also found even greater risk of multi-vessel disease (OR 4.16) in their large cohort comparison of fibrotic versus non-fibrotic lung disease when patients underwent cardiac catheterization for lung transplantation (54). Similar findings were noted by Izbicki and colleagues despite greater smoking history among chronic obstructive pulmonary disease (COPD) controls (55). Coronary calcification scoring as assessed during routine CT studies in patients with IPF has been proposed as a possible screening tool for detecting

CAD (56). Morbidity associated with acute ischaemia has not been well reported; only one study that compared CAD in IPF versus COPD patients noted worse survival in IPF from the time of cardiac catheterization (53). Prior speculation regarding possible benefits of statin use (52,57) as a treatment for fibrotic lung disease may, perhaps, reflect the increased risk of CAD (and statin use) among IPF patients. A recent large cohort assessment of IPF and ILD patients in Denmark that compared survival in statin users versus non-users found improved median survival in statin-treated patients for both disease groups with an overall reduced risk for all-cause mortality (HR 0.73) (58). Given the increased risk of CAD among ILD patients and related morbidity, evaluation for ACS should be considered at the time of an acute illness presentation.

The incidence and prevalence of congestive heart failure (CHF) are relatively unknown in ILD patients presenting with acute respiratory failure. Prior studies report an incidence of 1.1% at presentation in IPF patients (8) and 6% for all patients admitted with fibrotic ILD (13). Of note, updated guidelines for the diagnosis of AE emphasize the exclusion of CHF and volume overload as an initial first step, which follows a similar model in the diagnosis of acute respiratory distress syndrome (ARDS), where exclusion of pulmonary oedema initially leads to further assessment for other known causes or triggers of diffuse parenchymal infiltrates, (4). TTE may be the logical and least invasive assessment for cardiac dysfunction in the setting of suspected volume overload, although no specific approach has been recommended.

DEEP-VEIN THROMBOSIS/ PULMONARY EMBOLISM

Haemodynamic instability from massive PE in the setting of ILD may certainly lead to ICU admission. The incidence and prevalence of DVT/PE among patients with idiopathic interstitial pneumonia (IIP) have been previously described as 1.8 per 10,000 person-years with increased morbidity and mortality for those never treated previously with anticoagulants (HR 2.8) (59). Another large epidemiologic study suggested a 34% increased risk of DVT/PE in ILD patients compared to controls, which is greater than that associated with COPD or lung cancer (60). As patients with acute hypoxaemia may not be suspected of having DVT/PE, particularly when presenting with diffuse bilateral infiltrates, the true incidence of thromboembolic disease may be underestimated. A large cohort study of ILD patients noted that PE protocol CT was performed in only 43% of admitted patients, with PE diagnosed in 10% of patients subjected to a CT (13). The frequency of diagnosed

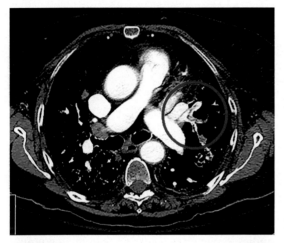

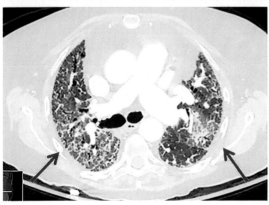

Figure 27.4 An 87-year-old female with previously established idiopathic NSIP presented with a three-week history of progressive dyspnoea and new-onset hypoxemia (>5 L of oxygen). A chest PE protocol CT revealed diffuse superimposed ground glass infiltrates (arrows in lower panel) and left segmental artery emboli (circle in upper panel). The ultrasound studies of the lower extremities were negative for DVT, and the patient was treated with antibiotics and therapeutic anticoagulation. She died on BiPAP support without mechanical ventilation on hospital day 12 after transition to comfort measures.

PE was no different between those with IPF and non-IPF disease. Comparatively, Song and colleagues found thromboembolic disease as a cause of acute respiratory worsening in less than 1% of hospitalized IPF patients (0.4%) (8). Finally, an autopsy study found PE in 17.3% of IPF patients dying from suspected AE (30). Directed management of DVT/PE in the setting of ILD is similar to that for other intrinsic lung diseases, but the impact of timely detection and directed treatment on survival is unclear (Figure 27.4).

DIAGNOSTIC EVALUATION OF CRITICAL ILLNESS IN ILD PATIENTS

CLINICAL PRESENTATION

Confounding the initial assessment of critically ill patients with underlying ILD is the non-specific nature of their clinical presentation. In particular, many may have slow or progressive decline in baseline symptoms with progressive hypoxaemia and fibrosis but do not meet criteria for AE because of a subacute presentation with a longer duration of decline (>30 days) or the absence of acute radiologic infiltrates superimposed on chronic changes of ILD. Such patients may have expected worsening in pulmonary hypertension or cor pulmonale, which is often the final cause of respiratory failure in patients with end-stage disease. Cough and fever were reported by Kondoh and colleagues in their original report of three patients presenting with suspected AE (1). In one large series reviewing the yield of diagnostic bronchoscopy for ILD patients hospitalized with respiratory failure, bronchoscopic findings, which were indicative of infection in only 12 of 106 patients, did not have a significant impact on management or outcome (29). Huie and colleagues also found a third of patients were febrile at the time of hospital presentation (27). In contrast, Song et al. noted greater prevalence of fever in those with confirmed infection than those meeting criteria for AE in their review of consecutive IPF patients presenting with respiratory worsening (51% versus 20%) (8). Other signs or symptoms such as lower extremity oedema or volume overload have not been previously reported among acutely ill ILD patients. Such findings may be reasonably attributed to either right- or left-sided heart disease. Asymmetric lower extremity oedema or swelling may prompt ultrasound assessment for DVT or the pursuit of a PE-protocol CT (based on presenting renal function), although in the presence of bilateral pulmonary infiltrates which is often atypical for PE in general, a high index of suspicion for possible thromboembolic disease is required. DVT/PE may often be diagnosed later during hospitalization (for example after initial poor response to empiric antibiotics or diuresis) or at post-mortem examination (30). Hypoxaemia with increased dyspnoea requiring higher oxygen support with invasive or non-invasive support is often the catalyst for ICU admission, but this alone is non-specific and can be attributed to multiple causes. No data exist on the severity of hypoxaemia as predictive of an underlying aetiology for acute respiratory failure.

An additional difficulty in the assessment of AE of ILD is that up to a third of patients have previously undiagnosed disease when they present with an AE event (13). While the identification of an underlying cause may be important for acute management, little is known about which specific testing is most likely to lead to an accurate ILD diagnosis. Indeed, many patients are too acutely ill to tolerate lung biopsy, though a surgical approach may provide greater yield. Auto-immune serologic studies and rheumatology consultation for an associated CTD may be indicated, especially if a clinical history is obtained that is suggestive, but benefit in terms of acute management or modification of treatment plans is limited. Whether diagnosing an associated CTD precludes lung transplant evaluation as rescue therapy is also unknown, as transplantation for patients with AE is rare, even when a diagnosis has been established, and the decision to offer transplant to patients with CTD-ILD is centre-dependent (61).

IMAGING STUDIES AND ECHOCARDIOGRAPHY

Current definition of AE requires bilateral, diffuse infiltrates superimposed on chronic changes of ILD. When superimposed infiltrates are present, the degree and pattern of underlying fibrosis may be difficult to assess, particularly in patients without previously established disease. The severity or extent of baseline radiologic fibrosis has not been found to be predictive of AE (8,10), but the extent and distribution of superimposed infiltrates have been associated with in-hospital mortality in IPF (62). Akira and colleagues confirmed that AE with more diffuse infiltrates portended worse in-hospital and follow-up mortality as compared to those with patchy or less extensive multifocal acute findings (63). Initial CT findings should be scrutinized for typical features of opportunistic infection such as *Pneumocystis jirovecii* pneumonia (PJP) or CHF. Findings such as interlobular septal thickening and pleural effusion may provide additional clues to a diagnosis of left ventricular dysfunction and CHF. Such findings which have also been reported in those with lone right-sided heart disease (64,65).

Performance of a PE protocol CT from two recent series ranged from 43% to 85% (13,27). Whether a PE protocol study performed at the time of ER assessment or admission is helpful or can be safely obtained may be dependent on presenting renal function and initial clinical suspicion for DVT/PE (such as asymmetric lower leg swelling, recent fall or trauma, associated malignancy, etc.). Indeed, of those patients who received screening studies in one series, only 10% had PE diagnosed, and these patients all had concomitant bilateral infiltrates (13). If infiltrates are minimal or absent, suspicion for worsening cor pulmonale or PE is reasonable, although PE may also be diagnosed in patients with parenchymal findings (66). Chest x-ray as a lone imaging study in the assessment of acute respiratory worsening to identify a specific aetiology is likely to be insufficient in defining subtle radiologic features of fibrosis or superimposed infiltrates, particularly in those with previously undiagnosed disease. With that in mind, admission or ER chest CT in patients with ILD and acute respiratory failure may be warranted, and, if safe to perform, may be obtained with contrast per a PE protocol for the same duration of scanner time.

Transthoracic echocardiography is commonly obtained during critical illness to assess both left- and right-ventricular dysfunction. Mean RVSP in one series of patients with fibrotic ILD was elevated at 56 mm Hg with a mean ejection fraction of 62% (13), but neither finding was predictive of in-hospital death from AE or secondary causes. Because RVSP is often elevated, TTE may be the best modality for detecting or excluding diastolic or systolic left ventricular dysfunction as contributing to pulmonary oedema, as emphasized by recent AE guidelines (4).

LABORATORY ASSESSMENTS

No specific laboratory studies can diagnose AE, but such testing may be helpful in the exclusion of secondary causes. A complete blood count to detect leucocytosis, an erythrocyte sedimentation rate (ESR) and C-reactive protein (CRP) as non-specific markers of inflammation or infection, sputum microbiology including culture and staining inclusive of PJP polymerase chain reaction (PCR) and blood cultures can all provide useful information, although these have not been independently assessed in terms of their yield or contribution to diagnosis. A metabolic panel with measurement of electrolytes, creatinine and blood urea nitrogen to assess renal function may be helpful to determine whether IV contrast for PE assessment can be safely given as well as guide diuresis in patients with suspected CHF. Brain natriuretic peptide (BNP) may be helpful in screening for CHF and PE, which may be present alone or together in the acutely hypoxaemic ILD patient. An elevated pro-BNP (>155 pg/mL) was found in 76% of acutely ill ILD patients in one case series when patients who had an admission TTE were found to have a mean RVSP of 53 mm Hg or higher. Although BNP can be non-specifically elevated in older patients, elevated BNP was not predictive of bronchoscopy findings or the presence of clinical heart failure (29).

Few data exist concerning the frequency of positive blood cultures among ILD patients with AE when assessed for infection. There are also no data on the contribution of bloodstream infection to morbidity or mortality versus infection diagnosed or suspected primarily in the lung. Arterial blood gas sampling may be more helpful in the assessment of hypercapnia than hypoxaemia, as a means of gauging respiratory failure and ventilation, but is non-specific in identifying an aetiology for acute respiratory worsening. Other laboratory assessments such as immunoglobulins or CTD serology panels, if clinically appropriate, may help in diagnosing infection or an undiagnosed CTD-ILD (if not previously established) as a cause of AE. In one series, the frequency of AE was greater in IPF than secondary ILD (CTD-ILD, chronic HP, etc.) (13,27), yet in-hospital mortality was similar due to the significant

morbidity associated with secondary causes such as infection or heart failure in non-IPF patients (13). In that regard, screening studies obtained during acute illness to detect the possibility of CTD-related diagnoses are unlikely to alter management or predict any incremental improvement in survival, and such testing should be obtained more on a case-by-case basis as defined by a reliable review of systems or suggestive history. Recent interest in procalcitonin as an indicator of acute bacterial infection has led to one small case series that examined its potential role in the differentiation of AE from acute infection in ILD. Significantly lower values were observed in AE compared to infected controls with acute respiratory distress syndrome (ARDS) (67) and infected ILD patients. Of note, depending on institutional cut-offs, mean serum procalcitonin was still positive in those with suspected AE (0.62 ± 1.30; normal range <0.15) though to a lesser degree. Also of interest, positive findings did not predict differences in survival at 30 days.

BRONCHOSCOPY

The first international consensus statement for diagnosis of AE specifically described performance of bronchoscopy as a means to rule out infection in those with known fibrosis and new infiltrates. While likely to provide the greatest diagnostic yield by direct lavage of the lung, little is known about historical yield in this population and its contribution to modifying care or acute management. Much anxiety exists in electively performing bronchoscopy in patients presenting with severe hypoxaemia and respiratory distress. In particular, there is concern that an invasive procedure may lead to sustained intubation and mechanical ventilation with its associated morbidity and mortality risks. Indeed, BAL has also been described as a trigger of AE (18,68). Consequently, yield may be affected by delayed performance of BAL as well as the institutional selection of screening studies or diagnostic tests when evaluating patients with acute respiratory compromise. Huie et al. noted that 85% of patients with acute respiratory worsening underwent bronchoscopy in their series, and 100% of definitive AE cases had the procedure performed (27). In a recent retrospective review of a large cohort of ILD patients with acute respiratory worsening undergoing bronchoscopy, the historical diagnostic yield was 13%, distributed nearly equally between infection and suspected alveolar haemorrhage (29). It was noted that a majority of procedures were performed after elective or with impending intubation, with elective procedures leading to escalation of care (including admission to ICU and inability to extubate after elective intubation) in 25% (29). Empiric management including antibiotics and steroids were also provided to nearly all patients, and changes in management as directed by positive bronchoscopy findings had negligible impact on immediate hospital mortality (29). BAL lymphocytosis appeared to be predictive of AE in IPF (8), while a larger ILD cohort study did not find similar utility for BAL cell differential counts in IPF or non-IPF patients (13). Viral studies have detected possible infection from the BAL of those with suspected AE (69,70), and the presence of pepsin in BAL (16) suggested reflux or aspiration as possible triggers of an AE event. While bronchoscopic findings may be helpful, the safety of bronchoscopy remains inconclusive. Many procedures are performed after expected intubation and mechanical ventilation, where true procedure-related complications may be underestimated. Other assessments such as nasotracheal suction or induced cough with nebulized saline have not been independently studied but may be reliable and safe approaches.

BIOPSY

Surgical biopsy is often recommended in the diagnostic assessment of ILD, but due to risk of complications and limited benefit when used in the acute setting, its performance has declined over time. Transbronchial biopsy may detect infectious or inflammatory aetiologies not seen on BAL alone, but its benefit in the ICU setting is limited, particularly with risk of pneumothorax and hastening further decline in those with already poor respiratory status. Surgical biopsy has also been previously reported as a trigger of AE (8,71). Although a recent epidemiologic assessment of surgical lung biopsy in ILD found in-hospital mortality to be only 1.7%, these procedures were performed electively and not during acute illness (20). Indeed, as autopsy studies in those dying from AE have found a predominance of histologic DAD, a non-specific injury pattern that does not identify a particular aetiology or require alteration in patient management, biopsy appears unwarranted in this setting.

MANAGEMENT OF CRITICALLY ILL PATIENTS WITH ILD

TREATMENT OF HYPOXAEMIA

Escalation of support for hypoxaemia ranges from supplemental oxygen delivery via nasal cannula to high-flow face mask and non-invasive positive pressure ventilation, all measures that can be taken before resorting to intubation and mechanical ventilation. As the underlying pathophysiology of lung injury is often unknown, proposed treatment strategies reflect those used in acute respiratory distress syndrome (ARDS) or non-specific lung injury and are titrated according to the severity of respiratory impairment. With worsening hypoxaemia and increased work of breathing, admission to a higher acuity setting with close monitoring is naturally pursued, although these interventions have not been adequately studied for their contribution to improving mortality or hospital survival. Recent trends in practice noting the significant morbidity and mortality of invasive mechanical ventilation have pushed providers towards using non-invasive high-flow nasal cannula with flows as high as 60 L/min and FiO_2 at 100% (72) with or without the use of positive airway pressure modalities of continuous positive airway pressure (CPAP) or bi-level positive airway pressure (BiPAP) to support increased work of breathing. Recent studies also suggest the utility of high-flow nasal cannula in those with advanced hypoxaemia, which can allow supportive oxygenation without the complications of invasive mechanical ventilation (73–75) and increase patient comfort while delaying or obviating the need to institute mechanical ventilatory support. Because there are no current, adequately validated treatment interventions for AE, avoiding sedation and mechanical ventilation, yet maintaining oxygen support and comfort are key principles for optimizing patient management.

TREATMENT OF SUSPECTED INFECTION

A review of several large series suggests that the empiric and directed treatment of infection occurs invariably in most ILD patients when hospitalized with acute respiratory decline. In the ICU setting, broad-spectrum antimicrobial coverage that is typically given for severe community-acquired pneumonia is often replicated for patients with suspected AE, and curtailment of such therapy can be considered after 48–72 hours of empiric treatment. There is no consensus for which antibiotics are best or evidence that this approach improves mortality even when infection is suspected, but given similar initial presentations in patients with AE and those who are ultimately diagnosed with infection, empiric treatment is reasonable. Empiric use of anti-viral or anti-fungal therapy has not been described or validated in AE, and most institutions avoid this except when immuno-compromised states exist or specific clinical presentations (nodular infiltrates or cavitations) are identified. In this setting, empiric trimethoprim-sulphamethoxazole at treatment doses for PJP may also be given, although evidence is lacking in the published literature and the incidence of PJP in this population is undefined.

USE OF HIGH-DOSE IV STEROIDS

Little data exist regarding the efficacy of high-dose or pulse IV steroids in the management of AE. While historically extrapolated from the management of exacerbations in CTD (76–80) or alveolar haemorrhage in patients with immunocompromised or cytokine-driven states (81,82), no validated evidence exists regarding its efficacy in AE. In a recent review of hospitalized ILD patients with acute respiratory failure, 30% were given protocol-directed treatment defined as methylprednisolone (or its equivalent) greater than 500 mg a day for at least 3 days or more, but no impact on survival was observed (13). Twenty-three percent of AE-IPF cases in another series were treated with pulsed dose steroids with or without an additional cytotoxic agent, but improved outcome was again not observed (8). Among IPF patients, use of high-dose IV steroids appeared to be associated with increased morbidity and in-hospital mortality, although this outcome may have been reflective of the greater morbidity and mortality associated with AE in patients with IPF rather than a direct complication of steroids themselves (13). While not predictive of greater mortality among non-IPF patients, no benefit was also found for corticosteroid administration (13). A review assessing consecutive IPF patients with suspected AE found

prior use of immunosuppressants contributed to worse survival during an AE event with no difference in survival in those receiving high-dose steroids during hospitalization (22). As no prior studies have supported the empiric use of IV steroids as beneficial for any ILD subtype or aetiology of acute respiratory decline, steroid therapy in this setting is likely unwarranted and of minimal benefit.

NON-INVASIVE AND INVASIVE MECHANICAL VENTILATION

Multiple studies have previously reported significant morbidity and mortality associated with intubation and mechanical ventilation in patients admitted with AE (25,26,83). Earlier series report a mortality of 85% (83) to 100% (25,26,84), with a more recent series suggesting 94% mortality (27). Mechanical ventilation was also independently predictive of in-hospital death in both IPF and non-IPF patients in one series (13). The morbidity associated with mechanical ventilation has not been correlated with either a greater severity of baseline disease (and therefore required support) or the direct consequences of ventilator-associated lung injury and its sequelae. No studies have identified an optimal mode of ventilator support, but given the similarity of an AE event to ARDS, a low tidal volume strategy is commonly applied (27). Recent cohort studies have suggested considerable variation in the duration of mechanical ventilation and its use as a predictor of hospital outcome (13,83,85), with some patients surviving for at least several weeks after planned tracheostomy and long-term ventilator weaning protocols. Indeed, given the poor outcome of patients requiring mechanical ventilation, it has been suggested that mechanical ventilation should only be used as a bridge to rescue transplantation (26,86), as it offers little short or long-term benefit.

OTHER TREATMENT STRATEGIES

Recent series have suggested benefit from haemoperfusion using polymyxin B-immobilized filters, which theoretically remove circulating pro-inflammatory cytokines and have been reported to improve survival in AE associated with IPF (87–89). The largest retrospective series to date of 160 patients treated at 18 Japanese institutions noted improved oxygenation and a 70% post-AE 1-month survival, as compared to the usually high mortality rate historically associated with hospitalization (23). While of interest, no comparison trials have occurred to date, and the practice has not been widely accepted. In two of three clinical trials assessing the efficacy of nintedanib as chronic therapy for IPF (12,90), frequency and time to an AE event appeared reduced compared to placebo, although this finding was not a primary indication for prescribing the drug. Lung transplantation is rarely performed as a rescue therapy in the setting of AE, and it cannot be reliably offered as a treatment strategy.

SHORT- AND LONG-TERM IMPLICATIONS OF ACUTE RESPIRATORY FAILURE: END-OF-LIFE AND PALLIATIVE CARE

Multiple small and large cohort series evaluating admission for critical illness in IPF and other fibrotic lung diseases report high rates of in-hospital morbidity and mortality (13,27,84,91–93). Mechanically ventilated patients have greater mortality that likely reflects a synergistic effect from both baseline disease and the additional complications of an AE event and its directed management. When patients are assessed based on disease

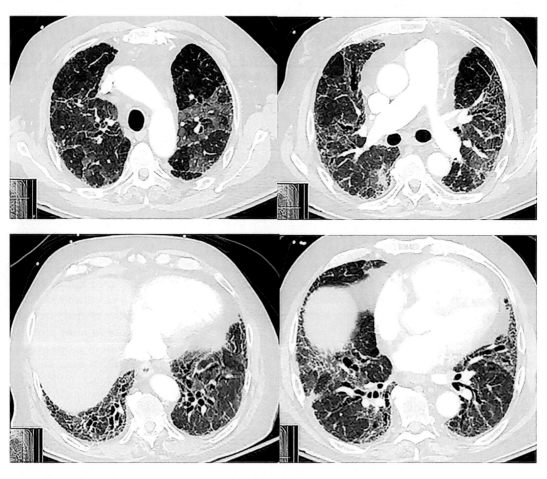

Figure 27.5 A 78-year-old male with biopsy proven IPF (UIP pathology without secondary aetiology) presented with a two-week history of progressive dyspnoea and dry cough. An admission chest CT revealed mild patchy ground glass infiltrates superimposed on early or possible UIP CT pattern. The patient was managed initially with high-flow oxygen support but eventually intubated and mechanically ventilated for six days, successfully undergoing extubation on hospital day 9 and discharged home on hospital day 16. The patient died 14 months later at home from progressive respiratory failure with hospice care support.

diagnosis (IPF versus non-IPF), in-hospital mortality appeared similar (13), though this was still greater in IPF patients admitted with suspected AE (8). Of note, post-discharge survival appeared dismal for both IPF and non-IPF patients regardless of the cause of the initial decompensation (8,13,27) (Figure 27.5). Inpatient and outpatient management strategies should reflect the overall scope of disease during an acute illness episode with a close assessment of expectations and patient-centred targets of symptom management and quality of life during and after ICU discharge. A recent study found that while more than half of IPF patients die in a hospital setting, only 13.7% received a formal palliative care referral, which was mostly obtained within a month of death (94). Indeed, challenges remain regarding the timing, location and appropriate provider (primary pulmonologist or intensivist) for patient–provider discussions of palliative measures or end-of-life decisions (95). Many patients admit to a lack of pre-hospital advisement on such issues and complete unawareness of the possibility of acute critical illness as a complication of their disease (96). Indeed, physicians are reluctant to take away hope unnecessarily due to the unpredictability of disease course and potential opportunities to participate in novel clinical trials or pursue currently available antifibrotic therapies (95). As current management of acutely ill patients with AE of underlying IPF is largely supportive with relatively little influence on acute and long-term survival post-ICU admission, a focus on patient realization of these expectations prior to and during critical illness are important steps in management.

CONCLUSIONS

Critical illness in ILD is dominated by AE and other related co-morbidities including advanced PH, CAD, DVT/PE and infection. Large studies assessing current morbidity and mortality in those presenting with acute respiratory failure suggest efforts to avoid invasive mechanical ventilation with high-flow oxygen support, the administration of empiric antibiotics and exclusion of cardiac dysfunction and thromboembolic disease. As morbidity and mortality remain high for patients presenting with AE, early involvement of palliative care during and after critical illness is important in maximizing patient quality of life and clarifying expectations.

REFERENCES

1. Kondoh Y, Taniguchi H, Kawabata Y, Yokoi T, Suzuki K, Takagi K. Acute exacerbation in idiopathic pulmonary fibrosis. Analysis of clinical and pathologic findings in three cases. *Chest.* 1993;103(6):1808–12.
2. Collard HR, Moore BB, Flaherty KR, Brown KK, Kaner RJ, King TE Jr., et al. Acute exacerbations of idiopathic pulmonary fibrosis. *Am J Respir Crit Care Med.* 2007;176(7):636–43.
3. Collard HR, Yow E, Richeldi L, Anstrom KJ, Glazer C. Suspected acute exacerbation of idiopathic pulmonary fibrosis as an outcome measure in clinical trials. *Respir Res.* 2013;14:73.
4. Collard HR, Ryerson CJ, Corte TJ, Jenkins G, Kondoh Y, Lederer DJ, et al. Acute Exacerbation of Idiopathic Pulmonary Fibrosis. An International Working Group Report. *Am J Respir Crit Care Med.* 2016;194(3):265–75.
5. Tachikawa R, Tomii K, Ueda H, Nagata K, Nanjo S, Sakurai A, et al. Clinical features and outcome of acute exacerbation of interstitial pneumonia: collagen vascular diseases-related versus idiopathic. *Respiration.* 2012;83(1):20–7.
6. Miyazaki Y, Tateishi T, Akashi T, Ohtani Y, Inase N, Yoshizawa Y. Clinical predictors and histologic appearance of acute exacerbations in chronic hypersensitivity pneumonitis. *Chest.* 2008;134(6):1265–70.
7. Hariri LP, Mino-Kenudson M, Shea B, Digumarthy S, Onozato M, Yagi Y, et al. Distinct histopathology of acute onset or abrupt exacerbation of hypersensitivity pneumonitis. *Hum Pathol.* 2012;43(5):660–8.
8. Song JW, Hong SB, Lim CM, Koh Y, Kim DS. Acute exacerbation of idiopathic pulmonary fibrosis: incidence, risk factors and outcome. *Eur Respir J.* 2011;37(2):356–63.
9. Ohshimo S, Ishikawa N, Horimasu Y, Hattori N, Hirohashi N, Tanigawa K, et al. Baseline KL-6 predicts increased risk for acute exacerbation of idiopathic pulmonary fibrosis. *Respir Med.* 2014;108(7):1031–9.

10. Kondoh Y, Taniguchi H, Katsuta T, Kataoka K, Kimura T, Nishiyama O, et al. Risk factors of acute exacerbation of idiopathic pulmonary fibrosis. *Sarcoidosis Vasc Diffuse Lung Dis*. 2010;27(2):103–10.

11. Sugino K, Nakamura Y, Ito T, Isshiki T, Sakamoto S, Homma S. Comparison of clinical characteristics and outcomes between combined pulmonary fibrosis and emphysema associated with usual interstitial pneumonia pattern and non-usual interstitial pneumonia. *Sarcoidosis Vasc Diffuse Lung Dis*. 2015;32(2):129–37.

12. Richeldi L, du Bois RM, Raghu G, Azuma A, Brown KK, Costabel U, et al. Efficacy and safety of nintedanib in idiopathic pulmonary fibrosis. *N Engl J Med*. 2014;370(22):2071–82.

13. Moua T, Westerly BD, Dulohery MM, Daniels CE, Ryu JH, Lim KG. Patients With Fibrotic Interstitial Lung Disease Hospitalized for Acute Respiratory Worsening: A Large Cohort *Analysis*. *Chest*. 2016;149(5):1205–14.

14. Parambil JG, Myers JL, Ryu JH. Histopathologic features and outcome of patients with acute exacerbation of idiopathic pulmonary fibrosis undergoing surgical lung biopsy. *Chest*. 2005;128(5): 3310–5.

15. Wootton SC, Kim DS, Kondoh Y, Chen E, Lee JS, Song JW, et al. Viral Infection in Acute Exacerbation of Idiopathic Pulmonary Fibrosis. *Am J Respir Crit Care Med*. 2011;183(12):1698–702.

16. Lee JS, Song JW, Wolters PJ, Elicker BM, King TE Jr., Kim DS, et al. Bronchoalveolar lavage pepsin in acute exacerbation of idiopathic pulmonary fibrosis. *Eur Respir J*. 2012;39(2):352–8.

17. Johannson KA, Vittinghoff E, Lee K, Balmes JR, Ji W, Kaplan GG, et al. Acute exacerbation of idiopathic pulmonary fibrosis associated with air pollution exposure. *Eur Respir J*. 2014;43(4):1124–31.

18. Sakamoto K, Taniguchi H, Kondoh Y, Wakai K, Kimura T, Kataoka K, et al. Acute exacerbation of IPF following diagnostic bronchoalveolar lavage procedures. *Respir Med*. 2012;106(3):436–42.

19. Kim DS, Park JH, Park BK, Lee JS, Nicholson AG, Colby T. Acute exacerbation of idiopathic pulmonary fibrosis: frequency and clinical features. *Eur Respir J*. 2006;27(1):143–50.

20. Hutchinson JP, Fogarty AW, McKeever TM, Hubbard RB. In-Hospital Mortality after Surgical Lung Biopsy for Interstitial Lung Disease in the United States. 2000 to 2011. *Am J Respir Crit Care Med*. 2016;193(10):1161–7.

21. Churg A, Muller NL, Silva CI, Wright JL. Acute exacerbation (acute lung injury of unknown cause) in UIP and other forms of fibrotic interstitial pneumonias. *Am J Surg Pathol*. 2007;31(2):277–84.

22. Papiris SA, Kagouridis K, Kolilekas L, Papaioannou AI, Roussou A, Triantafillidou C, et al. Survival in Idiopathic pulmonary fibrosis acute exacerbations: the non-steroid approach. *BMC Pulm Med*. 2015;15:162.

23. Abe S, Azuma A, Mukae H, Ogura T, Taniguchi H, Bando M, et al. Polymyxin B-immobilized fiber column (PMX) treatment for idiopathic pulmonary fibrosis with acute exacerbation: a multicenter retrospective analysis. *Intern Med*. 2012;51(12):1487–91.

24. Oishi K, Mimura-Kimura Y, Miyasho T, Aoe K, Ogata Y, Katayama H, et al. Association between cytokine removal by polymyxin B hemoperfusion and improved pulmonary oxygenation in patients with acute exacerbation of idiopathic pulmonary fibrosis. *Cytokine*. 2013;61(1):84–9.

25. Fumeaux T, Rothmeier C, Jolliet P. Outcome of mechanical ventilation for acute respiratory failure in patients with pulmonary fibrosis. *Intensive Care Med*. 2001;27(12):1868–74.

26. Stern JB, Mal H, Groussard O, Brugiere O, Marceau A, Jebrak G, et al. Prognosis of patients with advanced idiopathic pulmonary fibrosis requiring mechanical ventilation for acute respiratory failure. *Chest*. 2001;120(1):213–9.

27. Huie TJ, Olson AL, Cosgrove GP, Janssen WJ, Lara AR, Lynch DA, et al. A detailed evaluation of acute respiratory decline in patients with fibrotic lung disease: aetiology and outcomes. *Respirology*. 2010;15(6):909–17.

28. Collard HR, Brown KK, Martinez FJ, Raghu G, Roberts RS, Anstrom KJ. Study design implications of death and hospitalization as end points in idiopathic pulmonary fibrosis. *Chest.* 2014;146(5):1256–62.

29. Arcadu A, Moua T. Bronchoscopy assessment of acute respiratory failure in interstitial lung disease. *Respirology.* 2017;22(2):352–9.

30. Oda K, Ishimoto H, Yamada S, Kushima H, Ishii H, Imanaga T, et al. Autopsy analyses in acute exacerbation of idiopathic pulmonary fibrosis. *Respir Res.* 2014;15:109.

31. Acharya S, Mahajan SN, Shukla S, Diwan SK, Banode P, Kothari N. Rheumatoid interstitial lung disease presenting as cor pulmonale. *Lung India.* 2010;27(4):256–9.

32. Chang B, Wigley FM, White B, Wise RA. Scleroderma patients with combined pulmonary hypertension and interstitial lung disease. *J Rheumatol.* 2003;30(11):2398–405.

33. Koschel DS, Cardoso C, Wiedemann B, Hoffken G, Halank M. Pulmonary hypertension in chronic hypersensitivity pneumonitis. *Lung.* 2012;190(3):295–302.

34. Oliveira RK, Pereira CA, Ramos RP, Ferreira EV, Messina CM, Kuranishi LT, et al. A haemodynamic study of pulmonary hypertension in chronic hypersensitivity pneumonitis. *Eur Respir J.* 2014;44(2):415–24.

35. Lettieri CJ, Nathan SD, Barnett SD, Ahmad S, Shorr AF. Prevalence and outcomes of pulmonary arterial hypertension in advanced idiopathic pulmonary fibrosis. *Chest.* 2006;129(3):746–52.

36. Nathan SD, Shlobin OA, Ahmad S, Koch J, Barnett SD, Ad N, et al. Serial development of pulmonary hypertension in patients with idiopathic pulmonary fibrosis. *Respiration.* 2008;76(3):288–94.

37. Shorr AF, Wainright JL, Cors CS, Lettieri CJ, Nathan SD. Pulmonary hypertension in patients with pulmonary fibrosis awaiting lung transplant. *Eur Respir J.* 2007;30(4):715–21.

38. Nadrous HF, Pellikka PA, Krowka MJ, Swanson KL, Chaowalit N, Decker PA, et al. Pulmonary hypertension in patients with idiopathic pulmonary fibrosis. *Chest.* 2005;128(4):2393–9.

39. Papakosta D, Pitsiou G, Daniil Z, Dimadi M, Stagaki E, Rapti A, et al. Prevalence of pulmonary hypertension in patients with idiopathic pulmonary fibrosis: correlation with physiological parameters. *Lung.* 2011;189(5):391–9.

40. D'Andrea A, Stanziola A, Di Palma E, Martino M, D'Alto M, Dellegrottaglie S, et al. Right Ventricular Structure and Function in Idiopathic Pulmonary Fibrosis with or without Pulmonary Hypertension. *Echocardiography.* 2016;33(1):57–65.

41. Zisman DA, Karlamangla AS, Ross DJ, Keane MP, Belperio JA, Saggar R, et al. High-resolution chest CT findings do not predict the presence of pulmonary hypertension in advanced idiopathic pulmonary fibrosis. *Chest.* 2007;132(3):773–9.

42. Parra ER, David YR, da Costa LR, Ab'Saber A, Sousa R, Kairalla RA, et al. Heterogeneous remodeling of lung vessels in idiopathic pulmonary fibrosis. *Lung.* 2005;183(4):291–300.

43. Judge EP, Fabre A, Adamali HI, Egan JJ. Acute exacerbations and pulmonary hypertension in advanced idiopathic pulmonary fibrosis. *Eur Respir J.* 2012;40(1):93–100.

44. Farkas L, Gauldie J, Voelkel NF, Kolb M. Pulmonary hypertension and idiopathic pulmonary fibrosis: a tale of angiogenesis, apoptosis, and growth factors. *Am J Respir Cell Mol Biol.* 2011;45(1):1–15.

45. Nadrous HF, Pellikka PA, Krowka MJ, Swanson KL, Chaowalit N, Decker PA, et al. The impact of pulmonary hypertension on survival in patients with idiopathic pulmonary fibrosis. *Chest.* 2005;128(6 Suppl):616S–7S.

46. Kimura M, Taniguchi H, Kondoh Y, Kimura T, Kataoka K, Nishiyama O, et al. Pulmonary hypertension as a prognostic indicator at the initial evaluation in idiopathic pulmonary fibrosis. *Respiration.* 2013;85(6):456–63.

47. King TE Jr., Brown KK, Raghu G, du Bois RM, Lynch DA, Martinez F, et al. BUILD-3: a randomized, controlled trial of bosentan in idiopathic pulmonary fibrosis. *Am J Respir Crit Care Med.* 2011;184(1):92–9.

48. Raghu G, Behr J, Brown KK, Egan JJ, Kawut SM, Flaherty KR, et al. Treatment of idiopathic pulmonary fibrosis with ambrisentan: a parallel, randomized trial. *Ann Intern Med.* 2013;158(9):641–9.

49. Koschel DS, Kolditz M, Hoeffken G, Halank M. Combined vasomodulatory therapy for severe pulmonary hypertension in chronic hypersensitivity pneumonitis. *Med Sci Monit.* 2010;16(5):pCS55–7.

50. Mittoo S, Jacob T, Craig A, Bshouty Z. Treatment of pulmonary hypertension in patients with connective tissue disease and interstitial lung disease. *Can Respir J.* 2010;17(6):282–6.

51. Hubbard RB, Smith C, Le Jeune I, Gribbin J, Fogarty AW. The association between idiopathic pulmonary fibrosis and vascular disease: a population-based study. *Am J Respir Crit Care Med.* 2008;178(12): 1257–61.

52. Ponnuswamy A, Manikandan R, Sabetpour A, Keeping IM, Finnerty JP. Association between ischaemic heart disease and interstitial lung disease: a case-control study. *Respir Med.* 2009;103(4):503–7.

53. Nathan SD, Basavaraj A, Reichner C, Shlobin OA, Ahmad S, Kiernan J, et al. Prevalence and impact of coronary artery disease in idiopathic pulmonary fibrosis. *Respir Med.* 2010;104(7):1035–41.

54. Kizer JR, Zisman DA, Blumenthal NP, Kotloff RM, Kimmel SE, Strieter RM, et al. Association between pulmonary fibrosis and coronary artery disease. *Arch Intern Med.* 2004;164(5):551–6.

55. Izbicki G, Ben-Dor I, Shitrit D, Bendayan D, Aldrich TK, Kornowski R, et al. The prevalence of coronary artery disease in end-stage pulmonary disease: is pulmonary fibrosis a risk factor? *Respir Med.* 2009;103(9):1346–9.

56. Nathan SD, Weir N, Shlobin OA, Urban BA, Curry CA, Basavaraj A, et al. The value of computed tomography scanning for the detection of coronary artery disease in patients with idiopathic pulmonary fibrosis. *Respirology.* 2011;16(3):481–6.

57. Santana AN, Kairalla RA, Carvalho CR. Potential role of statin use in idiopathic pulmonary fibrosis. *Am J Respir Crit Care Med.* 2008;177(9):1048.

58. Vedel-Krogh S, Nielsen SF, Nordestgaard BG. Statin Use Is Associated with Reduced Mortality in Patients with Interstitial Lung Disease. *PLoS One.* 2015;10(10):e0140571.

59. Sode BF, Dahl M, Nielsen SF, Nordestgaard BG. Venous thromboembolism and risk of idiopathic interstitial pneumonia: a nationwide study. *Am J Respir Crit Care Med.* 2010;181(10):1085–92.

60. Sprunger DB, Olson AL, Huie TJ, Fernandez-Perez ER, Fischer A, Solomon JJ, et al. Pulmonary fibrosis is associated with an elevated risk of thromboembolic disease. *Eur Respir J.* 2012;39(1):125–32.

61. Takagishi T, Ostrowski R, Alex C, Rychlik K, Pelletiere K, Tehrani R. Survival and extrapulmonary course of connective tissue disease after lung transplantation. *J Clin Rheumatol.* 2012;18(6):283–9.

62. Fujimoto K, Taniguchi H, Johkoh T, Kondoh Y, Ichikado K, Sumikawa H, et al. Acute exacerbation of idiopathic pulmonary fibrosis: high-resolution CT scores predict mortality. *Eur Radiol.* 2012;22(1):83–92.

63. Akira M, Kozuka T, Yamamoto S, Sakatani M. Computed tomography findings in acute exacerbation of idiopathic pulmonary fibrosis. *Am J Respir Crit Care Med.* 2008;178(4):372–8.

64. Grosse C, Grosse A. CT findings in diseases associated with pulmonary hypertension: a current review. *Radiographics.* 2010;30(7):1753–77.

65. Alhamad EH, Al-Boukai AA, Al-Kassimi FA, Alfaleh HF, Alshamiri MQ, Alzeer AH, et al. Prediction of pulmonary hypertension in patients with or without interstitial lung disease: reliability of CT findings. *Radiology.* 2011;260(3):875–83.

66. Camera L, Campanile F, Imbriaco M, Ippolito R, Sirignano C, Santoro C, et al. Idiopathic pulmonary fibrosis complicated by acute thromboembolic disease: chest X-ray, HRCT and multi-detector row CT angiographic findings. *J Thorac Dis.* 2013;5(1):82–6.

67. Nagata K, Tomii K, Otsuka K, Tachikawa R, Nakagawa A, Otsuka K, et al. Serum procalcitonin is a valuable diagnostic marker in acute exacerbation of interstitial pneumonia. *Respirology.* 2013;18(3):439–46.

68. Hiwatari N, Shimura S, Takishima T, Shirato K. Bronchoalveolar Lavage as a Possible Cause of Acute Exacerbation in Idiopathic Pulmonary Fibrosis Patients. *Tohoku J Exp Med.* 1994;174(4):379–86.

69. Wootton SC, Kim DS, Kondoh Y, Chen E, Lee JS, Song JW, et al. Viral infection in acute exacerbation of idiopathic pulmonary fibrosis. *Am J Respir Crit Care Med.* 2011;183(12):1698–702.

70. Ushiki A, Yamazaki Y, Hama M, Yasuo M, Hanaoka M, Kubo K. Viral infections in patients with an acute exacerbation of idiopathic interstitial pneumonia. *Respir Investig.* 2014;52(1):65–70.

71. Kondoh Y, Taniguchi H, Kitaichi M, Yokoi T, Johkoh T, Oishi T, et al. Acute exacerbation of interstitial pneumonia following surgical lung biopsy. *Respir Med.* 2006;100(10):1753–9.

72. Papazian L, Corley A, Hess D, Fraser JF, Frat JP, Guitton C, et al. Use of high-flow nasal cannula oxygenation in ICU adults: a narrative review. *Intensive Care Med.* 2016.

73. Horio Y, Takihara T, Niimi K, Komatsu M, Sato M, Tanaka J, et al. High-flow nasal cannula oxygen therapy for acute exacerbation of interstitial pneumonia: A case series. *Respir Investig.* 2016;54(2):125–9.

74. Peters SG, Holets SR, Gay PC. High-flow nasal cannula therapy in do-not-intubate patients with hypoxemic respiratory distress. *Respir Care.* 2013;58(4):597–600.

75. Roca O, Hernandez G, Diaz-Lobato S, Carratala JM, Gutierrez RM, Masclans JR, et al. Current evidence for the effectiveness of heated and humidified high flow nasal cannula supportive therapy in adult patients with respiratory failure. *Crit Care.* 2016;20(1):109.

76. Weusten BL, Jacobs JW, Bijlsma JW. Corticosteroid pulse therapy in active rheumatoid arthritis. *Semin Arthritis Rheum.* 1993;23(3):183–92.

77. Adu D, Pall A, Luqmani RA, Richards NT, Howie AJ, Emery P, et al. Controlled trial of pulse versus continuous prednisolone and cyclophosphamide in the treatment of systemic vasculitis. *Qjm.* 1997;90(6):401–9.

78. Sharada B, Kumar A, Kakker R, Adya CM, Pande I, Uppal SS, et al. Intravenous dexamethasone pulse therapy in diffuse systemic sclerosis. A randomized placebo-controlled study. *Rheumatol Int.* 1994;14(3):91–4.

79. Badsha H, Edwards CJ. Intravenous pulses of methylprednisolone for systemic lupus erythematosus. *Semin Arthritis Rheum.* 2003;32(6):370–7.

80. Kreuter A, Gambichler T, Breuckmann F, Rotterdam S, Freitag M, Stuecker M, et al. Pulsed high-dose corticosteroids combined with low-dose methotrexate in severe localized scleroderma. *Arch Dermatol.* 2005;141(7):847–52.

81. Metcalf JP, Rennard SI, Reed EC, Haire WD, Sisson JH, Walter T, et al. Corticosteroids as adjunctive therapy for diffuse alveolar hemorrhage associated with bone marrow transplantation. University of Nebraska Medical Center Bone Marrow Transplant Group. *Am J Med.* 1994;96(4):327–34.

82. Raptis A, Mavroudis D, Suffredini A, Molldrem J, Rhee FV, Childs R, et al. High-dose corticosteroid therapy for diffuse alveolar hemorrhage in allogeneic bone marrow stem cell transplant recipients. *Bone Marrow Transplant.* 1999;24(8):879–83.

83. Mollica C, Paone G, Conti V, Ceccarelli D, Schmid G, Mattia P, et al. Mechanical ventilation in patients with end-stage idiopathic pulmonary fibrosis. *Respiration.* 2010;79(3):209–15.

84. Al-Hameed FM, Sharma S. Outcome of patients admitted to the intensive care unit for acute exacerbation of idiopathic pulmonary fibrosis. *Can Respir J.* 2004;11(2):117–22.

85. Paone G, Mollica C, Conti V, Vestri A, Cammarella I, Lucantoni G, et al. Severity of illness and outcome in patients with end-stage idiopathic pulmonary fibrosis requiring mechanical ventilation. *Chest.* 2010;137(1):241–2; author reply 2.

86. Disayabutr S, Calfee CS, Collard HR, Wolters PJ. Interstitial lung diseases in the hospitalized patient. *BMC Med.* 2015;13:245.

87. Noma S, Matsuyama W, Mitsuyama H, Suetsugu T, Koreeda Y, Mizuno K, et al. Two cases of acute exacerbation of interstitial pneumonia treated with polymyxin B-immobilized fiber column hemoperfusion treatment. *Intern Med.* 2007;46(17):1447–54.

88. Itai J, Ohshimo S, Kida Y, Ota K, Iwasaki Y, Hirohashi N, et al. A pilot study: a combined therapy using polymyxin-B hemoperfusion and extracorporeal membrane oxygenation for acute exacerbation of interstitial pneumonia. *Sarcoidosis Vasc Diffuse Lung Dis.* 2014;31(4): 343–9.

89. Enomoto N, Mikamo M, Oyama Y, Kono M, Hashimoto D, Fujisawa T, et al. Treatment of acute exacerbation of idiopathic pulmonary fibrosis with direct hemoperfusion using a polymyxin B-immobilized fiber column improves survival. *BMC Pulm Med.* 2015;15:15.

90. Richeldi L, Costabel U, Selman M, Kim DS, Hansell DM, Nicholson AG, et al. Efficacy of a tyrosine kinase inhibitor in idiopathic pulmonary fibrosis. *N Engl J Med.* 2011;365(12):1079–87.

91. Brown AW, Fischer CP, Shlobin OA, Buhr RG, Ahmad S, Weir NA, et al. Outcomes after hospitalization in idiopathic pulmonary fibrosis: a cohort study. *Chest.* 2015;147(1):173–9.

92. Saydain G, Islam A, Afessa B, Ryu JH, Scott JP, Peters SG. Outcome of patients with idiopathic pulmonary fibrosis admitted to the intensive care unit. *Am J Respir Crit Care Med.* 2002;166(6):839–42.

93. Zafrani L, Lemiale V, Lapidus N, Lorillon G, Schlemmer B, Azoulay E. Acute respiratory failure in critically ill patients with interstitial lung disease. *PLoS One.* 2014;9(8):e104897.

94. Lindell KO, Liang Z, Hoffman LA, Rosenzweig MQ, Saul MI, Pilewski JM, et al. Palliative care and location of death in decedents with idiopathic pulmonary fibrosis. *Chest.* 2015;147(2):423–9.

95. Lewis D, Scullion J. Palliative and end-of-life care for patients with idiopathic pulmonary fibrosis: challenges and dilemmas. *Int J Palliat Nurs.* 2012;18(7):331–7.

96. Bajwah S, Koffman J, Higginson IJ, Ross JR, Wells AU, Birring SS, et al. 'I wish I knew more …' the end-of-life planning and information needs for end-stage fibrotic interstitial lung disease: views of patients, carers and health professionals. *BMJ Support Palliat Care.* 2013;3(1):84–90.

Index